50% OFF

Online Adult-Gerontology Acute Care NP Prep Course!

By Mometrix University

Dear Customer,

We consider it an honor and a privilege that you chose our Adult-Gerontology Acute Care NP Practice Questions. As a way of showing our appreciation and to help us better serve you, we are offering **50% off our online Adult-Gerontology Acute Care NP Prep Course.** Many Adult-Gerontology courses cost hundreds of dollars and don't deliver enough value. With our course, you get access to the best prep material, and **you only pay half price**.

We have structured our online course to perfectly complement your printed practice questions. The course contains **in-depth lessons** that cover all the most important topics, **video reviews** that explain difficult concepts, over **600 online practice questions** to ensure you feel prepared, and more than **400 digital flashcards**, so you can study while you're on the go.

Online Adult-Gerontology Acute Care Nurse Practitioner Prep Course

Topics Covered:

- APRN Core Competencies
  - Advanced Pharmacology
  - Advanced Physiology/Pathophysiology
- Clinical Practice
  - Clinical Decision Making/Management
- Role-Professional Responsibilities
  - Scope and Standards of Practice
  - Research and Evidence-Based Practice
- Health Care Systems
  - Health Care Policy and Delivery

Course Features:

- Adult-Gerontology ACNP Study Guide
  - Get content that complements our best-selling study guide.
- Full-Length Practice Tests and Flashcards
  - With over 600 online practice questions and 400+ digital flashcards, you can test yourself again and again.
- Mobile Friendly
  - If you need to study on the go, the course is easily accessible from your mobile device.

To receive this discount, visit our website at mometrix.com/university/adult-gerontology-acnp or simply scan this QR code with your smartphone. At the checkout page, enter the discount code: **agnp50off**

If you have any questions or concerns, please don't hesitate to contact us at universityhelp@mometrix.com.

Sincerely,

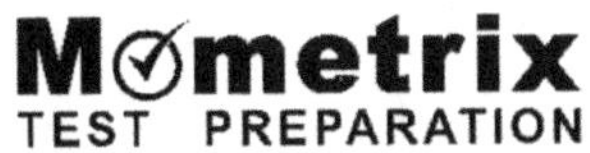

FREE Study Skills Videos/DVD Offer

Dear Customer,

Thank you for your purchase from Mometrix! We consider it an honor and a privilege that you have purchased our product and we want to ensure your satisfaction.

As a way of showing our appreciation and to help us better serve you, we have developed Study Skills Videos that we would like to give you for FREE. These videos cover our *best practices* for getting ready for your exam, from how to use our study materials to how to best prepare for the day of the test.

All that we ask is that you email us with feedback that would describe your experience so far with our product. Good, bad, or indifferent, we want to know what you think!

To get your FREE Study Skills Videos, you can use the **QR code** below, or send us an **email** at studyvideos@mometrix.com with *FREE VIDEOS* in the subject line and the following information in the body of the email:

- The name of the product you purchased.
- Your product rating on a scale of 1-5, with 5 being the highest rating.
- Your feedback. It can be long, short, or anything in between. We just want to know your impressions and experience so far with our product. (Good feedback might include how our study material met your needs and ways we might be able to make it even better. You could highlight features that you found helpful or features that you think we should add.)

If you have any questions or concerns, please don't hesitate to contact me directly.

Thanks again!

Sincerely,

Jay Willis
Vice President
jay.willis@mometrix.com
1-800-673-8175

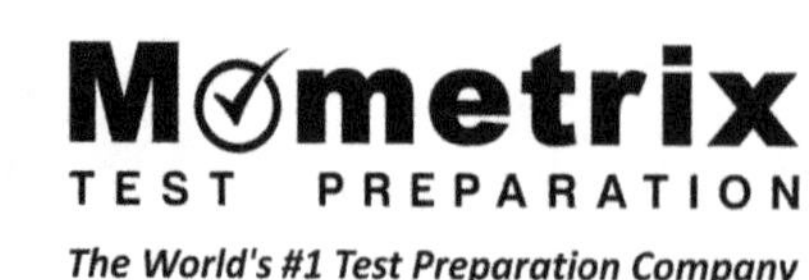

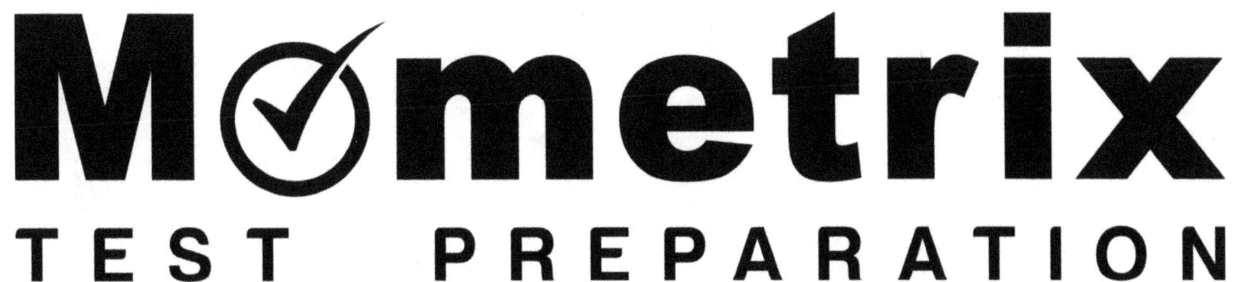

Adult-Gerontology Acute Care Nurse Practitioner Review Book

NP Certification Secrets Study Guide

Full-Length Practice Test

Nursing Review Video Tutorials

2nd Edition

Written and edited by Mometrix Test Prep

Printed in the United States of America

This paper meets the requirements of ANSI/NISO Z39.48-1992 (Permanence of Paper).

Paperback
ISBN 13: 978-1-5167-1847-4
ISBN 10: 1-5167-1847-X

Hardback
ISBN 13: 978-1-5167-1880-1
ISBN 10: 1-5167-1880-1

Dear Future Exam Success Story

First of all, **THANK YOU** for purchasing Mometrix study materials!

Second, congratulations! You are one of the few determined test-takers who are committed to doing whatever it takes to excel on your exam. **You have come to the right place.** We developed these study materials with one goal in mind: to deliver you the information you need in a format that's concise and easy to use.

In addition to optimizing your guide for the content of the test, we've outlined our recommended steps for breaking down the preparation process into small, attainable goals so you can make sure you stay on track.

We've also analyzed the entire test-taking process, identifying the most common pitfalls and showing how you can overcome them and be ready for any curveball the test throws you.

Standardized testing is one of the biggest obstacles on your road to success, which only increases the importance of doing well in the high-pressure, high-stakes environment of test day. Your results on this test could have a significant impact on your future, and this guide provides the information and practical advice to help you achieve your full potential on test day.

Your success is our success

We would love to hear from you! If you would like to share the story of your exam success or if you have any questions or comments in regard to our products, please contact us at **800-673-8175** or **support@mometrix.com**.

Thanks again for your business and we wish you continued success!

Sincerely,
The Mometrix Test Preparation Team

Need more help? Check out our flashcards at:
http://mometrixflashcards.com/NP

TABLE OF CONTENTS

Introduction

Thank you for purchasing this resource! You have made the choice to prepare yourself for a test that could have a huge impact on your future, and this guide is designed to help you be fully ready for test day. Obviously, it's important to have a solid understanding of the test material, but you also need to be prepared for the unique environment and stressors of the test, so that you can perform to the best of your abilities.

For this purpose, the first section that appears in this guide is the **Secret Keys**. We've devoted countless hours to meticulously researching what works and what doesn't, and we've boiled down our findings to the five most impactful steps you can take to improve your performance on the test. We start at the beginning with study planning and move through the preparation process, all the way to the testing strategies that will help you get the most out of what you know when you're finally sitting in front of the test.

We recommend that you start preparing for your test as far in advance as possible. However, if you've bought this guide as a last-minute study resource and only have a few days before your test, we recommend that you skip over the first two Secret Keys since they address a long-term study plan.

If you struggle with **test anxiety**, we strongly encourage you to check out our recommendations for how you can overcome it. Test anxiety is a formidable foe, but it can be beaten, and we want to make sure you have the tools you need to defeat it.

Secret Key #1 – Plan Big, Study Small

There's a lot riding on your performance. If you want to ace this test, you're going to need to keep your skills sharp and the material fresh in your mind. You need a plan that lets you review everything you need to know while still fitting in your schedule. We'll break this strategy down into three categories.

Information Organization

Start with the information you already have: the official test outline. From this, you can make a complete list of all the concepts you need to cover before the test. Organize these concepts into groups that can be studied together, and create a list of any related vocabulary you need to learn so you can brush up on any difficult terms. You'll want to keep this vocabulary list handy once you actually start studying since you may need to add to it along the way.

Time Management

Once you have your set of study concepts, decide how to spread them out over the time you have left before the test. Break your study plan into small, clear goals so you have a manageable task for each day and know exactly what you're doing. Then just focus on one small step at a time. When you manage your time this way, you don't need to spend hours at a time studying. Studying a small block of content for a short period each day helps you retain information better and avoid stressing over how much you have left to do. You can relax knowing that you have a plan to cover everything in time. In order for this strategy to be effective though, you have to start studying early and stick to your schedule. Avoid the exhaustion and futility that comes from last-minute cramming!

Study Environment

The environment you study in has a big impact on your learning. Studying in a coffee shop, while probably more enjoyable, is not likely to be as fruitful as studying in a quiet room. It's important to keep distractions to a minimum. You're only planning to study for a short block of time, so make the most of it. Don't pause to check your phone or get up to find a snack. It's also important to **avoid multitasking**. Research has consistently shown that multitasking will make your studying dramatically less effective. Your study area should also be comfortable and well-lit so you don't have the distraction of straining your eyes or sitting on an uncomfortable chair.

The time of day you study is also important. You want to be rested and alert. Don't wait until just before bedtime. Study when you'll be most likely to comprehend and remember. Even better, if you know what time of day your test will be, set that time aside for study. That way your brain will be used to working on that subject at that specific time and you'll have a better chance of recalling information.

Finally, it can be helpful to team up with others who are studying for the same test. Your actual studying should be done in as isolated an environment as possible, but the work of organizing the information and setting up the study plan can be divided up. In between study sessions, you can discuss with your teammates the concepts that you're all studying and quiz each other on the details. Just be sure that your teammates are as serious about the test as you are. If you find that your study time is being replaced with social time, you might need to find a new team.

Secret Key #2 – Make Your Studying Count

You're devoting a lot of time and effort to preparing for this test, so you want to be absolutely certain it will pay off. This means doing more than just reading the content and hoping you can remember it on test day. It's important to make every minute of study count. There are two main areas you can focus on to make your studying count:

Retention

It doesn't matter how much time you study if you can't remember the material. You need to make sure you are retaining the concepts. To check your retention of the information you're learning, try recalling it at later times with minimal prompting. Try carrying around flashcards and glance at one or two from time to time or ask a friend who's also studying for the test to quiz you.

To enhance your retention, look for ways to put the information into practice so that you can apply it rather than simply recalling it. If you're using the information in practical ways, it will be much easier to remember. Similarly, it helps to solidify a concept in your mind if you're not only reading it to yourself but also explaining it to someone else. Ask a friend to let you teach them about a concept you're a little shaky on (or speak aloud to an imaginary audience if necessary). As you try to summarize, define, give examples, and answer your friend's questions, you'll understand the concepts better and they will stay with you longer. Finally, step back for a big picture view and ask yourself how each piece of information fits with the whole subject. When you link the different concepts together and see them working together as a whole, it's easier to remember the individual components.

Finally, practice showing your work on any multi-step problems, even if you're just studying. Writing out each step you take to solve a problem will help solidify the process in your mind, and you'll be more likely to remember it during the test.

Modality

Modality simply refers to the means or method by which you study. Choosing a study modality that fits your own individual learning style is crucial. No two people learn best in exactly the same way, so it's important to know your strengths and use them to your advantage.

For example, if you learn best by visualization, focus on visualizing a concept in your mind and draw an image or a diagram. Try color-coding your notes, illustrating them, or creating symbols that will trigger your mind to recall a learned concept. If you learn best by hearing or discussing information, find a study partner who learns the same way or read aloud to yourself. Think about how to put the information in your own words. Imagine that you are giving a lecture on the topic and record yourself so you can listen to it later.

For any learning style, flashcards can be helpful. Organize the information so you can take advantage of spare moments to review. Underline key words or phrases. Use different colors for different categories. Mnemonic devices (such as creating a short list in which every item starts with the same letter) can also help with retention. Find what works best for you and use it to store the information in your mind most effectively and easily.

Secret Key #3 – Practice the Right Way

Your success on test day depends not only on how many hours you put into preparing, but also on whether you prepared the right way. It's good to check along the way to see if your studying is paying off. One of the most effective ways to do this is by taking practice tests to evaluate your progress. Practice tests are useful because they show exactly where you need to improve. Every time you take a practice test, pay special attention to these three groups of questions:

- The questions you got wrong
- The questions you had to guess on, even if you guessed right
- The questions you found difficult or slow to work through

This will show you exactly what your weak areas are, and where you need to devote more study time. Ask yourself why each of these questions gave you trouble. Was it because you didn't understand the material? Was it because you didn't remember the vocabulary? Do you need more repetitions on this type of question to build speed and confidence? Dig into those questions and figure out how you can strengthen your weak areas as you go back to review the material.

Additionally, many practice tests have a section explaining the answer choices. It can be tempting to read the explanation and think that you now have a good understanding of the concept. However, an explanation likely only covers part of the question's broader context. Even if the explanation makes sense, **go back and investigate** every concept related to the question until you're positive you have a thorough understanding.

As you go along, keep in mind that the practice test is just that: practice. Memorizing these questions and answers will not be very helpful on the actual test because it is unlikely to have any of the same exact questions. If you only know the right answers to the sample questions, you won't be prepared for the real thing. **Study the concepts** until you understand them fully, and then you'll be able to answer any question that shows up on the test.

It's important to wait on the practice tests until you're ready. If you take a test on your first day of study, you may be overwhelmed by the amount of material covered and how much you need to learn. Work up to it gradually.

On test day, you'll need to be prepared for answering questions, managing your time, and using the test-taking strategies you've learned. It's a lot to balance, like a mental marathon that will have a big impact on your future. Like training for a marathon, you'll need to start slowly and work your way up. When test day arrives, you'll be ready.

Start with the strategies you've read in the first two Secret Keys—plan your course and study in the way that works best for you. If you have time, consider using multiple study resources to get different approaches to the same concepts. It can be helpful to see difficult concepts from more than one angle. Then find a good source for practice tests. Many times, the test website will suggest potential study resources or provide sample tests.

Practice Test Strategy

When you're ready to start taking practice tests, follow this strategy:

Untimed and Open-Book Practice

Take the first test with no time constraints and with your notes and study guide handy. Take your time and focus on applying the strategies you've learned.

Timed and Open-Book Practice

Take the second practice test open-book as well, but set a timer and practice pacing yourself to finish in time.

Timed and Closed-Book Practice

Take any other practice tests as if it were test day. Set a timer and put away your study materials. Sit at a table or desk in a quiet room, imagine yourself at the testing center, and answer questions as quickly and accurately as possible.

Keep repeating timed and closed-book tests on a regular basis until you run out of practice tests or it's time for the actual test. Your mind will be ready for the schedule and stress of test day, and you'll be able to focus on recalling the material you've learned.

Secret Key #4 – Pace Yourself

Once you're fully prepared for the material on the test, your biggest challenge on test day will be managing your time. Just knowing that the clock is ticking can make you panic even if you have plenty of time left. Work on pacing yourself so you can build confidence against the time constraints of the exam. Pacing is a difficult skill to master, especially in a high-pressure environment, so **practice is vital**.

Set time expectations for your pace based on how much time is available. For example, if a section has 60 questions and the time limit is 30 minutes, you know you have to average 30 seconds or less per question in order to answer them all. Although 30 seconds is the hard limit, set 25 seconds per question as your goal, so you reserve extra time to spend on harder questions. When you budget extra time for the harder questions, you no longer have any reason to stress when those questions take longer to answer.

Don't let this time expectation distract you from working through the test at a calm, steady pace, but keep it in mind so you don't spend too much time on any one question. Recognize that taking extra time on one question you don't understand may keep you from answering two that you do understand later in the test. If your time limit for a question is up and you're still not sure of the answer, mark it and move on, and come back to it later if the time and the test format allow. If the testing format doesn't allow you to return to earlier questions, just make an educated guess; then put it out of your mind and move on.

On the easier questions, be careful not to rush. It may seem wise to hurry through them so you have more time for the challenging ones, but it's not worth missing one if you know the concept and just didn't take the time to read the question fully. Work efficiently but make sure you understand the question and have looked at all of the answer choices, since more than one may seem right at first.

Even if you're paying attention to the time, you may find yourself a little behind at some point. You should speed up to get back on track, but do so wisely. Don't panic; just take a few seconds less on each question until you're caught up. Don't guess without thinking, but do look through the answer choices and eliminate any you know are wrong. If you can get down to two choices, it is often worthwhile to guess from those. Once you've chosen an answer, move on and don't dwell on any that you skipped or had to hurry through. If a question was taking too long, chances are it was one of the harder ones, so you weren't as likely to get it right anyway.

On the other hand, if you find yourself getting ahead of schedule, it may be beneficial to slow down a little. The more quickly you work, the more likely you are to make a careless mistake that will affect your score. You've budgeted time for each question, so don't be afraid to spend that time. Practice an efficient but careful pace to get the most out of the time you have.

Secret Key #5 – Have a Plan for Guessing

When you're taking the test, you may find yourself stuck on a question. Some of the answer choices seem better than others, but you don't see the one answer choice that is obviously correct. What do you do?

The scenario described above is very common, yet most test takers have not effectively prepared for it. Developing and practicing a plan for guessing may be one of the single most effective uses of your time as you get ready for the exam.

In developing your plan for guessing, there are three questions to address:

- When should you start the guessing process?
- How should you narrow down the choices?
- Which answer should you choose?

When to Start the Guessing Process

Unless your plan for guessing is to select C every time (which, despite its merits, is not what we recommend), you need to leave yourself enough time to apply your answer elimination strategies. Since you have a limited amount of time for each question, that means that if you're going to give yourself the best shot at guessing correctly, you have to decide quickly whether or not you will guess.

Of course, the best-case scenario is that you don't have to guess at all, so first, see if you can answer the question based on your knowledge of the subject and basic reasoning skills. Focus on the key words in the question and try to jog your memory of related topics. Give yourself a chance to bring the knowledge to mind, but once you realize that you don't have (or you can't access) the knowledge you need to answer the question, it's time to start the guessing process.

It's almost always better to start the guessing process too early than too late. It only takes a few seconds to remember something and answer the question from knowledge. Carefully eliminating wrong answer choices takes longer. Plus, going through the process of eliminating answer choices can actually help jog your memory.

Summary: Start the guessing process as soon as you decide that you can't answer the question based on your knowledge.

How to Narrow Down the Choices

The next chapter in this book (**Test-Taking Strategies**) includes a wide range of strategies for how to approach questions and how to look for answer choices to eliminate. You will definitely want to read those carefully, practice them, and figure out which ones work best for you. Here though, we're going to address a mindset rather than a particular strategy.

Your chances of guessing an answer correctly depend on how many options you are choosing from.

How many choices you have	How likely you are to guess correctly
5	20%
4	25%
3	33%
2	50%
1	100%

You can see from this chart just how valuable it is to be able to eliminate incorrect answers and make an educated guess, but there are two things that many test takers do that cause them to miss out on the benefits of guessing:

- Accidentally eliminating the correct answer
- Selecting an answer based on an impression

We'll look at the first one here, and the second one in the next section.

To avoid accidentally eliminating the correct answer, we recommend a thought exercise called **the $5 challenge**. In this challenge, you only eliminate an answer choice from contention if you are willing to bet $5 on it being wrong. Why $5? Five dollars is a small but not insignificant amount of money. It's an amount you could afford to lose but wouldn't want to throw away. And while losing $5 once might not hurt too much, doing it twenty times will set you back $100. In the same way, each small decision you make—eliminating a choice here, guessing on a question there—won't by itself impact your score very much, but when you put them all together, they can make a big difference. By holding each answer choice elimination decision to a higher standard, you can reduce the risk of accidentally eliminating the correct answer.

The $5 challenge can also be applied in a positive sense: If you are willing to bet $5 that an answer choice *is* correct, go ahead and mark it as correct.

Summary: Only eliminate an answer choice if you are willing to bet $5 that it is wrong.

Which Answer to Choose

You're taking the test. You've run into a hard question and decided you'll have to guess. You've eliminated all the answer choices you're willing to bet $5 on. Now you have to pick an answer. Why do we even need to talk about this? Why can't you just pick whichever one you feel like when the time comes?

The answer to these questions is that if you don't come into the test with a plan, you'll rely on your impression to select an answer choice, and if you do that, you risk falling into a trap. The test writers know that everyone who takes their test will be guessing on some of the questions, so they intentionally write wrong answer choices to seem plausible. You still have to pick an answer though, and if the wrong answer choices are designed to look right, how can you ever be sure that you're not falling for their trap? The best solution we've found to this dilemma is to take the decision out of your hands entirely. Here is the process we recommend:

Once you've eliminated any choices that you are confident (willing to bet $5) are wrong, select the first remaining choice as your answer.

Whether you choose to select the first remaining choice, the second, or the last, the important thing is that you use some preselected standard. Using this approach guarantees that you will not be enticed into selecting an answer choice that looks right, because you are not basing your decision on how the answer choices look.

This is not meant to make you question your knowledge. Instead, it is to help you recognize the difference between your knowledge and your impressions. There's a huge difference between thinking an answer is right because of what you know, and thinking an answer is right because it looks or sounds like it should be right.

Summary: To ensure that your selection is appropriately random, make a predetermined selection from among all answer choices you have not eliminated.

Test-Taking Strategies

This section contains a list of test-taking strategies that you may find helpful as you work through the test. By taking what you know and applying logical thought, you can maximize your chances of answering any question correctly!

It is very important to realize that every question is different and every person is different: no single strategy will work on every question, and no single strategy will work for every person. That's why we've included all of them here, so you can try them out and determine which ones work best for different types of questions and which ones work best for you.

Question Strategies

Read Carefully

Read the question and answer choices carefully. Don't miss the question because you misread the terms. You have plenty of time to read each question thoroughly and make sure you understand what is being asked. Yet a happy medium must be attained, so don't waste too much time. You must read carefully, but efficiently.

Contextual Clues

Look for contextual clues. If the question includes a word you are not familiar with, look at the immediate context for some indication of what the word might mean. Contextual clues can often give you all the information you need to decipher the meaning of an unfamiliar word. Even if you can't determine the meaning, you may be able to narrow down the possibilities enough to make a solid guess at the answer to the question.

Prefixes

If you're having trouble with a word in the question or answer choices, try dissecting it. Take advantage of every clue that the word might include. Prefixes and suffixes can be a huge help. Usually they allow you to determine a basic meaning. Pre- means before, post- means after, pro - is positive, de- is negative. From prefixes and suffixes, you can get an idea of the general meaning of the word and try to put it into context.

Hedge Words

Watch out for critical hedge words, such as *likely*, *may*, *can*, *sometimes*, *often*, *almost*, *mostly*, *usually*, *generally*, *rarely*, and *sometimes*. Question writers insert these hedge phrases to cover every possibility. Often an answer choice will be wrong simply because it leaves no room for exception. Be on guard for answer choices that have definitive words such as *exactly* and *always*.

Switchback Words

Stay alert for *switchbacks*. These are the words and phrases frequently used to alert you to shifts in thought. The most common switchback words are *but*, *although*, and *however*. Others include *nevertheless*, *on the other hand*, *even though*, *while*, *in spite of*, *despite*, *regardless of*. Switchback words are important to catch because they can change the direction of the question or an answer choice.

FACE VALUE

When in doubt, use common sense. Accept the situation in the problem at face value. Don't read too much into it. These problems will not require you to make wild assumptions. If you have to go beyond creativity and warp time or space in order to have an answer choice fit the question, then you should move on and consider the other answer choices. These are normal problems rooted in reality. The applicable relationship or explanation may not be readily apparent, but it is there for you to figure out. Use your common sense to interpret anything that isn't clear.

Answer Choice Strategies

ANSWER SELECTION

The most thorough way to pick an answer choice is to identify and eliminate wrong answers until only one is left, then confirm it is the correct answer. Sometimes an answer choice may immediately seem right, but be careful. The test writers will usually put more than one reasonable answer choice on each question, so take a second to read all of them and make sure that the other choices are not equally obvious. As long as you have time left, it is better to read every answer choice than to pick the first one that looks right without checking the others.

ANSWER CHOICE FAMILIES

An answer choice family consists of two (in rare cases, three) answer choices that are very similar in construction and cannot all be true at the same time. If you see two answer choices that are direct opposites or parallels, one of them is usually the correct answer. For instance, if one answer choice says that quantity *x* increases and another either says that quantity *x* decreases (opposite) or says that quantity *y* increases (parallel), then those answer choices would fall into the same family. An answer choice that doesn't match the construction of the answer choice family is more likely to be incorrect. Most questions will not have answer choice families, but when they do appear, you should be prepared to recognize them.

ELIMINATE ANSWERS

Eliminate answer choices as soon as you realize they are wrong, but make sure you consider all possibilities. If you are eliminating answer choices and realize that the last one you are left with is also wrong, don't panic. Start over and consider each choice again. There may be something you missed the first time that you will realize on the second pass.

AVOID FACT TRAPS

Don't be distracted by an answer choice that is factually true but doesn't answer the question. You are looking for the choice that answers the question. Stay focused on what the question is asking for so you don't accidentally pick an answer that is true but incorrect. Always go back to the question and make sure the answer choice you've selected actually answers the question and is not merely a true statement.

EXTREME STATEMENTS

In general, you should avoid answers that put forth extreme actions as standard practice or proclaim controversial ideas as established fact. An answer choice that states the "process should be used in certain situations, if…" is much more likely to be correct than one that states the "process should be discontinued completely." The first is a calm rational statement and doesn't even make a definitive, uncompromising stance, using a hedge word *if* to provide wiggle room, whereas the second choice is a radical idea and far more extreme.

BENCHMARK

As you read through the answer choices and you come across one that seems to answer the question well, mentally select that answer choice. This is not your final answer, but it's the one that will help you evaluate the other answer choices. The one that you selected is your benchmark or standard for judging each of the other answer choices. Every other answer choice must be compared to your benchmark. That choice is correct until proven otherwise by another answer choice beating it. If you find a better answer, then that one becomes your new benchmark. Once you've decided that no other choice answers the question as well as your benchmark, you have your final answer.

PREDICT THE ANSWER

Before you even start looking at the answer choices, it is often best to try to predict the answer. When you come up with the answer on your own, it is easier to avoid distractions and traps because you will know exactly what to look for. The right answer choice is unlikely to be word-for-word what you came up with, but it should be a close match. Even if you are confident that you have the right answer, you should still take the time to read each option before moving on.

General Strategies

TOUGH QUESTIONS

If you are stumped on a problem or it appears too hard or too difficult, don't waste time. Move on! Remember though, if you can quickly check for obviously incorrect answer choices, your chances of guessing correctly are greatly improved. Before you completely give up, at least try to knock out a couple of possible answers. Eliminate what you can and then guess at the remaining answer choices before moving on.

CHECK YOUR WORK

Since you will probably not know every term listed and the answer to every question, it is important that you get credit for the ones that you do know. Don't miss any questions through careless mistakes. If at all possible, try to take a second to look back over your answer selection and make sure you've selected the correct answer choice and haven't made a costly careless mistake (such as marking an answer choice that you didn't mean to mark). This quick double check should more than pay for itself in caught mistakes for the time it costs.

PACE YOURSELF

It's easy to be overwhelmed when you're looking at a page full of questions; your mind is confused and full of random thoughts, and the clock is ticking down faster than you would like. Calm down and maintain the pace that you have set for yourself. Especially as you get down to the last few minutes of the test, don't let the small numbers on the clock make you panic. As long as you are on track by monitoring your pace, you are guaranteed to have time for each question.

DON'T RUSH

It is very easy to make errors when you are in a hurry. Maintaining a fast pace in answering questions is pointless if it makes you miss questions that you would have gotten right otherwise. Test writers like to include distracting information and wrong answers that seem right. Taking a little extra time to avoid careless mistakes can make all the difference in your test score. Find a pace that allows you to be confident in the answers that you select.

KEEP MOVING

Panicking will not help you pass the test, so do your best to stay calm and keep moving. Taking deep breaths and going through the answer elimination steps you practiced can help to break through a stress barrier and keep your pace.

Final Notes

The combination of a solid foundation of content knowledge and the confidence that comes from practicing your plan for applying that knowledge is the key to maximizing your performance on test day. As your foundation of content knowledge is built up and strengthened, you'll find that the strategies included in this chapter become more and more effective in helping you quickly sift through the distractions and traps of the test to isolate the correct answer.

Now it's time to move on to the test content chapters of this book, but be sure to keep your goal in mind. As you read, think about how you will be able to apply this information on the test. If you've already seen sample questions for the test and you have an idea of the question format and style, try to come up with questions of your own that you can answer based on what you're reading. This will give you valuable practice applying your knowledge in the same ways you can expect to on test day.

Good luck and good studying!

Core Competencies: Advanced Physical Assessment

Theories of Human Growth and Development

Issues of Human Development

Several issues of human development that are addressed by theory are described below:

- **Universality vs. Context Specificity**: Universality implies that all individuals will develop in the same way, no matter what culture they live in. Context Specificity implies that development will be influenced by the culture in which the individual lives.
- **Assumptions about human nature** (3 doctrines: original sin, innate purity, and tabula rasa):
  - Original sin says that children are inherently bad and must be taught to be good.
  - Innate purity says that children are inherently good.
  - Tabula rasa says that children are born without good or bad tendencies and can be taught right vs. wrong.
- **Behavioral Consistency**: Children either behave in the same manner no matter what the situation or setting, or they change their behavior depending on the setting and who is interacting with them.
- **Nature vs. Nurture**: Nature is the genetic influences on development. Nurture is the environment and social influences on development.
- **Continuity vs. Discontinuity**: Continuity states that development progresses at a steady rate and the effects of change are cumulative. Discontinuity states that development progresses in a stair-step fashion and the effects of early development have no bearing on later development.
- **Passivity vs. Activity**: Passivity refers to development being influenced by outside forces. Activity refers to development influenced by the child himself and how he responds to external forces.
- **Critical vs. Sensitive Period**: The critical period is that window of time when the child will be able to acquire new skills and behaviors. The sensitive period refers to a flexible time period when a child will be receptive to learning new skills, even if it is later than the norm.

Developmental Tasks According to Erickson

The developmental tasks according to **Erik Erikson**:

- **Trust vs. Mistrust (Birth to 1 year)**: Trust, faith and optimism develop if the needs of warmth, food and love are met. If not, this can result in mistrust.
- **Autonomy vs. Shame/Doubt (Ages 1-3)**: The child desires independence in basic self-care tasks and wants choice. If independence is not encouraged, this can lead to doubt and shame. Independence develops self-control and willpower.
- **Initiative vs. Guilt (Ages 3-6)**: The child engages in self-directed play and starts activities without outside influence. Imaginative play and competition are introduced. This can lead to guilt or direction and purpose based on how this initiative is supportive.

- **Industry vs. Inferiority (Ages 6-12)**: The child values feeling capable and competent, and develops a sense of pride and self-worth. They desire to do what is right and good. Social interactions between peers becomes more important, and comparing achievements can result in feelings of pride or feelings of inferiority if not properly guided.
- **Identity vs. Role Confusion (Ages 12-18)**: Parents, teachers, peers, family members, church, culture, and ethnicity all role model and pressure youth to adopt certain behaviors. The task of adolescents is to discover their own identity.
- **Intimacy vs. Isolation (Ages 18-40)**: Young people learn to commit to another person in a love or family relationship. They learn the behavior required to maintain this relationship.
- **Generativity vs. Stagnation (Ages 40-65)**: Adults have many tasks when they try to find their own interests and niche in the work world. Family, community, and work roles are defined.
- **Integrity vs. Despair (Ages 65+)**: Older people ponder their life experiences to put them into perspective. They learn to accept the aging process and begin to think about their own death.

Sigmund Freud's Stages of Psychosexual Development

Sigmund Freud's stages of psychosexual development are listed and described below:

- **Oral stage (Birth to 1 year)**: obsessed with oral activities and must have these needs met for proper psychosocial development, very attached to mother.
- **Anal stage (Ages 1-3)**: masters toilet training.
- **Phallic stage (Ages 3-6)**: child focuses on childbirth and differences between the sexes, develops sexual obsession with parent of opposite sex (Oedipal complex-boy drawn to mother, Electra complex-girl drawn to father).
- **Latency stage (Ages 6-11)**: Oedipal or Electra complex wanes, focus is now socialization, begins to gravitate toward the same sex parent to learn appropriate gender roles.
- **Genital stage (Ages 12 and older)**: puberty, attracted to opposite sex, learns to relate to opposite gender and control sexual drive.

Piaget's Theory of Cognitive Development

Piaget believed that development was progressive and followed a set pattern. He believed the child's environment, his interactions with others in that environment, and how the environment responds help to shape his cognitive development. **There are 4 stages to Piaget's theory:**

- The **sensorimotor stage (birth to age 2)** is when the child learns to work toward a goal, the relationship between cause and effect, that objects still exist even though they cannot see them, and a sense of self.
- In the **preoperational stage (ages 2-7)** language skills develop, the child only sees his point of view, he does not think abstractly, and has a difficult time telling fact from fantasy.
- The **concrete operations stage (ages 7-11)** is when children begin to understand relationships between objects and events, learn to classify and use patterns, understand that some occurrences are reversible, and see other's points of view.
- The **formal operations stage (ages 12 years and older)** is the stage of abstract thinking, better reasoning skills, and forward thinking.

Maslow's Hierarchy of Needs

Maslow defined human motivation in terms of needs and wants. His **hierarchy of needs** is classically portrayed as a pyramid sitting on its base divided into horizontal layers. He theorized that, as humans fulfill the needs of one layer, their motivation turns to the layer above. The layers consist of (from bottom to top):

- **Physiological**: The need for air, fluid, food, shelter, warmth, and sleep.
- **Safety**: A safe place to live, a steady job, a society with rules and laws, protection from harm, and insurance or savings for the future.
- **Love/Belonging**: A network consisting of a significant other, family, friends, co-workers, religion, and community.
- **Esteem or self-respect**: The knowledge that you are a person who is successful and worthy of esteem, attention, status, and admiration.
- **Self-actualization**: The acceptance of your life, choices, and situation in life and the empathetic acceptance of others, as well as the feeling of independence and the joy of being able to express yourself freely and competently.

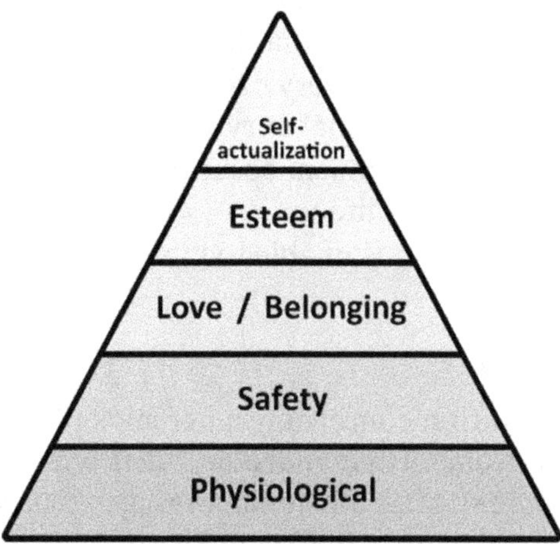

Review Video: Maslow's Hierarchy of Needs
Visit mometrix.com/academy and enter code: 461825

Behavioral Theories

Pavlov demonstrated classical conditioning when he found that a dog that would salivate when presented with food would also salivate when the person who normally fed him was present. He paired a bell ringing with the feeding and found that after a time, the dog would also salivate to the ringing of the bell. Consequently, his theory was that learning takes place when a behavior can be produced in response to something totally unrelated to that behavior.

Skinner demonstrated operant conditioning when he found that behavior can be changed depending on the response given to the behavior. If the response to the behavior was positive (praise, a hug) then the behavior would continue or increase in frequency. If the response was negative (a frown, words of criticism) then the behavior would decrease in frequency or cease altogether.

Biopsychosocial Theory of Patient Care

The biopsychosocial theory of patient care recognizes that **biology, psychology, and social circumstances** all interact in the development of an illness, the patient's perception of the illness, and the patient's ability to make a good recovery. In the biopsychosocial care model, a multidisciplinary healthcare team, including nurses, mental health professionals, social workers, and physicians, work together to address all aspects of a patient's health issue—the medical problem, psychological state, and social, cultural, and economic situation—in order to find an integrated solution. For example, adding stress-reduction, exercise, and nutritional programs to the standard medical treatment protocol for cardiovascular disease patients has been shown to be more effective. Many patients with chronic diseases or conditions may benefit from support groups that provide social and psychological benefits that may enhance the effects of drug therapy and surgery.

Biological Theories of Aging

There are a number of biological theories of aging:

- **Wearing down**: The body is compared to a machine that simply begins to wear down over time because of the damage caused by years of use.
- **Autoimmune reaction**: The body develops an autoimmune reaction against itself with aging, causing damage and destruction to tissues.
- **Free radical accumulation**: Chemicals that bring about aging accumulate in the body.
- **Cellular programming**: The cells of every organism have a pre-determined programmed life expectancy beyond which one cannot survive.
- **Mutation**: Mutations within the organism occur over time and these eventually make changes that are incompatible with life.
- **Homeostasis**: Over time, the body is unable to maintain stable levels of necessary chemicals in the body.

Selye's Theory of Adaptation

Selye developed a **theory of adaptation** concerning a person's physiologic response to stress called the general adaptation syndrome. This syndrome starts with the classic "fight or flight" response of the body to physiologic stress. Catecholamines are released and the adrenal cortical response begins. This is called the **alarm response** and is short-lived. This immediate response allows the person to respond quickly to stress. Since the alarm response cannot be sustained without resulting in death, the body next shifts into the **resistance stage**. Some cortisol is still being released as the body begins to adapt to the stressor. If the stressor persists, the body becomes exhausted. Changes then occur to the cardiovascular, gastrointestinal, and immune systems and death can occur. The **exhaustion stage** does not always occur in response to most life stressors. As the body ages, it loses some of its resistance and ability to adapt to stress. This results in exhaustion and death in the elderly more easily than it does in younger people.

History and Physical Assessment

Components of Health History

There are several different components that must be included in a nursing **health history**:

- The **biographic element** of the nursing health history includes the patient's name, age, physical address, sex, marital status, occupational status, religious preference, healthcare financing, and regular physician.
- The **chief complaint** is the next aspect of the history and involves the reason the patient is seeking care.
- Following this, the **history of the present illness** details the current health problem, including date of onset, description of symptoms, and any aggravating factors.

- **Past medical history** entails asking about the patient's usual health status, past medical or surgical problems, immunization status, current medications, allergies (including medication allergies), and family history.
- A detailed **family history** is important as it may reveal risk factors for certain medical conditions such as heart disease, diabetes, arthritis, hypertension, or mental disorders.
- The **review of systems** is used to obtain a full, systematic report by the patient on subjective symptoms. For example, in inquiring about the cardiovascular system, the nurse notes positive or negative answers regarding chest pain and other symptoms or problems that are pertinent to heart function and circulation.
- The patient's **lifestyle** is another important component of the nursing health history and includes habits, diet, sleep, hobbies, and the patient's ability to perform the activities of daily living.
- A **social history** is the component of the nursing health history that details family relationships, ethnicity, educational level, economic status, and the condition of the patient's home and environment.
- The nursing health history also includes the patient's **psychological status** and the patient's **usual means of obtaining healthcare.**

OBTAINING A HEALTH HISTORY

The **health history assessment** and **review of systems** help to identify nursing care needs:

- First, check the patient's chart for information gathered by other health professionals and note any areas that need clarification prior to the patient interview.
- Use the written tool provided by the facility to record the history, customizing it to the patient.
- Record any changes in this information during the patient's hospital stay.
- Plan the time of the interview with the patient when there are not critical care needs that must be met first.
- Take time to alleviate patient's anxiety and establish rapport and trust.
- Approach the patient with an attitude of respect and sincere caring.
- Listen to the patient and use effective therapeutic communication skills during the interview.
- Review all areas of the health history with the patient and then ask for any other information that may be important. The family may be able to fill in missing information if the patient is unable to do so.

NORMAL STRUCTURE AND FUNCTION ACROSS THE LIFESPAN

It is vital to understand the **normal structure and function** of anatomy and physiology across the lifespan, from infants to geriatric patients, when performing a nursing assessment. For example, normal pulse rates and blood pressure ranges for a newborn are vastly different from those for an adult. A healthy newborn will have a resting heartbeat of 70 to 190 beats per minute, but this standard changes to 60 to 100 beats per minute in adults. It is important to recognize the normal differences in skin color and hue, and the development of dentition and muscle function across the lifespan. There are standard developmental stages from infancy to adolescence, as well as documented normal changes in geriatric physiology.

Organs That Maintain Homeostasis in the Body

The **organs of homeostatic function** include the following:

- **Lungs**: The lungs help maintain acid-base balance by releasing CO_2. They also remove water via expired air.
- **Kidneys**: The kidneys maintain fluid balance in the body by filtering the blood and releasing fluid as needed. Electrolyte levels are maintained in the same way. Wastes and toxins are removed from the blood and body in the urine. The pH of the blood is maintained via the retention of hydrogen ions.
- **Heart:** The heart must pump blood with sufficient force to properly perfuse all organs and to push enough blood through the kidneys for filtering.
- **Adrenal glands**: Aldosterone and cortisol are produced by the adrenals to cause the kidneys to retain sodium and fluids.
- **Pituitary:** The pituitary stores and releases antidiuretic hormone (ADH) from the hypothalamus to direct the kidneys to retain fluids to maintain cellular osmotic pressure.
- **Parathyroid:** Parathyroid hormone maintains calcium and phosphate levels by causing calcium absorption by the intestines and renal tubules and from the bones as needed.

Daily Gain and Loss of Fluids

The body's fluid gains and losses should be about equal on a daily basis to maintain fluid and electrolyte balance. This can be monitored by measuring **intake** and **output** (I & O), but a number of other factors must be considered as well:

Fluid gains are as follows:

- Food people eat each day contains about 1000 mL of fluid.
- Fluids they drink average 1300 mL per day.
- Metabolic processes produce about 300 mL per day.

Fluid losses are as follows:

- Fluid is lost via the kidneys by production of 1-2 L of urine daily.
- The skin sweats and this evaporates an average of 600 mL daily, but this can increase up to 1000 mL/hr in hot and dry climates, during fever, or as a result of burns. Fluid loss can decrease in hot humid conditions.
- Exhaled air accounts for 300-400 mL of fluid loss daily.
- Fluids lost in stools total about 100-200 mL daily.

Physical Examination Techniques

The **physical exam** is an important element of nursing assessment. The physical assessment needs to be organized and systematic and should be age- and developmentally-appropriate. The physical exam may be a complete physical exam, a system-specific exam, or an exam of a specific body part. The basic **techniques** of a physical exam are inspection, palpation, auscultation, and percussion. The nurse makes a visual, aural, and olfactory assessment of the patient. This includes paying attention to the patient's skin tone, breathing sounds, and breath odor. Palpation includes techniques for touching the patient's body in order to get physical information such as temperature, skin tone and condition, or swelling in the glands. Auscultation is the examination of sounds within the body, such as heart tones, wheezing or crackling in the lungs, or bowel sounds. Auscultation is usually performed with a stethoscope. Percussion involves making quick taps to parts of the body with the fingers to ascertain the shape and condition of organs, identify areas of tenderness, or assess reflexes.

Palpation

Use of **palpation** can provide valuable details during physical assessment of the patient:

- Be sure to wash and warm the hands prior to touching the patient.
- Do not use gloves unless you anticipate contact with bodily fluids.
- Explain the process and how it will feel and instruct the patient to relax the muscles if appropriate. Provide warmth and privacy during palpation.
- Use light palpation to feel the cervical lymph nodes and thyroid glands and to feel the superficial blood vessels for thrills.
- Place your hands on the chest to detect heart vibrations and to feel tactile fremitus during speech.
- Palpate the relaxed abdomen to identify structures and their borders and any masses or nodules on otherwise smooth organ surfaces.
- Utilize both hands to palpate the female reproductive organs by pushing organs into the reach of the other hand.

Palpation to identify organs and structures takes practice. Each patient is different but after you palpate many patients, the similarities in organ borders and consistency can be determined.

Palpating for Tactile Fremitus

The act of speaking causes the chest wall to vibrate. This vibration can be felt by placing your hands lightly on the chest wall over a section of the lungs bilaterally while the patient repeats the letter "e" or the numbers "99." The amount of vibration felt depends on the weight of the patient, the muscle mass of the chest and back, gender, deepness of the voice, and condition of the lungs. **Tactile fremitus** is greater over major airways and normal lung tissue. It is less over lungs full of air or with emphysema or a pneumothorax. Lung consolidation will produce increased fremitus. The nurse should not feel for fremitus over the sternum or scapula. The areas above and below the breasts and above, medial to, and below the scapulae should be tested.

Percussion

Percussion is striking part of the body to set the chest or abdominal wall into motion, producing sound that helps to locate underlying organs and reveal whether they are dense or filled with air or fluid. The sounds produced include:

- **Tympany**: Hollow drum sound produced when the organ contains air (stomach, intestines).
- **Resonance**: Hollow, low-pitched sound of normal lungs.
- **Hyperresonance**: Low-pitched sound of lungs with emphysema or pneumothorax (louder than resonance).
- **Dullness**: "thud" heard over dense structures such as the liver.
- **Flatness**: sound heard over muscles or bones such as in the thigh.

Percussion is performed by placing the middle finger of one hand over the area and striking it with the middle finger of the opposite hand. It can be used to find the margins of an organ or area of pathology by repeatedly striking areas near to each other and listening for changes in sound representing the edge of the organ. The extent of lung consolidation can be determined in this manner.

AUSCULTATION

Auscultation is listening to sounds within the body through either the bell or the diaphragm of the stethoscope. These sounds differ in the following ways:

- **Intensity**: The level of sound in terms of loudness.
- **Frequency**: Low or high pitch of the sound.
- **Quality**: Helps to distinguish between rumbling and musical-type sounds.

The **bell** of the stethoscope is best when listening for the lower frequency sounds of heart murmurs or bruit, with the bell placed lightly on the skin. The **diaphragm** is best for high-pitched sounds, such as heart or lung sounds or bowel sounds, with the diaphragm placed firmly on the skin. The nurse should not touch the tubing or place the end of the stethoscope in contact with cloth or hair, or extra sounds will be heard that may obscure the sounds transmitted.

Cardiovascular Assessment

Assessment of the Cardiovascular System

Cardiovascular assessment includes questioning the patient for any family history of death at a young age or other cardiovascular diseases. Elderly African-American males are at highest risk for cardiovascular problems. One must question the patient about edema, chest pain, dyspnea, fatigue, vertigo, syncope or other changes in consciousness, weight gain, and leg cramps or pain. If chest pain is a symptom, one must ask about the intensity, timing, location, any radiation, quality, meaning to the patient, factors that aggravate or alleviate the pain, nausea, dyspnea, diaphoresis, or any other accompanying symptoms. Physical assessment includes assessment of vital signs, heart and lung sounds, skin assessment, radial, popliteal, and pedal pulses, circulation and sensation of extremities, and auscultation of the aorta, renal, iliac, and femoral arteries for bruits. Blood should be taken for a lipid profile and electrolytes. The patient must be helped to modify risk factors such as hypertension, smoking, diabetes, obesity, hyperlipidemia, inactivity, and stress.

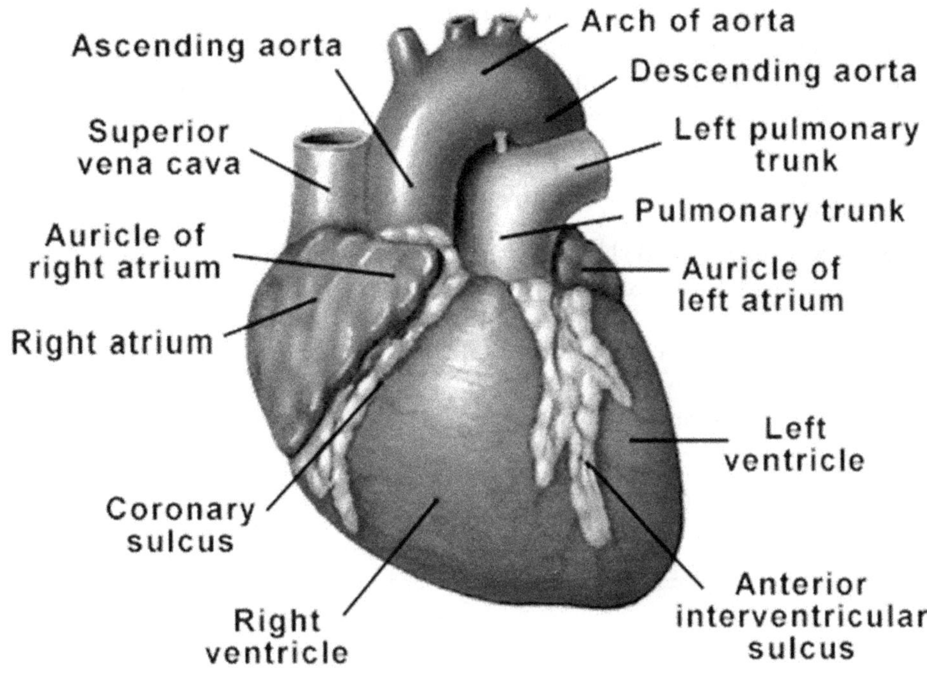

Review Video: Cardiovascular Assessment
Visit mometrix.com/academy and enter code: 323076

Assessment of Heart Sounds

Auscultation of **heart sounds** can help to diagnose different cardiac disorders. Areas to auscultate include the aortic area, pulmonary area, Erb's point, tricuspid area, and the apical area. The normal heart sounds represent closing of the valves.

- The **first heart sound** (S1) "lub" is closure of the mitral and tricuspid valves (heard at apex/left ventricular area of the heart).
- The **second heart sound** (S2) "dub" is closure of the aortic and pulmonic valves (heard at the base of the heart). There may be a slight splitting of the S2.

The time between S1 and S2 is systole and the time between S2 and the next S1 is diastole. Systole and diastole should be silent although ventricular disease can cause gallops, snaps, or clicks and stenosis of the valves or failure of the valves to close can cause murmurs. Pericarditis may cause a friction rub.

Additional **heart sounds**:

- **Gallop rhythms**: S3 commonly occurs after S2 in children and young adults but may indicate heart failure or left ventricular failure in older adults (when heard with patient lying on left side). S4 occurs before S1, during the contracting of the atria when there is ventricular hypertrophy, found in coronary artery disease, hypertension, or aortic valve stenosis.
- **Opening snap**: Unusual high-pitched sound occurring after S2 with stenosis of mitral valve from rheumatic heart disease
- **Ejection click**: Brief high-pitched sound after S1; aortic stenosis
- **Friction rub**: Harsh, grating holosystolic sound; pericarditis
- **Murmur**: Sound caused by turbulent blood flow from stenotic or malfunctioning valves, congenital defects, or increased blood flow. Murmurs are characterized by location, timing in the cardiac cycle, intensity (rated from Grade I to Grade VI), pitch (low to high-pitched), quality (rumbling, whistling, blowing) and radiation (to the carotids, axilla, neck, shoulder, or back).

Electrocardiogram

The **electrocardiogram** records and shows a graphic display of the electrical activity of the heart through a number of different waveforms, complexes, and intervals:

- **P wave**: Start of electrical impulse in the sinus node and spreading through the atria, muscle depolarization
- **QRS complex:** Ventricular muscle depolarization and atrial repolarization
- **T wave**: Ventricular muscle repolarization (resting state) as cells regain negative charge
- **U wave**: Repolarization of the Purkinje fibers

A modified lead II ECG is often used to monitor basic heart rhythms and dysrhythmias:

- Typical placement of leads for 2-lead ECG is 3 to 5 cm inferior to the right clavicle and left lower ribcage. Typical placement for a 3-lead ECG is (RA) right arm near shoulder, (LA) V_5 position over 5th intercostal space, and (LL) left upper leg near groin.

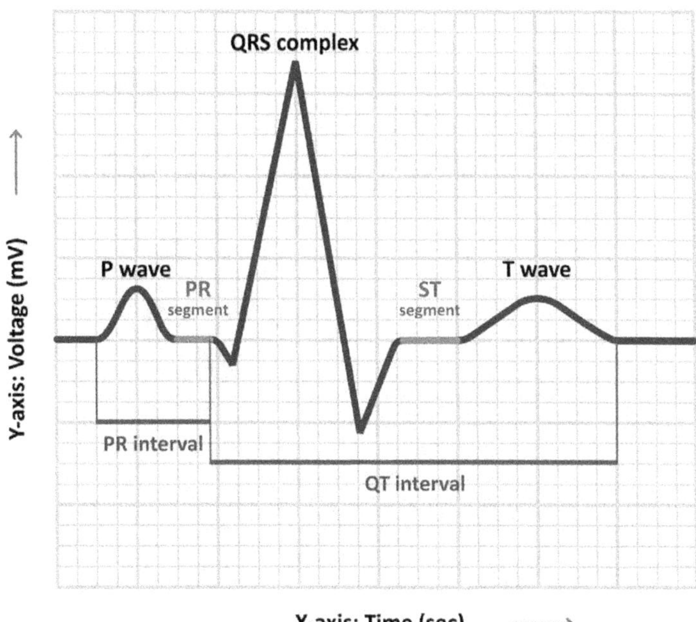

Administration of 12-Lead ECG

The **electrocardiogram** provides a graphic representation of the electrical activity of the heart. It is indicated for chest pain, dyspnea, syncope, acute coronary syndrome, pulmonary embolism, and possible MI. The standard 12 lead ECG gives a picture of electrical activity from 12 perspectives through placement of 10 body leads:

- 4 limb leads are placed distally on the wrists and ankles (but may be placed more proximally if necessary).
- Precordial leads:
  - V1: Right sternal border at 4th intercostal space.
  - V2: Left sternal border at 4th intercostal space.
  - V3: Midway between V2 and V4.
  - V4: Left midclavicular line at 5th intercostal space.
  - V5: Horizontal to V4 at left anterior axillary line.
  - V6: Horizontal to V5 at left midaxillary line.

In some cases, additional leads may be used:

- Right-sided leads are placed on the right in a mirror image of the left leads, usually to diagnose right ventricular infarction through ST elevation.

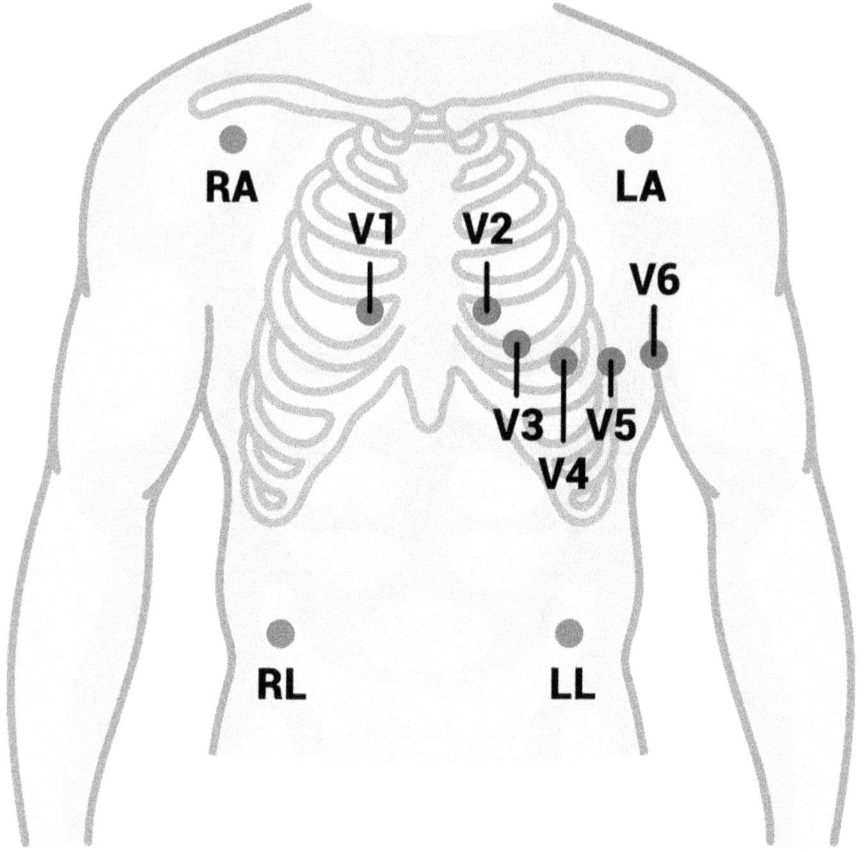

Review Video: 12 Lead ECG
Visit mometrix.com/academy and enter code: 962539

Cardiac Monitoring

Cardiac monitoring includes the evaluation of different intervals and segments on the electrocardiogram:

- **QT interval:** This is the complete time of ventricular depolarization and repolarization, which being with the QRS segment and ends when the Y wave is completed. Typically, duration usually ranges from 0.36 to 0.44 seconds, but this may vary depending on the heart rate. If the heat rate is rapid, the duration is shorter and vice versa. Certain medications can prolong the QT interval, in such cases monitoring this is critical. A prolonged QT interval puts the patient at risk for R-on-T phenomenon, which can result in dangerous arrhythmias.
- **ST segment:** This is an isoelectric period when the ventricles are in a plateau phase, completely depolarized and beginning recovery and repolarization. Deflection is usually isoelectric, but may range from -0.5 to +1mm. If the ST segment is ≥0.5 mm below the baseline, it is considered depressed and may be an indication of myocardial ischemia. Depression may also indicate digitalis toxicity. If the ST segment is elevated ≥1 mm above baseline, this is an indication of myocardial injury.

MAP

The **MAP (mean arterial pressure)** is most commonly used to evaluate perfusion as it shows pressure throughout the cardiac cycle. Systole is one-third and diastole two-thirds of the normal cardiac cycle. The MAP for a blood pressure of 120/60 is calculated as follows:

$$\text{MAP} = \frac{\text{Diastole} \times 2 + \text{Systole}}{3}$$

Example: Blood pressure 120/60

$$\text{MAP} = \frac{60 \times 2 + 120}{3} = \frac{240}{3} = 80$$

Normal range for mean arterial pressure is 70-100 mmHg. A MAP of greater than 60 mmHg is required to perfuse vital organs, including the heart, brain, and kidneys.

Oxygen Saturation as It Relates to Hemodynamic Status

Hemodynamic monitoring includes monitoring **oxygen saturation** levels, which must be maintained for proper cardiac function. The central venous catheter often has an oxygen sensor at the tip to monitor oxygen saturation in the right atrium. If the catheter tip is located near the renal veins, this can cause an increase in right atrial oxygen saturation; and near the coronary sinus, a decrease.

- Increased oxygen saturation may result from left atrial to right atrial shunt, abnormal pulmonary venous return, increased delivery of oxygen or decrease in extraction of oxygen.
- Decreased oxygen saturation may be related to low cardiac output with an increase in oxygen extraction or decrease in arterial oxygen saturation with normal differences in the atrial and ventricular oxygen saturation.

Cardiac Output

Cardiac output (CO) is the amount of blood pumped through the ventricles during a specified period. Normal cardiac output is about 5 liters per minutes at rest for an adult. Under exercise or stress, this volume may multiply 3 or 4 times with concomitant changes in the heart rate (HR) and stroke volume (SV). The basic formulation for calculating cardiac output is the heart rate (HR) per minute multiplied by the stroke volume (SR), which is the amount of blood pumped through the ventricles with each contraction. The stroke volume is controlled by preload, afterload, and contractibility.

$$\text{CO}\left(\frac{\text{mL}}{\text{min}}\right) = \text{HR}\left(\frac{\text{beats}}{\text{min}}\right) \times \text{SV (mL)}$$

The heart rate is controlled by the autonomic nervous system. Normally, if the heart rate decreases, stroke volume increases to compensate. The exception to this would be cardiomyopathies, so bradycardia results in a sharp decline in cardiac output.

Cardiac Index

Cardiac index (CI) is the cardiac output (CO) divided by the body surface area (BSA). This is essentially a measure of cardiac output tailored to the individual, based on height and weight, measured in liters/min per square meter of BSA.

- Normal value: 2.2–4.0 L/min/m^2

Stroke Volume

Stroke volume (SV) is the amount of blood pumped through the left ventricle with each contraction, minus any blood remaining inside the ventricle at the end of systole.

- Normal values: 60–70 mL
- Formula:

$$SV\ (mL) = CO\left(\frac{mL}{min}\right) \div HR\left(\frac{beats}{min}\right)$$

Pulmonary Vascular Resistance and Ejection Fraction

Pulmonary vascular resistance (PVR) is the resistance in the pulmonary arteries and arterioles against which the right ventricle has to pump during contraction. It is the mean pressure in the pulmonary vascular bed divided by blood flow. If PVR increases, SV decreases.

- Normal value: 1.2–3.0 units or 100–250 dynes/sec/cm^5

Ejection Fraction (EF) is the percentage of the total blood volume of the heart that is pumped out with each beat. Dramatically decreased values indicate heart failure.

- Normal value: 60–70%

Preload and Afterload

Preload refers to the amount of elasticity in the myocardium at the end of diastole when the ventricles are filled to their maximum volume and the stretch on the muscle fibers is the greatest. The preload value is based on the volume in the ventricles. The amount of preload (stretch) affects stroke volume because as stretch increases, the resultant contraction also increases (Frank-Starling Law). Preload may decrease because of dehydration, diuresis, or vasodilation. Preload may increase because of increased venous return, controlling fluid loss, transfusion, or intravenous fluids.

Afterload refers to the amount of systemic vascular resistance to left ventricular ejection of blood and pulmonary vascular resistance to right ventricular ejection of blood. Determinants of afterload include the size and elasticity of the great vessels and the functioning of the pulmonic and aortic valves. Afterload increases with hypertension, stenotic valves, and vasoconstriction.

Minimally/Non-Invasive Hemodynamic Monitoring

Hemodynamic monitoring and evaluation of cardiac function is an important component of the care of the critically ill patient. **Minimally or non-invasive** alternatives to traditional invasive means of hemodynamic monitoring (such as the use of a pulmonary artery catheter) include esophageal Doppler, arterial pressure based cardiac output monitoring, and impedance cardiography. **Esophageal Doppler** is a minimally invasive option used in surgical patients to monitor descending aortic blood flow and estimate cardiac output. A probe is inserted into the esophagus and then connected to a monitor, where waveform shapes produced by aortic blood flow are displayed.

Arterial pressure based cardiac output monitors (APCO's) use an algorithm to estimate cardiac output through the analysis of the arterial pressure waveform. The radial or femoral artery is accessed using a standard arterial catheter and no external calibration is needed.

Impedance cardiography is a non-invasive method of hemodynamic monitoring in which sensors placed on the body use electrical signals to measure the level of change in impedance in the thoracic fluid. A waveform is generated and is then used to calculate cardiac output and stroke volume, as well as ten additional hemodynamic parameters.

Intraarterial Blood Pressure Monitoring

Intraarterial blood pressure monitoring uses a catheter to measure systolic, diastolic, and mean arterial pressures (MAP) continuously. Before catheter insertion, collateral circulation must be assessed by Doppler or the Allen test (radial). Complications include arterial vasospasm, hematoma formation, hemorrhage (accidental disconnect), catheter occlusion, compartment syndrome, retroperitoneal bleed (femoral site), and thrombus/embolus.

Set up: The line should be connected to the monitor as well as a pressure bag set at 300 mmHg with no longer than 3 feet of stiff, noncompliant tubing to ensure accuracy. The transducer is leveled at the phlebostatic axis of the patient. The line should be kept free of any air or bubbles, and re-zeroed every four hours and with a change of patient position.

Waveform: A normal ABP waveform should be smooth and regular, with a dicrotic notch. To test, perform a "square-wave" or "Fast Flush" test; flush the line while watching the monitor. There should be a square shape, followed by two oscillations and a return to normal waves. A missing dicrotic notch indicates a blockage of some kind (thrombus, plaque, and vasospasm) or low pressure in the bag. Too many oscillations or an increased sharpness of the wave indicates under dampening and is caused by increased SVR or too long of tubing.

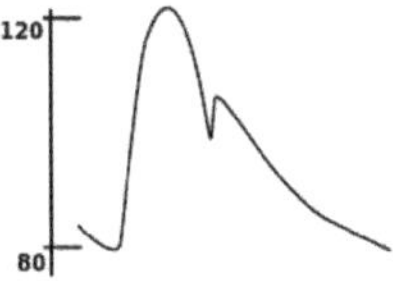

Assessing Jugular Venous Pressure

Jugular venous pressure (neck-vein) is used to assess the cardiac output and pressure in the right heart as the pulsations relate to changes in pressure in the right atrium. This procedure is usually not accurate if the pulse rate is >100. This is a non-invasive estimation of central venous pressure and waveform. Measurement should be done with the internal jugular if possible; if not, the external jugular may be used.

- **Elevate** the patient's head to 45° (and to 90° if necessary) with patient's head turned to the right.
- Position a **light** at an angle to illuminate veins and shadows.
- Measure the height of the **jugular vein pulsation** above the sternal joint, using a ruler.
    - Normal height is ≤4 cm above sternal angle.

Increased pressure (>4 cm) indicates increased pressure in the right atrium, and right heart failure. It may also indicate pericarditis or tricuspid stenosis. Laughing or coughing may trigger the Valsalva response and also cause an increase in pressure.

Additional Cardiac Assessments

The **stress test**, also called an exercise tolerance test, is a commonly used assessment to screen for ischemic heart disease. In this test, the patient is put through exercise with increasing rigor, generally on a treadmill, while attached to an ECG to monitor their heart's rhythm. The patient is assessed for chest pain and dizziness as the rigor level is increased, which is a reflection of the heart's capacity to handle increasing workloads effectively. The stress test is not diagnostic on its own, but provides feedback on the direction of additional testing.

Water-hammer pulse is characterized by the alternation between a bounding heartbeat that is strong and forceful, and then collapse. This could be the result of a heightened stroke volume, decreased peripheral resistance, or these two factors together. To assess for this pulse, the patient is seated and one arm is raised vertically. Upon palpation of the radial pulse in the raised arm, the pulse resembles a tapping in the muscles of the forearm. This is often an indication of aortic regurgitation.

Perfusion Pressure and Pulse Pressure

Perfusion pressure directly affects coronary blood flow, and coronary perfusion occurs during diastole. Coronary artery perfusion pressure is equal to the diastolic blood pressure minus the pulmonary artery occlusion pressure. Normal values are 60–80 mmHg. During the cardiac cycle, *aortic pressure* causes the coronaries to be perfused, while *ventricular pressure* compresses the coronaries during systole, decreasing perfusion.

The **pulse pressure** is the difference between systolic and diastolic pressures, and this can be an important indicator. For example, with a decrease in cardiac output, vasoconstriction takes place in the body's attempt to maintain the blood pressure. In this case, the MAP may remain unchanged, but the pulse pressure narrows. Patients should be assessed for changes in pulse pressure that may be precipitated by medications, such as diuretics that alter fluid volume.

Assessment of Lower Extremities

Assessment of lower extremities includes a number of different elements:

- **Appearance** includes comparing limbs for obvious differences or changes in skin or nails as well as evaluating for edema, color changes in skin, such as pallor or rubor. Legs that are thin, pale, shiny, and hairless indicate peripheral arterial disease.
- **Perfusion** should be assessed by checking venous filling time and capillary refill, skin temperature (noting changes in one limb or between limbs), bruits (indicating arterial narrowing), pulses (comparing both sides in a proximal to distal progression), ankle-brachial index and toe-brachial index.
- **Sensory function** includes the ability to feel pain, temperature, and touch.
- **Range of motion** of the ankle must be assessed to determine if the joint flexes past 90° because this is necessary for unimpaired walking and aids venous return in the calf.
- **Pain** is an important diagnostic feature of peripheral arterial disease, so the location, intensity, duration, and characteristics of pain are important.

Assessment of Pulse and Bruit

Evaluation of the pulses of the **lower extremities** is an important part of assessment for peripheral arterial disease/trauma. Pulses should be first evaluated with the patient in supine position and then again with the legs dependent, checking bilaterally and proximal to distal to determine if intensity of pulse decreases distally. Pedal pulses should be examined at both the posterior tibialis and the dorsalis pedis. The pulse should be evaluated as to the rate, rhythm, and intensity, which is usually graded on a 0 to 4 scale:

0 = pulse absent
1 = weak, difficult to palpate
2 = normal as expected
3 = full
4 = strong and bounding

Pulses may be **palpable** or **absent** with peripheral arterial disease. Absence of pulse on both palpation and Doppler probe does indicate peripheral arterial disease.

Bruits may be noted by auscultating over major arteries, such as femoral, popliteal, peroneal, and dorsalis pedis, indicating peripheral arterial disease.

Assessing Perfusion of Lower Extremities

Assessment of **perfusion** can indicate venous or arterial abnormalities:

- **Venous refill time**: Begin with the patient lying supine for a few moments and then have the patient sit with the feet dependent. Observe the veins on the dorsum of the foot and count the seconds before normal filling. Venous occlusion is indicated with times greater than 20 seconds.
- **Capillary refill**: Grasp the toenail bed between the thumb and index finger and apply pressure for several seconds to cause blanching. Release the nail and count the seconds until the nail regains normal color. Arterial occlusion is indicated with times of more than 2 to 3 seconds. Check both feet and more than one nail bed.
- **Skin temperature**: Using the palm of the hand and fingers, gently palpate the skin, moving distally to proximally and comparing both legs. Arterial disease is indicated by decreased temperature (coolness) or a marked change from proximal to distal. Venous disease is indicated by increased temperature about the ankle.

ABI

PROCEDURE

The ankle-brachial index **(ABI) examination** is done to evaluate peripheral arterial disease of the lower extremities.

1. Apply BP cuff to one arm, palpate brachial pulse, and place conductivity gel over the artery.
2. Place the tip of a Doppler device at a 45-degree angle into the gel at the brachial artery and listen for the pulse sound.
3. Inflate the cuff until the pulse sound ceases and then inflate 20 mmHg above that point.
4. Release air and listen for the return of the pulse sound. This reading is the brachial systolic pressure.
5. Repeat the procedure on the other arm and use the higher reading for calculations.
6. Repeat the same procedure on each ankle with the cuff applied above the malleoli and the gel over the posterior tibial pulse to obtain the ankle systolic pressure.
7. Divide the ankle systolic pressure by the brachial systolic pressure to obtain the ABI.

Sometimes, readings are taken both before and after 5 minutes of walking on a treadmill.

INTERPRETING RESULTS

Once the **ABI examination** is completed, the ankle systolic pressure must be divided by the brachial systolic pressure. Ideally, the BP at the ankle should be equal to that of the arm or slightly higher. With peripheral arterial disease the ankle pressure falls, affecting the ABI. Additionally, some conditions that cause calcification of arteries, such as diabetes, can cause a false elevation.

Calculation is simple:

$$\text{ABI} = \frac{\text{Ankle systolic}}{\text{Brachial systolic}}$$

The degree of disease relates to the **score**:

- >1.4: Abnormally high, may indicate calcification of vessel wall.
- 1.0–1.4: Normal reading, asymptomatic.
- 0.9–1.0: Low reading, but acceptable unless there are other indications of PAD.
- 0.8–0.9: Likely some arterial disease is present.
- 0.5–0.8: Moderate arterial disease
- < 0.5: Severe arterial disease.

Respiratory Assessment

Assessment of the Respiratory System

If significant respiratory distress is present, one must stabilize the patient before doing a **respiratory history** or ask family if available:

- Question the patient about risk factors, such as smoking, exposure to smoke or other inhaled toxins, past lung problems, and allergies.
- Ask the patient about symptoms of respiratory problems, such as dyspnea, cough, sputum production, fatigue, ability to do ADLs and IADLs, and chest pain.
- Determine how long symptoms have been present, the length of periods of dyspnea, aggravating and alleviating factors, and the severity of symptoms.

When performing a **physical assessment**, one should assess vital signs, posture, pulse oximetry, check nails for clubbing, do a skin assessment, listen to lung sounds via auscultation and percussion, and look for accessory muscle use, signs of anxiety, and edema. Depending on condition, blood may be drawn for arterial blood gases, electrolytes, and CBC. Sputum cultures may be obtained.

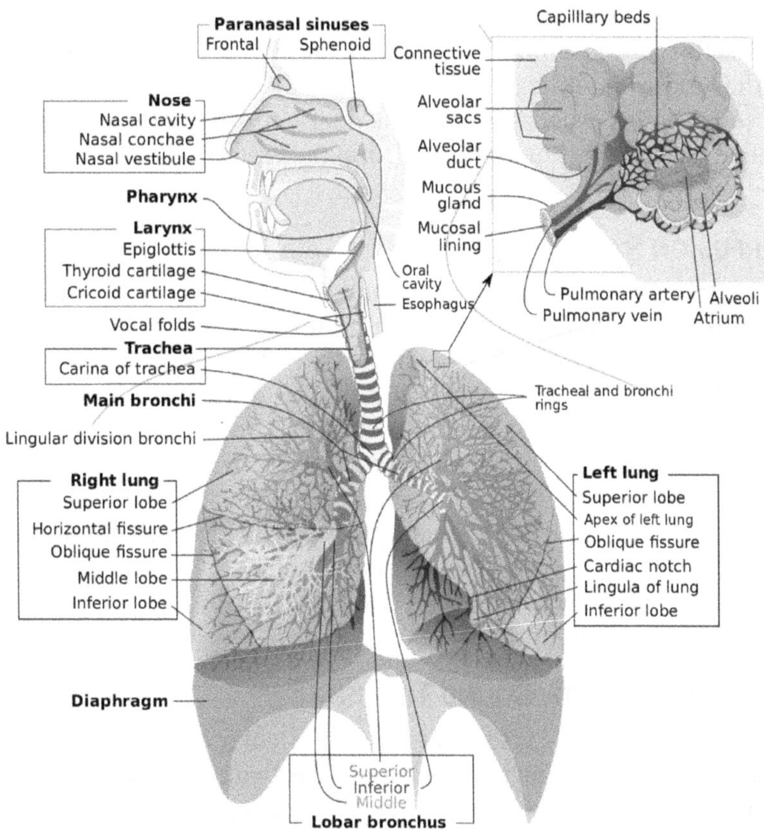

Review Video: Respiratory System
Visit mometrix.com/academy and enter code: 783075

PRIMARY AND SECONDARY MUSCLES USED FOR BREATHING

Muscles used for breathing are separated into primary and secondary muscle groups.

- The **primary muscle groups** are those that are used in normal, quiet breathing. When patients are in respiratory distress and breathing is more difficult, secondary muscle groups become activated. The muscles considered primary for breathing are the diaphragm and the external intercostal muscles. These muscles act by changing the pressure gradient, allowing the lungs to expand and air to flow in and out.
- The **secondary muscle groups** include the sternocleidomastoid, scaleni, internal intercostals, obliques, and abdominal muscles. These secondary muscle groups work when breathing is difficult, both in inspiration and expiration, in cases such as obstructions or bronchoconstriction. Use of these secondary muscle groups can often be seen on exam and may be described as see-saw or abdominal breathing (when the abdominal muscles are being used during exhalation) or retractions as the muscles activate and can be seen between rigid structures such as bone.

NORMAL PHYSIOLOGICAL AIRWAY CLEARANCE

Normal airway clearance is caused by various aspects of the respiratory system. A thin layer of mucus lines the airways as a protective mechanism against debris and helps trap foreign objects before they enter the lower airways. Proper hydration keeps the mucosa adequately moist so it can trap foreign debris. As this debris lands in the mucus, the cilia in the respiratory tract act as an "elevator" to push the debris up to the larynx, where it can either be coughed up or swallowed and digested. An intact cough reflex is necessary for the debris to stimulate the cough, and normal muscle strength and nerve innervation of the diaphragm is required to produce a sufficiently forceful cough.

VENTILATION/PERFUSION RATIO

In order to maintain homeostasis, the respiratory and cardiac systems need to maintain a careful balance. The **ventilation/perfusion ratio** indicates that ventilation of the lungs and perfusion to the lungs are within a normal balance. A normal ventilation/perfusion ratio is equal to 0.8. A ventilation/perfusion ratio higher than normal is indicative of ventilation that is too high, perfusion that is too low, or some combination of the two. This can occur because of hyperventilation (either physiological or caused by healthcare practitioners due to incorrect ventilator settings), pulmonary embolism, or hypotension. Essentially, a high ventilation/perfusion ratio means that there is more ventilation than perfusion. If the ventilation/perfusion ratio is lower than normal, then ventilation is too low, perfusion is too high, or some combination of the two. This can be caused by atelectasis, pneumonia, or lung disease. Whatever the cause, a low ventilation/perfusion ratio indicates that there is more perfusion than ventilation.

NORMAL AND ABNORMAL BREATH SOUND TERMS

Normal breath sounds can be divided into three types. Vesicular breath sounds are low, soft sounds that can normally be heard over the peripheral lung space. Bronchovesicular breath sounds are moderate pitch breath sounds that are normally heard in the upper lung fields. Tracheal breath sounds are higher in pitch and heard over the trachea. Abnormal breath sounds are also known as adventitious lung sounds. Wheezes are high-pitched, expiratory sounds caused by air flowing through an obstructed airway. Stridor is also high-pitched, but is usually heard on inspiration in the upper airways. Coarse crackles are caused by an excessive amount of secretions in the airway and can be heard on inspiration and expiration. Fine crackles occur late in the expiratory phase and usually occur when the peripheral airways are being "popped" back open.

Review Video: Lung Sounds
Visit mometrix.com/academy and enter code: 765616

Diagnostic Procedures and Tools Used During Assessment of Pulmonary Trauma/Disease

The diagnostic procedures and tools used during assessment of **pulmonary and thoracic trauma/disease** will vary according to the type and degree of injury/disease, but may include:

- **Thorough physical examination** including cardiac and pulmonary status, assessing for any abnormalities.
- **Electrocardiogram** to assess for cardiac arrhythmias.
- **Chest x-ray** should be done for all those with injuries to check for fractures, pneumothorax, major injuries, and placement of intubation tubes. X-rays can be taken quickly and with portable equipment so they can be completed quickly during the initial assessment.
- **Computerized tomography** may be indicated after initial assessment, especially if there is a possibility of damage to the parenchyma of the lungs.
- **Oximetry and atrial blood gases** as indicated.
- **12-lead electrocardiogram** may be needed if there are arrhythmias for more careful observation.
- **Echocardiogram** should be done if there is apparent cardiac damage.

Capnography with End-Tidal CO_2 Detector

Capnometry utilizes an **end-tidal CO_2 (ETCO) detector** that measures the concentration of CO_2 in expired air, usually through pH sensitive paper that changes color (commonly purple to yellow). Typically, the capnometer is attached to the ETT and a bag-valve-mask (BVM) ventilator attached. The capnogram provides data in the shape of a waveform that represents the partial pressure of exhaled gas. It is often used to confirm placement of endotracheal tubes as clinical assessment is not always sufficient, and it is a noninvasive mode of monitoring carbon dioxide in the respiratory cycle. Information provided by the capnogram includes:

- $PaCO_2$ level
- Type and degree of bronchial obstruction, such as COPD (waveform changes from rectangular to a fin-like)
- Air leaks in the ventilation system
- Rebreathing precipitated by need for new CO_2 absorber
- Cardiac arrest
- Hypothermia or reduced metabolism

Normal Capnogram

The normal capnogram is a waveform which represents the varying CO_2 level throughout the breath cycle.

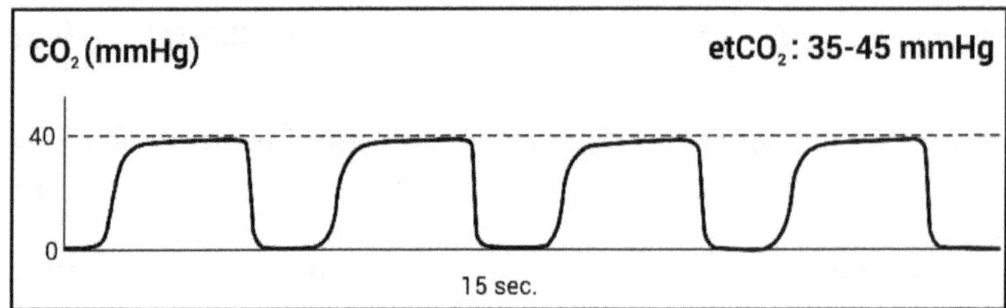

Arterial Blood Gases

Arterial blood gases (ABGs) are monitored to assess effectiveness of oxygenation, ventilation, and acid-base status and to determine oxygen flow rates. Partial pressure of a gas is that exerted by each gas in a mixture of gases, proportional to its concentration, based on total atmospheric pressure of 760 mmHg at sea level. Normal values include:

- Acidity/alkalinity (pH): 7.35-7.45.
- Partial pressure of carbon dioxide ($PaCO_2$): 35-45 mmHg.
- Partial pressure of oxygen (PaO_2): ≥80 mg Hg.
- Bicarbonate concentration (HCO_3^-): 22-26 mEq/L.
- Oxygen saturation (SaO_2): ≥95%.

The relationship between these elements, particularly the $PaCO_2$ and the PaO_2 indicates respiratory status. For example, $PaCO_2$ >55 and the PaO_2 <60 in a patient previously in good health indicates respiratory failure. There are many issues to consider. Ventilator management may require a higher $PaCO_2$ to prevent barotrauma and a lower PaO_2 to reduce oxygen toxicity.

Neurological Assessment

Assessment of the Neurological System

Assessment of the neurological system includes:

- Assess the **health history** for any trauma, falls, alcoholism, drug abuse, medications taken, and family history of neurological problems.
- Ask about any presenting **neurological symptoms**, the circumstances in which they occur, whether they fluctuate, and any associated factors, such as seizures, pain, vertigo, weakness, abnormal sensations, visual problems, loss of consciousness, changes in cognition, and motor problems.

Assessment includes determining the level of consciousness and cognition. Posture and movements are assessed for abnormalities. Facial expression and movement are noted. Cranial nerve assessment is done. The patient is assessed for strength, coordination, and balance and the ability to perform ADLs. One should assess for clonus and test all reflexes, including Babinski, gag, blink, swallow, upper and lower abdominal, cremasteric in males, plantar, perianal, biceps, triceps, brachioradialis, patellar and ankle. Peripheral sensation is tested by touching the patient with cotton balls and the sharp and dull ends of a broken tongue blade.

Review Video: Nervous System
Visit mometrix.com/academy and enter code: 708428

Assessing Functional Status

Functional abilities include the acts needed to meet basic needs and perform *activities of daily living* (ADLs), such as eating and elimination, as well as those *activities that are essential to independent living* (IADLs), such as shopping. A thorough assessment of the patient's functional abilities will identify areas that should be concentrated upon during rehabilitation. One should observe the patient as he/she performs these functions and record the following:

- Degree of independence shown
- Ability to complete activity without rest
- Nerve function
- Muscle function and strength
- Motion
- Coordination
- Cardiac status
- Respiratory status
- Assistance required to complete activity

The facility usually provides one of the tools available to record a functional assessment. The most common tool used is the Functional Independence Measure (FIM). Other tools available include the Barthel Index, the PULSES Profile, and the Patient Evaluation Conference System.

Cranial Nerves

	Name	Function	PE Test
I	Olfactory	Smell	Test olfaction
II	Optic	Visual acuity	Snellen eye chart; Accommodation
III	Oculomotor	Eye movement/ pupil	Pupillary reflex; Eye/eyelid motion
IV	Trochlear	Eye movement	Eye moves down & out
V	Trigeminal	Facial motor/ sensory	Corneal reflex; Facial sensation; Mastication
VI	Abducens	Eye movement	Lateral eye motion
VII	Facial	Facial expression; Taste	Moves forehead, closes eyes, smile/frown, puffs cheeks; Taste
VIII	Vestibulo-cochlear (Acoustic)	Hearing; Balance	Hearing (Weber/Rinne tests); Nystagmus
IX	Glosso-pharyngeal	Pharynx motor/sensory	Gag reflex; Soft palate elevation
X	Vagus	Visceral sensory, motor	Gag, swallow, cough
XI	Accessory	Sternocleidomastoid and trapezius (motor)	Turns head & shrugs shoulders against resistance
XII	Hypoglossal	Tongue movement	Push out tongue; move tongue from side to side

American Stroke Association Classification System for the Extent of Brain Attack Injury

The American Stroke Association developed a **brain attack outcome classification system** to standardize descriptions of stroke injuries:

- **Number of impaired domains** (Potentially affected neurological domains: motor, sensory, vision, language, cognition, and affect): Level 0: no domains impaired; Level 1: one domain impaired; Level 2: two domains impaired; Level 3: greater than 2 domains impaired.
- **Severity of impairment**: A (minimal or no neurological deficit due to stroke); B (mild/moderate deficit); or C (severe deficit). Note: When more than one domain is affected, severity is measured by the domain with the most impairment.

Assessment of function determines the ability to **live independently**:

- **I**: Independent in basic activities of daily living (BADL), such as bathing, eating, toileting, and walking; and instrumental activities of daily living (IADL), such as telephoning, shopping, maintaining a household, socializing, and using transportation.
- **II**: Independent in BADL but partially dependent in IADL.
- **III**: Partially dependent in BADL (less than 3 areas) and IADL.
- **IV**: Partially dependent in BADL (3 or more areas).
- **V**: Completely dependent in BADL (5 or more areas) and IADL.

Level III requires much assistance and Levels IV and V cannot live independently.

Administration of the NIHSS

The **National Institutes of Health Stroke Scale (NIHSS)** is administered with careful attention to directions. The examiner should record the answers and avoid coaching or repeating requests, although demonstration may be used with aphasic patients. The scale comprises 11 sections, with scores for each section ranging from 0 (normal) to 2 to 4:

- **Level of consciousness**: Response to noxious stimulation (0 to 3), request for month and his/her age (0 to 2), request to open and close eyes, grip and release unaffected hand (0 to 2).
- **Best gaze**: Horizontal eye movement (0 to 2).
- **Visual**: Visual fields (0 to 3).
- **Facial palsy**: Symmetry when patient shows teeth, raises eyebrows, and closes eyes (0 to 3).
- **Motor, arm**: Drift while arm extended with palms down (0 to 4).
- **Motor, leg**: Leg drift at 30 degrees while patient supine (0 to 4).
- **Limb ataxia**: Finger-nose and heel-shin (0 to 2).
- **Sensory**: Grimace or withdrawal from pinprick (0 to 2).
- **Best language**: Describes action of pictures (0 to 3).
- **Dysarthria**: Reads or describes words on list (0 to 2).
- **Distinction and inattention**: Visual spatial neglect (0 to 2).

Glasgow Coma Scale

The **Glasgow coma scale** (GCS) measures the depth and duration of coma or impaired level of consciousness and is used for post-operative assessment. The GCS measures three parameters: best eye response, best verbal response, and best motor response, with a total possible score that ranges from 3 to 15:

Eye opening	4: Spontaneous 3: To verbal stimuli 2: To pain (not of face) 1: No response
Verbal	5: Oriented 4: Conversation confused, but can answer questions 3: Uses inappropriate words 2: Speech incomprehensible 1: No response
Motor	6: Moves on command 5: Moves purposefully respond pain 4: Withdraws in response to pain 3: Decorticate posturing (flexion) in response to pain 2: Decerebrate posturing (extension) in response to pain 1: No response

Injuries/conditions are classified according to the total score: 3-8 Coma; ≤8 Severe head injury likely requiring intubation; 9-12 Moderate head injury; 13-15 Mild head injury.

ICP and Monroe-Kellie Hypothesis

Increasing **intracranial pressure (ICP)** is a frequent complication of brain injuries, tumors, or other disorders affecting the brain, so monitoring the ICP is very important. Increased ICP can indicate cerebral edema, hemorrhage, and/or obstruction of cerebrospinal fluid. The **Monroe-Kellie hypothesis** states that in order to maintain a normal ICP, a change in volume in one compartment must be compensated by a reciprocal change in volume in another compartment. There are 3 compartments in the brain: the brain tissue, cerebrospinal fluid (CSF), and blood.The

CSF and blood can change more easily to accommodate changes in pressure than tissue, so medical intervention focuses on cerebral blood flow and drainage. Normal ICP is 1-15 mmHg on transducer or 13.6–203.9 mmH_2O on manometer. As intracranial pressure increases, **symptoms** include:

- Headache.
- Alterations in level of consciousness.
- Restlessness.
- Slowly reacting or nonreacting dilated or pinpoint pupils.
- Seizures.
- Motor weakness.
- Cushing's triad (late sign):
    - Increased systolic pressure with widened pulse pressure.
    - Bradycardia in response to increased pressure.
    - Decreased respirations.

ICP Monitoring Devices

The **intracranial pressure (ICP) monitoring device** may be placed during surgery or a ventriculostomy performed in which a burr hole is drilled into the frontal area of the scalp and an **intraventricular catheter** threaded into the lateral ventricle. The intraventricular catheter may be used to monitor ICP and to drain excess CSF. Other monitoring devices include:

- **Intracranial pressure monitor bolt** (subarachnoid bolt) is applied through a burr hole with the distal end of the monitor probe resting in the subarachnoid space.
- **Epidural monitors** are placed into the epidural space.
- **Fiberoptic monitors** may be placed inside the brain.

The intraventricular catheter is the most accurate. CSF may be drained continuously or intermittently and must be monitored hourly for amount, color, and character. For ICP measurement, the patient's head must be elevated to 30-45° and the transducer leveled to the tragus of the ear or outer canthus of the eye, depending on facility policy.

Cerebral Blood Flow, MAP, and CPP

Cerebral blood flow, or the blood supply to the brain at any given moment, is influenced directly by one's **mean arterial pressure** (MAP). A MAP of greater than 60 mmHg is required to perfuse vital organs, including the brain. A MAP that falls below 60 mmHg risks ischemia and infarction. An excessively high MAP (greater than 100 mmHg) can also cause damage. A high MAP can result in increased oxygen demands by the heart, vascular injury, end organ damage, and stroke.

Cerebral perfusion pressure (CPP) is the pressure required to maintain adequate blood flow to the brain. CPP is based on mean arterial pressure (MAP) and intracranial pressure (ICP). Elevated ICP can be associated with a reduction in CPP.

$$CPP = MAP - ICP$$

- Normal CPP: 60-100 mmHg.
- <60 mmHg: Hypoperfusion occurs , resulting in focal or global ischemia.
- <30 mmHg: Hypoperfusion is marked and incompatible with life.
- >100 mmHg: Leads to hypertensive encephalopathy and cerebral edema (particularly if CPP >120 mmHg); Patients with chronic hypertension tolerate a higher level of CPP.

NEUROLOGICAL MOTOR TESTING AND TESTING FOR NUCHAL RIGIDITY

Neurological motor testing requires careful observation for involuntary or spastic movements and examination of muscles for lack of symmetry or atrophy with observation of gait. Muscle tone is examined by flexing and extending the upper and lower extremities, observing for flaccid or spastic changes. Muscle strength is examined by having the patient press fingers, wrists, elbows, hips, knees, ankles, and plantar area against resistance, graded 0 (no movement) to 5 (normal).

Pronator drift is an indication of disease of the upper motor neurons. The patient stands with eyes closed and both arms extended horizontally in front with the palms facing upwards (supination). The patient should be told to hold the arms still and not move them while the examiner taps downward on the arm. If motor neuron disease is present, the patient's arms will drift downward and hands will drift toward pronation.

Nuchal rigidity is tested by placing the hands behind the patient's head and flexing the neck gently to determine if there is increased resistance.

Endocrine Assessment

ASSESSING FOR ENDOCRINE DISORDERS

The **endocrine system** comprises organs that produce hormones that are critical to growth, sexual development, and metabolism, so changes in these areas are suggestive of endocrine disorders. While symptoms may vary widely, there are often generalized symptoms that can be associated with most endocrine disorders. One should question the patient about fatigue and ability to perform ADLs, heat or cold intolerance, changes in sexual libido, sexual functioning, and secondary sexual characteristics, weight fluctuation, sleep problems, decreased concentration and memory, and mood changes. During the physical exam, one should assess the patient for edema, "moon" face or "buffalo hump," exophthalmos, hair loss, female facial hair, enlarged trunk with thin extremities, and enlarged hands and feet. Vital signs should be assessed for hypo or hypertension, and one should assess for changes in skin appearance and vision.

THYROID IMAGING

Thyroid imaging plays a critical role in assessment of many thyroid diseases. This test may be used to determine the uptake characteristics of the thyroid gland in addition to the size and shape of the gland. In addition, thyroid imaging may determine how much iodine-131 is needed in order to safely ablate the gland when necessary. The radioactive iodine uptake scan (RAIU) is basically administration of iodine-123 with imaging performed 8 and 24 hours later:

Uptake of radioactive iodine is increased in disorders such as Graves' disease, "hot" nodules of various etiologies (including toxic multinodular goiter), TSH-secreting pituitary tumor, and iodine deficiency.

Uptake of radioactive iodine is decreased in the setting of thyroiditis and iodine excess.

Ultrasound imaging is used in thyroid disease to determine the size and structure of a thyroid nodule, such as to determine uniformity of shape, irregular contour, solid/cystic structure, and depth.

Immunologic and Oncologic Assessment

Cancer

Cancer is a potentially life-threatening disease that occurs due to irregular cell growth and reproduction. These cells can develop into a tumor that can occupy an area where normal body cells are usually found. Cancer cells also have the ability to metastasize, or extend, into other areas of the body. Cells within the body are constantly being replaced by normal cells. During this process, an abnormality in a cell's DNA can occur which causes it to become a malignant cancer cell. The body's immune system will usually attack and destroy this cell, but sometimes there can be a failure of the immune system to do this or the immune system is not able to destroy the cell. When this happens, the cancer cell can continue to reproduce itself until a tumor is formed. Some cancers can even attack normal, healthy cells within the body and alter their DNA so they will begin to reproduce as cancer cells.

Stages of Cancer Development

There are three stages of the development of cancer:

- **Initiation** is the action of a cancer-causing substance entering the body, reacting with DNA, and causing DNA mutation. Examples include cigarette smoke, radiation exposure, etc. The effects of initiation are irreversible; it results in permanent genetic change. Any daughter cells produced from the division of the mutated cell will also carry the mutation.
- **Promotion** is the process in which the body is repeatedly exposed to the cancer-causing substance. This repeats the process mentioned above and increases the likelihood of cancer cells being reproduced.
- **Progression** occurs when the malignant cancer cells begin to outnumber the normal, healthy cells because of continued replication within the body. At this point, the body is no longer able to attempt to repair the damage done to DNA by the cancer-causing agents and the normal cells continue to replicate as cancer cells.

Causes of Cancer

There are five main **causes of cancer**:

- **Radiation** can cause cancer by altering a cell's DNA. If the body is not able to repair the damages, the cell can reproduce as a cancer cell. Radiation exposure can be accidental or from diagnostic testing. UV light exposure is a form of radiation, also, and it causes skin cancer. Asbestos is considered a form of radiation, also, and causes mesothelioma tumors within the lungs.
- **Chemical carcinogens** can alter a cell's DNA to cause cancer. An example of this is cigarette smoke and exposure to tar within cigarettes.
- **Viruses** can cause cancer. Viruses that alter a cell's genetic material can stimulate the production of cancer cells.
- **The immune system** may be unsuccessful in repairing or destroying cells with altered DNA, which can lead to cancer. Certain cancer cells have the ability to alter the immune system so that it cannot recognize the formation of malignant cells within normal tissues.
- Cancer can also occur because of **inherited factors**. A person can inherit oncogenes responsible for causing certain types of cancer.

Cancer Cells Characteristics

Cancer cells have certain unique and defining **characteristics**:

- **Pleomorphism** means that the cells are of different dimensions and forms.
- **Hyperchromatism** refers to chromatin within the cell's nucleus that is seen clearly when staining is done for studies.
- **Polymorphism** is the ability of the cell's nucleus to expand and change its form.
- **Translocations** are changes in the chromosomes in which genetic information is swapped.
- **Deletions** occur when portions of a chromosomes' genetic information is obliterated.
- **Amplification** refers to multiple reproductions of a section of DNA.
- **Aneuploidy** refers to an atypical quantity of chromosomes.

Just like normal cells, cancer cells are constantly changing, dying, and reproducing. Different types of tumors grow at different rates. A tumor's growth rate, or **growth fraction**, is measured in a percentage of cells that are actively being reproduced at any given time. Tumor growth can also be measured in the amount of time it takes for tumor cells to double in quantity. This is called the **tumor volume doubling time**.

Tumors require proper nutrition in order to thrive and continue to grow. To receive the necessary nutrients, there must be blood supply to the tumor. This blood supply is produced through angiogenesis. If the blood supply is not available to the tumor, the tumor cells will die.

Gompertzian growth is a term that refers to a generality that is made regarding tumor growth. It is thought that tumors grow rapidly early on, but then growth slows down as the tumor enlarges. This most likely occurs because of not having the nutrients necessary to thrive.

Immunology

Immunology is the field of medicine that examines the body's ability to fight off infection. The body has a complicated system of cells and certain substances that react when an unknown agent attempts to cause an infectious process within the body. When a cell is altered to form a cancer cell, the body usually recognizes it as abnormal and attacks it. This prevents its replication and the development of more cancer cells. If immune cells are not functioning properly, the cancer cell could go on to reproduce more cells to eventually form a tumor that can potentially invade the surrounding tissues. Immunology also focuses on treatment research and ways in which the immune system can function more effectively in preventing cancer cell formation.

Review Video: Immune System
Visit mometrix.com/academy and enter code: 622899

Tumor Staging and Tumor Grading

Tumor staging and grading are two types of tumor severity assessment. They are assigned by the surgical pathologist. Tumor staging is a measurement of the size or extent of spread of a tumor. It is based on three parameters, known collectively as **TNM**. T stands for the size of the original local tumor, N specifies whether there is regional lymph node involvement, and M indicates whether there is distant metastatic spread. There is also a distinction between clinical staging prior to treatment and pathological staging after surgical resection. On the other hand, tumor grading is a histopathologic evaluation of the extent of differentiation of the tumor. Grading assesses the difference between the tumor and the surrounding tissues. Grade 1 tumors do not differ much in appearance from the normal tissue and are said to be well-differentiated. When the histopathological variation between normal and tumor tissues is large, graded as 3 or 4, the tumors are considered poorly differentiated (and more aggressive).

Important Terms

- **Invasion** is the process in which cancer cells continue to reproduce and effectively take over an area of the body's normal, healthy tissue.
- **Angiogenesis** is the process in which a tumor causes the body to produce blood vessels that enable the tumor to survive and grow.
- **Metastasis** is the extension of cancer cells to other parts of the body. This occurs when the cancer cells continue to reproduce and spread into other tissues in the area where the original cancer started. It can also occur through the blood or lymph stream by carrying cancer cells to other tissues within the body. Certain cancers have a propensity for metastasizing to specific areas of the body. For example, prostate and breast cancers are more likely to metastasize to the spine.
- **Tumor heterogeneity** is the term used to describe the dissimilarities found between cancer cells within a tumor. The more heterogeneous a tumor is, the more difficult it can be to treat and the more types of treatments may be required to treat it.
- **Hyperplasia** is the process in which the quantity of cells within a certain tissue multiplies. This occurs in healthy tissue and in cancerous tissue.
- **Metaplasia** is when one type of cell is interchanged with another within a specific tissue. This occurs in response to chronic damage inflicted on a certain type of cell.
- **Dysplasia** is a change in normal cells. This can involve a change in any of the cell's characteristics.
- **Anaplasia** is used to explain cancer cells. It means that certain cells hold the characteristics that are seen with cancer cells.

Gastrointestinal Assessment

Assessment of the Gastrointestinal System

Assessment of the gastrointestinal system includes:

- Ask about personal and family history of gastrointestinal problems and risk factors, such as alcoholism, smoking, drug and medicine use, and poor dietary habits.
- Ask about symptoms, such as GI discomfort, flatus, nausea, vomiting, diarrhea, and abdominal pain.
- Determine the defecation pattern and ask about weight fluctuations.

When performing a **physical assessment**, one must assess oral mucosa, tongue, teeth, pharynx, thyroid and parathyroid glands, skin color, moisture, turgor, nodules or lesions, bruises, scars, abdominal shape, and bowel sounds, assessing the abdomen in all 4 quadrants using the stethoscope diaphragm. The number of sounds heard determine if the intestines are functioning:

- **Absent**: no sounds in 3-5 minutes.
- **Hypoactive**: only one sound in 2 minutes.
- **Normal**: sounds heard every 5-20 seconds.
- **Hyperactive**: 5-6 sounds in <30 seconds.

One should examine the anal region for fissures, inflammation, tears, and dimples. Blood may be drawn for liver function studies, lipid profile, iron studies, CBC.

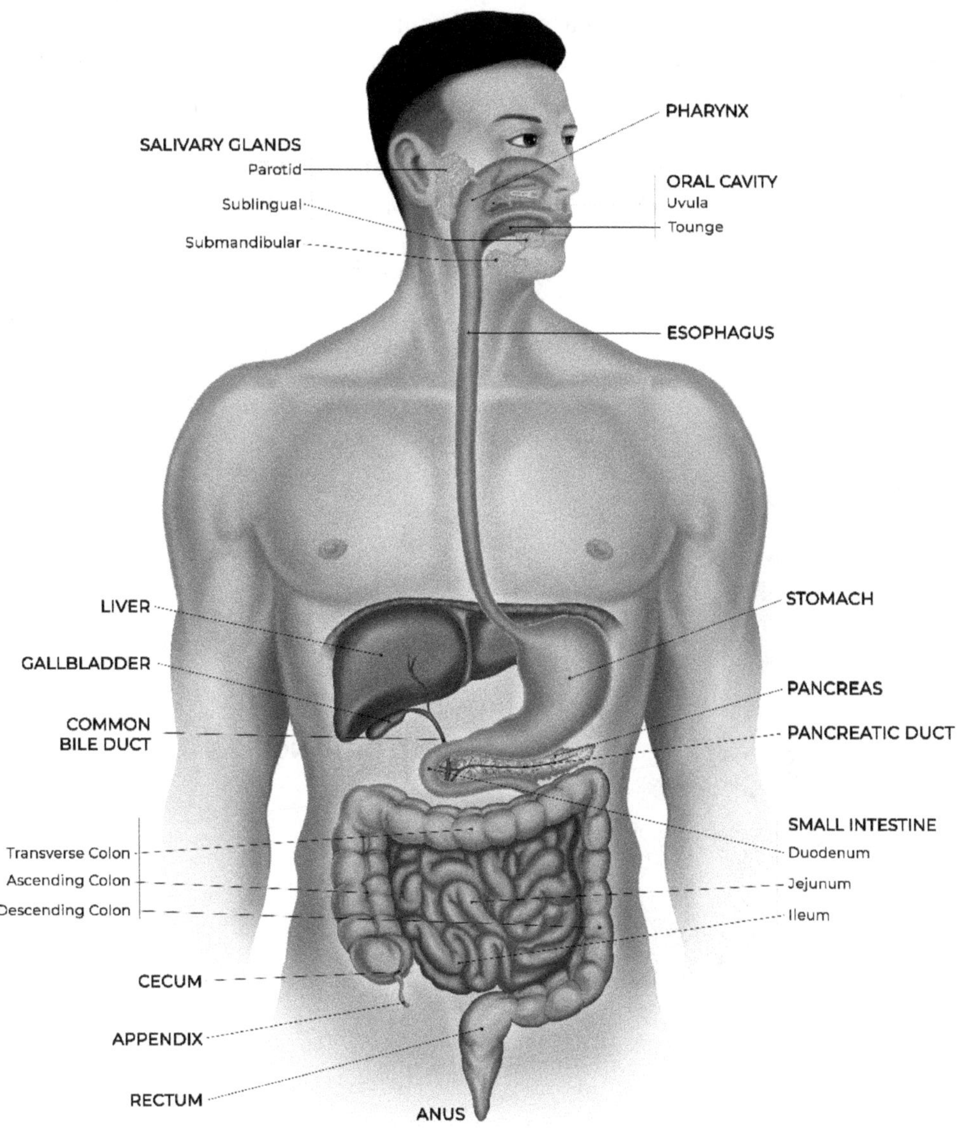

Review Video: Gastrointestinal System
Visit mometrix.com/academy and enter code: 378740

Assessment for Gallbladder and Pancreatic Disease

Gallbladder and pancreatic assessments are prompted by the appearance of symptoms. Symptoms of gallbladder disease include epigastric discomfort following fatty food intake, abdominal distention, right upper quadrant pain, which may be colicky, nausea, and vomiting. Pain may occur intermittently. The patient with pancreatitis may have acute onset of severe abdominal pain, back pain, extensive vomiting, and dyspnea. Pancreatitis is most often related to gallstones or alcoholism, so history of alcohol use and examination for gallstones must be done:

- Assess for RUQ tenderness and mass, bowel sounds, and abdominal guarding.
- Assess the vital signs for hypotension, tachycardia, or fever and note any anxiety, agitation, or confusion.
- Note signs of hypoxia.
- Assess the skin for jaundice and bruising on the flanks and near the umbilicus.
- Blood is drawn to assess amylase and lipase, CBC, calcium, glucose, and bilirubin.

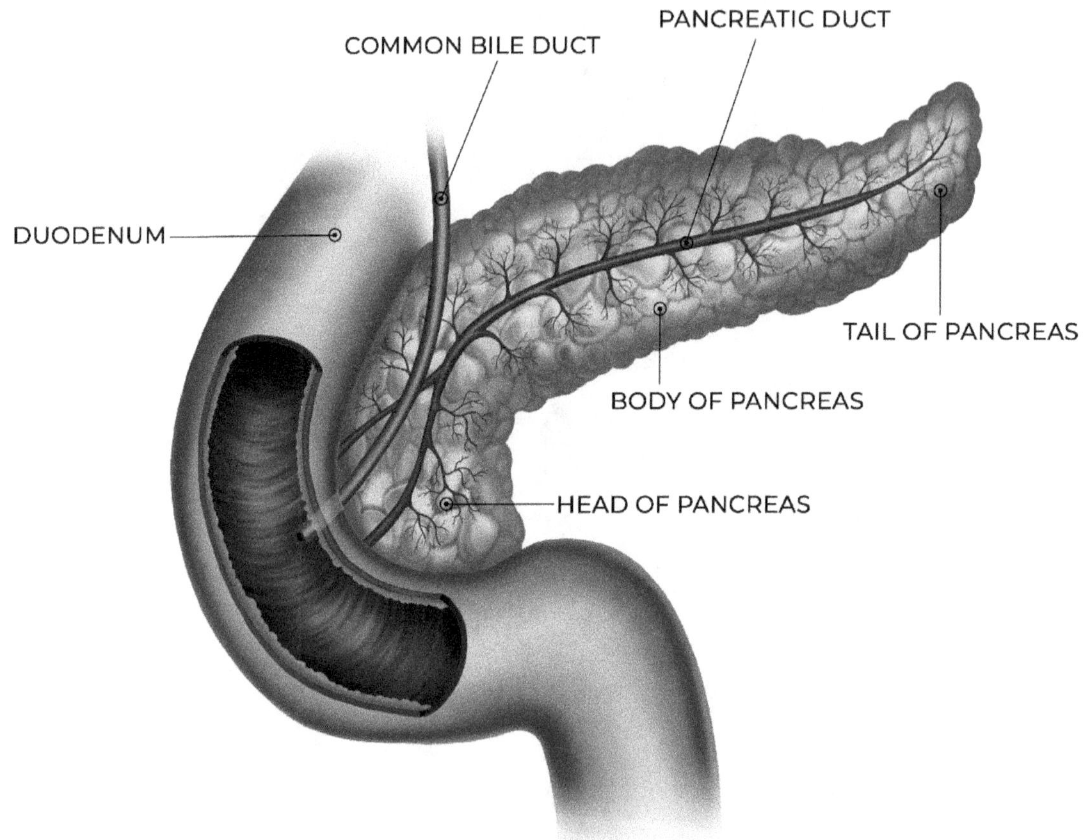

Assessment for Liver Disease

The liver must be 70% damaged before lab tests show abnormalities. Assessment of risk factors and early symptoms are important to identify early disease. Risk factors for **liver disease** include alcoholism and drug abuse, risky sexual practices, exposure to infection or environmental toxins, and travel to countries with poor sanitation. One should question the patient about symptoms of liver disease, such as fatigue, itching, abdominal pain, anorexia, weight gain, fever, blood in stools or black stools, sleep problems, lack of menstruation, and lack of libido. Physical assessment includes checking vital signs and skin for scratches, pallor, jaundice, dryness, bruising, petechiae, abdominal veins and spider angiomas, and red palms:

- Assess for gynecomastia, abdominal distension, fluid waves, bowel sounds, liver margins, tenderness, consistency, and hardness and sharpness of the edge.
- Examine extremities for wasting, edema, and weakness.

- Assess neurological system for cognitive status, tremors, balance problems, slurred speech.
- Identify testicular atrophy.
- Blood should be drawn for serum enzymes and proteins, bilirubin, ammonia, clotting factors, and lipid profile.

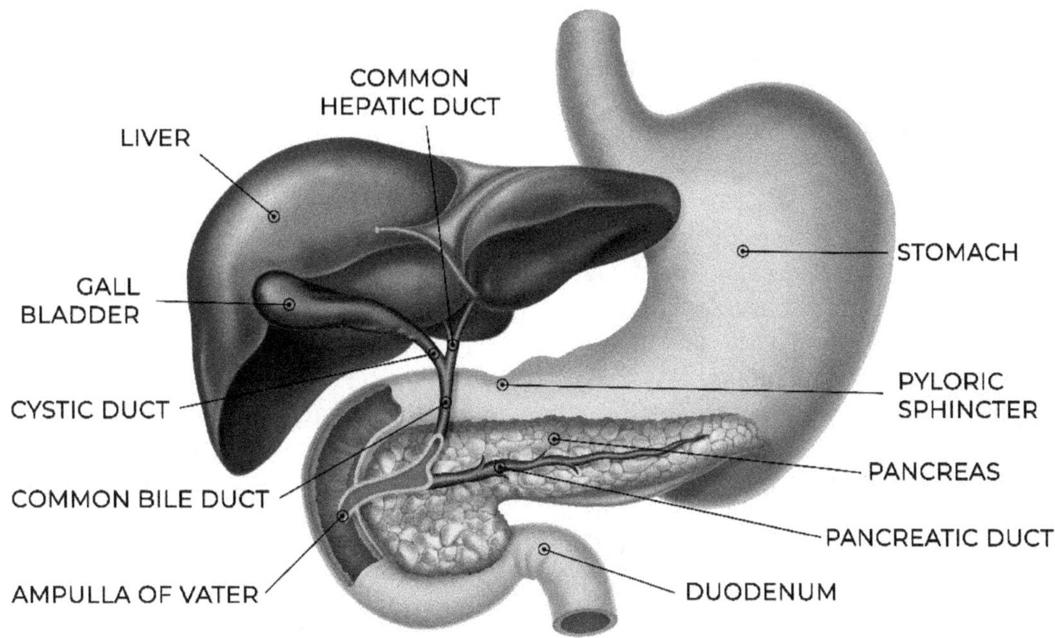

Assessment of Nutritional Status

Assessment of **nutritional status** begins with an assessment of the patient's intake. The patient is asked to report intake for the previous 24 hours. This may indicate the need for a **food diary** over a period of time:

- Compare the patient's nutritional intake with the requirements of the USDA's MyPlate.
- Measure height and weight and check against a BMI table to help determine nutritional status.
- Measure waist circumference.
- Assess the patient for physical signs of poor nutrition such as muscle wasting, obesity, hair breakage and loss, poor skin turgor, ulcers, bruising, and loss of subcutaneous tissue.
- Assess mucous membranes and condition of teeth, abdomen, extremities, and thyroid gland.

Nutritional status is connected to endocrine disease, infections, other acute and chronic diseases, digestion, absorption, excretion, and storage of nutrients so these areas must also be assessed. Blood testing should include proteins, transferrin, electrolytes, vitamins A and C, carotene, and CBC. Test urine for creatinine, thiamine, riboflavin, niacin, albumin, and iodine.

Assessing Nutritional Status of Hospitalized Patients

Assessing the nutritional status of the hospital inpatient is an important part of forming a care plan. The two screening tools that are most commonly used are the **Subjective Global Assessment (SGA)** and the **Prognostic Nutritional Index (PNI)**. The SGA provides a nutritional assessment based on both the patient history and current symptoms. The patient is asked about any changes in weight and is also asked questions about his or her diet. The presence of symptoms that may lead to weight loss and poor nutritional status, such as diarrhea, nausea, and vomiting, as well as water retention (edema) and muscle wasting (cachexia), is also included in the SGA. The PNI is also used as an indicator of malnutrition and is especially helpful in determining how well a patient will recover from surgery. The PNI assesses nutritional status through the measurement of serum proteins such as albumin and transferrin combined with a skinfold measurement and a cutaneous hypersensitivity test as an indicator of immune function.

Genitourinary Assessment

Assessment of Kidneys and Urinary Tract

Assessment of kidneys and urinary tract includes:

- Assess the health history for family urinary system disease and risk factors, such as previous urinary disease, increased age, immobility, hypertension, diabetes, chemical exposure, chronic disease, radiation to the pelvis, STDs, alcohol or drug use, and complications of pregnancy and delivery.
- Determine daily fluid intake.
- Question symptoms such as flank or abdominal pain, hesitancy, urgency, difficulty or straining with voiding, difficulty emptying the bladder, urinary incontinence, fatigue, SOB, exercise intolerance from anemia, fever, chills, blood in the urine, and GI symptoms.

Physical assessment includes vital signs, kidney and bladder palpation, and percussion over the bladder after urination:

- Palpate for ascites and edema.
- Measure the DTRs and check gait and ability to walk heel-to-toe.
- Examine the genitalia and check the urethra and vagina for herniation, irritation, or tears.

Urine specimen is obtained via clean catch midstream technique for analysis and culture if indicated. Blood is taken for a CBC, and in males, prostate specific antigen (PSA) levels will also be measured via blood specimen.

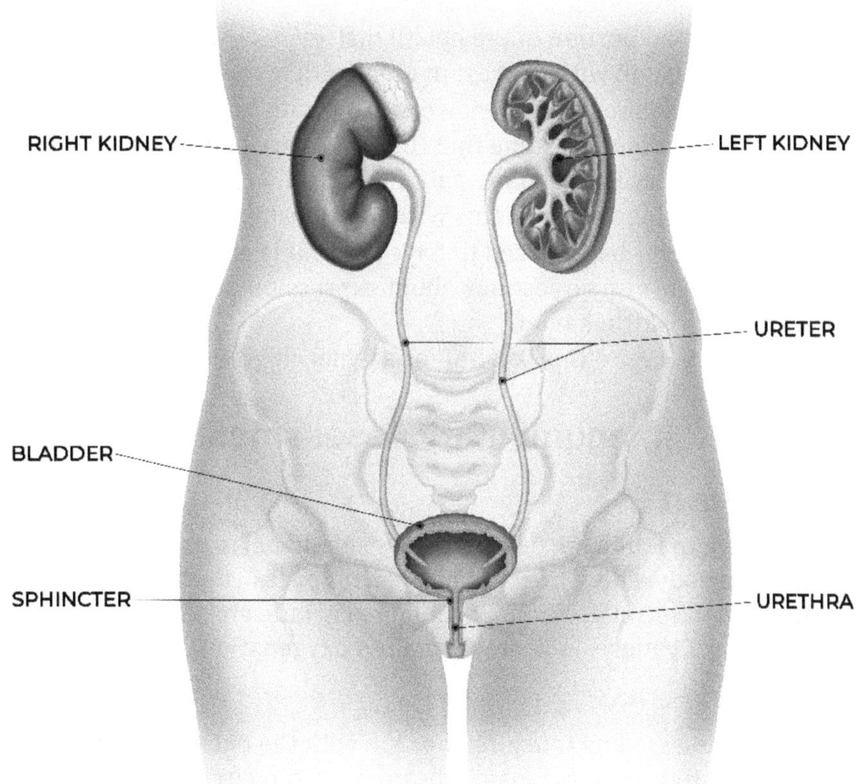

Review Video: Urinary System
Visit mometrix.com/academy and enter code: 601053

Kidney Regulatory Functions Regarding Fluid Balance

Kidney regulatory functions include maintaining **fluid balance.** Fluid excretion balances intake with output so increased intake results in a large output and vice versa:

- **Osmolality** (the number of electrolytes and other molecules per kg/urine) measures the concentration or dilution. With dehydration, osmolality increases; with fluid retention, osmolality decreases. With kidney disease, urine is dilute and the osmolality is fixed.
- **Specific gravity** compares the weight of urine (weight of particles) to distilled water (1.000). Normal urine is 1.010-1.025 with normal intake. High intake lowers the specific gravity and low intake raises it. In kidney disease, it often does not vary.
- **Antidiuretic hormone** (ADH/vasopressin) regulates the excretion of water and urine concentration in the renal tubule by varying water reabsorption. When fluid intake decreases, blood osmolality rises and this stimulates release of ADH, which increases reabsorption of fluid to return osmolality to normal levels. ADH is suppressed with increased fluid intake, so less fluid is reabsorbed.

Assessing Sexual Health and Preferences

Bringing up the topic of sex gives a patient permission to ask questions and openly discuss **sexual concerns**:

- Ask for permission to ask questions about sexual health and preferences during the gynecological/urological portion of the health history.
- If the patient refuses, go on with the rest of the health history, otherwise continue.
- Ask first if the person has sex with men, women, or both.
- Be nonjudgmental and do not assume that those who are elderly or disabled do not have sex. Use layman terms according to the patient's age and education level.
- Ask if the person is having any problems with relationships or sexual intercourse.
- Ask if the person has ever been forced to have sex or if is afraid of anyone close to them.
- End by asking if there are any questions about expression of sexual feelings, contraception, safe sex practices, or risky behavior.
- Refer those with problems to their doctor, or a gynecologist, urologist, or sex therapist.

Integumentary Assessment

General Skin Assessment

Skin color varies according to ethnicity. Color changes should be assessed to determine if they are local or extend over entire body, and if they are permanent or transient. Pallor may indicate stress, impaired oxygenation, and vasoconstriction. Erythema may indicate vasodilation, local inflammation, and blushing. Cyanosis indicates impaired oxygenation, and jaundice indicates increased bilirubin.

Temperature is typically assessed by touching the skin with the back of the hand. Skin should be warm and equal bilaterally. Hypothermia may indicate impaired circulation, intravenous infusion, and immobilized limb (such as in a cast). Hyperthermia may indicate fever, infection, and excessive exercise.

Review Video: Skin Assessment
Visit mometrix.com/academy and enter code: 794925

Effects of Age on Skin

Age is an important consideration when evaluating the skin because the characteristics of the skin change as people age.

- An **infant's** skin is thinner than an adult's because, while the epidermis is developed, the dermis layer is only about 60% of that of an adult and continues to develop after birth. The skin of premature infants is especially friable, allowing for transepidermal water loss and evaporative heat loss.
- During **adolescence**, the hair follicles activate, the thickness of the dermis decreases about 20%, and epidermal turnover time increases, so healing slows.

- As people **continue to age**, Langerhans' cells decrease in number, making the skin more prone to cancer, and the inflammatory reactions decrease. The sweat glands, vascularity, and subcutaneous fat all decrease, interfering with thermoregulation and contributing to dryness and irritation of the skin. The epidermal-dermal junction flattens, resulting in skin prone to tearing. The elastin in the skin degrades with age and solar exposure. The thinning of the hypodermis can lead to pressure ulcers.

Review Video: Integumentary System
Visit mometrix.com/academy and enter code: 655980

Braden Scale

The **Braden scale** is a risk assessment tool that has been validated clinically as predictive of the risk of patient's developing pressure sores. It was developed in 1988 by Barbara Braden and Nancy Bergstrom and is in wide use. The scale scores six different areas with five areas scored 1-4 points, and one area 1-3 points. The lower the score, the greater the risk.

Area	Score of 1	Score of 2	Score of 3	Score of 4
Sensory perception	Completely limited	Very limited	Slightly limited	No impairment
Moisture	Constantly moist	Very moist	Occasionally moist	Rarely moist
Activity	Bed	Chair	Occasional walk	Frequent walk
Mobility	Immobile	Limited	Slightly limited	No limitations
Nutritional pattern	Very poor	Inadequate	Adequate	Excellent
Friction and shear	Problem	Potential problem	No apparent problem	

Evaluating Wounds for Etiology

Wounds should be evaluated for **etiology** during the initial assessment to ensure proper treatment. Wounds can arise from a number of different causes:

- **Pressure**: Wounds that occur over bony prominences, such as the heels and coccyx, may be related to pressure, shear, or friction. The skin should be carefully examined for discolorations or changes in texture that might indicate compromise.
- **Arterial**: Arterial insufficiency is associated with a decrease in pedal pulses, and cool atrophic (shiny, dry) skin. It may result in small punctate-type ulcers, frequently on the dorsum of foot.
- **Venous stasis**: A decrease in venous circulation often results in hemoglobin leaking into the tissues of the lower leg, giving a brown discoloration. Tissue is often edematous, and ulcers are most common near the medial malleolus.
- **Diabetic neuropathy/ischemia**: Neuropathy can result in a lack of sensation to pain so that injuries to the feet may go unnoticed. Diabetes may also cause damage to small vessels, resulting in ischemia that can lead to ulcerations.

- **Trauma**: Injuries resulting from accidents or other types of trauma may vary considerably with some resulting in extensive damage to bones, tissues, organs, and circulation. Additionally, the wounds may be contaminated. Each wound must be assessed individually for multiple factors.
- **Burns**: Burn wounds may be chemical or thermal and should be assessed according to the area, the percentage of the body burned, and the depth of the burn. First-degree burns are superficial and affect the epidermis only. Second-degree burns extend through the dermis. Third degree burns affect underlying tissue, including vasculature, muscles, and nerves.
- **Infection**: An infected surgical or wound site can result in pain, edema, cellulitis, drainage, erosion of the sutures and ulceration of the tissue. Surgical sites must be assessed carefully and laboratory findings reviewed.

Elements of Wound Assessment

Location and Size

Wound location should be described in terms of anatomic position using landmarks (such as sternal notch, umbilicus, lateral malleolus), correct medical terminology, and directional terms:

- Anterior (in front)
- Posterior (behind)
- Superior (above)
- Inferior (below)

Wound size should be carefully described through actual measurement rather than association (the size of a dime). Measurements should be done with a disposable ruler in millimeters or centimeters. The current standard for measurement:

$$\text{Length} \times \text{width} \times \text{depth} = \text{dimension}$$

However, a clear description requires more detail. The measurement should be done at the greatest width and greatest length. More than 2 measurements may be needed if the wound is very irregularly shaped. The depth of the wound should be measured by inserting a sterile applicator and grasping or marking the applicator at skin level and then measuring the length below. Ideally, the wound should be photographed as well, following protocols for photography.

Wound Bed Tissue

Wound bed tissue should be described as completely as possible, including color and general appearance:

- **Granulation tissue** is slightly granular in appearance and deep pink to bright red and moist, bleeding easily if disturbed.
- **Clean non-granular tissue** is smooth and deep pink or red and is not healing.
- **Hypergranulation** is excessive soft flaccid granulating tissue that is raised above the level of the periwound tissue, preventing proper epithelization, and may reflect excess moisture in the wound.
- **Epithelization** should appear at wound edges first and then eventually cover the wound. It is dry and light pink or violet in color.
- **Slough** is necrotic tissue that is viscous, soft and yellow-gray in appearance and adheres to the wound.
- **Eschar** is hard dark brown or black leathery necrotic tissue that accumulates with death of the tissue.

Wound Margins

Wound margins and the tissue surrounding the wound should be described carefully and with correct terminology:

- **Color** should be described using color descriptions and such terms as blanched, erythematous (red), or ecchymosed (purple, green, yellow).
- **Skin texture** may be normal, indurated (hardened), or edematous (swollen). Note if there is cellulitis or maceration evident.
- **Wound edges** may be diffuse (without clear margins), well defined, or rolled. A healing ridge may be evident if granulation has begun. Note if the wound is closed (as with a surgical incision) or open (as with dehiscence or ulcerations). Note if wound edges are attached or unattached (indicating undermining or tunneling).
- **Tunneling or undermining** should be assessed by probing the wound margins with a moist sterile cotton applicator, using clock face locators (toward the head is 12 o'clock, for example). Tunneling may be described as extending from 3 o'clock to 4 o'clock. A large area is usually described as undermining. The size should be measured or estimated as closely as possible.

Distribution, Drainage, and Odor

Distribution of lesions should be clearly delineated if there is more than one lesion over an area. The arrangement of the lesions can be helpful for diagnosis and treatments.

- Linear (in a line).
- Satellites (small lesions around a larger one).
- Diffuse (scattered freely over an area).

Drainage may vary considerably from nothing at all to copious outpourings of discharge.

- Serous drainage is usually clear to slightly yellow.
- Serosanguinous drainage is a combination of serous drainage and blood.
- Sanguinous drainage is bloody.
- Purulent discharge may be thick and milky, yellow, brownish, or green, depending upon the infective agent.

Odor requires more subjective assessment, but the odor and type of discharge together can provide useful information. Some infective agents, such as *Pseudomonas,* produce distinctive odors, which may be described in various ways: Musty, Foul, Sweet.

Assessment Characteristics of Arterial, Neuropathic, and Venous Ulcers

The assessment process is important in delineating between the arterial, neuropathic or venous origin of the ulcer. Characteristics of each must be known and closely examined:

Location

- **Arterial**: Ends of toes, pressure points, traumatic nonhealing wounds
- **Neuropathic**: Plantar surface, metatarsal heads, toes, and sides of feet
- **Venous**: Between knees and ankles, medial malleolus

Wound Bed

- **Arterial**: Pale, necrotic
- **Neuropathic**: Red (or ischemic)
- **Venous**: Dark red, fibrinous slough

Exudate

- **Arterial**: Slight amount, infection common
- **Neuropathic**: Moderate to large amounts, infection common
- **Venous**: Moderate to large amounts

Wound Perimeter

- **Arterial**: Circular, well-defined
- **Neuropathic**: Circular, well-defined, often with callous formation
- **Venous**: Irregular, poorly-defined

Pain

- **Arterial**: Very painful
- **Neuropathic**: Pain often absent because of reduced sensation
- **Venous**: Pain varies

Skin

- **Arterial**: Pale, friable, shiny, and hairless, with dependent rubor and elevational pallor
- **Neuropathic**: Ischemic signs (as in arterial) may be evident with co-morbidity
- **Venous**: Brownish discoloration of ankles and shin, edema common

Pulses

- **Arterial**: Weak or absent
- **Neuropathic**: Present and palpable, diminished in neuroischemic ulcers
- **Venous**: Present and palpable

Musculoskeletal Assessment

Assessment to Establish Mechanism of Injury

Assessment to establish the **mechanism of injury** for an injury to the musculoskeletal system includes:

- **Question/Listen**: Reports from the patient (if responsive and cognitively aware), family or friends, and first responders often can establish how, when, and where an injury occurred. Police reports may be available in some cases. The trauma nurse should ask questions to clarify any information provided.
- **Observation**: The patient's general appearance (clean, soiled, unkempt, well-dressed, sporting clothes/uniform), obvious injuries (bruises, swelling, and bleeding), and odor (fruity, alcohol, urine, feces) may provide clues as to the mechanism of injury or the patient's general health and living situation.
- **Physical examination**: The trauma nurse should look for typical patterns of injury associated with different mechanisms of injury. For example, a fall from a height may result in fractures of both feet and back injuries. Hip and wrist fractures are common with falls. Blistering, redness, and sloughing of tissue may suggest burns.

Review Video: Muscular System
Visit mometrix.com/academy and enter code: 967216

Review Video: Skeletal System
Visit mometrix.com/academy and enter code: 256447

Assessing Risk of Falling

Many factors must be examined and combined to determine the **fall risk** status of a patient. They include age, sensory deficits, mobility problems, neurological disorders, past history of falling, cognitive impairment, and depression. Some medications, such as those associated with postural hypotension and psychotropic medications, may increase the danger of falls. The presence of dizziness, acute or chronic illness, poor physical status, elimination requirements, medications, and environmental concerns contribute to the risk for falls.

Multiple factors increase risk, so careful history and physical exam are necessary as part of assessment. When the presence of risk factors shows a risk for falls, this information should be communicated to other caregivers by wristband, colored markers on doors, care plans, or other effective means. The factors are then modified as much as possible. The patient should be re-evaluated as their condition changes or after a fall to determine the cause.

Assessing Patients with Disabilities

A patient with **disabilities** may find it very difficult to obtain screening for health problems due to inaccessibility:

- Work with the patient to resolve barriers to obtain weight, mammography, bone density tests, and pap/pelvic exams on a regular basis.
- Ask how to best assist the patient during the assessment.
- Observe the patient carefully for nonverbal communication, such as grimacing.
- If sensation is affected, warn the patient before touching any part of the body.
- Always address all areas of the patient's history, including sexual history.
- Use an interpreter that is not a family member if needed.

- Give the patient extra time to respond to questions when there is aphasia or other communication problems.
- Address the impact of the disability on the ability to perform ADLs, health status in general, access to healthcare, financial status, emotional status, work, community roles, and family wellbeing.

FAST Assessment

Focused abdominal sonography for trauma (FAST) assessment is a non-invasive ultrasound procedure that is part of the ATLS protocol for assessment of trauma and is generally now used in place of peritoneal lavage to detect free fluid (generally blood). FAST is about 85% to 90% effective in diagnosing intraperitoneal bleeding (usually associated with hepatic or splenic injury) as well as pneumo- and hemothorax (can detect as small a volume as 20 mL, depending on the sonographer's skill), and pericardial effusion associated with blunt or penetrating cardiac trauma. FAST may help to prioritize treatment when a patient presents with multiple penetrating injuries (especially involving inferior chest and superior abdomen). However, FAST is less effective in identifying bowel injuries. In some cases where a patient's condition is not clear, observation and a series of FAST assessments may help to identify problems, such as a slow bleed.

Psychosocial Assessment

Elements of the Psychosocial Assessment

A **psychosocial assessment** should provide additional information to the physical assessment to guide the patient's plan of care and should include:

- Previous hospitalizations and experience with healthcare
- Psychiatric history: Suicidal ideation, psychiatric disorders, family psychiatric history, history of violence and/or self-mutilation
- Chief complaint: Patient's perception
- Complementary therapies: Acupuncture, visualization, and meditation
- Occupational and educational background: Employment, retirement, and special skills
- Social patterns: Family and friends, living situation, typical activities, support system
- Sexual patterns: Orientation, problems, and sex practices
- Interests/abilities: Hobbies and sports
- Current or past substance abuse: Type, frequency, drinking pattern, use of recreational drugs, and overuse of prescription drugs
- Ability to cope: Stress reduction techniques
- Physical, sexual, emotional, and financial abuse: Older adults are especially vulnerable to abuse and may be reluctant to disclose out of shame or fear
- Spiritual/Cultural assessment: Religious/Spiritual importance, practices, restrictions (such as blood products or foods), and impact on health/health decisions

Cognitive Assessment

Individuals with evidence of dementia, delirium, or short-term memory loss should have cognition assessed. The **mini-mental state exam (MMSE)** or the **mini-cog test** are both commonly used. These tests require the individual to carry out specified tasks and are used as a baseline to determine change in mental status.

MMSE:

- Remembering and later repeating the names of 3 common objects
- Counting backward from 100 by 7s or spelling "world" backward
- Naming items as the examiner points to them
- Providing the location of the examiner's office, including city, state, and street address
- Repeating common phrases
- Copying a picture of interlocking shapes
- Following simple 3-part instructions, such a picking up a piece of paper, folding it in half, and placing it on the floor

A score of ≥24/30 is considered a normal functioning level.

Mini-cog:

- Remembering and later repeating the names of 3 common objects
- Drawing the face of a clock, including all 12 numbers and the hands, and indicating the time specified by the examiner

A score of 3-5 (out of 5) indicates a lower chance of dementia but does not rule it out.

Confusion Assessment Method

The **Confusion Assessment Method** is an assessment tool intended to be used by those without psychiatric training in order to assess the progression of delirium in patients. The tool covers 9 factors, some factors have a range of possibilities, and others are rated only as to whether the characteristic is present, not present, uncertain, or not applicable. The tool also provides room to describe abnormal behavior. Factors indicative of delirium include:

1. **Onset**: Acute change in mental status
2. **Attention**: Inattentive, stable, or fluctuating
3. **Thinking**: Disorganized, rambling conversation, switching topics, illogical
4. **Level of consciousness**: Altered, ranging from alert to coma
5. **Orientation**: Disoriented (person, place, and time)
6. **Memory**: Impaired
7. **Perceptual disturbances**: Hallucinations, illusions
8. **Psychomotor abnormalities**: Agitation (tapping, picking, moving) or retardation (staring, not moving)
9. **Sleep-wake cycle**: Awake at night and sleepy in the daytime

**The Confusion Assessment Method indicates delirium if there is an acute onset, fluctuating inattention, and disorganized thinking OR altered level of consciousness.*

Hamilton Anxiety Scale

The **Hamilton Anxiety Scale** (HAS or HAMA) is utilized to evaluate the anxiety related symptomatology that may be present in adults as well as children. It provides an evaluation of overall **anxiety** and its degree of severity. This includes **somatic anxiety** (physical complaints) and **psychic anxiety** (mental agitation and distress). This scale consists of 14 items based on anxiety produced symptoms. Each item is ranked 0-4 with 0 indicating no symptoms present and 4 indicating severe symptoms present. This scale is frequently utilized in psychotropic drug evaluations. If performed before a particular medication has been started and then again at later visits, the HAS can be helpful in adjusting medication dosages based in part on the individual's score. It is often utilized as an outcome measure in clinical trials.

Beck Depression Inventory

The **Beck Depression Inventory (BDI)** is a widely utilized, self-reported, multiple-choice questionnaire consisting of 21 items, which measures the **degree of depression**. This tool is designed for use in adults ages 17-80. It evaluates physical symptoms such as weight loss, loss of sleep, loss of interest in sex, fatigue, and attitudinal symptoms such as irritability, guilt, and hopelessness. The items rank in four possible answer choices based on an increasing severity of symptoms. The test is scored with the answers ranging in value from 0 to 3. The total score is utilized to determine the degree of depression. The usual ranges include: 0-9 no signs of depression, 10-18 mild depression, 19-29 moderate depression, and 30-63 severe depression.

Evaluation for Suicidal or Homicidal Thoughts

During a risk assessment two of the most important areas to evaluate are the patient's **risk for self-harm or harm to others**. The staff member performing the assessment should very closely evaluate for any descriptions or thoughts the patient may have concerning these risks. Direct questioning on these subjects should be performed and documented. Close evaluation of any delusional thoughts the patient may be having should be carefully evaluated. Does the patient believe he or she is being instructed by others to perform either of these acts? Safety of the patient and others needs to be a top priority and carefully documented. If the patient indicates that they are having these thoughts or ideas, they must be placed in either suicidal or assault precautions with close monitoring per facility protocol.

Suicide Risk Assessment

A **suicide risk assessment** should be completed and documented upon admission, with each shift change, at discharge, or any time suicidal ideations are suggested by the patient. This risk assessment should evaluate some of the following criteria:

- Would the patient sign a contract for safety?
- Is there a suicide plan? How lethal is the plan?
- What is the elopement risk?
- How often are the suicidal thoughts, and have they attempted suicide before?

Any associated symptoms of hopelessness, guilt, anger, helplessness, impulsive behaviors, nightmares, obsessions with death, or altered judgment should also be assessed and documented. The higher the score the higher the risk for suicide.

Alcohol Use Assessment

The **Clinical Instrument for Withdrawal for Alcohol (CIWA)** is a tool used to assess the severity of alcohol withdraw. Each category is scored 0-7 points based on the severity of symptoms, except #10, which is scored 0-4. A score <5 indicates mild withdrawal without need for medications; for scores ranging 5-15, benzodiazepines are indicated to manage symptoms. A score >15 indicates severe withdrawal and the need for admission to the unit.

1. Nausea/Vomiting
2. Tremor
3. Paroxysmal Sweats
4. Anxiety
5. Agitation
6. Tactile Disturbances
7. Auditory Disturbances
8. Visual Disturbances
9. Headache
10. Disorientation or Clouding of Sensorium

The **CAGE** tool is used as a quick assessment to identify problem drinkers. Moderate drinking, (1-2 drinks daily or one drink a day for older adults) is usually not harmful to people in the absence of other medical conditions. However, drinking more can lead to serious psychosocial and physical problems. One drink is defined as 12 ounces of beer/wine cooler, 5 ounces of wine, or 1.5 ounces of liquor.

- **C** - *Cutting Down*: "Do you think about trying to cut down on drinking?"
- **A** - *Annoyed at Criticism*: "Are people starting to criticize your drinking?"
- **G** - *Guilty feeling*: "Do you feel guilty or try to hide your drinking?"
- **E** - *Eye opener*: "Do you increasingly need a drink earlier in the day?

"Yes" on one question suggests the possibility of a drinking problem. "Yes" on ≥2 indicates a drinking problem

Screening for Risk-Taking Behavior

The ability to assess outcomes and respond appropriately to risks are part of the decision-making process. Decision making can be impaired in patients with mental health disorders such as depression, anxiety, bipolar disorder, and personality disorders, as well as in patients who have experienced a brain injury or have a dependence on drugs or alcohol. Health care providers should screen patients for the presence of high-risk behaviors. This may be accomplished through a self-administered questionnaire or through a patient interview with a trained clinician. Examples of **high-risk behaviors** include substance use/abuse, high risk sexual behaviors, high risk driving behaviors such as drinking and driving, speeding or riding with a drunk driver, and violence related behaviors. Patients with an increased response to risk taking may exhibit signs of impulsivity and sensation seeking. Conversely, other patients may exhibit abnormally cautious behavior.

Assessment of Unique Needs of Veterans

Assessment of **veterans** must include not only the standard assessments appropriate for the patient's age and gender but also assessment of combat-associated injuries and illnesses:

- Shrapnel and/or gunshot injuries: Associated physical limitations, pain
- Amputations: Mobility and prosthesis issues; body image issues
- PTSD: Extent, frequency of attacks, limiting factors, triggers
- Depression, suicidal ideation
- Substance abuse: Type and extent

Because a large number of veterans are among the homeless population, the veteran's living arrangements should be explored and appropriate referrals made if the patient is in need of housing. Veterans may be unaware of programs offered through the U.S. Department of Veterans Affairs and should be provided information about these programs as appropriate for the patient's needs.

Pain Assessment

Pathophysiology of Pain

Nociceptors

Nociceptors are the primary neurons, or **sensory receptors**, responding to stimuli in the skin, muscle, and joints, as well as the stomach, bladder, and uterus. These neurons have specialized responses for mechanical, thermal, or chemical stimuli. The **neuron stimulation** is a direct result of tissue injury and follows four stages: **transduction** where a change occurs, **transmission** where the impulse is transferred along the neural path, **modulation** or translation of the signal, and **perception** by the patient. When injury occurs, the nociceptors initiate the process that begins **depolarization of the peripheral nerve**. Nociceptors may consist of either A-fiber axons or C-fiber axons. The message travels along the neural pathway and creates a perception of pain. A-fiber axons carry these pain messages at a much faster rate than C-fiber axons.

Nociceptive Pain

Nociceptive pain is an umbrella term for pain caused by **stimulation of the neuroreceptor**. This stimulation is a direct result of tissue injury. The severity of pain is proportionate to the extent of the injury. Nociceptive pain can be subdivided into two classifications: somatic and visceral pain. **Somatic pain** is located in the cutaneous tissues, bone joints, and muscle tissues. **Visceral pain** is specific to internal organs protected by a layer of viscera, such as the cardiovascular, respiratory, gastrointestinal, or genitourinary systems. Both types are treatable with opioids.

Visceral Pain

Visceral pain is associated with the internal organs. It can be very different depending on the affected organ. Not all internal organs are sensitive to pain (some lack **nociceptors**, such as the spleen, kidney, and pancreas), and may withstand a great deal of damage without causing pain. Other internal organs, such as the stomach, bladder, and ureters, can create significant pain from even the slightest damage. Visceral pain generally has a **poorly defined area**. It is also capable of referring pain to other remote locations away from the area of injury. It is described as a squeezing or cramping: a deep ache within the internal organs. The patient may complain of a generalized sick feeling or have nausea and vomiting. Visceral pain generally responds well to treatment with **opioids**.

Somatic Pain

Somatic pain refers to messages from pain receptors located in the **cutaneous or musculoskeletal tissues**. When the pain occurs within the musculoskeletal tissue, it is referred to as **deep somatic pain**. Metastasizing cancers commonly cause deep somatic pain. **Surface pain** refers to pain concentrated in the **dermis and cutaneous layers** such as that caused by a surgical incision. Deep somatic pain is generally described as a dull, throbbing ache that is well focused on the area of trauma. It responds well to **opioids**. Surface somatic pain is also directly focused on the injury. It is frequently described as sharper than deep somatic pain. It may also present as a burning or pricking sensation.

Neuropathic Pain

Neuropathic pain results from injury to the **nervous system**. This can result from cancer cells compressing the nerves or spinal cord, from actual cancerous invasion into the nerves or spinal cord, or from chemical damage to the nerves caused by chemotherapy and radiation. Other causes include diabetes- and alcohol-related damage, trauma, neuralgias, or other illnesses affecting the neural path either centrally or peripherally. When the nerves become damaged, they are unable to carry accurate information. This results in more severe, distinct **pain messages**. The nerves may also relay pain messages long after the original cause of the pain is resolved. It can be described as sharp, burning, shooting, shocking, tingling, or electrical in nature. It may travel the length of the nerve path from the spine to a distal body part such as a hand, or down the buttocks to a foot. NSAIDs and opioids are generally ineffective against neuropathic pain, though adjuvants may enhance the therapeutic effect of opioids. Nerve blocks may also be used.

Adverse Systemic Effects of Pain

Acute pain causes **adverse systemic effects** that can negatively affect many body systems.

- **Cardiovascular**: Tachycardia and increased blood pressure is a common response to pain, causing increased cardiac output and systemic vascular resistance. In those with pre-existing cardiovascular disease, such as compromised ventricular function, cardiac output may decrease. The increased myocardial need for oxygen may cause or worsen myocardial ischemia.
- **Respiratory**: Increased need for oxygen causes an increase in minute ventilation and splinting due to pain, which may compromise pulmonary function. If the chest wall movement is constrained, tidal volume falls, impairing the ability to cough and clear secretions. Bed rest further compromises ventilation.
- **Gastrointestinal**: Sphincter tone increases and motility decreases, sometimes resulting in ileus. There may be an increased secretion of gastric acids, which irritates the gastric lining and can cause ulcerations. Nausea, vomiting, and constipation may occur. Reflux may result in aspiration pneumonia. Abdominal distention may occur.
- **Urinary**: Increased sphincter tone and decreased motility result in urinary retention.
- **Endocrine**: Hormone levels are affected by pain. Catabolic hormones such as catecholamine, cortisol, and glucagon increase, and anabolic hormones such as insulin and testosterone decrease. Lipolysis increases along with carbohydrate intolerance. Sodium retention can occur because of increased ADH, aldosterone, angiotensin, and cortisol. This in turn causes fluid retention and a shift to extracellular space.
- **Hematologic**: There may be reduced fibrinolysis, increased adhesiveness of platelets, and increased coagulation.
- **Immune**: Leukocytosis and lymphopenia may occur, increasing risk of infection.

- **Emotional**: Patients may experience depression, anxiety, anger, decreased appetite, and sleep deprivation. This type of response is most common in those with chronic pain, who usually have different systemic responses from those with acute pain.

Core Principles of Pain Assessment and Management

According to the Joint Commission, assessing pain should be a priority in patient care, and organizations must establish **policies** for assessment and treatment of pain and must educate staff members about these policies. The Joint Commission considers a **plan of care** regarding pain control an essential patient right. Hospitals should be consistent in the use of the same assessment tools throughout the organization, specific to different patient populations (for example, pediatrics and geriatrics). The latest standards (2018) of evidence-based practice include the following:

- Organizations must establish a clinical leadership team to oversee pain management and safe prescription of opioids.
- Patients must be involved in planning and setting goals and should receive education regarding safe use of opioid and non-opioid medications.
- Patients should be screened for pain in all assessments, including visits to the emergency department.
- Patients at high risk for opioid misuse or adverse effects must be identified and monitored.
- Healthcare providers should have access to prescription drug monitoring safety databases, such as the prescription databases provided by most states.
- Organizations must provide performance improvement educational programs regarding pain assessment and management and must collect and analyze data on its pain assessment and management.

Areas Addressed When Assessing Pain

Information concerning a patient's pain can be gathered from a variety of sources, including observations, interviews with the patient and family, medical records, and observations of other health care providers. However, it is important to remember that each patient's pain is **subjective** and **personal**. Pain is defined as whatever the patient says it is. Having the patient give parameters of quality, location, duration, speed of onset, and intensity can all be beneficial in forming a treatment plan based on the patient's needs. Pain is also influenced by psychological, social, and spiritual factors. Behavioral, psychological, and subjective assessment information such as physical demeanor and vital signs can be helpful in further defining a patient's pain parameters.

Physical Signs of Pain

The best assessment of the patient's pain is **the patient's own report**. All other information is assessed as supporting this report. However, when this method is restricted or unavailable, **physical signs and symptoms** can help the nurse's assessment capabilities. It is important to be familiar with the patient's **baseline** or resting information to give a clear picture of the changes the body may go through when experiencing significant pain. Systolic blood pressure, heart rate, and respirations may all increase above the patient's normal parameters. Tightness or tension may be felt in major muscle groups. Posturing can also occur: the patient may guard areas of the body, curl themselves up into a fetal position, or hold only certain body portions rigid. Calling out, increased volume in speech, and moaning can also be indicators. Facial expressions, such as flat affect or grimacing, and distraction from their surroundings also indicate a significant increase in stressful stimuli.

Importance of Pain Assessments in Advanced Disease

As many as 90% of all **advanced disease patients** will experience some level of pain. The hospice and palliative care philosophy focuses on the relief of pain and provision for comfort measures for all patients who desire it to improve quality of life. Each patient has the right to accept or refuse treatment for their pain. This becomes difficult when the patient is unable to **communicate** their desires and pain level. It can be assumed that if a patient was experiencing pain when able to communicate, they will continue to experience pain when the ability to communicate has been compromised—pain will be present even in an unconscious state. Changes from previous behavioral, psychological, and subjective and objective assessment data provide the supporting information for continued pain assessments in a nonverbal patient.

Pain Assessment Tools

ABCDE Mnemonic Approach to Pain Assessment

The Agency for Healthcare Policy and Research recommends use of the **ABCDE method** for assessing and managing pain:

- **Asking** the patient about the extent of pain and assessing systematically.
- **Believing** that the degree of pain the patient reports is accurate.
- **Choosing** the appropriate method of pain control for the patient and circumstances.
- **Delivering** pain interventions appropriately and in a timely, logical manner.
- **Empowering** patients and family by helping them to have control of the course of treatment.

The **5 key elements of pain assessment** include:

- **Quality**: Words are used to describe pain, such as *burning*, *stabbing*, *deep*, *shooting*, and *sharp*. Some may complain of pressure, squeezing, and discomfort rather than pain.
- **Intensity**: Use of a 0-10 scale or other appropriate scale to quantify the degree of pain.
- **Location**: Where the patient indicates pain.
- **Duration**: Constant or comes and goes, breakthrough pain.
- **Aggravating/alleviating factors**: Those things that increase the intensity of pain and those that relieve the pain.

Unidimensional Tools for Pain Assessment

Unidimensional tools for pain assessment focus on one aspect only: the patient's level of pain. Tools include:

- **Visual analog/Numeric rating scale**: A 1-10 rating scale presented visually or verbally from which the patient chooses a number to describe the degree of pain the patient is experiencing. Zero represents no pain, 1 very mild pain, and 10 the most severe pain the patient can imagine.
- **Descriptive**: Pain is described in simple terms that a patient can choose from: mild, moderate, or severe. This may be especially helpful for patients from other countries or cultures where the 1-10 scale is not generally used.
- **FACES**: A chart shows a facial expression scale of simple drawings showing faces with different emotions, such as happiness, fear, and pain. Used primarily for children over age 3 and for nonverbal adults, although both a child's and an adult's version are available. A revised version applies numeric values to expressions so that pain can be assessed according to a numeric rating scale as well.

Multidimensional Tools for Pain Assessment

Multidimensional tools used for pain assessment include:

- **Multidimensional Pain Inventory**: The patient begins by identifying a significant other and then answering 20 questions (rating scale 0-6) about the current rate of pain, the degree of interference in daily life, the ability to work, satisfaction from social/recreational activities, support level of the significant other, mood, pain during the previous week, changes brought about by pain, concerns of the significant other, ability to deal with pain, irritability, and anxiety.
- **Brief pain inventory**: Patients are assessed on the severity of pain (on a 1-10 scale), location of pain, impact of pain on daily function, pain medication, and amount of pain relief in the past 24 hours or the past week. They are asked if the pain interferes with general activity, walking, normal work, mood, interpersonal relations, sleep, or enjoyment of life.
- **McGill pain questionnaire**: The patient marks areas of internal and external pain on body diagrams and selects appropriate adjectives for 20 different sections regarding sensory, affective, and evaluative perceptions. For example, the questionnaire allows the patient to indicate if the pain is "flickering, quivering, pulsing, throbbing, beating, or pounding." The patient also rates present pain intensity (PPI) from 0 (none) to 5 (excruciating).

Assessment Tools for Cognitively Impaired or Nonverbal Patients

The following are types of assessment tools available for use with cognitively impaired or nonverbal patients:

- **Discomfort Scale for Dementia of the Alzheimer Type (DS-DAT)**: For use with elderly persons experiencing dementia, decreased cognition, and decreased verbalization.
- **Assessment of Discomfort in Dementia Protocol (ADD)**: Particularly designed for use with patients exhibiting difficult behaviors.
- **Checklist of Nonverbal Pain Indicators (CNPI)**: Pain measurement with cognitive impairment.
- **Noncommunicative Patient's Pain Assessment Instrument (NOPPAIN)**: Specifically for use by nursing assistants.
- **Pain Assessment for the Dementing Elderly (PADE)**: Assessing physical pain behaviors.
- **Pain Assessment Tool in Confused Older Adults (PATCOA)**: Focuses on the observation of nonverbal cues.
- **Pain Assessment in Advanced Dementia (PAINAD)**: Adapted from the DS-DAT.
- **Pain Assessment Checklist for Seniors with Limited Ability to Communicate (PACSLAC)**: To assess common and subtle symptoms.
- **Abbey Pain Scale**: For late-stage dementia in nursing home environments.

Neuropathic Pain Scale

The **Neuropathic Pain Scale** (NPS) is the first tool designed specifically to assess the types of pain associated with neuropathy. The NPS comprises 10 sections with 9 assessed with a 0 to 10 (not unpleasant to intolerable) scale:

- Intensity of pain.
- Sharpness of pain.
- Heat of pain.
- Dullness of pain.
- Coldness of pain.

- Skin sensitivity to touch, clothing.
- Itchiness.
- Overall unpleasantness of pain.
- Intensity of deep and surface pain.

The 10th section asks for narrative descriptions of the **time quality** of pain. The patient chooses from three options: (1) feeling background pain all of the time with occasional flare-ups, (2) feeling a single type of pain all the time, and (3) feeling a single type of pain sometimes while having some pain-free periods. The patient then is asked to describe the pain experienced.

Barriers to Optimal Pain Assessments

Barriers to optimal pain assessments include:

- **Professional**: Health care providers may lack knowledge about pain assessment and management of different patient populations or may carry out assessments based on personal perceptions rather than validated pain assessment instruments. Some may be concerned about managing adverse effects or the patient's development of tolerance or addiction. In other cases, healthcare providers may lack empathy for patients' suffering. Lack of cultural awareness may affect interpretation of pain. For example, patients in cultures that encourage expression of pain may be assessed as having more pain than patients from cultures that value stoicism.
- **System**: The organization may lack clear policies regarding pain assessment and management, and may not have established clear guidelines for consistent use of pain assessment instruments. Additionally, supervision and accountability may be inadequate, and the organization may be concerned about costs and reimbursement for treatment.
- **Patient**: For personal or cultural reasons, patients may minimize or overstate the degree of pain, interfering with assessment. Some patients may be concerned about addiction or the effects of drugs on cognition (confusion, disorientation, lethargy) or other side effects (constipation, nausea, itching). Some may want to protect family from knowing the extent of pain.
- **Family**: Cultural biases may influence how the family responds to a patient's pain, and this can influence the patient's response as well. Families may lack understanding of the role of pain assessment and management. Some lack understanding about the difference between addiction and pain control at the end of life.
- **Society**: Concerns about drug abuse and addiction often permeate society and influence societal attitudes toward pain control and appropriate drugs to use. Laws and regulations may make access to certain drugs, such as those derived from marijuana, difficult or impossible to obtain.

Influential Factors in Pain Perception

Factors that can influence the perception of pain include:

- **Emotional state/Attitude**: Patients who are extremely upset or anxious may be so overwhelmed they don't feel the pain, or they may experience pain as more severe than those who are relaxed and calm. If patients expect to suffer from pain, they are also more likely to report severe pain than patients who expect that their pain will be controlled.

- **Cultural expectations**: Perception may vary according to cultural beliefs about pain. For example, if a patient believes that pain is punishment, the patient may agonize over past sins. If a patient believes that pain is fate and reflects karma, then the patient may feel that bearing pain is necessary.
- **Pain threshold**: Different patients simply perceive and experience pain to different degrees. What may be a minor pain to one individual may be severe to another.

Effects of Gender on Pain Experience

Gender can affect pain sensitivity, tolerance, distress, and exaggeration of pain, and the patient's willingness to report pain, as well as displayed nonverbal cues concerning the pain experience. Studies indicate that women generally have **lower pain thresholds** and **less tolerance** for noxious stimuli or pain factors that hinder them from doing things they enjoy. Women seek help for pain-related problems sooner than men and respond better to therapy. Women also experience more **visceral pain** than men. Men are more prone to experience **somatic pain** and show more stoicism regarding pain experiences than women. **Neuropathic pain** seems to be experienced equally between men and women. Nurses need to be careful that biases concerning gender experiences with pain do not skew their assessments of pain. However, they need to be aware that pain experiences are always individual and may differ between the sexes.

Psychological Factors in Experience of Pain

Psychological factors that may influence a patient's experience of pain include:

- **Fear**: The fear of pain and the anticipation of having pain are factors in how much pain a person feels, because the fear stimulates areas of the brain that focus attention on the body so that the patient experiences an increased sensation of pain. Fear also causes muscles to tense, blood pressure to increase, and the heart rate to increase, and all of these can exacerbate the perception of pain. While pain medications may be necessary, practicing relaxation and mindfulness exercises may help to reduce anxiety and have a positive effect.
- **Depression**: The same neurotransmitters that transmit sensations of pain are also those that transmit moods, so many people with depression present first with complaints of pain or discomfort, and this can result in chronic pain if the depression is not resolved. In some cases, pain may lead to depression, but then the depression worsens the pain so it becomes a cycle of worsening discomfort. Patients may benefit from cognitive behavioral therapy or medication such as SSRIs.

Pain Documentation in Medical Records

Recommendations for **pain documentation** in the medical record include:

- Describe the time of onset, the location of pain, the character of the pain, and the degree of pain, using a validated pain assessment instrument (either a self-reporting instrument, such as the visual analog scale, or one based on observation, such as PAINAD).
- Document all interventions, both pharmacological (opioids, adjuvants) and nonpharmacological (positioning, massage, relaxation exercises), including the time, the dosage, and the method of administration.
- Assess and document the initial response to the medication based on the expected response time. For example, an IV medication should take effect almost immediately, but oral medications may take up to 20 minutes to take effect.

- Assess and document the duration of response based on the expected duration of the medication. For example, if a medication response is expected to last for 6 hours, the patient's pain level should be assessed at least every 2 hours and more frequently if the rate of pain increases.
- Describe any adverse effects, such as itching or nausea.

Geriatric Assessment

Age Categories of the Elderly

The elderly population can be divided into three groups. The age group ranging from 65-74 years are considered the **young-old**, from 75-84 are considered the **middle-old**, and 85 and older are considered **old-old**. There are many physical and psychological changes that occur as someone moves through these age groups. As this population increases in size, so does the number of those with physical and mental illnesses.

Factors That Influence Presentation of Illness in Older Adults

There are three major factors that influence **how an illness will present in an older patient.** These factors, either alone or in combination with one another, have the potential to make an ordinarily standard clinical presentation confusing for the clinician.

- The first of these factors is **underreporting of illness or the symptoms associated** with illness. There are a number of reasons that illnesses are not reported: the patient may fear hospitalization, institutionalization, or loss of control, or the patient may be convinced that there really is no problem.
- Another factor is the **pattern of distribution of illness** amongst the elderly population. This affects presentation because there are a number of diseases and problems that are prevalent among older adults, including congestive heart failure, arthritis, osteoporosis, and pneumonia, therefore identifying and differentiating the primary diagnosis may be difficult.
- The last factor is an **altered response to illness**. This can make diagnosis and treatment very difficult because symptoms may be exaggerated by other problems, or they may be nonexistent.

Age-Related Considerations When Evaluating Adult Patients

Because each individual patient is exposed to different environmental, psychological and physical stressors that can affect the aging process, it is important to consider that some patients may experience adverse health problems, while other patients of the same age may not be affected. As individuals age, the amount of wear on the body, as well as the likelihood of pathological changes, increases at different rates for every individual. Factors affecting the aging process include proper nutrition (or the lack thereof), level of physical activity, smoking, alcohol consumption, environmental or occupational exposures, and socioeconomic standing. Also, remember that as an individual ages, a disease or problems with one organ or organ system will have a marked effect on other systems, because the body is not able to compensate as it once was. Symptoms may not be noticeable until other functions begin to decline. Most often, health issues manifest in the elderly as confusion, so close attention must be given to this symptom and investigated when present.

Changes Associated with Aging

Biological Changes

As people move from the young-old to the old-old, many **physical and biological changes** occur throughout their bodies. Organs and tissues such as the kidneys, liver, heart, GI tract, and brain begin to decline, and some, such as the ovaries and uterus, fall into disuse and atrophy. Dysfunction of the **kidneys and liver** is of particular importance because these organs are responsible for drug metabolism. This population may also experience peripheral neuropathy, decreased reaction times, and decreased balance due to changes in the nervous system. There can also be a decline in the five senses. Changes in vision and hearing can affect performance on many of the assessment tools used to evaluate this population for mental health issues such as depression, delirium, dementia, or anxiety.

Psychological Changes

Psychological changes can occur in cognition, learning capacity, and memory. These changes can lead to **decreased continued development** and can **change relationships** with family and friends. Many of the cognitive changes are brought about by a general atrophy of the brain. The aging process does not impair a person's state of consciousness, however, there can be a generalized decrease in concentration, attention span, and reaction times, leading to poor performance on many assessment tools. Learning may be diminished simply because the elderly person may lack motivation.

Memory loss does not go hand in hand with the aging process. Memory loss can occur for a variety of reasons such as disease processes, medications, substance abuse, or depression.

Sociocultural Changes

The elderly may experience many **social changes** such as change in functional independence, employment, and social experiences with groups and friends. As the individual moves from young-old to old-old, many of the things that they were able to **do for themselves** will diminish. This can range from fixing household problems to basic activities of daily living (ADLs) such as bathing and dressing. This population also enters retirement and daily life may become less organized and they may experience financial stress and anxiety. With retirement, this population may also have a reduction in healthcare benefits inhibiting them from seeking needed assistance. Debilitating medical conditions may also inhibit their social activities and they may experience feelings of isolation.

Basic Patient Safety Assessments When Evaluating a Patient

There are **4 basic assessments** that the nurse should make when **assessing a patient's safety** and identifying possible safety concerns:

- The first of these is the **mobility assessment**; different safety risks apply to patients who are mobile as opposed to those who are not. An immobile patient, for example, has a tendency to form pressure ulcers, or bedsores.
- The next assessment is the evaluation of the patient's **level of awareness**; is the patient able to communicate to the nursing staff when something is wrong? If not, certain measures should be undertaken to ensure that the nursing staff is aware of a change in the patient's condition.
- An extension of this assessment is determining whether the patient is in **critical condition**; these patients must be monitored more closely for changes.
- An assessment of the patient's **mental status** is also important because the patient may not be able to make safe decisions on his or her own.

Functional Evaluation of Elderly Patient

A **functional evaluation of the elderly patient** examines the patient's ability to carry out activities of daily living (ADL) that are critical in gauging the patient's ability to care for oneself without the need of assistance. Use the **Index of Independence in Activities of Daily Living Scale** to check foundational tasks such as taking a shower, getting dressed, eating, and going to the bathroom. Aged patients will be more likely to overstate what they are able to do and understate their limitations, while the patient's family will likely understate what the patient is able to handle. Assess mental ability with the following exams:

- Short Portable Mental Status Questionnaire (SPMSQ)
- Mini-Mental State Exam (MMSE)

The **Tinetti Balance and Gait Evaluation** exams are also important elements of the functional evaluation of an elderly patient. These tests, along with the simple **Up-and-Go test,** are used to assess the balance and gait issues that elderly patients have. The patient has to complete certain actions, such as sitting down and standing up from a chair, turning around, bending over, etc. The entire assessment takes approximately 15–20 minutes. The **Lawton and Brody: Instrumental Activities of Daily Learning** test is used to check whether the patient can do more complex activities important to daily living, second to the ADL's required for basic function. Examples of IADLs include the ability to go shopping, wash clothes, cook, etc. The **Index of Independence of Activities of Daily Living** is utilized to find what the patient is able do independently on a regular basis.

Depression and Suicide in the Elderly

Depression commonly goes unidentified in an aging patient. Cognitive changes are often wrongly identified as dementia, confusion, or natural aging changes, rather than depression. It is important to be cognizant of the prevalence of this issue among the elderly, and treat appropriately.

Suicide rates for elderly patients are higher than any other age group. The compounding stress and emotional burden of losing loved ones, mobility, and independence often contribute to suicidal ideations. Other factors include seemingly unbearable psychological anguish, dissatisfaction, and unmet requirements. Suicide is more commonly seen in elderly males (seven times higher rate), Caucasians, unmarried individuals (divorced, separated, single), individuals who are poor and/or out of work, individuals with mental problems, the very sick, individuals with substance additions, individuals that are grieving (particularly in the first year of loss or retirement), those without friends or community relationships, or those who have tried suicide before. Suicidal thoughts and attempts may be overt or covert.

As with patients of other age ranges, if an elderly patient hints at suicidal ideations or thoughts, this must be addressed directly by the nurse.

Indications and Assessments for Delirium

Delirium (acute confusion) presents in a variety of indications. The patient may experience mental issues, including inattention or short attention span, difficulty remembering, trouble with perception, bafflement, and lack of decision-making. There may be changing moods, faulty ability to manage whims, stress, slight to moderate depression, visual or auditory hallucinations, confabulation, changing intellectual ability that worsens at night (sun-downing) and is more frequently seen in patients that have had prior dementia, psychomotor agitation including inability to sleep, tachycardia, enlarged pupils, and perspiration. The patient may appear restless, overcautious, not cautious enough, or appear lost/stunned. There may be tachycardia, high blood pressure, fever, rapid breathing, and there might be focal neurological indications.

Physical assessments include a complete history, physical examination, check of mind and neurological issues to determine what is causing the problem, foundation of lab work such as CBC, electrocardiogram, chest radiograph, urinalysis, urine toxicology, and other assessments that are deemed necessary, such as EED, CT, or blood work for drugs.

Core Competencies: Advanced Pathophysiology

Cardiovascular Pathophysiology

Acute Coronary Syndromes

Acute coronary syndrome (ACS) is the impairment of blood flow through the coronary arteries, leading to ischemia of the cardiac muscle. Angina frequently occurs in ACS, manifesting as crushing pain substernally, radiating down the left arm or both arms. However, in females, elderly, and diabetics, symptoms may appear less acute and include nausea, shortness of breath, fatigue, pain/weakness/numbness in arms, or no pain at all (*silent ischemia*). There are multiple classifications of angina:

- **Stable angina:** Exercise-induced, short lived, relieved by rest or nitroglycerin. Other precipitating events include decrease in environmental temperature, heavy eating, strong emotions (such as fright or anger), or exertion, including coitus.
- **Unstable angina** (preinfarction or crescendo angina): A change in the pattern of stable angina, characterized by an increase in pain, not responding to a single nitroglycerin or rest, and persisting for >5 minutes. May cause a change in EKG, or indicate rupture of an atherosclerotic plaque or the beginning of thrombus formation. Treat as a medical emergency, indicates impending MI.
- **Variant angina** (Prinzmetal's angina): Results from spasms of the coronary arteries. Associated with or without atherosclerotic plaques and is often related to smoking, alcohol, or illicit stimulants, but can occur cyclically and at rest. Elevation of ST segments usually occurs with variant angina. Treatment is nitroglycerin or calcium channel blockers.

Myocardial Infarctions

NSTEMI and STEMI

Non–ST-segment elevation MI (NSTEMI): ST elevation on the electrocardiogram (ECG) occurs in response to myocardial damage resulting from infarction or severe ischemia. The absence of ST elevation may be diagnosed as unstable angina or NSTEMI, but cardiac enzyme levels increase with NSTEMI, indicating partial blockage of coronary arteries with some damage. Symptoms are consistent with unstable angina, with chest pain or tightness, pain radiating to the neck or arm, dyspnea, anxiety, weakness, dizziness, nausea, vomiting, and heartburn. Initial treatment may include nitroglycerin, β-blockers, antiplatelet agents, or antithrombotic agents. Ongoing treatment may include β-blockers, aspirin, statins, angiotensin-converting enzyme inhibitors, angiotensin-receptor blockers, and clopidogrel. Percutaneous coronary intervention is not recommended.

ST-segment elevation MI (STEMI): This more severe type of MI involves complete blockage of one or more coronary arteries with myocardial damage, resulting in ST elevation. Symptoms are those of acute MI. As necrosis occurs, Q waves often develop, indicating irreversible myocardial damage, which may result in death, so treatment involves immediate reperfusion before necrosis can occur.

Q-Wave and Non-Q-Wave Myocardial Infarctions

Formerly classified as transmural or non-transmural, myocardial infarctions are now classified as Q-wave or non-Q-wave:

- **Q-Wave:**
  - Characterized by a series of abnormal Q waves (wider and deeper) on ECG, especially in the early morning (related to adrenergic activity).
  - Infarction is usually prolonged and results in necrosis.
  - Coronary occlusion is complete in 80-90% of cases.
  - Q-wave MI is often, but not always, transmural.
  - Peak CK levels occur in about 27 hours.
- **Non-Q-Wave**
  - Characterized by changes in ST-T wave with ST depression (usually reversible within a few days).
  - Usually reperfusion occurs spontaneously, so infarct size is smaller. Contraction necrosis related to reperfusion is common.
  - Non-Q-wave MI is usually non-transmural.
  - Coronary occlusion is complete in only 20-30%.
  - Peak CK levels occur in 12-13 hours.
  - Reinfarction is common.

Locations and Types

Myocardial infarctions are also classified according to their location and the extent of injury. Q-wave infarctions involve the full thickness of the heart muscle, often producing a series of Q waves on ECG. While an MI most frequently damages the left ventricle and the septum, the right ventricle may be damaged as well, depending upon the area of the occlusion:

- **Anterior** (V_2 to V_4): Occlusion in the proximal left anterior descending (LAD) or left coronary artery. Reciprocal changes found in leads II, III, aV_F.
- **Lateral** (I, aV_L, V_5, V_6): Occlusion of the circumflex coronary artery or branch of left coronary artery. Often causes damage to anterior wall as well; Reciprocal changes found in leads II, III, aV_F.
- **Inferior/diaphragmatic** (II, III, aV_F): Occlusion of the right coronary artery and causes conduction malfunctions. Reciprocal changes found in leads I and aV_L.
- **Right ventricular** (V_{4R}, V_{5R}, V_{6R}): Occlusion of the proximal section of the right coronary artery and damages in the right ventricle and the inferior wall. No reciprocal changes should be noted on an ECG.
- **Posterior** (V_8, V_9)**:** Occlusion in the right coronary artery or circumflex artery and may be difficult to diagnose. Reciprocal changes found in V_1-V_4.

Clinical Manifestations and Diagnosis

Clinical manifestations of myocardial infarction may vary considerably. More than half of all patients present with acute MIs with no prior history of cardiovascular disease.

Signs/symptoms: Angina with pain in chest that may radiate to neck or arms, palpitations, hypertension or hypotension, dyspnea, pulmonary edema, dependent edema, nausea/vomiting, pallor, skin cold and clammy, diaphoresis, decreased urinary output, neurological/psychological disturbances: anxiety, light-headed, headache, visual abnormalities, slurred speech, and fear.

Diagnosis is based on the following:

- ECG obtained immediately to monitor heart changes over time. Typical changes include T-wave inversion, elevation of ST segment, abnormal Q waves, tachycardia, bradycardia, and dysrhythmias.
- Echocardiogram: decreased ventricular function is possible, especially for transmural MI.
- Labs:
    - **Troponin**: Increases within 3–6 hours, peaks 14–20; elevated for up to 1-2 weeks.
    - **Creatinine kinase (CK-MB):** Increases 4–8 hours and peaks at about 24 hours (earlier with thrombolytic therapy or PTCA).
    - **Ischemia Modified Albumin (IMA):** Increase within minutes, peak 6 hours and return to baseline; verify with other labs.
    - **Myoglobin**: Increases in 30 minutes–4 hours, peaks 6–7 hours. While an increase is not specific to an MI, a failure to increase can be used to rule out an MI.

Papillary Muscle Rupture

Papillary muscle rupture is a rare but often deadly complication of myocardial ischemia/infarct. It most commonly occurs with inferior infarcts. The papillary muscles are part of the cardiac wall structure. Attached to the lower portion of the ventricles, they are responsible for the opening and closing of the tricuspid and mitral valve and preventing prolapse during systole. Rupture of the papillary muscle can occur with myocardial infarct or ischemia in the area of the heart surrounding the papillary muscle. Since the papillary muscles support the mitral valve, rupture will cause severe mitral regurgitation that may result in cardiogenic shock and subsequent death. Rupture of the papillary muscle may be partial or complete and is considered a life-threatening emergency.

Signs and symptoms: Acute heart failure, pulmonary edema, and cardiogenic shock (tachycardia, diaphoresis, loss of consciousness, pallor, tachypnea, mental status changes, weak or thready pulse, and decreased urinary output).

Diagnosis: Transesophageal echocardiography (TEE) to visualize the papillary muscles, color flow Doppler, echocardiogram and physical assessment. In patients with papillary muscle rupture, a holosystolic murmur starting at the apex and radiating to the axilla may be present.

Treatment: Emergent surgical intervention to repair the mitral valve.

In the cases of complete rupture, patients often experience the rapid development of cardiogenic shock and subsequent death.

Carotid Artery Stenosis

The common carotid artery branches from the subclavian artery and then bifurcates into the external carotid and internal carotid arteries. This point of bifurcation is a common site for the development of plaques, causing **carotid artery stenosis** that interferes with cranial blood flow. When stenosis develops slowly, collateral vessels may form to aid circulation, but sudden occlusion can cause permanent brain damage and death. Most stenosis is caused by atherosclerosis, with increasing incidence with age. Most ischemia relates to an embolism or thrombus formation.

Symptoms of occlusion are often asymptomatic; however, they include severe pain, anxiety, and those symptoms common to brain attacks (hemiparesis, confusion, aphasia, and diplopia).

Diagnosis: Duplex ultrasound (combining conventional ultrasound with Doppler, determines blood flow and obstruction), CT scan, MRA or angiogram (will indicate degree of blockage).

Treatment may include:

- Medications: Anticoagulants and thrombolytics.
- Carotid endarterectomy (recommended if stenosis >60%): poses the danger of a post-procedure stroke due to plaque dislodgement or increased blood flow to narrowed vessels, so the benefits must be carefully weighed.
- Carotid stents/angioplasty (newer non-invasive approaches).

Aortic Aneurysms

Types

A **dissecting aortic aneurysm** occurs when the wall of the aorta is torn and blood flows between the layers of the wall, dilating and weakening it until it risks rupture (which has a 90% mortality). Aortic aneurysms are more than twice as common in males as females, but females have a higher mortality rate, possibly due to increased age at diagnosis.

Abdominal aortic aneurysms (AAA) are usually related to atherosclerosis, but may also result from Marfan syndrome, Ehlers-Danlos disease, and connective tissue disorders. Rupture usually does not allow time for emergent repair, so identifying and correcting before rupture is essential. Different classification systems are used to describe the type and degree of dissection. Common classification:

- **DeBakey classification** uses anatomic location as the focal point:
  - *Type I* begins in the ascending aorta but may spread to include the aortic arch and the descending aorta (60%). This is also considered a proximal lesion or Stanford type A.
  - *Type II* is restricted to the ascending aorta (10-15%). This is also considered a proximal lesion or Stanford type A.
  - *Type III* is restricted to the descending aorta (25-30%). This is considered a distal lesion or Stanford type B.
- Types I and II are thoracic and type III is abdominal.

Diagnosis and Treatment

Aortic aneurysms are often asymptomatic, but when symptomatic, patients present with substernal pain, back pain, dyspnea and/or stridor (from pressure on trachea), cough, distention of neck veins, palpable and pulsating abdominal mass, edema of neck and arms.

Diagnosis: X-ray, CT, MRI, Cardiac catheterization, TEE/transthoracic echocardiogram.

Treatment includes:

- **Anti-hypertensives** to reduce systolic BP, such as β-blockers (esmolol) or Alpha-β-blocker combinations (labetalol) to reduce force of blood as it leaves the ventricle to reduce pressure against the aortic wall. IV vasodilators (sodium nitroprusside) may also be needed.
- **Intubation and ventilation** may be required if the patient is hemodynamically unstable.
- **Analgesia/sedation** to control anxiety and pain.

- **Surgical repair:** *Type I and II* are usually repaired surgically because of the danger of rupture and cardiac tamponade. *Type III (abdominal)* is often followed medically and surgically only if the aneurysm is >5.5cm or rapidly expanding. There are two types of surgical repair:
  - *Open*: Patient is placed on cardiopulmonary bypass, and through an abdominal incision the damaged portion is removed, and a graft is sutured in place.
  - *Endovascular*: A stent graft is fed through the arteries to line the aorta and exclude the aneurysm.

Complications: Myocardial infarction, renal injury, and GI hemorrhage/ischemic bowel, which may occur up to years after surgery. Endo-leaks can occur with a stent graft, increasing risk of rupture.

Aortic Rupture

Aortic rupture is a catastrophic breakage of the aorta, generally as the result of trauma or rupture of an aortic aneurysm. Aortic rupture (spontaneous) most commonly occurs in the abdominal aorta. The patient typically experiences a severe tearing pain and loses consciousness from hypovolemic shock as the blood pours out of the aorta. Tachycardia occurs and the patient may exhibit cyanosis. An ecchymotic area may appear in the flank area because of retroperitoneal pooling of blood. Diagnostic tests include ultrasound or CT. Survival depends on the size of the tear, the amount of blood loss, and the length of time until surgical repair. About 90% of patients die prior to surgery. An aortic occlusion balloon to stem bleeding may be placed temporarily in order to stabilize the patient. Surgical repair may be via an open procedure of endovascular therapy. Risk factors include male gender, older age, smoking, history of MI, family history of abdominal aortic aneurysm, peripheral arterial disease, and hypertension.

Cardiogenic Shock

In **cardiogenic shock,** the heart fails to pump enough blood to provide adequate circulation and oxygen to the body. The primary cause of cardiogenic shock is acute myocardial infarction, especially an anterior wall MI. Other causes include papillary muscle/ventricular septal rupture, pericarditis/myocarditis, prolonged tachyarrhythmia, and hypotensive medications.

Signs/Symptoms: Hypotension, altered mental status secondary to decreased cerebral circulation, oliguria, tachypnea or tachycardia, cool extremities, jugular venous distension, and pulmonary edema possible.

Diagnosis: ABGs: metabolic acidosis, hypoxia, hypocapnia; lactic acidosis, BNP, BUN and K elevated; EKG: arrhythmias, specifically SVT/V-tach, Sinus bradycardia, AV block and IVCDs possible; however, the EKG may be normal.

- Arterial Line Values: CI <1.8 L/min, PCWP >18 mmHg, SBP <90, MAP <60, Increased CVP and PAP.

Treatment includes:

- Dobutamine IV to increase cardiac contractility.
- Norepinephrine IV if SBP <70.
- Morphine can be given for pain; while potential for hypotension, it will decrease SNS response and decrease HR and MVO_2.
- Treat underlying cause (e.g., papillary rupture = valve replacement)
- Intra-aortic Balloon Pump (IABP): Increases cardiac blood flow.
- Re-vascularization if secondary to acute MI (CABG or PCI).

Obstructive Shock

Obstructive shock occurs when the preload (diastolic filling of the RV) of the heart is obstructed in one or several ways. There can be obstruction to the great vessels of the heart (such as from pulmonary embolism), there can be excessive afterload because the flow of blood out of the heart is obstructed (resulting in decreased cardiac output), or there can be direct compression of the heart, which can occur when blood or air fills the pericardial sac with cardiac tamponade or tension pneumothorax. Other causes include aortic dissection, vena cava syndrome, systemic hypertension, and cardiac lesions. Obstructive shock is often categorized with cardiogenic shock because of their similarities. **Signs and symptoms** of obstructive shock may vary depending on the underlying cause but typically include:

- Decrease in oxygen saturation
- Hemodynamic instability with hypotension and tachycardia, muffled heart sounds
- Chest pain
- Neurological impairment (disorientation, confusion)
- Dyspnea
- Impaired peripheral circulation (cool extremities, pallor)
- Generalized pallor and cyanosis

Treatment depends on the cause and may include oxygen, pericardiocentesis, needle thoracostomy or chest tube, and fluid resuscitation.

Cardiac Tamponade

Cardiac tamponade occurs with pericardial effusion, causing pressure against the heart. It may be a complication of trauma, pericarditis, cardiac surgery, pneumothorax, or heart failure. About 50 mL of fluid normally circulates in the pericardial area to reduce friction, and a sudden increase in this volume or air in the pericardial sac can compress the heart, causing a number of cardiac responses such as:

- Increased end-diastolic pressure in both ventricles
- Decrease in venous return
- Decrease in ventricular filling

Symptoms may include pressure or pain in the chest, dyspnea, and pulsus paradoxus >10 mmHg. Beck's triad (increased CVP, distended neck veins, muffled heart sounds, and hypotension) is common. A sudden decrease in chest tube drainage can occur as fluid and clots accumulate in the pericardial sac, preventing the blood from filling the ventricles and decreasing cardiac output and perfusion of the body, including the kidneys (resulting in decreased urinary output). X-ray may show change in cardiac silhouette and mediastinal shift (in 20%). Treatment includes pericardiocentesis with large bore needle or surgical repair to control bleeding and relieve cardiac compression. Risk factors include cardiac surgery, cardiac tumors, MI, and chest trauma.

CARDIOMYOPATHY

DILATED CARDIOMYOPATHY

Dilated cardiomyopathy (DCM) occurs when some precipitating factor leads to decreased cardiac perfusion. The resulting ischemic cardiac tissue is replaced with scar tissue, and the healthy cells are forced to over-compensate, causing hypertrophy and over stretching. Eventually, the muscle cells become stretched beyond compensation, and dilated and weak chamber results, unable to properly contract. This causes a decrease in stroke volume and cardiac output, with the end result being enlargement of the mitral and tricuspid valves and severe valve regurgitation. While DCM is the most common form of cardiomyopathy, causes include:

- **Vascular**: Cardiac ischemia, hypertension, atherosclerosis
- **Metabolic:** Diabetes, uremia, thyrotoxicosis, and acromegaly, muscular dystrophy
- **Genetics** (familial DCM), and childbirth (peripartum DCM)
- **Viral infections,** particularly adenovirus, Varicella zoster, HIV, and Hepatitis C may cause DCM
- **Alcohol poisoning or cocaine addiction**
- **Radiation or heavy metal poisoning**, specifically cobalt

Signs/Symptoms: Dyspnea, SOB, tachycardia, S3/S4 heart sounds, holosystolic murmur, wheezes/crackles, pleural effusions, edema, JVD, ascites

Diagnosis: EKG (tachycardia/T wave changes), chest X-ray (cardiomegaly), 2D Echocardiogram (valve regurgitation/EF).

Treatment includes:

- Treat underlying cause if possible; supportive care
- Heart transplant if patient is a candidate and damage is permanent

HYPERTROPHIC CARDIOMYOPATHY

Hypertrophic cardiomyopathy (HCM) is a genetic disorder that causes idiopathic thickening of the heart muscle, primarily involving the ventricular septum and portions of the left ventricle. Patients with HCM produce abnormal sarcomeres and misalignment of muscle cells (myocardial disarray). Basically, HCM is characterized by ventricular hypertrophy, an asymmetrical septum, forceful systole, cardiac dysrhythmias, and myocardial disarray. Because the abnormal cells develop over time, it is common for HCM to remain undiagnosed until middle or late adulthood.

Signs/Symptoms: Exertional or atypical chest pain, dyspnea at rest, syncope, frequent palpitations (common due to reoccurring dysrhythmias).

Diagnosis: 2D echo (structure and EF), EKG (pathological Q waves and dysrhythmias), Xray (cardiomegaly), Family history (especially cardiac death, reoccurring dysrhythmias, or myocardial hypertrophy).

Treatment includes:

- **Surgery:** Septal myectomy is gold standard: high mortality (3-10%), but increases cardiac output and quality of life.
- **Alcohol-based septal ablation:** Ethanol 100% injected into a branch of the LAD, creating a controlled area of infarction and consequentially thinning the septum.

Restrictive Cardiomyopathy

Restrictive cardiomyopathy (RCM) occurs when the ventricles become stiff and noncompliant, resulting in decreased end-diastolic cardiac refill volume. The ventricular stiffening is caused by the infiltration of fibroelastic tissue into the cardiac muscle (such as in amyloidosis or sarcoidosis). Atrial enlargement can be seen in most cases of RCM as a result of the increased effort required to push blood from the atria into the ventricles. It is not uncommon for a patient to be in atrial fibrillation secondary to atrial enlargement. In advanced cases, ventricular dysrhythmias may also be seen.

Signs/Symptoms: Exercise intolerance/fatigue, edema, crackles, elevated CVP, S3/S4, murmur, SOB at rest

Diagnosis: 2D echo (enlarged atria, decreased compliance of ventricle), hemodynamic monitoring (increased right atrial pressure and pulmonary wedge pressure, and SVR), X-Ray (cardiomegaly), EKG (atrial fibrillation), endomyocardial biopsy (to differentiate from constrictive pericarditis).

Treatment includes:

- **Medications**: β-blockers increase ventricular filling; antiarrhythmics may be ordered
- **Surgical**: Heart transplant, if patient is a candidate

Dysrhythmias

Sinus Bradycardia

There are 3 primary types of **sinus node dysrhythmias**: sinus bradycardia, sinus tachycardia, and sinus arrhythmia. **Sinus bradycardia (SB)** is caused by a decreased rate of impulse from sinus node. The pulse and ECG usually appear normal except for a slower rate.

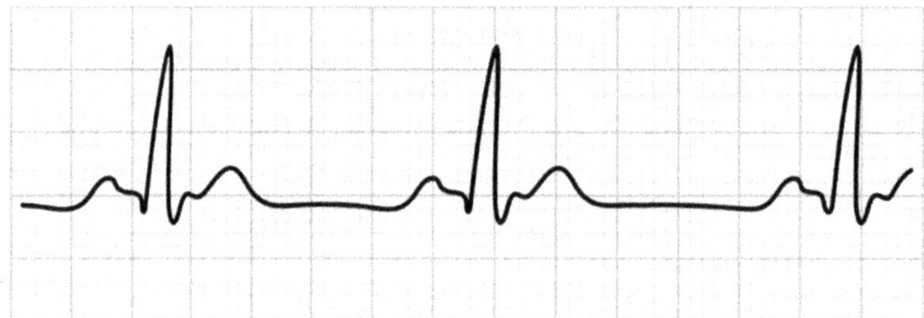

SB is characterized by a regular pulse <50-60 bpm with P waves in front of QRS, which are usually normal in shape and duration. PR interval is 0.12-0.20 seconds, QRS interval is 0.04-0.11 seconds, and P:QRS ratio of 1:1. SB may be caused by several factors:

- May be normal in athletes and older adults; generally not treated unless symptomatic
- Conditions that lower the body's metabolic needs, such as hypothermia or sleep
- Hypotension and decrease in oxygenation
- Medications such as calcium channel blockers and β-blockers

- Vagal stimulation that may result from vomiting, suctioning, defecating, or certain medical procedures (carotid stent placement, etc.)
- Increased intracranial pressure
- Myocardial infarction

Treatment: involves eliminating cause if possible, such as changing medications. Atropine 0.5-1.0 mg may be given IV to block vagal stimulation or increase rate if symptomatic.

Sinus Tachycardia

Sinus tachycardia (ST) occurs when the sinus node impulse increases in frequency. ST is characterized by a regular pulse >100 with P waves before QRS but sometimes part of the preceding T wave. QRS is usually of normal shape and duration (0.04-0.11 seconds) but may have consistent irregularity. PR interval is 0.12-0.20 seconds and P:QRS ratio of 1:1.

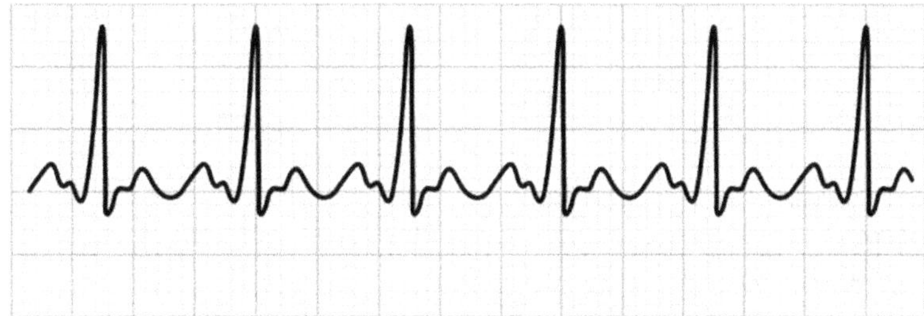

The rapid pulse decreases diastolic filling time and causes reduced cardiac output with resultant hypotension. Acute pulmonary edema may result from the decreased ventricular filling if untreated. ST may be **caused** by a number of factors:

- Acute blood loss, shock, hypovolemia, anemia
- Sinus arrhythmia, hypovolemic heart failure
- Hypermetabolic conditions, fever, infection
- Exertion/exercise, anxiety, stress
- Medications, such as sympathomimetic drugs

Treatment: eliminating precipitating factors, calcium channel blockers and β-blockers to reduce heart rate.

Supraventricular Tachycardia

Supraventricular tachycardia (SVT) (>100 BPM) may have a sudden onset and result in congestive heart failure. Rate may increase to 200–300 BMP, which will significantly decrease cardiac output due to decreased filling time. SVT originates in the atria rather than the ventricles but is controlled by the tissue in the area of the AV node rather than the SA node. Rhythm is usually rapid but regular. The P wave is present but may not be clearly defined as it may be obscured by the preceding T wave, and the QRS complex appears normal. The PR interval is 0.12-0.20 seconds and the QRS interval is 0.04-0.11 seconds with a P:QRS ratio of 1:1.

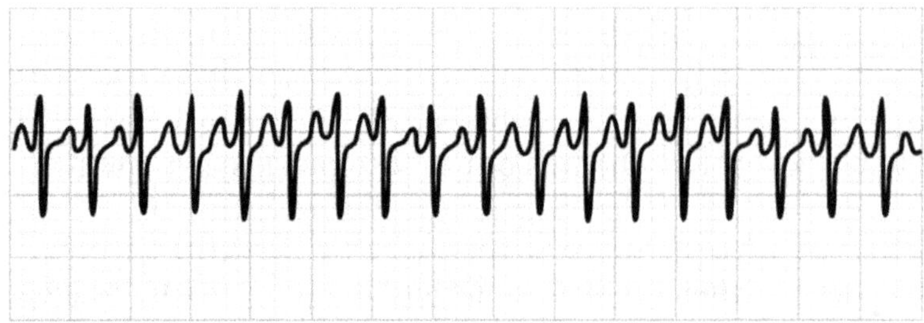

SVT may be episodic with periods of normal heart rate and rhythm between episodes of SVT, so it is often referred to as paroxysmal SVT (PSVT).

Treatment: Adenosine, digoxin (Lanoxin®), Verapamil (Calan®, Verelan®), vagal maneuvers, cardioversion.

Sinus Arrhythmia

Sinus arrhythmia (SA) results from irregular impulses from the sinus node, often paradoxical (increasing with inspiration and decreasing with expiration) because of stimulation of the vagal nerve during inspiration and rarely causes a negative hemodynamic effect. These cyclic changes in the pulse during respiration are quite common in both children and young adults and often lesson with age but may persist in some adults. Sinus arrhythmia can, in some cases, relate to heart or valvular disease and may be increased with vagal stimulation for suctioning, vomiting, or defecating. Characteristics of SA include a regular pulse 50-100 BPM, P waves in front of QRS with duration (0.04-0.11 seconds) and shape of QRS usually normal, PR interval of 0.12-0.20 seconds, and P:QRS ratio of 1:1.

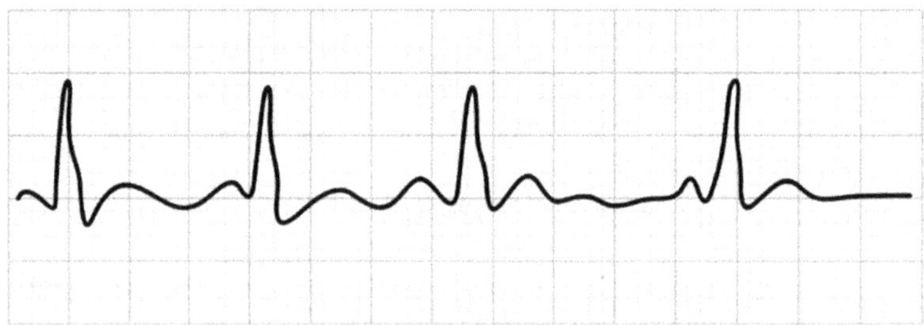

Treatment is usually not necessary unless it is associated with bradycardia.

Premature Atrial Contraction

There are 3 primary types of **atrial dysrhythmias**: premature atrial contraction, atrial flutter, and atrial fibrillation. Premature atrial contraction (PAC) is essentially an extra beat precipitated by an electrical impulse to the atrium before the sinus node impulse. The extra beat may be caused by alcohol, caffeine, nicotine, hypervolemia, hypokalemia, hypermetabolic conditions, atrial ischemia, or infarction. Characteristics include an irregular pulse because of extra P waves, the shape and duration of QRS is usually normal (0.04-0.11 seconds) but may be abnormal, PR interval remains between 0.12-0.20, and P:QRS ratio is 1:1. Rhythm is irregular with varying P-P and R-R intervals.

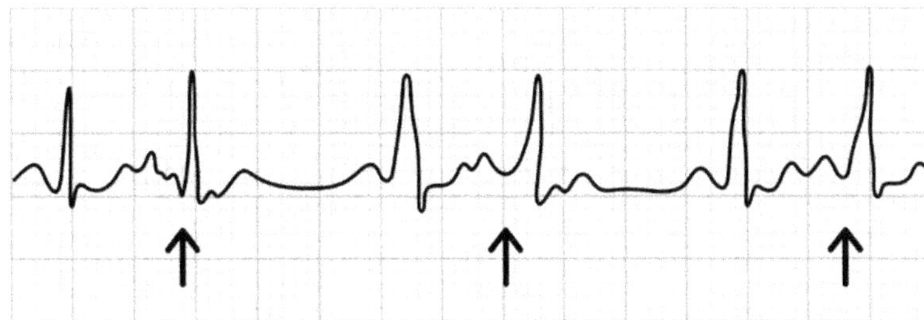

PACs can occur in an essentially healthy heart and are not usually cause for concern unless they are frequent (>6 hr) and cause severe palpitations. In that case, atrial fibrillation should be suspected.

Atrial Flutter

Atrial flutter (AF) occurs when the atrial rate is faster, usually 250-400 beats per minute, than the AV node conduction rate so not all of the beats are conducted into the ventricles. The beats are effectively blocked at the AV node, preventing ventricular fibrillation although some extra ventricular impulses may pass though. AF is caused by the same conditions that cause A-fib: coronary artery disease, valvular disease, pulmonary disease, heavy alcohol ingestion, and cardiac surgery. AF is characterized by atrial rates of 250-400 with ventricular rates of 75-150, with ventricular rate usually being regular. P waves are saw-toothed (referred to as F waves), QRS shape and duration (0.04-0.11 seconds) are usually normal, PR interval may be hard to calculate because of F waves, and the P:QRS ratio is 2:1 to 4:1. Symptoms include chest pain, dyspnea, and hypotension.

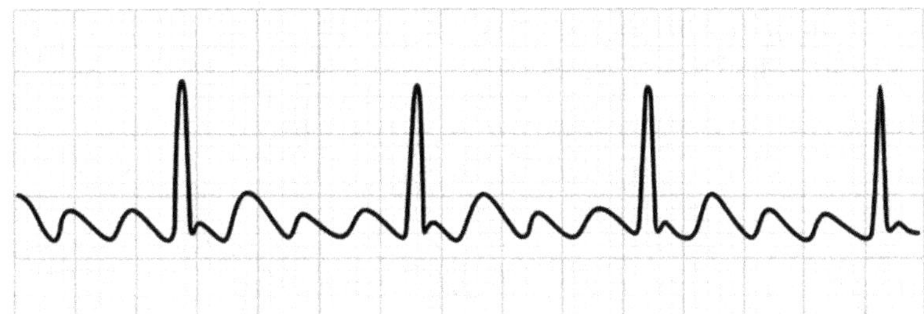

Treatment includes:

- Emergent cardioversion if condition is unstable
- Medications to slow ventricular rate and conduction through AV node: non-dihydropyridine calcium channel blockers (Cardizem®, Calan®) and beta blockers
- Medications to convert to sinus rhythm: Corvert®, Tikosyn, Amiodarone; also used in practice: Cardioquin®, Norpace®, Cordarone®

Atrial Fibrillation

Atrial fibrillation (A-fib) is rapid, disorganized atrial beats that are ineffective in emptying the atria, so that blood pools in the chambers. This can lead to thrombus formation and emboli. The ventricular rate increases with a decreased stroke volume, and cardiac output decreases with increased myocardial ischemia, resulting in palpitations and fatigue. A-fib is caused by coronary artery disease, valvular disease, pulmonary disease, heavy alcohol ingestion, infection, and cardiac surgery; however, it can also be idiopathic. A-fib is characterized by a very irregular pulse with atrial rate of 300-600 and ventricular rate of 120-200, shape and duration (0.04-0.11 seconds) of QRS is usually normal. Fibrillatory (F) waves are seen instead of P waves. The PR interval cannot be measured and the P:QRS ratio is highly variable.

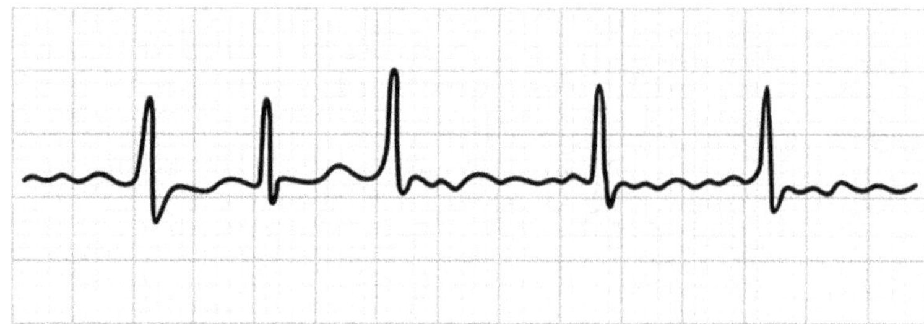

Treatment is the same as atrial flutter.

Review Video: EKG Interpretation: Afib and Aflutter
Visit mometrix.com/academy and enter code: 263842

Premature Junctional Contraction

The area around the AV node is the junction, and dysrhythmias that arise from that area are called junctional dysrhythmias. Premature junctional contraction (PJC) occurs when a premature impulse starts at the AV node before the next normal sinus impulse reaches the AV node. PJC is similar to premature atrial contraction (PAC) and generally requires no treatment although it may be an indication of digoxin toxicity. The ECG may appear basically normal with an early QRS complex that is normal in shape and duration (0.04-0.11 seconds). The P wave may be absent or it may precede, be part of, or follow the QRS with a PR interval of 0.12 seconds. The P:QRS ratio may vary from <1:1 to 1:1 (with inverted P wave). The underlying rhythm is usually regular at a heart rate of 60-100. Significant symptoms related to PJC are rare.

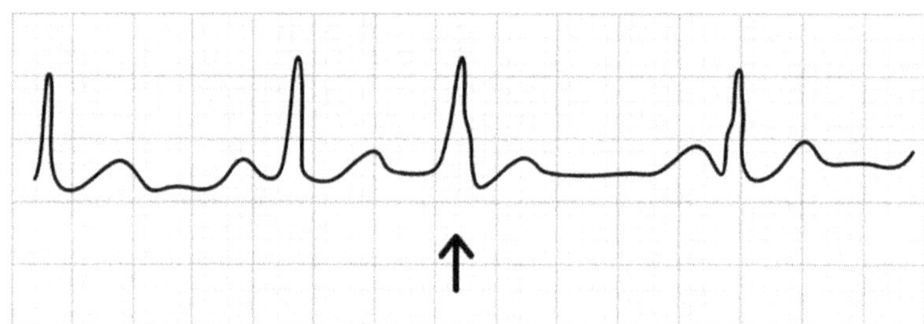

Junctional Rhythms

Junctional rhythms occur when the AV node becomes the pacemaker of the heart. This can happen because the sinus node is depressed from increased vagal tone or a block at the AV node prevents sinus node impulses from being transmitted. While the sinus node normally sends impulses 60-100 beats per minute, the AV node junction usually sends impulses at 40-60 beats per minute. The QRS complex is of usual shape and duration (0.04-0.11 seconds). The P wave may be inverted and may be absent, hidden or after the QRS. If the P wave precedes the QRS, the PR interval is <0.12 seconds. The P:QRS ratio is <1:1 or 1:1. The junctional escape rhythm is a protective mechanism preventing asystole with failure of the sinus node. An **accelerated**

junctional rhythm is similar, but the heart rate is 60-100. **Junctional tachycardia** occurs with heart rate of >100.

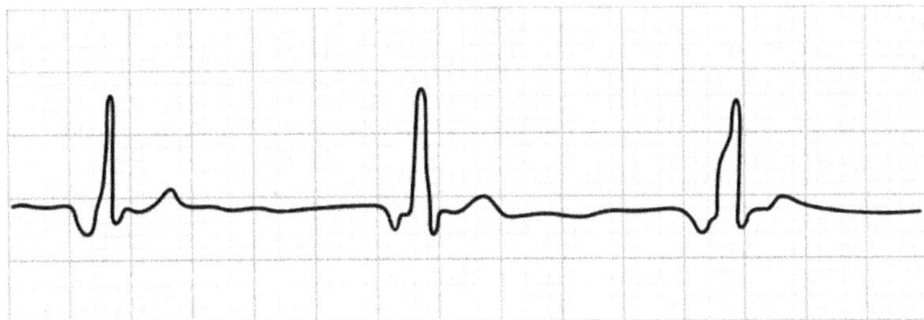

AV Nodal Reentry Tachycardia

AV nodal reentry tachycardia occurs when an impulse conducts to the area of the AV node and is then sent in a rapidly repeating cycle back to the same area and to the ventricles, resulting in a fast ventricular rate. The onset and cessation are usually rapid. AV nodal reentry tachycardia (also known as paroxysmal atrial tachycardia or supraventricular tachycardia if there are no P waves) is characterized by atrial rate of 150-250 with ventricular rate of 75-250, P wave that is difficult to see or absent, QRS complex that is usually normal and a PR interval of <0.12 if a P wave is present. The P:QRS ratio is 1-2:1. Precipitating factors include nicotine, caffeine, hypoxemia, anxiety, underlying coronary artery disease and cardiomyopathy. Cardiac output may be decreased with a rapid heart rate, causing dyspnea, chest pain, and hypotension.

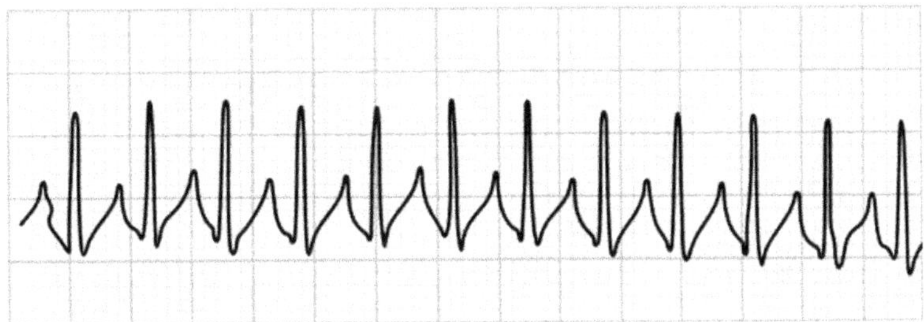

Treatment includes:

- Vagal maneuvers (carotid sinus massage, gag reflex, holding breath/bearing down)
- Medications (adenosine, verapamil, or diltiazem)
- Cardioversion if other methods unsuccessful

Premature Ventricular Contractions

Premature ventricular contractions (PVCs) are those in which the impulse begins in the ventricles and conducts through them prior to the next sinus impulse. The ectopic QRS complexes may vary in shape, depending upon whether there is one site (unifocal) or more (multifocal) that stimulates the ectopic beats. PVCs usually cause no morbidity unless there is underlying cardiac disease or an acute MI. PVCs are characterized by an irregular heartbeat, QRS that is ≥0.12 seconds and oddly shaped. PVCs are often not treated in otherwise healthy people. PVCs may be precipitated by electrolyte imbalances, caffeine, nicotine, or alcohol. Because PVCs may occur with any supraventricular dysrhythmia, the underlying rhythm must be noted as well as the PVCs. If there are more than six PVCs in an hour, that is a risk factor for developing ventricular tachycardia.

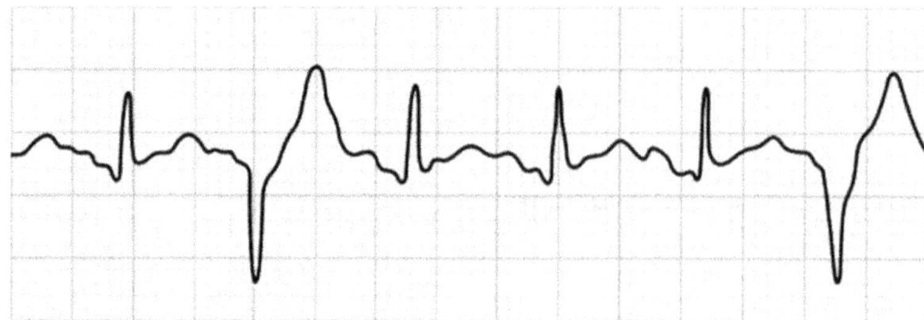

Bigeminy is a rhythm where every other beat is a PVC. **Trigeminy** is a rhythm where every third beat is a PVC.

Ventricular bigeminy is a rhythm where every other beat is a PVC. **Ventricular trigeminy** is a rhythm where every third beat is a PVC.

Treatment: Lidocaine (affects the ventricles, may cause CNS toxicity with nausea and vomiting), Procainamide (affects the atria and ventricles and may cause decreased BP and widening of QRS and QT); treat underlying cause.

Ventricular Tachycardia

Ventricular tachycardia (VT) is greater than 3 PVCs in a row with a ventricular rate of 100-200 beats per minute. Ventricular tachycardia may be triggered by the same factors as PVCs and often is related to underlying coronary artery disease. The rapid rate of contractions makes VT dangerous as the ineffective beats may render the person unconscious with no palpable pulse. A detectable rate is usually regular and the QRS complex is ≥0.12 seconds and is usually abnormally shaped. The P wave may be undetectable with an irregular PR interval if P wave is present. The P:QRS ratio is often difficult to ascertain because of the absence of P waves.

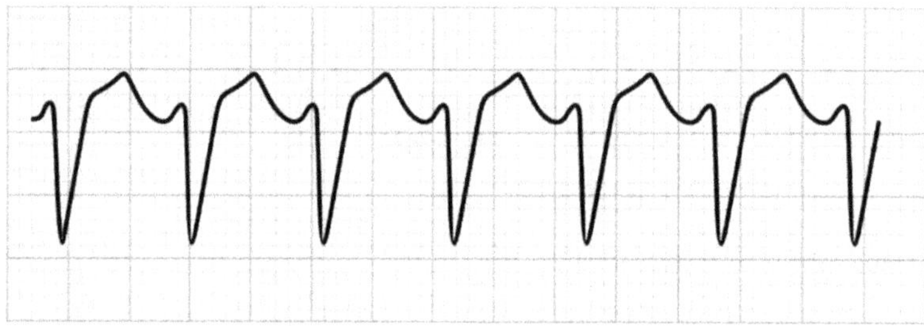

Treatment is as follows:

- With pulse: Synchronized cardioversion, adenosine
- No pulse: Same as ventricular fibrillation

Narrow Complex and Wide Complex Tachycardias

Tachycardias are classified as narrow complex or wide complex. Wide and narrow refer to the configuration of the QRS complex.

- **Wide complex tachycardia (WCT)**: About 80% of cases of WCT are caused by ventricular tachycardia. WCT originates at some point below the AV node and may be associated with palpitations, dyspnea, anxiety, diaphoresis, and cardiac arrest. Wide complex tachycardia is diagnosed with more than 3 consecutive beats at a heart rate >100 BPM and QRS duration ≥0.12 seconds.

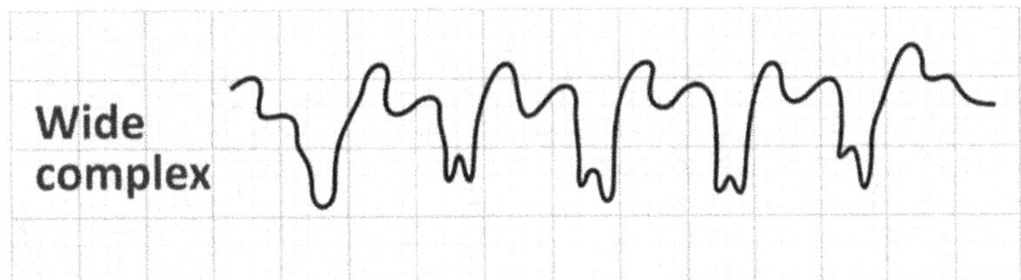

- **Narrow complex tachycardia (NCT)**: NCT is associated with palpitations, dyspnea, and peripheral edema. NCT is generally supraventricular in origin. Narrow complex tachycardia is diagnosed with ≥3 consecutive beats at heart rate of >100 BPM and QRS duration of <0.12 seconds.

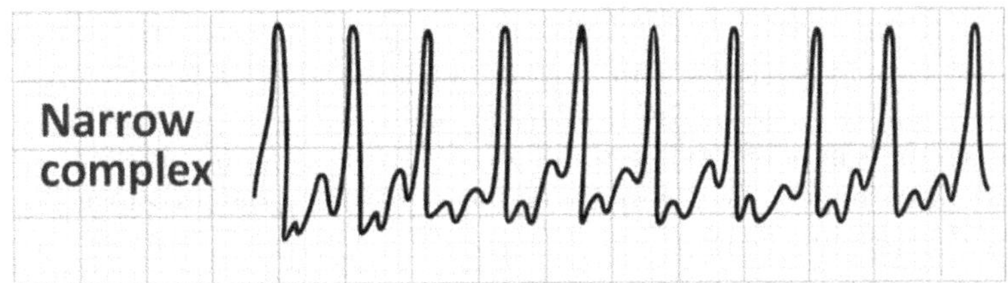

Ventricular Fibrillation

Ventricular fibrillation (VF) is a rapid, very irregular ventricular rate >300 beats per minute with no atrial activity observable on the ECG, caused by disorganized electrical activity in the ventricles. The QRS complex is not recognizable as ECG shows irregular undulations. The causes are the same as for ventricular tachycardia and asystole. VF is accompanied by lack of palpable pulse, audible pulse, and respirations and is immediately life threatening without defibrillation.

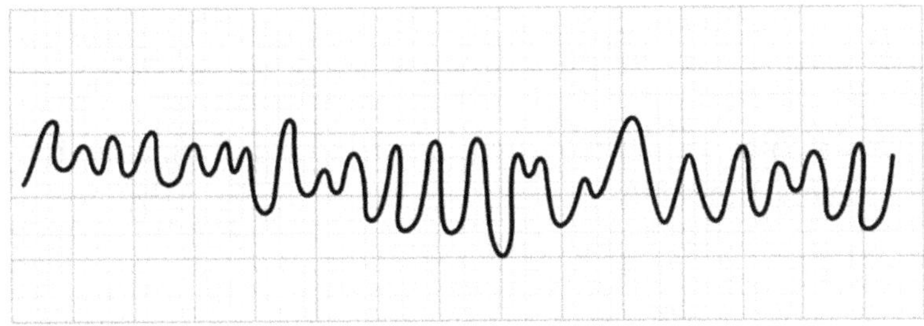

Treatment includes:

- Emergency defibrillation, the cause should be identified and treated
- Epinephrine 1 mg q 3-5minutes then amiodarone 300mg (2nd dose: 150mg) IV push

Review Video: EKG Interpretation: Ventricular Arrythmias
Visit mometrix.com/academy and enter code: 933152

Idioventricular Rhythm

Ventricular escape rhythm (idioventricular) occurs when the Purkinje fibers below the AV node create an impulse. This may occur if the sinus node fails to fire or if there is blockage at the AV node so that the impulse does not go through. Idioventricular rhythm is characterized by a regular ventricular rate of 20-40 BPM. Rates >40 BPM are called accelerated idioventricular rhythm. The P wave is missing and the QRS complex has a very bizarre and abnormal shape with duration of ≥0.12 seconds. The low ventricular rate may cause a decrease in cardiac output, often making the patient lose consciousness. In other patients, the idioventricular rhythm may not be associated with reduced cardiac output.

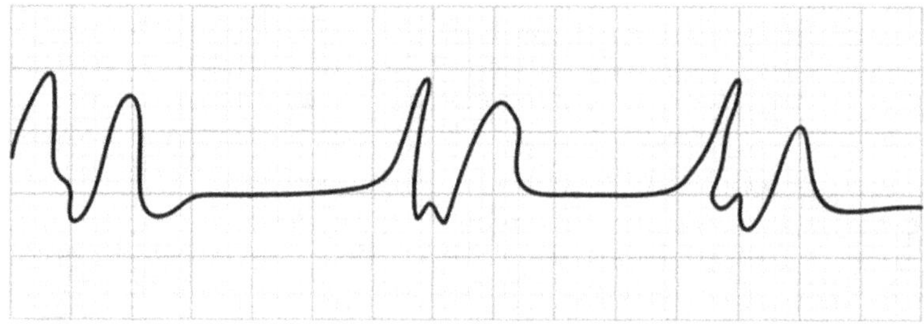

Ventricular Asystole

Ventricular asystole is the absence of audible heartbeat, palpable pulse, and respirations, a condition often referred to as "cardiac arrest." While the ECG may show some P waves initially, the QRS complex is absent although there may be an occasional QRS "escape beat" (agonal rhythm). Cardiopulmonary resuscitation is required with intubation for ventilation and establishment of an intravenous line for fluids. Without immediate treatment, the patient will suffer from severe hypoxia and brain death within minutes. Identifying the cause is critical for the patient's survival. Consider the "Hs & Ts": hypovolemia, hypoxia, hydrogen ions (acidosis), hypo/hyperkalemia, hypothermia, tension pneumothorax, tamponade (cardiac), toxins, and thrombosis (pulmonary or coronary). Even with immediate treatment, the prognosis is poor and ventricular asystole is often a sign of impending death.

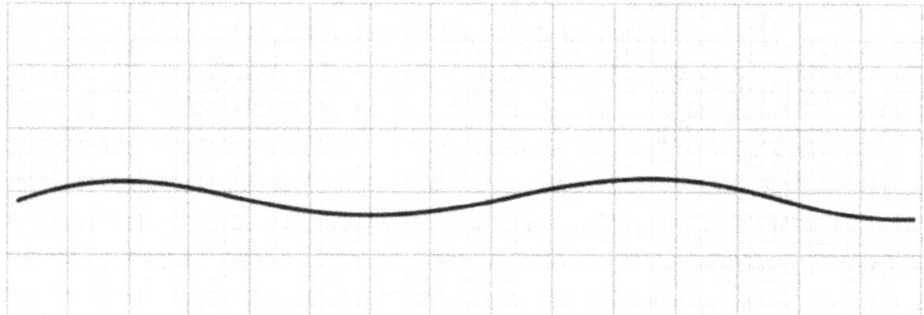

Treatment includes:

- CPR only; Asystole is not a shockable rhythm therefore defibrillation is not indicated
- Epinephrine 1 mg q 3-5 minutes

Sinus Pause

Sinus pause occurs when the sinus node fails to function properly to stimulate heart contractions, so there is a pause on the ECG recording that may persist for a few seconds to minutes, depending on the severity of the dysfunction. A prolonged pause may be difficult to differentiate from cardiac arrest. During the sinus pause, the P wave, QRS complex and PR and QRS intervals are all absent. P:QRS ratio is 1:1 and the rhythm is irregular. The pulse rate may vary widely, usually 60-100 BPM. Patients with frequent pauses may complain of dizziness or syncope. The patient may need to undergo an electrophysiology study and medication reconciliation to determine the cause. If measures such as decreasing medication are not effective, a pacemaker is usually indicated (if symptomatic).

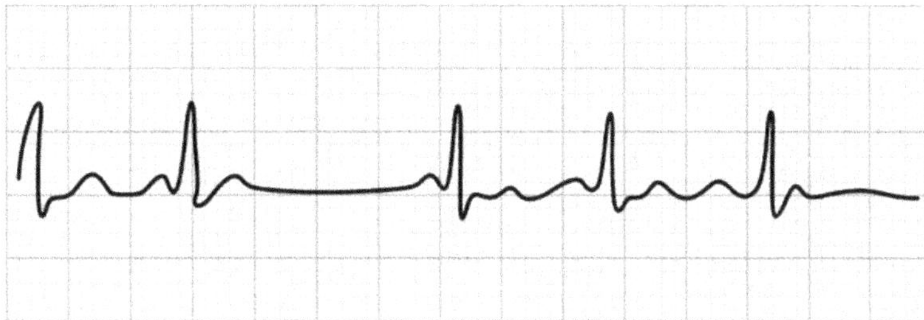

First-Degree AV Block

First-degree AV block occurs when the atrial impulses are conducted through the AV node to the ventricles at a rate that is slower than normal. While the P and QRS are usually normal, the PR interval is >0.20 seconds, and the P:QRS ratio is 1:1. A narrow QRS complex indicates a conduction abnormality only in the AV node, but a widened QRS indicates associated damage to the bundle branches as well. *Chronic* first-degree block may be caused by fibrosis/sclerosis of the conduction system related to coronary artery disease, valvular disease, cardiac myopathies and carries little morbidity, thus is often left untreated. *Acute* first-degree block, on the other hand, is of much more concern and may be related to digoxin toxicity, β-blockers, amiodarone, myocardial infarction, hyperkalemia, or edema related to valvular surgery.

Treatment: involves eliminating cause if possible, such as changing medications. Atropine 0.5-1.0 mg may be given IV if rate falls.

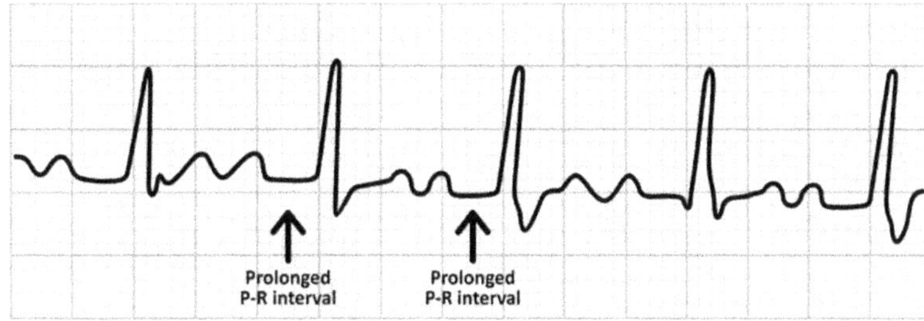

Second-Degree AV Block

Second-degree AV block occurs when some of the atrial beats are blocked. Second-degree AV block is further subdivided according to the patterns of block.

Type I

Mobitz type I block (Wenckebach) occurs when each atrial impulse in a group of beats is conducted at a lengthened interval until one fails to conduct (the PR interval progressively increases), so there are more P waves than QRS complexes, but the QRS complex is usually of normal shape and duration. The sinus node functions at a regular rate, so the P-P interval is regular, but the R-R interval usually shortens with each impulse. The P:QRS ratio varies, such as 3:2, 4:3, 5:4. This type of block by itself usually does not cause significant morbidity unless associated with an inferior wall myocardial infarction.

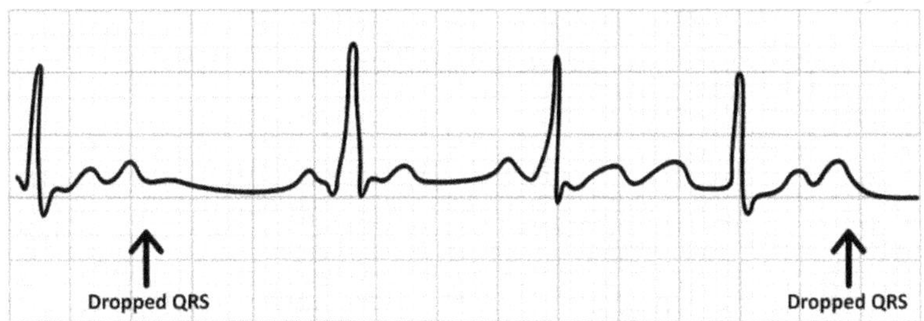

TYPE II

In Mobitz type II, only some of the atrial impulses are conducted unpredictably through the AV node to the ventricles, and the block always occurs below the AV node in the bundle of His, the bundle branches, or the Purkinje fibers. The PR intervals are the same if impulses are conducted, and the QRS complex is usually widened. The P:QRS ratio varies 2:1, 3:1, and 4:1. Type II block is more dangerous than Type I because it may progress to complete AV block and may produce Stokes-Adams syncope. Additionally, if the block is at the Purkinje fibers, there is no escape impulse. Usually, a transcutaneous cardiac pacemaker and defibrillator should be at the patient's bedside. **Symptoms** may include chest pain if the heart block is precipitated by myocarditis or myocardial ischemia.

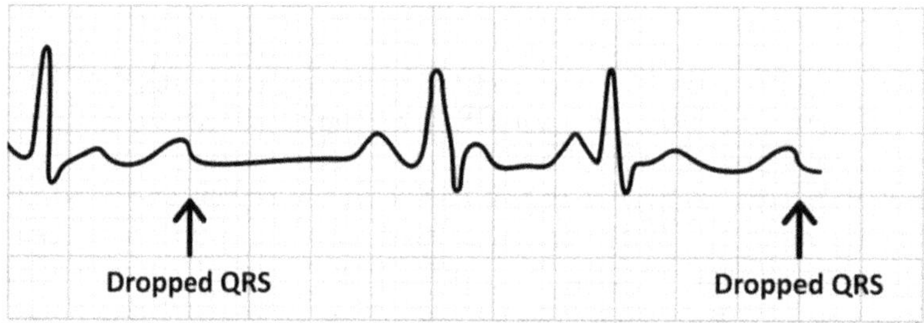

THIRD-DEGREE

With third-degree AV block, there are more P waves than QRS complexes, with no clear relationship between them. The atrial rate is 2-3 times the pulse rate, so the PR interval is irregular. If the SA node malfunctions, the AV node fires at a lower rate, and if the AV node malfunctions, the pacemaker site in the ventricles takes over at a bradycardic rate; thus, with complete AV block, the heart still contracts, but often ineffectually. With this type of block, the atrial P (sinus rhythm or atrial fibrillation) and the ventricular QRS (ventricular escape rhythm) are stimulated by different impulses, so there is AV dissociation.

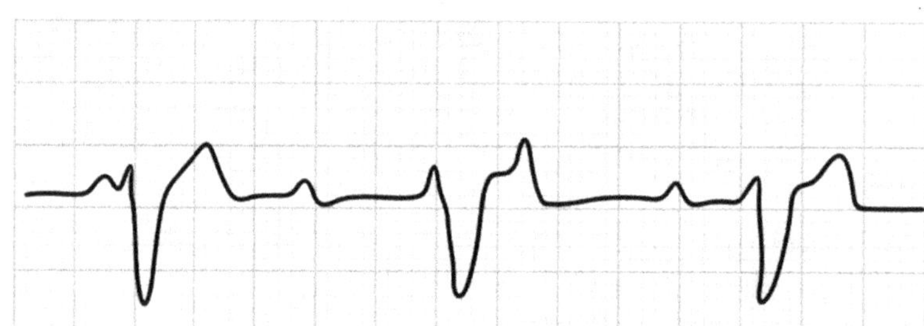

The heart may compensate at rest but can't keep pace with exertion. The resultant bradycardia may cause congestive heart failure, fainting, or even sudden death, and usually conduction abnormalities slowly worsen. **Symptoms** include dyspnea, chest pain, and hypotension, which are treated with IV atropine. Transcutaneous pacing may be needed. Complete persistent AV block normally requires implanted pacemakers, usually dual chamber.

> **Review Video: AV Heart Blocks**
> Visit mometrix.com/academy and enter code: 487004

BUNDLE BRANCH BLOCKS

A **right bundle branch block (RBBB)** occurs when conduction is blocked in the right bundle branch that carries impulses from the Bundle of His to the right ventricle. The impulse travels through the left ventricle instead, and then reaches the right ventricle, but this causes a slight delay in contraction of the right ventricle. A RBBB is characterized by normal P waves (as the right atrium still contracts appropriately), but the QRS complex is widened and notched (referred to as an "RSR pattern" that resembles the letter "M") in lead V1, which is a reflection of the asynchronous ventricular contraction. The PR interval is normal or prolonged, and the QRS interval is > 0.12 seconds. P:QRS ratio remains 1:1 with regular rhythms.

A **left bundle branch block (LBBB)** occurs when there is a delay in conduction between the left atrium and left ventricle. It is also characterized by normal or inverted P waves, but the QRS complex may be widened with a deep S wave and an interval of >0.12 seconds (in lead V1) that resembles a "W." The PR interval may be normal or prolonged. The P:QRS ratio is 1:1 and the rhythm is regular.

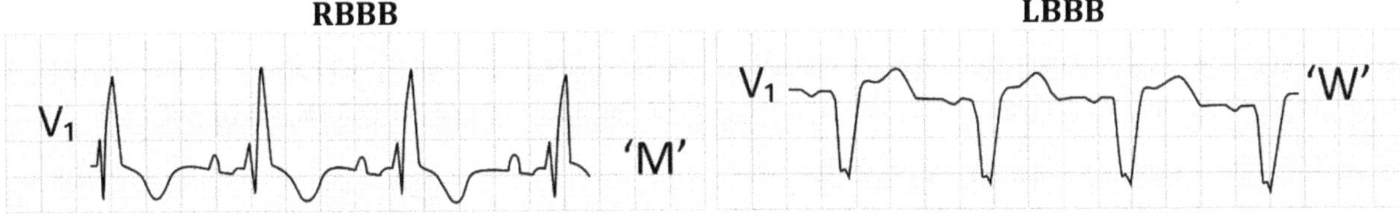

Heart Failure

Heart failure (formerly congestive heart failure) is a cardiac disease that includes disorders of contractions (systolic dysfunction) or filling (diastolic dysfunction) or both and may include pulmonary, peripheral, or systemic edema. The most common causes are coronary artery disease, systemic or pulmonary hypertension, cardiomyopathy, and valvular disorders. The incidence of chronic heart failure correlates with age. The 2 main types of HF are systolic and diastolic. HF is classified according to symptoms and prognosis:

- **Class I**: The patient is essentially asymptomatic during normal activities with no pulmonary congestion or peripheral hypotension. There is no restriction on activities, and prognosis is good.
- **Class II**: Symptoms appear with physical exertion but are usually absent at rest, resulting in some limitations of activities of daily living (ADLs). Slight pulmonary edema may be evident by basilar rales. Prognosis is good.
- **Class III**: Obvious limitations of ADLs and discomfort on any exertion. Prognosis is fair.
- **Class IV**: Symptoms at rest. Prognosis is poor.

Treatment may include:

- Careful monitoring of **fluid** balance and **weight** to determine changes in fluid retention
- Low sodium diet
- Restriction of activity
- **Medications** may include diuretics, vasodilators, or ACE inhibitors to decrease the heart's workload, digoxin may be given to increase contractibility
- **Anticoagulant therapy** if distended atria, enlarged ventricles, or atrial fibrillation to decrease the danger of thromboembolic

Review Video: Congestive Heart Failure
Visit mometrix.com/academy and enter code: 924118

Systolic Heart Failure

Systolic heart failure is the typical "left-sided" failure and reduces the amount of blood ejected from the ventricles during contraction (decreased ejection fraction). This stimulates the SNS to produce catecholamines to support the myocardium, which eventually causes down regulation, the destruction of beta and adrenergic receptor sites, and ultimately further myocardial damage. Because of reduced perfusion, the R-A-A pathway (renin, angiotensin I&II, aldosterone) is initiated by the kidneys, causing sodium and fluid retention. The end result of these processes is increased preload and afterload, thus increased workload on the ventricles. They begin to lose contractibility and blood begins to pool inside, stretching the myocardium (ventricular remodeling). The heart compensates by thickening the muscle (hypertrophy) without an adequate increase in capillary blood supply, leading to ischemia.

Symptoms: Activity intolerance, dyspnea/orthopnea (sleeping in a recliner is a classic symptom), cough (frothy sputum), edema, heart sounds S3 and S4, hepatomegaly, JVD, LOC changes, and tachycardia.

Treatment includes:

- Medication
- **Surgery**: Heart transplant (if a candidate)
- **Lifestyle modification**: Low-sodium diet, supplemental oxygen, daily weights (report >3 lb/day or 5 lb/week weight gain to physician)

Diastolic Heart Failure

Diastolic heart failure may be difficult to differentiate from systolic heart failure based on clinical symptoms, which are similar. With diastolic heart failure, the myocardium is unable to sufficiently relax to facilitate filling of the ventricles. This may be the end result of systolic heart failure as myocardial hypertrophy stiffens the muscles, and the causes are similar. Diastolic heart failure is more common in females >75. Typically, intra-cardiac pressures at rest are within normal range but increase markedly on exertion. Because the relaxation of the heart is delayed, the ventricles do not expand enough for the fill-volume, and the heart cannot increase stroke volume during exercise, so symptoms (dyspnea, fatigue, pulmonary edema) are often pronounced on exertion. Ejection fractions are usually >40-50% with increase in left ventricular end-diastolic pressure (LVEDP) and decrease in left ventricular end-diastolic volume (LVEDV).

The major goal with all types of heart failure is to prevent further damage and remodeling, prevent exacerbations, and improve the patient's long-term prognosis.

Acute Heart Failure

Acute decompensated heart failure occurs when the body cannot compensate for the heart's inability to provide adequate perfusion. Cardiac output is no longer sufficient to meet the metabolic demands of the body. Acute heart failure occurs suddenly and can be precipitated by dysrhythmias, illness, noncompliance with medications, acute ischemia, fluid overload or hypertensive crisis. Acute heart failure is most commonly related to left ventricular systolic or diastolic dysfunction. It requires immediate treatment to restore adequate perfusion and is often life-threatening.

Signs and symptoms: Dyspnea, cough, edema, ascites and elevated jugular venous pressure, fatigue, cool extremities, hypotension and altered mental status

Diagnostic testing: Chest X-ray, electrocardiogram, physical exam; labs—basic metabolic panel, BUN, creatinine, and B-natriuretic peptide (BNP)

Treatment: Rapid assessment and stabilization of the patient. The physical assessment should include a thorough evaluation of the patient's respiratory status and supplemental oxygen and potentially ventilator support may be necessary. Medications: Diuretics to decrease fluid volume; vasodilators to decrease pulmonary congestion. Cardiac monitoring, urine output monitoring, sodium restriction, and venous thromboembolism prophylaxis may also be utilized.

Acute Cardiac-Related Pulmonary Edema

Acute cardiac-related pulmonary edema occurs when heart failure results in fluid overload, leading to third-spacing of fluid into the interstitial spaces of the lungs. Pulmonary edema may result from MI, chronic HF, volume overload, ischemia, or mitral stenosis.

Symptoms include severe dyspnea, cough with blood-tinged frothy sputum, wheezing/rales/crackles on auscultation, cyanosis, and diaphoresis.

Diagnosis: Auscultation, chest x-ray, and echocardiogram.

Treatment includes:

- Sitting position with 100% oxygen by mask to achieve PO_2 >60%
- Non-invasive pressure support ventilation (BiPAP) or endotracheal intubation and mechanical ventilation
- Morphine sulfate 2-8 mg (IV for severe cases), repeated every 2-4 hours as needed–decreases pre-load and anxiety
- IV diuretics (furosemide ≥40 mg or bumetanide ≥1 mg) to provide venous dilation and diuresis
- Nitrates as a bolus with an infusion – decrease pre-load
- Inhaled β-adrenergic agonists or aminophylline for bronchospasm
- Digoxin IV for tachycardia
- ACE inhibitors, nitroprusside to reduce afterload

Hypertensive Crises

Hypertensive crises are marked elevations in blood pressure that can cause severe organ damage if left untreated. Hypertensive crises may be caused by endocrine/renal disorders (pheochromocytoma), dissection of an aortic aneurysm, pulmonary edema, subarachnoid hemorrhage, stroke, eclampsia, and medication noncompliance. There are 2 classifications:

- **Hypertensive emergency** occurs when acute hypertension, usually >220 systolic and 120 mmHg diastolic, must be treated immediately to lower blood pressure in order to prevent damage to vital organs.
- **Hypertensive urgency** occurs when acute hypertension must be treated within a few hours but the vital organs are not in immediate danger. Blood pressure is lowered more slowly to avoid hypotension, ischemia of vital organs, or failure of autoregulation.
    - 1/3 reduction in 6 hours
    - 1/3 reduction in next 24 hours
    - 1/3 reduction over days 2-4

Symptoms: Basilar HA, blurred vision, chest pain, N/V, SOB, seizures, ruddy pallor, and anxiety

Diagnostics: ECG, Chest x-ray, CBC, BMP, Urinalysis (+ blood and casts)

Treatment includes:

- Medications: Vasodilators (Cardene, Nitro, etc.) and diuretics
- Nursing Interventions: Raise HOB to 90°, supplemental O_2, frequent neuro checks, teach concerning medication compliance

Myocardial Conduction System Abnormalities

Prolonged QT Interval

The normal **QT interval** is 400-460 ms in females and 400-440 ms in males. QT interval value greater than 500 ms increases risk of cardiac abnormalities. If the QT interval extends greater than half the RR, it is prolonged. Long QT syndrome occurs when depolarization and repolarization is prolonged between beats and can result in torsades de points or VT. "R-on-T" phenomenon can trigger these dangerous arrhythmias and is a serious risk with long QT intervals, as the chance of a PVC (specifically the ventricular depolarization of the PVC) falling on the t-wave is what induces the arrhythmia. The longer the QT interval, the greater the chance of this phenomenon occurring. Long QT syndrome may be a genetic condition or may be acquired and associated with electrolyte imbalances, some medications (antidepressants, diuretics, antibiotics), and some conditions (anorexia nervosa). Continuous QT interval monitoring measures from the QRS complex (depolarization) to the end of the T wave (repolarization). Indications (AHA recommendations) include patients:

- Newly diagnosed with bradyarrhythmia
- Receiving anti-arrhythmic drugs or other drugs associated with torsade de pointes (a life-threatening dysrhythmia)
- Overdosing on agents or receiving antipsychotics or drugs that may cause arrhythmias
- With electrolyte imbalances (hypokalemia, hypomagnesemia) that may cause arrhythmias
- With acute neurological events, such as stroke

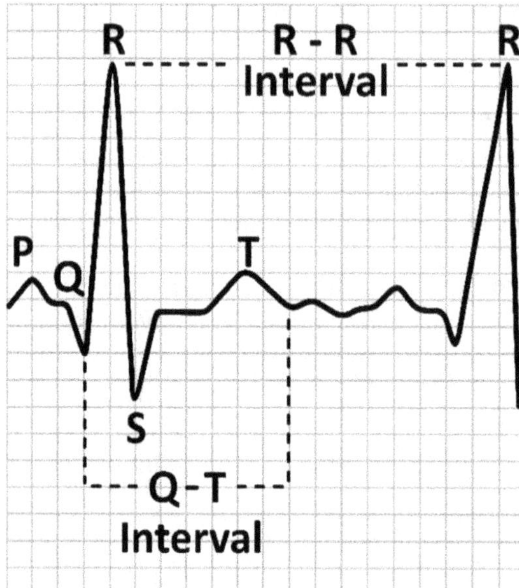

Wolff-Parkinson-White Syndrome

The Wolff-Parkinson-White syndrome (a preexcitation syndrome) is characterized by a short PR interval and a delta wave, which appears as a slurred upstroke into the QRS complex, so the PR interval is missing. The QRS complex is prolonged because of the delta wave. The rhythm is very irregular and the rate is often 250-300 bpm. The delta wave is produced because of premature depolarization of part of the ventricles. With preexcitation syndromes, electrical stimulation of the ventricles occurs through an accessory (in this case Kent's bundle) pathway while the impulse also travels through the AV node, and this can lead to rapid paroxysmal tachyarrhythmias (usually AV reentry tachycardia—AVRT). About 40% develop atrial fibrillation. Medications, such as amiodarone and sotalol may be used to slow conduction, but cardioversion may be necessary. WPW syndrome is most common in children and young adults.

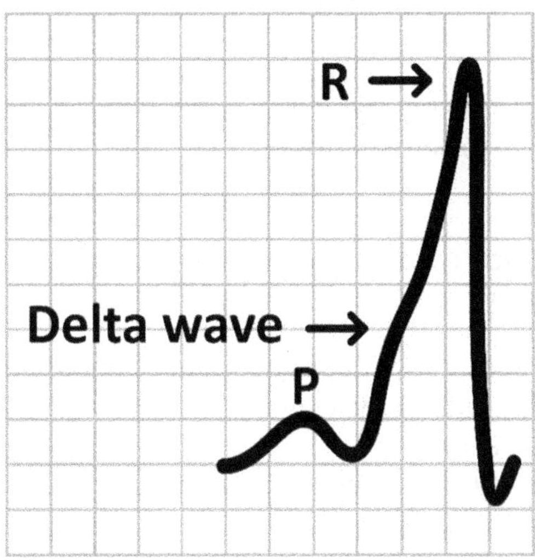

Endocarditis

Endocarditis is an infection of the lining of the heart that covers the heart valves and contains Purkinje fibers, known as the endocardium. Risk factors include being over 60 years of age, being male, IV drug use, and dental infections. Staphylococcal aureus is the most common cause of infective endocarditis. Etiology includes subacute bacterial endocarditis (often related to dental procedures), prosthetic valvular endocarditis (following valve replacement), and right sided endocarditis (often related to catheter infections and IV drug use). Organisms enter the bloodstream from portals of entry (surgery, catheterization, IV drug abuse) and migrate to the heart, growing on the endothelial tissue and forming vegetations (verrucae), collagen deposits, and platelet thrombi. With endocarditis, the valves frequently become deformed, but the pathogenic agents may also invade other tissues, such as the chordae tendineae. The lesions may invade adjacent tissue and break off, becoming emboli. The mitral valve is the most common valve affected, followed by aortic, tricuspid, and the pulmonary valve being the least often affected. Positive blood cultures, widened pulse pressures, ECG, murmurs, and vegetations seen on a transesophageal echocardiogram are used to make the diagnosis. After diagnosis is made, antibiotics are used for treatment, and when unsuccessful or when heart failure is present, valve repair may be warranted. Serious complications from endocarditis include emboli, sepsis, and heart failure. Untreated endocarditis is fatal.

Diagnosis and Treatment

Diagnosis of **endocarditis** is made on the basis of clinical presentation and diagnostic procedures that may include:

- **Blood cultures** should be done with 3 sets for both aerobic and anaerobic bacteria. Diagnosis is definitive if 2 cultures are positive, but a negative culture does not preclude bacterial endocarditis.
- **Echocardiogram** may identify vegetation on valves or increasing heart failure

- **ECG** may demonstrate prolonged PR interval
- **Anemia** (normochromic, normocytic)
- Elevated **white blood cell** count
- Elevated **erythrocyte sedimentation rate (ESR)** and **C-reactive protein (CRP)**

Treatment includes general management of symptoms and the following:

- **Antimicrobials** specific to the pathogenic organism, usually administered IV for 4 to 6 weeks
- **Surgical replacement** of aortic and/or mitral valves may be necessary (in 30% to 40% of cases) if there is no response to treatment and/or after infection is controlled if there are severe symptoms related to valve damage

Clinical Symptoms

Clinical symptoms of **endocarditis** usually relate to the response to infection, the underlying heart disease, emboli, or immunological response. Typical symptoms include:

- Slow onset with unexplained low-grade and often intermittent **fever**
- **Anorexia** and weight loss, difficulty feeding
- General **lassitude** and malaise
- **Splenomegaly** present in 60% of patients; **hepatomegaly** may also be present
- **Anemia** is present in almost all patients
- Sudden **aortic valve insufficiency** or mitral valve insufficiency
- **Cyanosis** with clubbing of fingers
- **Embolism** of other body organs (brain, liver, bones)
- **Congestive heart failure**
- **Dysrhythmias**
- New or change in **heart murmur**
- **Immunological responses**
- **Janeway lesions**: painless areas of hemorrhage on palms of hands and soles of feet
- **Splinter hemorrhages**: thin, brown-black lines on nails of fingers and toes
- **Petechiae**: pinpoint-sized hemorrhages on oral mucous membranes, as well as hands and trunk
- **Roth spots**: retinal hemorrhagic lesions caused by emboli on nerve fibers
- **Glomerulonephritis**: microscopic hematuria

Myocarditis

Myocarditis is inflammation of the cardiac myocardium (muscle tissue), usually triggered by a viral infection, such as the influenza virus, Coxsackie virus, and HIV. Myocarditis can also be caused by bacteria, fungi, or parasites, or an allergic response to medications. In some cases, it is also a complication of endocarditis. It may also be triggered by chemotherapy drugs and some antibiotics. Myocarditis can result in dilation of the heart, development of thrombi on the heart walls (known as mural thrombi), and infiltration of blood cells around the coronary vessels and between muscle fibers, causing further degeneration of the muscle tissue. The heart may become enlarged and weak, as the ability to pump blood is impaired, leading to congestive heart failure. Symptoms depend upon the extent of damage but may include fatigue, dyspnea, pressure and discomfort in chest or epigastric area, and palpitations.

Diagnosis and Treatment

Diagnosis of **myocarditis** depends upon the clinical picture, as there is no test specific for myocarditis, although a number of tests may be done to verify the clinical diagnosis:

- **Chest radiograph** may indicate cardiomegaly or pulmonary edema.
- **ECG** may show nonspecific changes.
- **Echocardiogram** may indicate cardiomegaly and demonstrate defects in functioning.
- **Cardiac catheterization** and **cardiac biopsy** will yield confirmation in 65% of cases, but not all of the heart muscle may be affected, so a negative finding does not rule out myocarditis.
- **Viral cultures** of nasopharynx and rectal may help to identify organism.
- **Viral titers** may increase as disease progresses.
- **Polymerase chain reaction** (PCR) of biopsy specimen may be most effective for diagnosis.

Treatment:

- As indicated for underlying cause (such as antibiotics)
- Restriction of activities
- Careful **monitoring** for heart failure and medical treatment as indicated (e.g., diuretics, digoxin)
- **Oxygen** as needed to maintain normal oxygen saturation
- **IV gamma globulin** for acute stage

Acute Pericarditis

Pericarditis is inflammation of the pericardial sac with or without increased pericardial fluid. It may be an isolated process or the effect of an underlying disease. If the underlying cause is autoimmune or related to malignancy of some sort, the patient usually presents with symptoms that relate to that disorder. However, most cases are related to a viral etiology, and therefore usually present with flu-like symptoms. Patients that have idiopathic pericarditis or viral pericarditis have a good prognosis with medication alone.

Signs/Symptoms: Sharp chest pain, worsened with inspiration and relieved by leaning forward or sitting up (most common symptom; "Mohammad's Sign"), pericardial effusion, respiratory distress, auscultated friction rub, ST elevation/PR depression (progresses to flattened T, inverted T, then return to normal); risk of pericardial effusion.

Diagnosis: Echocardiogram, ECG, pericardiocentesis or pericardial biopsy, cardiac enzymes (may be mildly elevated), WBC/ESR/CRP all elevated.

Treatment includes:

- **Medications**: NSAIDs for pain/inflammation, Colchicine 0.5 mg twice a day for six months is often prescribed in adjunct to NSAID therapy, as it decreases the incidence of recurrence
- **Surgery**: Pericardiectomy only in extreme cases

Mitral Stenosis

Mitral stenosis is a narrowing of the mitral valve that allows blood to flow from the left atrium to the left ventricle. Pressure in the left atrium increases to overcome resistance, resulting in enlargement of the left atrium and increased pressure in the pulmonary veins and capillaries of the lung (pulmonary hypertension). Mitral stenosis can be caused by infective endocarditis, calcifications, or tumors in the left atrium.

Signs/Symptoms: Exertional dyspnea, orthopnea/nocturnal dyspnea, right-sided heart failure, loud S_1 and S_2, and mid-diastolic murmur.

Diagnosis: Cardiac catheterization, chest x-ray, echocardiogram, ECG.

Treatment includes:

- **Medications**: Antiarrhythmic, anticoagulant, and antihypertensive medications
- **Surgical**: Open/closed commissurotomy, balloon valvuloplasty, and mitral valve replacement

Mitral Valve Insufficiency

Mitral valve insufficiency occurs when the mitral valve fails to close completely so that there is backflow into the left atrium from the left ventricle during systole, decreasing cardiac output. It may occur with mitral stenosis or independently. Mitral valve insufficiency can result from damage caused by rheumatic fever, myxomatous degeneration, infective endocarditis, collagen vascular disease (Marfan's syndrome), or cardiomyopathy/left heart failure. There are **3 phases** of the disease:

- **Acute:** May occur with rupture of a chordae tendineae or papillary muscle causing sudden left ventricular flooding and overload.
- **Chronic compensated:** Enlargement of the left atrium to decrease filling pressure, and hypertrophy of the left ventricle.
- **Chronic decompensated:** Left ventricle fails to compensate for the volume overload; ↓stroke volume & ↓ cardiac output.

Symptoms: Orthopnea/dyspnea, split S_2/S_3/S_4 heart sounds, systolic murmur, palpitations, right-sided heart failure, fatigue, angina (rare).

Diagnosis: Cardiac catheterization, chest x-ray, echocardiogram, ECG.

Treatment includes:

- **Medications**: Antiarrhythmic, anticoagulant, and antihypertensive medications.
- **Surgical**: Annuloplasty or valvuloplasty, and mitral valve replacement.

Aortic Stenosis

Aortic stenosis is a stricture (narrowing) of the aortic valve that controls the flow of blood from the left ventricle. This causes the left ventricular wall to thicken as it increases pressure to overcome the valvular resistance, increasing afterload and increasing the need for blood supply from the coronary arteries. This condition may result from a birth defect or childhood rheumatic fever, and tends to worsen over the years as the heart grows.

Symptoms: Angina, exercise intolerance, dyspnea, split S_1 and S_2, systolic murmur at base of carotids, hypotension on exertion, syncope, left-sided heart failure; sudden death can occur.

Diagnosis: Cardiac catheterization, chest x-ray, echocardiogram, ECG.

Treatment includes:

- **Medications**: Antiarrhythmic, anticoagulant, and antihypertensive medications
- **Surgical**: Balloon valvuloplasty, and aortic valve replacement

Pulmonic Stenosis

Pulmonic stenosis is a stricture of the pulmonary blood that controls the flow of blood from the right ventricle to the lungs, resulting in right ventricular hypertrophy as the pressure increases in the right ventricle and decreased pulmonary blood flow. The condition may be asymptomatic or symptoms may not be evident until adulthood, depending upon the severity of the defect. Pulmonic stenosis may be associated with a number of other heart defects.

Symptoms: May be asymptomatic; dyspnea on exertion, systolic heart murmur, right-sided heart failure.

Diagnosis: Cardiac catheterization, chest x-ray, echocardiogram, ECG.

Treatment includes:

- **Medications**: Antiarrhythmic, anticoagulant, and antihypertensive medications
- **Surgical**: Balloon valvuloplasty, valvotomy, valvectomy with or without transannular patch, and pulmonary valve replacement

Blunt Cardiac Trauma and Traumatic Injury to the Great Vessels

Blunt cardiac trauma most often occurs as the result of motor vehicle accidents, falls, or other blows to the chest. This can result in respiratory distress, rupture of the great vessels, and cardiac tamponade/increasing intrathoracic pressure. The right atrium and right ventricle are the most commonly injured because they are anterior to the rest of the heart. While not definitive, echocardiogram in conjunction with CPK MB levels is useful in predicting complications. Because diagnosis is challenging until complications appear, every patient with suspected blunt chest trauma should receive an ECG upon admission/STAT. If abnormalities are present, continuous cardiac monitoring should be done for 24-48 hours. Decreased cerebral perfusion/anoxia may result in severe agitation with combative behavior.

Traumatic injuries to the great vessels most commonly result from severe decelerating blunt force or penetrating injuries, with aortic trauma the most common. If the aorta is torn, it will result in almost instant death, but in some cases, there is an incomplete laceration to the intimal lining (innermost membrane) of the aorta, causing an aortic hematoma or bulging. This lining, the adventitia, is quite strong and often will contain the rupture long enough to allow surgical repair.

Diagnosis: Chest x-ray or CT; transesophageal echocardiogram to verify

Treatment: STAT surgical repair to avoid eventual rupture, during which other vessels are examined for clotting or internal injuries

Penetrating Cardiac Injuries

The incidence of **penetrating cardiac injuries** has been on the rise, primarily associated with gunshot injuries and stabbings. The extent of damage caused by a stab wound is often easier to assess than gunshot wounds, which may be multiple and often result in unpredictable and widespread damage not only to the heart but other structures. Mortality rates are very high in the first hour after a penetrating cardiac injury, so it is imperative that the patient be taken immediately to a trauma center rather than attempts be made to stabilize the person at the site. NEVER attempt to remove the object in the field/without a physician present.

The primary complications:

- **Exsanguination** is frequently related to gunshot wounds, and prognosis is very poor. This may lead to hemothorax and hemorrhagic shock.
- **Cardiac tamponade** is more common with knife wounds, but prognosis is fairly good with surgical repair. Cardiac tamponade often presents with three classic symptoms, known as Beck's triad that should be quickly recognized: muffled heart sounds, low arterial blood pressure, and jugular vein distention.
- **Pneumothorax**: Deviated trachea, increasing SVR, tachypnea and anxiety all may indicate tension pneumothorax, which is a medical emergency. It is treated by emergent insertion of a chest tube or needle aspiration of trapped air. Open wounds can be emergently dressed with a three-sided dressing until a chest tube can be inserted to create a "flutter valve" effect and allow trapped air to escape.

Nursing Considerations: Management includes controlling bleeding, giving fluids and vasopressors for blood pressure, preparing patient for surgery, and monitoring for the above-mentioned complications.

Congenital Heart Defects Seen in Adulthood

Congenital heart defects are often identified in infancy or early childhood; however, diagnosis may be delayed until adulthood due to the lack of signs and symptoms. Atrial septal and ventricular septal defects are common congenital anomalies that can present at any age. An atrial septal defect occurs when part of the atrial septum does not form properly, leaving a hole in the septum. A ventricular septal defect results from a hole in the septum separating the ventricles. Patent ductus arteriosus, coarctation of the aorta and Ebstein's anomaly are other types of congenital defects that are less commonly diagnosed in adulthood.

Signs and symptoms: Murmurs, cyanosis, clubbing of the fingernails, shortness of breath, fatigue, syncope, palpitations, and edema. Heart failure and endocarditis may also occur.

Diagnosis: Physical assessment, EKG, Chest X-ray, transesophageal echocardiogram, CT, and MRI.

Treatment: Treatment options depend on the size and location of the defect. Most commonly the anomaly will be corrected by open surgical repair; however percutaneous intervention may be an option in some patients.

Peripheral Arterial and Venous Insufficiency

Characteristics of **peripheral arterial and venous insufficiency** are listed below:

- **Arterial Insufficiency:**
    - **Pain:** Ranging from intermittent claudication to severe and constant shooting pain
    - **Pulses:** Weak or absent
    - **Skin:** Rubor on dependency, but pallor of foot on elevation; pale, shiny, and cool skin with loss of hair on toes and foot; nails thick and ridged
    - **Ulcers:** Painful, deep, circular, often necrotic ulcers on toe tips, toe webs, heels, or other pressure areas
    - **Edema:** Minimal

- **Venous Insufficiency:**
  - **Pain:** Aching/cramping
  - **Pulses:** Strong/present
  - **Skin:** Brownish discoloration around ankles and anterior tibial area
  - **Ulcers:** Varying degrees of pain in superficial, irregular ulcers on medial or lateral malleolus and sometimes the anterior tibial area
  - **Edema:** Moderate to severe

ACUTE PERIPHERAL VASCULAR INSUFFICIENCY

Acute peripheral arterial insufficiency can occur when sudden occlusion of a blood vessel causes tissue ischemia, ultimately leading to cellular death and necrosis. This can occur as a result of traumatic injury or non-traumatic events such as arterial thrombus or embolism, vasospasm, or severe swelling (compartment syndrome). Risk factors for acute peripheral arterial insufficiency include age, tobacco use, diabetes mellitus, hyperlipidemia, and hypertension.

- **Signs and symptoms**: Classic 6 P's: Pain (extreme, unrelieved by narcotics), pallor, pulselessness, poikilothermia (the inability to regulate body temperature; extremity is room temperature), paresthesias, and paralysis (late).
- **Diagnosis**: Ultrasound, angiography, and physical exam; labs—coagulation studies, CBC, BMP, creatinine phosphokinase.
- **Treatment**: Re-establishment of blood flow to the affected area.
- **Arterial thrombus or embolism**: Mechanical thrombolysis may be performed to remove the clot occluding the vessel.
  - *Trauma*: Surgical repair of the severed/injured vessels. Fasciotomy may be performed in the event of compartment syndrome to relieve pressure.
  - *Other treatment options:* Hyperbaric oxygen therapy, anti-platelet therapy for the prevention of arterial thrombosis and anti-coagulant therapy for the prevention of venous thrombosis.

ACUTE VENOUS THROMBOEMBOLISM

Acute venous thromboembolism (VTE) is a condition that includes both deep vein thrombosis (DVT) and pulmonary emboli (PE). VTE may be precipitated by invasive procedures, lack of mobility, and inflammation, so it is a common complication in critical care units. **Virchow's triad** comprises common risk factors: blood stasis, injury to endothelium, and hypercoagulability. Some patients may be initially asymptomatic, but **symptoms** may include:

- Aching or throbbing pain
- Positive Homan's sign (pain in calf when foot is dorsiflexed)
- Unilateral erythema and edema
- Dilation of vessels
- Cyanosis

Diagnosis: ultrasound and/or D-dimer test, which tests the serum for cross-linked fibrin derivatives. A CT scan, pulmonary angiogram, and ventilation-perfusion lung scan may be used to diagnose pulmonary emboli.

Treatment includes:

- Medications: IV heparin, tPA, or other anticoagulation; analgesia for pain
- Surgical: May have to surgically remove clot if large
- Bed rest, elevation of affected limb; stockings on ambulation

Prevention: Use of sequential compression devices (SCDs) or foot pumps, routine anticoagulant use for those at highest risk (Heparin SQ), early and frequent ambulation

Respiratory Pathophysiology

Acute Pulmonary Embolism

Acute pulmonary embolism occurs when a pulmonary artery or arteriole is blocked, cutting off blood supply to the pulmonary vessels and subsequent oxygenation of the blood. While most pulmonary emboli are from thrombus formation, they can also be caused by air, fat, or septic embolus (from bacterial invasion of a thrombus). Common originating sites for thrombus formation are the deep veins in the legs, the pelvic veins, and the right atrium. Causes include stasis related to damage to endothelial wall and changes in blood coagulation factors. Atrial fibrillation poses a serious risk because blood pools in the right atrium, forming clots that travel directly through the right ventricle to the lungs. The obstruction of the artery/arteriole causes an increase in alveolar dead space in which there is ventilation but impairment of gas exchange because of the ventilation/perfusion mismatching or intrapulmonary shunting. This results in hypoxia, hypercapnia, and the release of mediators that cause bronchoconstriction. If more than 50% of the vascular bed becomes excluded, pulmonary hypertension occurs.

Symptoms and Diagnosis

Clinical manifestations of **acute pulmonary embolism** (PE) vary according to the size of the embolus and the area of occlusion.

Symptoms include:

- Dyspnea with tachypnea
- Cyanosis; may turn grey or blue from nipple line up (massive PE)
- Anxiety and restlessness, feeling of doom
- Chest pain, tachycardia, may progress to arrhythmias (PEA)
- Fever
- Rales
- Cough (sometimes with hemoptysis)
- Hemodynamic instability

Diagnostic tests are as follows:

- ABG analysis may show hypoxemia (decreased PaO_2), hypocarbia (decreased $PaCO_2$) and respiratory alkalosis (increased pH).
- D-dimer will show elevation with PE but is not definitively diagnostic without a CT scan.
- ECG may show sinus tachycardia or other abnormalities.
- Echocardiogram can show emboli in the central arteries and can assess the hemodynamic status of the right side of the heart.
- Spiral CT may provide definitive diagnosis.

- V/Q scintigraphy can confirm diagnosis.
- Pulmonary angiograms also can confirm diagnosis.

Medical Management

Medical management of **pulmonary embolism** starts with preventive measures for those at risk, including leg exercises, elastic compression stockings, and anticoagulation therapy. Most pulmonary emboli present as medical emergencies, so the immediate task is to stabilize the patient. **Medical management** may include:

- **Oxygen** to relieve hypoxemia
- **Intravenous infusions:** Dobutamine (Dobutrex®) or dopamine (Intropin®) to relieve hypotension
- **Cardiac monitoring** for dysrhythmias and issues due to right sided heart failure
- **Medications** as indicated: digitalis glycosides, diuretic, and antiarrhythmics
- Intubation and mechanical ventilation may be required
- **Analgesics** (such as morphine sulfate) or sedation to relieve anxiety
- **Anticoagulants** to prevent recurrence (although it will not dissolve clots already present), including heparin and warfarin (Coumadin®)
- **Placement of percutaneous venous filter** (Greenfield) in the inferior vena cava to prevent further emboli from entering the lungs, if anticoagulation therapy is contraindicated
- **Thrombolytic therapy,** recombinant tissue-type plasminogen activator (rt-PA) or streptokinase, for those severely compromised, but these treatments have limited success and pose the danger of bleeding

Traumatic Asphyxia

Asphyxia may relate to a number of different injuries:

- **Traumatic asphyxia** most commonly involves a crush injury of the thorax and possibly traumatic injuries to multiple organs. Crush injuries are characterized by petechiae in the area of compression although tight-fitting clothing, such as a woman's bra, may prevent petechiae from forming.
- **Manual strangulation** may involve crush injuries to the throat, such as hyoid fracture. Often the face appears cyanotic while the rest of the body does not. Petechiae may be present on the face as well. Bruising may be noted about the throat.
- **Ligature strangulation** is similar to manual although throat markings are different, with an indented area surrounding the neck.
- **Hanging** produces a V-shaped marking on the throat and does not encircle the neck.
- **Choking** obstructs the airway. (May require bronchoscopy to remove foreign object).

In all cases, immediate establishment of airway, breathing, and circulation (ABCs) takes precedence. Surgical intervention may be needed for traumatic crush injuries.

Submersion Asphyxia

Submersion asphyxiation (near-drowning) can cause profound damage to the central nervous system, pulmonary dysfunction related to aspiration, cardiac hypoxia with life-threatening arrhythmias, fluid and electrolyte imbalances, and multi-organ damage, so treatment can be complex. Hypothermia related to near drowning has some protective affect because blood is shunted to the brain and heart.

Treatment includes:

- Immediate establishment of airway, breathing and circulation (ABCs)
- NG tube and gastric decompression to reduce risk of aspiration
- Neurological evaluation
- Pulmonary management includes monitoring for ≥72 hours for respiratory deterioration. Ventilation may need positive-end expiratory pressure (PEEP), but this poses danger to cardiac output and can cause barotrauma, so use should be limited.
- In patients that are symptomatic but do not yet need intubation, use supplemental oxygen to keep $SpO_2 > 94\%$
- Monitoring of cardiac output and function
- Neurological care to reduce cerebral edema and increased intracranial pressure and prevent secondary injury
- Rewarming if necessary (0.5-1.0 °C/hr)

Acute Lung Injury and Acute Respiratory Distress Syndrome

Acute lung injury (ALI) comprises a syndrome of respiratory distress culminating in **acute respiratory distress syndrome (ARDS).** ARDS is a dangerous, potentially fatal respiratory condition, always caused by an illness or injury to the lungs. Lung injury causes fluid to leak into the spaces between the alveoli and capillaries, increasing pressure on the alveoli, causing them to collapse. With increased fluid accumulation in the lungs, the ability of the lungs to move oxygen into the blood is decreased, resulting in hypoxemia. Lung injury also causes a release of cytokines, a type of inflammatory protein, which then brings neutrophils to the lung. These proteins and cells leak into nearby blood vessels and cause inflammation throughout the body. This immune response, in combination with low levels of blood oxygen, can lead to organ failure. Symptoms are characterized by respiratory distress within 72 hours of surgery or a serious injury to a person with otherwise normal lungs and no cardiac disorder. Untreated, the condition results in respiratory failure, MODS, and a mortality rate of 5-30%.

Symptoms include:

- Refractory hypoxemia (hypoxemia not responding to increasing levels of oxygen)
- Crackling rales/wheezing in lungs
- Decrease in pulmonary compliance which results in increased tachypnea with expiratory grunting
- Cyanosis/skin mottling
- Hypotension and tachycardia
- Symptoms associated with volume overload are missing (3rd heart sound or JVD)
- Respiratory alkalosis initially but, as the disease progresses, replaced with hypercarbia and respiratory acidosis
- Normal X-ray initially but then diffuse infiltrates in both lungs, while the heart and vessels appear normal

Management

The management of **acute respiratory distress syndrome (ARDS)** involves providing adequate gas exchange and preventing further damage to the lung from forced ventilation.

Treatment includes:

- Mechanical ventilation to maintain oxygenation and ventilation
- Corticosteroids (may increase mortality rates in some patient populations, though this is the most commonly given treatment), nitrous oxide, inhaled surfactant, and anti-inflammatory medications
- Treatment of the underlying condition is the only proven treatment, especially identifying and treating an infection with appropriate antibiotics, as sepsis is most common etiology for ARDS, but prophylactic antibiotics are not indicated.
- Conservative fluid management is indicated to reduce days on the ventilator, but does not reduce overall mortality.

Pharmacologic preventive care: Enoxaparin 40 mg subcutaneously QD, sucralfate 1 g NGT four times daily or omeprazole 40 mg IV QD, and enteral nutrition support within 24 hours of ICU admission or intubation.

Ventilation Management

Ventilation management in ARDS consists of the following:

- O_2 therapy by nasal prongs, cannula, or mask may be sufficient in very mild cases to maintain oxygen saturation above 90%. Oxygen should be administered at 100% because of the mismatch between ventilation (V) and perfusion (Q), which can result in hypoxia on position change.
- ARDS oxygenation goal is PaO_2 55-80 mmHg or SpO_2 88-95%.
- Endotracheal intubation may be needed if SpO_2 falls or CO_2 levels rise.
- The ARDS Network recommends low tidal volumes (6 mL/kg) and higher PEEP (12 cmH_2O or more).
- The low tidal volume ventilation described above is referred to as lung protective ventilation, and it has been shown to reduce mortality in patients with ARDS.
- Placing patients with severe ARDS in prone position for 18-24 hours per day with chest and pelvis supported and abdomen unsupported allows the diaphragm to move posteriorly, increasing functional residual capacity (FRC) in many patients.

Acute Respiratory Failure

Cardinal Signs

The **cardinal signs of respiratory failure** include:

- Tachypnea
- Tachycardia
- Anxiety and restlessness
- Diaphoresis

Symptoms may vary according to the cause. An obstruction may cause more obvious respiratory symptoms than other disorders.

- Early signs may include changes in the depth and pattern of respirations with flaring nares, sternal retractions, expiratory grunting, wheezing, and extended expiration as the body tries to compensate for hypoxemia and increasing levels of carbon dioxide.
- Cyanosis may be evident.

- Central nervous depression, with alterations in consciousness occurs with decreased perfusion to the brain.
- As the hypoxemia worsens, cardiac arrhythmias, including bradycardia, may occur with either hypotension or hypertension.
- Dyspnea becomes more pronounced with depressed respirations.
- Eventually stupor, coma, and death can occur if the condition is not reversed.

Hypoxemic and Hypercapnic Respiratory Failure

Hypoxemic respiratory failure occurs suddenly when gaseous exchange of oxygen for carbon dioxide cannot keep up with demand for oxygen or production of carbon dioxide:

- PaO_2 <60 mmHg
- $PaCO_2$ >40 mmHg
- Arterial pH <7.35

Hypoxemic respiratory failure can be the result of low inhaled oxygen, as at high elevations or with smoke inhalation. The following ventilatory mechanisms may be involved:

- Alveolar hypotension
- Ventilation-perfusion mismatch (the most common cause)
- Intrapulmonary shunts
- Diffusion impairment

Hypercapnic respiratory failure results from an increase in $PaCO_2$ >45-50 mmHg associated with respiratory acidosis and may include:

- Reduction in minute ventilation, total volume of gas ventilated in one minute (often related to neurological, muscle, or chest wall disorders, drug overdoses, or obstruction of upper airway.
- Increased dead space with wasted ventilation (related to lung disease or disorders of chest wall, such as scoliosis)
- Increased production of CO_2 (usually related to infection, burns, or other causes of hypermetabolism)
- Oxygen saturation may be normal or below normal.

Underlying Causes

There are a number of underlying causes for **respiratory failure:**

- **Airway obstruction:** Obstruction may result from an inhaled object or from an underlying disease process, such as cystic fibrosis, asthma, pulmonary edema, or infection.
- **Inadequate respirations:** This is a common cause among adults, especially related to obesity and sleep apnea. It may also be induced by an overdose of sedation medications such as opioids.
- **Neuromuscular disorders:** Those disorders that interfere with the neuromuscular functioning of the lungs or the chest wall, such as muscular dystrophy or spinal cord injuries can prevent adequate ventilation.
- **Pulmonary abnormalities:** Those abnormalities of the lung tissue, found in pulmonary fibrosis, burns, ARDS, and reactions to drugs, can lead to failure.
- **Chest wall abnormalities:** Disorders that impact lung parenchyma, such as severe scoliosis or chest wounds can interfere with lung functioning.

Nursing interventions to help prevent respiratory issues:

- Turn, position, and ambulate the patient.
- Have the patient cough and breathe deeply.
- Use vibration and percussion treatments.
- Hydrate the patient to help hydrate the airway secretions, and incentive spirometry.

Management

Respiratory failure must be **treated** immediately before severe hypoxemia causes irreversible damage to vital organs.

- **Identifying and treating** the underlying cause should be done immediately because emergency medications or surgery may be indicated. Medical treatments will vary widely depending upon the cause; for example, cardiopulmonary structural defects may require surgical repair, pulmonary edema may require diuresis, inhaled objects may require surgical removal, and infections may require aggressive antimicrobials.
- **Intravenous lines/central lines** are inserted for testing, fluids and medications.
- **Oxygen therapy** should be initiated to attempt to reverse hypoxemia; however, if refractory hypoxemia occurs, then oxygen therapy alone will not suffice. Oxygen levels must be titrated carefully.
- **Intubation and mechanical ventilation** are frequently required to maintain adequate ventilation and oxygenation. Positive end expiratory pressure (PEEP) may be necessary with refractory hypoxemia and collapsed alveoli.
- **Respiratory status** must be monitored constantly, including arterial blood gases and vital signs.

Pneumonia

Pneumonia is inflammation of the lung parenchyma, filling the alveoli with exudate. It is common throughout childhood and adulthood. Pneumonia may be a primary disease or may occur secondary to another infection or disease, such as lung cancer. Pneumonia may be caused by bacteria, viruses, parasites, or fungi. Common causes for community-acquired pneumonia (CAP) include:

- *Streptococcus pneumoniae*
- *Legionella* species
- *Haemophilus influenzae*
- *Staphylococcus aureus*
- *Mycoplasma pneumoniae*
- Viruses

Pneumonia may also be caused by chemical damage. Pneumonia is characterized by **location**:

- **Lobar** involves one or more lobes of the lungs. If lobes in both lungs are affected, it is referred to as bilateral or double pneumonia.
- **Bronchial/lobular** involves the terminal bronchioles, and exudate can involve the adjacent lobules. Usually the pneumonia occurs in scattered patches throughout the lungs.
- **Interstitial** involves primarily the interstitium and alveoli where white blood cells and plasma fill the alveoli, generating inflammation and creating fibrotic tissue as the alveoli are destroyed.

Hospital-Acquired Pneumonia

Hospital-acquired pneumonia (HAP) is defined as pneumonia that did not appear to be present on admission that occurs at least 48 hours after admission to a hospital. **Healthcare-associated pneumonia (HCAP)** is defined as pneumonia that occurs in a patient within 90 days of being hospitalized for 2 or more days at an acute care hospital or LTAC. **Ventilator-associated pneumonia (VAP)** is one type of hospital acquired pneumonia that a patient acquires more than 48 hours after having an ETT placed. The most common way that the patient is infected is via aspiration of bacteria that is colonized in the upper respiratory tract. It is estimated that close to 75% of patients that are critically ill will be colonized with multidrug resistant bacteria within 48 hours of entering an ICU. Aspiration occurs at a rate of about 45% in patients with no health problems and the rate is much higher in those with HAP, HCAP, and VAP. The frequency of patients developing these types of pneumonia is increasing, with those at highest risk being those with immunosuppression, septic shock, currently hospitalized for more than five days, and those who have had antibiotics for another infection within the previous three months. These types of pneumonia should be considered if a patient already hospitalized has purulent sputum or a change in respiratory status such as deoxygenating, in combination with a worsening or new chest x-ray infiltrate.

Treatment includes:

- Antibiotic therapy.
- Using appropriate isolation and precautions with infected patients.
- Preventive measures include maintaining ventilated patients in 30° upright positions, frequent oral care for vent patients, and changing ventilator circuits as per protocol.

Antibiotic treatment options for HAP, HCAP, and VAP should take into account many factors, including culture data (when available), patient's comorbidities, flora in the unit, any recent antibiotics by the patient, and whether the patient is at high risk for having multidrug resistant bacteria. As most critical care patients are at high risk, due to factors such as being in an ICU setting, ventilators, and comorbidities, antibiotic recommendations to follow are for coverage for patients with risk factors for multidrug resistant bacteria.

One of the following:

- Ceftazidime 2 g every 8 hours IV **OR**
- Cefepime 2 g every 8 hours IV **OR**
- Imipenem 500 mg every 6 hours IV **OR**
- Piperacillin-tazobactam 4.5 g every 6 hours IV

AND:

- Ciprofloxacin 400 mg every 8 hours IV **OR**
- Levaquin 750 mg every 24 hours IV

Aspiration Pneumonitis/Pneumonia

Aspiration pneumonitis/pneumonia may occur as the result of any type of aspiration, including foreign objects. The aspirated material creates an inflammatory response, with the irritated mucous membrane at high risk for bacterial infection secondary to the aspiration, causing pneumonia. Gastric contents and oropharyngeal bacteria are commonly aspirated. Gastric contents can cause a severe chemical pneumonitis with hypoxemia, especially if the pH is <2.5. Acidic food particles can cause severe reactions. With acidic damage, bronchospasm and atelectasis occur rapidly with tracheal irritation, bronchitis, and alveolar damage with interstitial edema and hemorrhage. Intrapulmonary shunting and V/Q mismatch may occur. Pulmonary artery pressure increases. Non-acidic liquids and food particles are less damaging, and symptoms may clear within 4 hours of liquid aspiration or granuloma may form about food particles in 1-5 days. Depending upon the type of aspiration, pneumonitis may clear within a week, ARDS or pneumonia may develop, or progressive acute respiratory failure may lead to death.

There are a number of risk factors that can lead to **aspiration pneumonitis/pneumonia:**

- Altered level of consciousness related to illness or sedation
- Depression of gag, swallowing reflex
- Intubation or feeding tubes
- Ileus or gastric distention
- Gastrointestinal disorders, such as gastroesophageal reflux disorders (GERD)

Diagnosis is based on clinical findings, ABGs showing hypoxemia, infiltrates observed on x-ray, and ↑ WBC if infection is present.

Symptoms: Similar to other pneumonias:

- Cough often with copious sputum
- Respiratory distress, dyspnea
- Cyanosis
- Tachycardia
- Hypotension

Treatment includes:

- Suctioning as needed to clear upper airway
- Supplemental oxygen
- Antibiotic therapy as indicated after 48 hours if symptoms not resolving
- Symptomatic respiratory support

Foreign Body Aspiration

Foreign body aspiration can cause obstruction of the pharynx, larynx or trachea, leading to acute dyspnea or asphyxiation, and the object may also be drawn distally into the bronchial tree. With adults, most foreign bodies migrate more readily down the right bronchus. Food is the most frequently aspirated, but other small objects, such as coins or needles, may also be aspirated. Sometimes the object causes swelling, ulceration, and general inflammation that hampers removal.

Symptoms include:

- **Initial***:* Severe coughing, gagging, sternal retraction, wheezing. Objects in the larynx may cause inability to breathe or speak and lead to respiratory arrest. Objects in the bronchus cause cough, dyspnea, and wheezing.
- **Delayed***:* Hours, days, or weeks later, an undetected aspirant may cause an infection distal to the aspirated material. Symptoms depend on the area and extent of the infection.

Treatment includes:

- Removal with laryngoscopy or bronchoscopy (rigid is often better than flexible)
- Antibiotic therapy for secondary infection
- Surgical bronchotomy (rarely required)
- Symptomatic support

Chronic Bronchitis

Chronic bronchitis is a pulmonary airway disease characterized by severe cough with sputum production for at least 3 months a year for at least 2 consecutive years. Irritation of the airways (often from smoke or pollutants) causes an inflammatory response, increasing the number of mucus-secreting glands and goblet cells while ciliary function decreases so that the extra mucus plugs the airways. Additionally, the bronchial walls thicken, alveoli near the inflamed bronchioles become fibrotic, and alveolar macrophages cannot function properly, increasing susceptibility to infections. Chronic bronchitis is most common in those >45 years old and occurs twice as frequently in females as males.

Symptoms include:

- Persistent cough with increasing sputum
- Dyspnea
- Frequent respiratory infections

Treatment includes:

- Bronchodilators
- Long term continuous oxygen therapy or supplemental oxygen during exercise
- Pulmonary rehabilitation to improve exercise and breathing
- Antibiotics during infections
- Corticosteroids for acute episodes

Emphysema

Emphysema, the primary component of COPD, is characterized by abnormal distention of air spaces at the ends of the terminal bronchioles, with destruction of alveolar walls so that there is less and less gaseous exchange and increasing dead space with resultant hypoxemia, hypercapnia, and respiratory acidosis. The capillary bed is damaged as well, altering pulmonary blood flow and raising pressure in the right atrium (cor pulmonale) and pulmonary artery, leading to cardiac failure. Complications include respiratory insufficiency and failure. There are 2 primary types of emphysema (and both forms may be present):

- **Centrilobular** (the most common form) involves the central portion of the respiratory lobule, sparing distal alveoli, and usually affects the upper lobes. Typical symptoms include abnormal ventilation-perfusion ratios, hypoxemia, hypercapnia, and polycythemia with right-sided heart failure.
- **Panlobular** involves enlargement of all air spaces, including the bronchiole, alveolar duct, and alveoli, but there is minimal inflammatory disease. Typical symptoms include hyperextended rigid barrel chest, marked dyspnea, weight loss, and active expiration.

COPD

Stages

Functional dyspnea, body mass index (BMI), and spirometry are used to assess the **stages of chronic obstructive pulmonary disease (COPD)**. Spirometry measures used are the ratio of forced expiratory volume in the first second of expiration (FEV_1) after full inhalation to total forced vital capacity (FVC). Normal lung function decreases after age 35; so normal values are adjusted for height, weight, gender, and age:

- **Stage I** (mild): Minimal dyspnea with or without cough and sputum. FEV_1 is ≥80% of predicted rate and FEV_1:FVC <70%.
- **Stage 2** (moderate): Moderate to severe chronic exertional dyspnea with or without cough and sputum. FEV_1 is 50-80% of predicted rate and FEV_1:FVC <70%.
- **Stage 3** (severe): Same as stage 2 but with repeated episodes with increased exertional dyspnea and condition impacting quality of life. FEV_1 is 30-50% of predicted rate and FEV_1:FVC <70%.
- **Stage 4** (very severe): Severe dyspnea and life-threatening episodes that severely impact quality of life. FEV_1 is 30% of predicted rate or <50% with chronic respiratory failure and FEV_1:FVC <70%.

Management

COPD is not reversible, so management aims at slowing its progression, relieving symptoms, and improving quality of life:

- Smoking cessation is the primary means to slow progression and may require smoking cessation support in the form of classes or medications, such as Zyban®, nicotine patches or gum, clonidine, or nortriptyline.
- Bronchodilators, such as albuterol (Ventolin®) and salmeterol (Serevent), relieve bronchospasm and airway obstruction.
- Corticosteroids, both inhaled (Pulmicort®, Vanceril®) and oral (prednisone) may improve symptoms but are used mostly for associated asthma.
- Oxygen therapy may be long term continuous or used during exertion.
- Bullectomy (for bullous emphysema) to remove bullae (enlarged airspaces that do not ventilate).
- Lung volume reduction surgery may be done if involvement in the lung is limited; however, mortality rates are high.
- Lung transplantation is a definitive high-risk option.
- Pulmonary rehabilitation includes breathing exercises, muscle training, activity pacing, and modification of activities.

Chronic Ventilatory Failure

Chronic ventilatory failure occurs when alveolar ventilation fails to increase in response to increasing levels of carbon dioxide, usually associated with chronic pulmonary diseases, such as asthma and COPD, drug overdoses, or diseases that impair respiratory effort, such as Guillain-Barré and myasthenia gravis. Normally, the ventilatory system is able to maintain PCO_2 and pH levels within narrow limits, even though PO_2 levels may be more variable, but with ventilatory failure, the body is not able to compensate for the resultant hypercapnia and pH falls, resulting in respiratory acidosis. Symptoms include increasing dyspnea with tachypnea, gasping respirations, and use of accessory muscles. Patients may become confused as hypercapnia causes increased intracranial pressure. If pH is <7.2, cardiac arrhythmias, hyperkalemia, and hypotension can occur as pulmonary arteries constrict and the peripheral vascular system dilates. Diagnosis is per symptoms, ABGs consistent with respiratory acidosis (PCO_2 >50 and pH <7.35), pulse oximetry, and chest x-ray. Treatment can include non-invasive PPV (BiPAP), endotracheal mechanical ventilation, corticosteroids, and bronchodilators.

Chronic Asthma

The 3 primary symptoms of **chronic asthma** are cough, wheezing, and dyspnea. In cough-variant asthma, a severe cough may be the only symptom, at least initially. Chronic asthma is characterized by recurring bronchospasm and inflammation of the airways resulting in airway obstruction. Asthma affects the bronchi and not the alveoli. While no longer considered part of COPD because airway obstruction is not constant and is responsive to treatment, over time fibrotic changes in the airways can result in permanent obstruction, especially if asthma is not treated adequately. Symptoms of chronic asthma include nighttime coughing, exertional dyspnea, tightness in the chest, and cough. Acute exacerbations may occur, sometimes related to triggers, such as allergies, resulting in increased dyspnea, wheezing, cough, tachycardia, bronchospasm, and rhonchi. Treatment of chronic asthma includes chest hygiene, identification and avoidance of triggers, prompt treatment of infections, bronchodilators, long-acting β-2 agonists, and inhaled glucocorticoids.

Status Asthmaticus

Pathophysiology

Status asthmaticus is a severe acute attack of asthma that does not respond to conventional therapy. An acute attack of asthma is precipitated by some stimulus, such as an antigen that triggers an allergic response, resulting in an inflammatory cascade that causes edema of the mucous membranes (swollen airway), contraction of smooth muscles (bronchospasm), increased mucus production (cough and obstruction), and hyperinflation of airways (decreased ventilation and shunting). Mast cells and T lymphocytes produce cytokines, which continue the inflammatory response through increased blood flow coupled with vasoconstriction and bronchoconstriction, resulting in fluid leakage from the vasculature. Epithelial cells and cilia are destroyed, exposing nerves and causing hypersensitivity. Sympathetic nervous system receptors in the bronchi stimulate bronchodilation.

Clinical Symptoms

The person with **status asthmaticus** will often present in acute distress, non-responsive to inhaled bronchodilators. Symptoms include:

- Signs of airway obstruction
- Sternal and intercostal retractions
- Tachypnea and dyspnea with increasing cyanosis
- Forced prolonged expirations
- Cardiac decompensation with increased left ventricular afterload and increased pulmonary edema resulting from alveolar-capillary permeability. Hypoxia may trigger an increase in pulmonary vascular resistance with increased right ventricular afterload.
- Pulsus paradoxus (decreased pulse on inspiration and increased on expiration) with extra beats on inspiration detected through auscultation but not detected radially. Blood pressure normally decreases slightly during inspiration, but this response is exaggerated. Pulsus paradoxus indicates increasing severity of asthma.
- Hypoxemia (with impending respiratory failure)

- Hypocapnia followed by hypercapnia (with impending respiratory failure)
- Metabolic acidosis

Indications for Mechanical Ventilation for Status Asthmaticus

Mechanical ventilation (MV) for status asthmaticus should be avoided, if possible, because of the danger of increased bronchospasm as well as barotrauma and decreased circulation. However, there are some absolute indications for the use of intubation and ventilation and a number of other indications that are evaluated on an individual basis.

The following are **absolute indications for MV:**

- Cardiac and/or pulmonary arrest
- Markedly depressed mental status (obtundation)
- Severe hypoxia and/or apnea

The following are **relative indications for MV:**

- Exhaustion/muscle fatigue from exertion of breathing
- Sharply diminished breath sounds and no audible wheezing
- Pulse paradoxus >20-40 mmHg; absent = imminent respiratory arrest
- PaO_2 <70 mmHg on 100% oxygen
- Dysphonia
- Central cyanosis
- Increased hypercapnia
- Metabolic/respiratory acidosis: pH <7.20

In this patient population, ventilator goal is to minimize airway pressures while oxygenating the patient. Vent settings include: low tidal volume (6-8 mL/kg), low respiratory rate (10-14 respirations/minute), and high inspiratory flow rate (80-100 L/min).

Air Leak Syndromes

Air leak syndromes may result in significant respiratory distress. Leaks may occur spontaneously or secondary to some type of trauma (accidental, mechanical, iatrogenic) or disease. As pressure increases inside the alveoli, the alveolar wall pulls away from the perivascular sheath and subsequent alveolar rupture allows air to follow the perivascular planes and flow into adjacent areas. There are two categories:

- **Pneumothorax:**
    - Air in the pleural space causes a lung to collapse.
- **Barotrauma/volutrauma** with air in the interstitial space (usually resolve over time):
    - Pneumoperitoneum is air in the peritoneal area, including the abdomen and occasionally the scrotal sac of male infants.
    - Pneumomediastinum is air in the mediastinal area between the lungs.
    - Pneumopericardium is air in the pericardial sac that surrounds the heart.
    - Subcutaneous emphysema is air in the subcutaneous tissue planes of the chest wall.
    - Pulmonary interstitial emphysema (PIE) is air trapped in the interstitium between the alveoli.

Pneumothorax

Pneumothorax occurs when there is a leak of air into the pleural space, resulting in complete or partial collapse of a lung.

Symptoms: Vary widely depending on the cause and degree of the pneumothorax and whether or not there is an underlying disease. Symptoms include acute pleuritic pain (95%), usually on the affected side, and decreased breath sounds. In a *tension pneumothorax,* symptoms include tracheal deviation and hemodynamic compromise.

Diagnosis: Clinical findings; radiograph: 6-foot upright posterior-anterior; ultrasound may detect traumatic pneumothorax.

Treatment: Chest-tube thoracostomy with underwater seal drainage is the most common treatment for all types of pneumothorax.

- Tension pneumothorax: Immediate needle decompression and chest tube thoracostomy
- Small pneumothorax, patient stable: Oxygen administration and observation for 3-6 hours. If no increase is shown on repeat x-ray, patient may be discharged with another x-ray in 24 hours.
- Primary spontaneous pneumothorax: Catheter aspiration or chest tube thoracostomy

Pleural Effusion and Empyema

Pleural effusion is the accumulation of fluid in the pleural space, usually secondary to other disease processes, such as heart failure, TB, neoplasms, nephrotic syndrome, and viral respiratory infections. The fluid may be serous, bloody, or purulent (empyema) and transudative or exudative. Signs and symptoms depend on underlying condition but includes dyspnea, from mild to severe. Tracheal deviation away from affected side may be evident. Diagnosis includes chest x-ray, lateral decubitus x-ray, CT, thoracentesis, and pleural biopsy. Treatment includes treating underlying cause, thoracentesis to remove fluid, insertion of chest tube, pleurodesis, or pleurectomy or pleuroperitoneal shunt (primarily with malignancy).

Empyema is a pleural effusion in which the collection of pleural fluid is thick and purulent, usually as a result of bacterial pneumonia or penetrating chest trauma. Empyema may also occur as a complication of thoracentesis or thoracic surgery. Signs and symptoms include acute illness with fever, chills, pain, cough, and dyspnea. Diagnosis is per chest CT and thoracentesis with culture and sensitivity. Treatment includes antibiotics and drainage of pleural space per needle aspiration, tube thoracostomy, or open chest drainage with thoracotomy.

Pulmonary Fibrosis

Pulmonary fibrosis is a progressive disease of the lungs in which scarring of the tissue causes the lining of the lungs to thicken. This thickening prevents adequate oxygen exchange from occurring. The cause of pulmonary fibrosis is unknown, however environmental toxins such as asbestos, infections, smoking and occupational exposure to wood or metal dust may be contributing factors. The disease is more prevalent in males and the average age at the time of diagnosis is between 40 and 70. There may also be a genetic predisposition in the development of pulmonary fibrosis. The median survival for patients diagnosed with pulmonary fibrosis is less than five years.

Signs and symptoms: Shortness of breath, dry cough, fatigue, weight loss, and clubbing of the finger tips and nails.

Diagnosis: Physical assessment, chest x-ray and/or computed tomography, pulmonary function tests, arterial blood gases and lung biopsy.

Treatment: There is no cure for pulmonary fibrosis and treatment options are minimal. Anti-inflammatory medications such as corticosteroids may be used for symptom management as well as supplemental oxygen therapy. Lung transplantation may be an option for some patients based on age and advancement of disease. Some patients may be eligible for participation in a clinical trial, as there are research efforts focused on treatment options to halt the progression of the disease.

Pulmonary Hypertension and Pulmonary Arterial Hypertension

Pulmonary arterial hypertension (PAH) is a progressive disease of the pulmonary arteries that can severely compromise cardiovascular patients. It may involve multiple processes. Usually the pulmonary vasculature adjusts easily to accommodate blood volume from the right ventricle. If there is increased blood flow, the low resistance causes vasodilation and vice versa. However, sometimes the pulmonary vascular bed is damaged or obstructed, and this can impair the ability to handle changing volumes of blood. In that case, an increase in flow will increase the pulmonary arterial pressure, increasing pulmonary vascular resistance (PVR). This in turn, increases pressure on the right ventricle (RV) with increased RV workload and eventually causes RV hypertrophy with displacement of the intraventricular septum and tricuspid regurgitation (cor pulmonale). Over time, this leads to right heart failure and death. Pulmonary hypertension is usually diagnosed by right-sided heart catheterization and is indicated by systolic pulmonary artery pressure >30 mmHg and mean pulmonary artery pressure >25 mmHg. Non-invasive testing may include echocardiogram to look for cardiac changes.

Types

Pulmonary hypertension or pulmonary arterial hypertension (PAH) may be classified as primary (idiopathic) or secondary.

- **Primary (idiopathic) PAH** may result from changes in immune responses, pulmonary emboli, sickle cell disease, collagen diseases, Raynaud's, and the use of contraceptives. The cause may be unknown or genetic.
- **Secondary PAH** may result from pulmonary vasoconstriction brought on by hypoxemia related to COPD, sleep-disordered breathing, kyphoscoliosis, obesity, smoke inhalation, altitude sickness, interstitial pneumonia, and neuromuscular disorders. It may also be caused by a decrease in pulmonary vascular bed of 50-75%, which may result from pulmonary emboli, vasculitis, tumor emboli, and interstitial lung disease, such as sarcoidosis. Primary cardiac disease, such as congenital defects in infants, and acquired disorders, such as rheumatic valve disease, mitral stenosis, and left ventricular failure may also contribute to PAH.

Treatment Options for PAH

Medical treatment for **pulmonary arterial hypertension (PAH)** aims to identify and treat any underlying cardiac or pulmonary disease, control symptoms, and prevent complications:

- **Oxygen therapy** may be needed, especially supplemental oxygen during exercise.
- **Calcium channel blockers** may provide vasodilation for some patients.
- **Pulmonary vascular dilators**, such as IV epoprostenol (Flolan®) and subcutaneous treprostinil sodium (Remodulin®) and oral bosentan (Tracleer®) help to control symptoms and prolong life.

- **Anticoagulants**, such as warfarin (Coumadin®) are an important part of therapy because of recurrent pulmonary emboli. Studies have shown that anticoagulation increases survival rates.
- **Diuretics**, such as furosemide (Lasix®) may be needed to relieve edema and restrict fluids, especially with right ventricular hypertrophy.

In some patients who cannot be managed adequately through medical treatment, a heart-lung transplant may be considered as the only effective treatment for long-term survival.

Management of Pulmonary and Thoracic Trauma

Pulmonary Hemorrhage

Pulmonary hemorrhage is an acute life-threatening injury that often results in death prior to arrival at the hospital; however, those presenting with traumatic pulmonary hemorrhage, as from a blunt or penetrating injury, require immediate surgical repair. Even with immediate surgery, survival after serious injury to a major pulmonary vessel is rare. It is important that a large bore IV be immediately inserted and fluid replacement begun while blood is typed and cross matched. The patient should be evaluated for shock and treatment, including colloid solutions, crystalloids, or blood, provided as indicated. Pulmonary hemorrhage may result in hemothorax. In some cases, pneumothorax may also be present, resulting in mediastinal shift that increases the difficulty of identifying and repairing the bleeding vessel. If the patient is stabilized, computed tomography may provide accurate diagnosis to isolate the area of hemorrhage.

Tracheal Perforation/Injury

Tracheal perforation/injury may result from external injury, such as from trauma from a vehicle accident or from an assault, such as a gunshot or knife wound, or in some cases a laceration as a complication of percutaneous dilation tracheostomy (PDT) or other endotracheal tubes. In some cases, an inhaled foreign object may become lodged in the trachea and eventually erode the tissue. If the injury is severe, respiratory failure may cause death in a very short period of time, so rapid diagnosis and treatment is critical.

Symptoms include:

- Severe respiratory distress
- Hemoptysis
- Strider with progressive dysphonia
- Pneumothorax, pneumomediastinum
- Subcutaneous emphysema from air leaking from the pleural space into the tissues of the chest wall, neck, face, and even into the upper extremities

Treatment includes:

- Intubation and non-surgical healing for small lacerations
- Surgical repair for larger wounds or severe respiratory distress

Pulmonary Contusion

Pulmonary contusion is the result of direct force to the lung, resulting in parenchymal injury, bleeding, and edema that impact the capillary-alveoli juncture, resulting in intrapulmonary shunting as the alveoli and interstitium fill with fluid. Parenchymal injury reduces compliance and impairs ventilation. Diagnosis may be more difficult if other injuries, such as fractured ribs or pneumothorax, are also present because they may all contribute to respiratory distress. CT scans provide the best diagnostic tool.

Symptoms vary widely depending upon the degree of injury:

- Mild dyspnea
- Severe progressive dyspnea
- Hemoptysis
- Acute respiratory failure

Treatment varies according to the injury:

- Close monitoring of arterial blood gases and respiratory status
- Supplemental oxygen
- Intubation and mechanical ventilation with positive-end expiratory pressure (PEEP) for more severe respiratory distress
- Fluid management and diuretics to control pulmonary edema
- Respiratory physiotherapy to clear secretions

Fractured Ribs

Fractured ribs are usually the result of severe trauma, such as blunt force from a motor vehicle accident or physical abuse. Underlying injuries should be expected according to the area of fractures:

- Upper 2 ribs: Injuries to trachea, bronchi, or great vessels
- Right-sided ≥ rib 8: Trauma to liver
- Left-sided ≥ rib 8: Trauma to spleen

Pain, often localized or experienced on respirations or compression of chest way may be the primary symptom of rib fractures, resulting in shallow breathing that can lead to atelectasis or pneumonia.

Diagnosis: Chest x-ray or CT scan.

Treatment is primarily supportive as rib fractures usually heal in about 6 weeks: however, preventing pulmonary complications (pneumothorax, hemothorax) often necessitates adequate pain control. Underlying injuries are treated according to the type and degree of injury:

- Supplemental oxygen
- Analgesia may include NSAIDs, intercostal nerve blocks, and narcotics
- Pulmonary physiotherapy
- Rib belts
- Surgical fixation (ORIF) only in those requiring thoracotomy for underlying injuries
- Splinting

Flail Chest

Flail chest is a more common injury in adults and older teens than children. It occurs when at least 3 adjacent ribs are fractured, both anteriorly and posteriorly, so that they float free of the rib cage. There may be variations, such as the sternum floating with ribs fractured on both sides. Flail chest results in a failure of the chest wall to support changes in intrathoracic pressure so that paradoxical respirations occur with the flail area contracting on inspiration and expanding on expiration. The lungs are not able to expand properly, decreasing ventilation, but the degree of respiratory distress may relate to injury to underlying structures more than the flail chest alone. **Treatment**:

- Initial stabilization with tape, one side only, don't wrap chest
- Give analgesia for pain relief
- Respiratory physiotherapy is done to prevent atelectasis
- Mechanical ventilation is usually not indicated unless needed for underlying injuries
- Surgical fixation is usually done only in those who require thoracotomy for underlying injuries

HEMOTHORAX

Hemothorax occurs with bleeding into the pleural space, usually from major vascular injury such as tears in intercostal vessels, lacerations of great vessels, or trauma to lung parenchyma. A small bleed may be self-limiting and seal, but a tear in a large vessel can result in massive bleeding, followed quickly by hypovolemic shock. The pressure from the blood may result in the inability of the lung to ventilate and a mediastinal shift. Often a hemothorax occurs with a pneumothorax, especially in severe chest trauma. Further symptoms include severe respiratory distress, decreased breath sounds, and dullness on auscultation.

Treatment includes placement of a chest tube to drain the hemothorax, but with large volumes, the pressure may be preventing exsanguination, which can occur abruptly as the blood drains and the pressure is reduced, so a large bore intravenous line should be in place before placement of the chest tube and typed and cross-matched blood immediately available. Autotransfusion may be used, but it is contraindicated if the wound is older than three hours and has the possibility of bowel/stomach contamination, liver failure, and malignancy. Thoracotomy may be indicated after chest tube insertion if there is still hemodynamic instability, tension hemothorax, more than 1500 mL blood initially on insertion, or bleeding continues at a rate of >300 mL/hr.

Neurological Pathophysiology

ENCEPHALOPATHIES

HYPERTENSIVE ENCEPHALOPATHY WITH CEREBRAL EDEMA

Hypertensive encephalopathy can occur as part of a hypertensive crisis. With chronic hypertension, the brain adapts to higher pressures to regulate blood flow, but in a hypertensive crisis, autoregulation of the blood-brain barrier is overwhelmed and the capillaries leak fluid into the tissue and vasodilation takes place with resultant cerebral edema. Damage to arterioles occurs, causing increasing neurological deficits and papilledema. Hypertensive encephalopathy is relatively rare, but carries a high mortality rate and is most common in middle-aged males with long-standing hypertension. **Symptoms** usually develop over 1-2 days and include:

- Non-specific neurological deficits, such as weakness and visual abnormalities
- Alterations in mental status, including confusion
- Headache, often constant
- Nausea and vomiting
- Seizures
- Coma

Treatment for Hypertensive Encephalopathy with Cerebral Edema

Hypertensive encephalopathy with cerebral edema requires prompt treatment in order to prevent neurological damage.

Treatment includes identifying and treating the underlying causes for the hypertensive crisis and taking steps to lower the blood pressure:

- **Nitroprusside sodium (Nitropress®)** is usually used initially to lower BP. However, caution must be used not to lower the blood pressure too quickly, as this can lead to cerebral ischemia.
- **Positioning** of the patient to prevent obstruction of venous return from the head
- **Monitoring blood gas** and maintaining $PaCO_2$ at 33-37 mmHg to facilitate vasoconstriction of cerebral arteries
- **Preventing hyperthermia** with antipyretics and cooling devices
- **BP monitoring** and maintenance
- **Seizure control** with phenobarbital and/or phenytoin
- **Lidocaine** through endotracheal tube or intravenously prior to nasotracheal suctioning
- **Diuretics**, such as osmotic agents (mannitol) and loop diuretics (furosemide) to control fluid volume
- **Controlling metabolic demand** by measures to increase pain control and reduce stimulation
- **Barbiturates** (pentobarbital, thiopental) in high doses may be used if other treatments fail to decrease intracranial pressure

Hypoxic Encephalopathy

Cerebral hypoxia (hypoxic encephalopathy) occurs when the oxygen supply to the brain is decreased. If hypoxia is mild, the brain compensates by increasing cerebral blood flow, but it can only double in volume and cannot compensate for severe hypoxic conditions. Hypoxia may be the result of insufficient oxygen in the environment, inadequate exchange at the alveolar level of the lungs, or inadequate circulation to the brain. Brain cells may begin dying within 5 minutes if deprived of adequate oxygenation, so any condition or trauma that interferes with oxygenation can result in brain damage:

- Near-drowning
- Asphyxia
- Cardiac arrest
- High altitude sickness
- Carbon monoxide
- Diseases that interfere with respiration, such as myasthenia gravis and amyotrophic lateral sclerosis
- Anesthesia complications

Symptoms include increasing neurological deficits, depending upon the degree and area of damage, with changes in mentation that range from confusion to coma. Prompt identification of the cause and increase in perfusion to the brain is critical for survival.

Metabolic Encephalopathy

Metabolic encephalopathy (hepatic encephalopathy) is damage to the brain resulting from a disturbance in metabolism, primarily hepatic failure to remove toxins from the blood. There may be impairment in cerebral blood flow, cerebral edema, or increased intracranial pressure. It can occur as the result of the ingestion of drugs or toxins which can have a direct toxic effect on neurons, but it can also occur with liver disease, especially when stressed by co-morbidities, such as hemorrhage, hypoxemia, surgery, trauma, renal failure with dialysis, or electrolyte imbalances.

Symptoms may vary:

- Irritability and agitation
- Alterations in consciousness
- Dysphonia
- Lack of coordination, spasticity
- Seizures are common and may be the presenting symptom
- Disorientation progressing to coma

Prompt diagnosis is important because the condition may be reversible if underlying causes are identified and treated before permanent neuronal damage occurs.

Treatment varies according to the underlying cause.

Infectious Encephalopathy

Infectious encephalopathy is an encompassing term describing encephalopathies caused by a wide range of bacteria, viruses, or prions. Common to all infections are altered brain function that results in alterations in consciousness and personality, cognitive impairment, and lethargy. A wide range of neurological symptoms may occur: myoclonus, seizures, dysphagia, and dysphonia, neuromuscular impairment with muscle atrophy and tremors or spasticity. **Treatment** depends on the underlying cause and response to treatment. Prion infections are not treatable, but bacterial infections may respond to antibiotic therapy, and viral infections may be self-limiting. HIV-related encephalopathy results from opportunistic infections as immune responses decrease, usually indicated by CD4 counts <50. Aggressive antiretroviral treatment and treatment of the infection may reverse symptoms if permanent damage has not occurred for HIV-related encephalopathy. Treatment for other infectious encephalopathies varies according to the type of infection and underlying causes.

Cerebral Aneurysms

Cerebral aneurysms, the weakening and dilation of a cerebral artery, are usually congenital (90%) while the remaining (10%) result from direct trauma or infection. Aneurysms are usually 2-7 mm in size and occur in the Circle of Willis at the base of the brain. A rupturing aneurysm may decrease perfusion as well as increasing pressure on surrounding brain tissue. Cerebral aneurysms are classified as follows:

- **Berry/saccular:** The most common congenital type occurs at a bifurcation and grows from the base on a stem, usually at the Circle of Willis.
- **Fusiform**: Large and irregular (>2.5 cm) and rarely ruptures but causes increased intracranial pressure. Usually involves the internal carotid or vertebrobasilar artery.
- **Mycotic**: Rare type that occurs secondary to bacterial infection and aseptic emboli.
- **Dissecting**: Wall is torn apart and blood enters layers. This may occur during angiography or secondary to trauma or disease.
- **Traumatic Charcot-Bouchard (pseudoaneurysm):** Small lesion resulting from chronic hypertension.

Arteriovenous Malformation

Arteriovenous malformation (AVM) is a congenital abnormality within the brain consisting of a tangle of dilated arteries and veins without a capillary bed. AVMs can occur anywhere in the brain and may cause no significant problems. Usually the AVM is "fed" by one or more cerebral arteries, which enlarge over time, shunting more blood through the AVM. The veins also enlarge in response to increased arterial blood flow because of the lack of a capillary bridge between the two. Because vein walls are thinner and lack the muscle layer of an artery, the veins tend to rupture as the AVM becomes larger, causing a subarachnoid hemorrhage. Chronic ischemia that may be related to the AVM can result in cerebral atrophy. Sometimes small leaks, usually accompanied by headache and nausea and vomiting, may occur before rupture. AVMs may cause a wide range of neurological symptoms, including changes in mentation, dizziness, sensory abnormalities, confusion, increasing ICP, and dementia.

Treatment includes:

- Supportive management of symptoms
- Surgical repair or focused irradiation (definitive treatments)

Intracranial/Intraventricular Hemorrhage

Epidural and Subdural

Epidural hemorrhage is bleeding between the dura and the skull that pushes the brain downward and inward. The hemorrhage is usually caused by arterial tears, so bleeding is often rapid, leading to severe neurological deficits and respiratory arrest.

Subdural hemorrhage is bleeding between the dura and the cerebrum, usually from tears in the cortical veins of the subdural space. It tends to develop more slowly than epidural hemorrhage and can result in a subdural hematoma. If the bleeding is acute and develops within minutes or hours of injury, the prognosis is poor. Subacute hematomas that develop more slowly cause varying degrees of injury. Subdural hemorrhage is a common injury related to trauma but it can also result from coagulopathies or aneurysms. Symptoms of acute injury may occur within 24-48 hours, but subacute bleeding may not be evident for up to 2 weeks after injury. Chronic hemorrhage occurs primarily in the elderly. Symptoms vary and may include bradycardia, tachycardia, hypertension, and alterations in consciousness. Older children and adults usually require surgical evacuation of the hematoma.

Subarachnoid

Subarachnoid hemorrhage (SAH) may occur after trauma but is a common result of rupture of a berry aneurysm or an arteriovenous malformation (AVM). However, there are a number of disorders that may be implicated: neoplasms, sickle cell disease, infection, hemophilia, and leukemia. The first presenting symptom may be complaints of severe headache, nausea and vomiting, nuchal rigidity, palsy related to cranial nerve compression, retinal hemorrhages, and papilledema. Late complications include hyponatremia and hydrocephalus. **Symptoms** worsen as intracranial pressure rises. SAH from aneurysm is classified as follows:

- **Grade I:** No symptoms or slight headache and nuchal rigidity
- **Grade II:** Moderate to severe headache with nuchal rigidity and cranial nerve palsy
- **Grade III**: Drowsy, progressing to confusion or mild focal deficits
- **Grade IV:** Stupor, with hemiparesis (moderate to severe), early decerebrate rigidity, and vegetative disturbances
- **Grade V**: Coma state with decerebrate rigidity

Treatment includes:

- Identifying and treating underlying cause
- Observing for re-bleeding
- Anti-seizure medications (such as levetiracetam or phenytoin) to control seizures
- Antihypertensives
- Surgical repair if indicated

Cerebral Vasospasm

Cerebral vasospasm, a luminal narrowing of cerebral arteries, occurs in about 70% of patients after aneurysmal subarachnoid hemorrhage, resulting in ischemic stroke or death in about 15-20%. Onset is usually 4-12 days after initial rupture. The most common sign of vasospasm is new onset lethargy, which requires a STAT transcranial doppler. If progressive neurological decline is noted, a STAT angiogram will be needed. The cause is unclear but may relate to narrowing caused by pressure of the clot on the arteries. The large arteries are usually affected, causing decreased perfusion to large cerebral areas. A number of therapies are under study, but three common approaches include:

- **Hypertensive hypervolemic hemodilution therapy** (HHH) involves using vasoactive drugs to increase systolic BP to 150-160 while diluting the blood with intravenous fluids and volume expanders in order to improve perfusion. However, if done prior to clipping of the aneurysm, this poses a danger of rebleeding. Cerebral edema, increased intracranial pressure, cardiac failure, and electrolyte imbalance may also occur.
- **Nimodipine** every 4 hours for 21 days reduces/prevents vasospasm. IV magnesium and milrinone may also be used.
- **Cerebral angioplasty** may be done if medical approaches fail but poses a danger of perforation, thromboembolism, and stenosis.

Hydrocephalus

Communicating and Noncommunicating

The ventricular system produces and circulates cerebrospinal fluid (CSF). The right and left lateral ventricles open into the third ventricle at the interventricular foramen (foramen of Monro). The aqueduct of Sylvius connects the third and fourth ventricles. The fourth ventricle, anterior to the cerebellum, supplies CSF to the subarachnoid space and the spinal cord (dorsal surface). The CSF circulates and then returns to the brain and is absorbed in the arachnoid villi. **Hydrocephalus** occurs when there is an imbalance between production and absorption of cerebrospinal fluid in the ventricles, resulting from impaired absorption or obstruction, which may be congenital or acquired. There are two common types of hydrocephalus:

- **Communicating:** CSF flows (communicates) between the ventricles but is not absorbed in the subarachnoid space (arachnoid villi).
- **Noncommunicating:** CSF is obstructed (non-communicating) between the ventricles, with the obstruction most often due to stenosis of the aqueduct of Sylvius.

Symptoms

Symptoms of hydrocephalus depend on the age of onset. In *early infancy*, before closure of cranial sutures, head enlargement is the most common presentation, but in adults with less elasticity in the skull, neurological symptoms usually relate to increasing pressure on structures of the brain. Hydrocephalus may occur at any age, but the type that occurs in *young/middle-aged adults* is different than that common in children or those >50. Hydrocephalus in young and middle-aged adults may result from a congenital defect, hydrocephalus of infancy with shunt failure, or trauma and is characterized by:

- Headache relieved by vomiting
- Papilledema
- Lack of bladder control
- Strabismus and other visual disorders
- Ataxia
- Irritability
- Lethargy
- Confusion and impairment of cognitive abilities

With **adult-onset normal pressure hydrocephalus** (>50) cerebrospinal fluid increases and dilates the ventricles, but frequently without increasing intracranial pressure. The cause is often unclear. Symptoms include gait disturbance, bladder control issues, and mild dementia

Treatment

Hydrocephalus is diagnosed through CT and MRI scans, which help to determine the cause. **Treatment** may vary somewhat depending upon the underlying disorder. For example, if obstruction is caused by a tumor, surgical excision to directly remove the obstruction is required. Generally, however, most hydrocephalus is treated with shunts:

- **Ventricular-peritoneal shunt:** This procedure is the most common and consists of placing a ventricular catheter directly into the ventricles (usually lateral) at one end with the other end in the peritoneal area to drain away excess CSF. There is a one-way valve near the proximal end that prevents backflow but opens when pressure rises to drain fluid. In some cases, the distal end drains into the right atrium.
- **Third ventriculostomy:** A small opening is made in the base of the third ventricle so CSF can bypass an obstruction. This procedure is not common and is done with a small endoscope.

Acute Spinal Cord Injury

Spinal cord injuries may result from blunt trauma (such as automobile accidents), falls from a significant height, sports injuries, and penetrating trauma (such as gunshot or knife wounds). Damage results from mechanical injury and secondary responses resulting from hemorrhage, edema, and ischemia. The type of symptoms relates to the area and degree of injury. About 50% of spinal cord injuries involve the cervical spine between C4 and C7 with a 20% mortality rate, and 50% of injuries result in quadriplegia. Neurogenic shock may occur with injury above T6, with bradycardia, hypotension, and autonomic instability. Patients may develop hypoxia because of respiratory dysfunction. With high injuries, up to 70% of patients will require a tracheostomy (especially at or above C3). Patients with paralysis are at high risk for pressure sores, urinary tract infections (from catheterization), and constipation and impaction. Management varies according to the level of injury but may include mobilization, mechanical ventilation, support surfaces, ROM, assisted mobility, rehabilitation therapy, analgesia, psychological counseling, bowel training, and skin care.

Neurologic Infectious Disease

Bacterial Meningitis

Bacterial meningitis may be caused by a wide range of bacteria, including *Streptococcus pneumoniae* and *Neisseria meningitidis.* Bacteria can enter the CNS from distant infection, surgical wounds, invasive devices, nasal colonization, or penetrating trauma. The infective process includes inflammation, exudates, WBC accumulation, and brain tissue damage with hyperemia and edema. Purulent exudate covers the brain and invades and blocks the ventricles, obstructing CSF and leading to increased intracranial pressure. **Symptoms** include abrupt onset, fever, chills, severe headache, nuchal rigidity, and alterations of consciousness with seizures, agitation, and irritability. Antibodies specific to bacteria don't cross the blood brain barrier, so immune response is poor. Some may have photophobia, hallucinations, and/or aggressive behavior or may become stuporous and lapse into coma. Nuchal rigidity may progress to opisthotonos. Reflexes are variable but Kernig and Brudzinski signs are often positive. Signs may relate to particular bacteria, such as rashes, sore joints, or a draining ear. **Diagnosis** is usually based on lumbar puncture examination of cerebrospinal fluid and symptoms. **Treatment** includes IV antibiotics and supportive care: fluids, a dark and calm environment, measures to reduce ICP, etc.

Fungal Meningitis

Fungal meningitis is the least common cause of meningitis. It occurs when a fungal organism enters into the subarachnoid space, cerebral spinal fluid, and meninges. Immune deficient patients such as those with HIV, cancer, or immunodeficiency syndromes are most at risk for the development of fungal meningitis. The most common organisms causing fungal meningitis are candida albicans and Cryptococcus neoformans. Fungal meningitis caused by candida may occur in immunosuppressed patients, in those who have had a ventricular shunt placed, or in those that have had a lumbar puncture performed. Cryptococcus is a fungus found in soil throughout the world and does not usually affect people with a healthy immune system. Cryptococcal meningitis is most commonly seen in patients with HIV/AIDS and is one of the leading causes of death in HIV/AIDS patients in certain parts of Africa.

Signs and symptoms: Headache, fever, nausea and vomiting, stiff neck, photophobia and mental status changes.

Diagnosis: Lumbar puncture with subsequent culture of cerebral spinal fluid. In addition, blood cultures may be obtained as well as a CT of the head.

Treatment: The treatment of fungal meningitis involves a long course of anti-fungal medications, including Amphotericin B, flucytosine, and fluconazole. Anticonvulsants may be administered for seizure control.

Viral Infections That Can Impact the Neurological System

Many different types of **viral infections** can impact the neurological system either by direct infection transmitted through the bloodstream or by spreading along the nerve pathways (such as rabies). Common viral infections affecting the neurological system include:

- **Viral encephalitis**: Arboviral infections are transmitted from an animal host to an arthropod (typically a mosquito or tick) to humans, who are typically dead-end hosts. Arboviral infections include western equine encephalitis, eastern equine encephalitis, St. Louis encephalitis, Powassan encephalitis, Colorado tick fever and La Crosse encephalitis. West Nile virus may also invade the CNS and cause encephalitis.
- **Viral meningitis**: Viral meningitis is usually self-limiting within 7 to 10 days and is less severe than bacterial meningitis.
- **Herpes virus**: Herpes simplex virus can invade the nervous system and cause herpes simplex encephalitis, which has a high mortality rate.
- **HIV**: Inflammation may affect the CNS and interfere with neuronal functions.

Neuromuscular Disorders

Multiple Sclerosis

Multiple sclerosis is an autoimmune disorder of the CNS in which the myelin sheath around the nerves is damaged and replaced by scar tissue that prevents conduction of nerve impulses.

Symptoms vary widely and can include problems with balance and coordination, tremors, slurring of speech, cognitive impairment, vision impairment, nystagmus, pain, and bladder and bowel dysfunction. Symptoms may be relapsing-remitting, progressive, or a combination. Onset is usually at 20 to 30 years of age, with incidence higher in females. Patient may initially present with problems walking or falling or optic neuritis (30%) causing loss of central vision. Males may complain of sexual dysfunction as an early symptom. Others have dysuria with urinary retention.

Diagnosis is based on clinical and neurological examination and MRI. **Treatment** is symptomatic and includes treatment to shorten duration of episodes and slow progress.

- **Glucocorticoids**: Methylprednisolone
- **Immunomodulator**: Interferon beta, glatiramer acetate, natalizumab
- **Immunosuppressant**: Mitoxantrone
- **Hormone**: Estriol (for females)

ALS

Amyotrophic lateral sclerosis (ALS) is a progressive degenerative disease of the upper and lower motor neurons, resulting in progressively severe symptoms such as spasticity, hyperreflexia, muscle weakness, and paralysis that can cause dysphagia, cramping, muscular atrophy, and respiratory dysfunction. ALS may be sporadic or familial (rare). Speech may become monotone; however, cognitive functioning usually remains intact. Eventually, patients become immobile and cannot breathe independently.

Diagnosis is based on history, electromyography, nerve conduction studies, and MRI. Treatment includes riluzole to delay progression of the disease. Patients in the ED usually have been diagnosed and have developed an acute complication, such as acute respiratory failure, aspiration pneumonia, or other trauma.

Treatment includes:

- Nebulizer treatments with bronchodilators and steroids
- Antibiotics for infection
- Mechanical ventilation

If **ventilatory assistance** is needed, it is important to determine if the patient has a living will expressing the wish to be ventilated or not or has assigned power of attorney for health matters to someone to make this decision.

Parkinson's Disease

Parkinson's disease (PD) is an extrapyramidal movement motor system disorder caused by loss of brain cells that produce dopamine. Typical symptoms include tremor of face and extremities, rigidity, bradykinesia, akinesia, poor posture, and a lack of balance and coordination causing increasing problems with mobility, talking, and swallowing. Some may suffer depression and mood changes. Tremors usually present unilaterally in an upper extremity.

Diagnosis includes:

- **Cogwheel rigidity test**: The extremity is put through passive range of motion, which causes increased muscle tone and ratchet-like movements.
- Physical and neurological exam
- Complete history to rule out drug-induced Parkinson akinesia

Treatment includes:

- Symptomatic support
- Dopaminergic therapy: Levodopa, amantadine, and carbidopa
- Anticholinergics: Trihexyphenidyl, benztropine
- Drug-induced Parkinson disease: Terminate drugs

Drug therapy tends to decrease in effectiveness over time, and patients may present with a marked increase in symptoms. Discontinuing the drugs for 1 week may exacerbate symptoms initially, but functioning may improve when drugs are reintroduced.

Guillain-Barré Syndrome

Guillain-Barré syndrome (GBS) is an autoimmune disorder of the myelinated motor peripheral nervous system, causing ascending and descending paralysis. GBS is often triggered by a viral infection, but may be idiopathic in origin. Diagnosis is by history, clinical symptoms, and lumbar puncture, which often show increased protein with normal glucose and cell count although protein may not increase for a week or more.

Review Video: Guillain-Barre Syndrome
Visit mometrix.com/academy and enter code: 742900

Symptoms include:

- Numbness and tingling with increasing weakness of lower extremities that may become generalized, sometimes resulting in complete paralysis and inability to breathe without ventilatory support.
- Deep tendon reflexes are typically absent and some people experience facial weakness and ophthalmoplegia (paralysis of muscles controlling movement of eyes).

Treatment includes:

- Supportive: Fluids, physical therapy, and antibiotics for infections
- Patients should be hospitalized for observation and placed on ventilator support if forced vital capacity is reduced.
- While there is no definitive treatment, plasma exchange or IV immunoglobulin may shorten the duration of symptoms.

Muscular Dystrophy

Muscular dystrophies are genetic disorders with gradual degeneration of muscle fibers and progressive weakness and atrophy of skeletal muscles and loss of mobility. Pseudohypertrophic (Duchenne) muscular dystrophy is the most common form and the most severe. It is an X-linked disorder in about 50% of the cases with the rest sporadic mutations, affecting males almost exclusively. Children typically have some delay in motor development with difficulty walking and have evidence of muscle weakness by about age 3. Pseudohypertrophic refers to enlargement of muscles by fatty infiltration associated with muscular atrophy, which causes contractures and deformities of joints. Abnormal bone development results in spinal and other skeletal deformities. The disease progresses rapidly, and most children are wheelchair bound by about 12 years of age. As the disease progresses, it involves the muscles of the diaphragm and other muscles needed for respiration. Mild to frank mental deficiency is common. Facial, oropharyngeal, and respiratory muscles weaken late in the disease. Cardiomegaly commonly occurs. Death most often relates to respiratory infection or cardiac failure by age 25. Treatment is supportive.

Cerebral Palsy

Cerebral palsy (CP) is a non-progressive motor dysfunction related to CNS damage associated with congenital, hypoxic, or traumatic injury before, during, or ≤2 years after birth. It may include visual defects, speech impairment, seizures and mental retardation. There are 4 types of motor dysfunction:

- **Spastic**: Damage to the cerebral cortex or pyramidal tract. Constant hypertonia and rigidity lead to contractures and curvature of the spine.
- **Dyskinetic**: Damage to the extrapyramidal, basal ganglia. Tremors and twisting with exaggerated posturing and impairment of voluntary muscle control.
- **Ataxic**: Damage to the extrapyramidal cerebellum. Atonic muscles in infancy with lack of balance, instability of muscles, and poor gait.
- **Mixed**: Combinations of all three types with multiple areas of damage.

Characteristics of CP include:

- Hypotonia or hypertonia with rigidity and spasticity
- Athetosis (constant writhing motions)
- Ataxia
- Hemiplegia (one-sided involvement, more severe in upper extremities)
- Diplegia (all extremities involved, but more severe in lower extremities)
- Quadriplegia (all extremities involved with arms flexed and legs extended)

Myasthenia Gravis

Myasthenia gravis is an autoimmune disorder that results in sporadic, progressive weakness of striated (skeletal) muscles because of impaired transmission of nerve impulses. Myasthenia gravis usually affects muscles controlled by the cranial nerves although any muscle group may be affected. Many patients also have thymomas.

Signs and symptoms include weakness and fatigue that worsens throughout the day. Patients often exhibit ptosis and diplopia. They may have trouble chewing and swallowing and often appear to have masklike facies. If respiratory muscles are involved, patients may exhibit signs of respiratory failure. Myasthenic crisis occurs when patients can no longer breathe independently.

Diagnosis includes electromyography and the Tensilon test (an IV injection of edrophonium or neostigmine, which improves function if the patient has myasthenia gravis, but does not improve function if the symptoms are from a different cause). CT or MRI to diagnose thymoma.

Treatment includes anticholinesterase drugs (neostigmine, pyridostigmine) to relieve some muscle weakness, but these drugs lose effectiveness as the disease progresses. Corticosteroids may be used. Thymectomy is performed if thymoma is present. Tracheotomy and mechanical ventilation may be needed for myasthenic crisis.

Seizure Disorders

Partial Seizures

Partial seizures are caused by electrical discharges to a localized area of the cerebral cortex, such as the frontals, temporal, or parietal lobes with seizure characteristics related to the area of involvement. They may begin in a focal area and become generalized, often preceded by an aura.

- **Simple partial:** Unilateral motor symptoms including somatosensory, psychic, and autonomic
  - Aversive: Eyes and head turned away from focal side
  - Sylvan (usually during sleep): Tonic-clonic movements of the face, salivation, and arrested speech
- **Special sensory:** Various sensations (numbness, tingling, prickling, or pain) spreading from one area. May include visual sensations, posturing or hypertonia.
- **Complex (Psychomotor):** No loss of consciousness, but altered consciousness and non-responsive with amnesia. May involve complex sensorium with bad tastes, auditory or visual hallucinations, feeling of déjà vu, strong fear. May carry out repetitive activities, such as walking, running, smacking lips, chewing, or drawling. Rarely aggressive. Seizure usually followed by prolonged drowsiness and confusion. Most common ages 3 through adolescence.

Generalized Seizures

Generalized seizures lack a focal onset and appear to involve both hemispheres, usually presenting with loss of consciousness and no preceding aura.

- **Tonic-clonic (Grand Mal)**: Occurs without warning
  - Tonic period (10-30 seconds): Eyes roll upward with loss of consciousness, arms flexed; stiffen in symmetric tonic contraction of body, apneic with cyanosis and salivating
  - Clonic period (10 seconds to 30 minutes, but usually 30 seconds). Violent rhythmic jerking with contraction and relaxation. May be incontinent of urine and feces. Contractions slow and then stop.

Following seizures, there may be confusion, disorientation, and impairment of motor activity, speech and vision for several hours. Headache, nausea, and vomiting may occur. Person often falls asleep and awakens more lucid.

- **Absence (Petit Mal):** Onset between 4-12 and usually ends in puberty. Onset is abrupt with brief loss of consciousness for 5-10 seconds and slight loss of muscle tone but often appears to be daydreaming. Lip smacking or eye twitching may occur.

Epilepsy

Epilepsy is diagnosed based on a history of seizure activity as well as supporting EEG findings. Treatment is individualized. First line treatments include antiepileptic medications for partial and generalized tonic-clonic seizures. Usually treatment is started with one medication, but this may need to be changed, adjusted, or an additional medication added until the seizures are under control or to avoid adverse effects, which include allergic reactions, especially skin irritations and acute or chronic toxicity. Milder reactions often subside with time or adjustment in doses. Toxic reactions may vary considerably, depending upon the medication and duration of use, so close monitoring is essential. Severe rash and hepatotoxicity are common toxic reactions that occur with many of the antiepileptic drugs. Dosages of drugs may need to be adjusted to avoid breakthrough seizures during times of stress, such as during illness or surgery. Alcohol/drug abuse and sleep deprivation may also cause breakthrough seizures. Most anticonvulsant drugs are teratogenic.

Status Epilepticus

Status epilepticus (SE) is usually generalized tonic-clonic seizures that are characterized by a series of seizures with intervening time too short for regaining of consciousness. The constant assault and periods of apnea can lead to exhaustion, respiratory failure with hypoxemia and hypercapnia, cardiac failure, and death.

Causes: Uncontrolled epilepsy or non-compliance with anticonvulsants, infections such as encephalitis, encephalopathy or stroke, drug toxicity (isoniazid), brain trauma, neoplasms, and metabolic disorders.

Treatment includes:

- Anticonvulsants usually beginning with a fast-acting benzodiazepine (lorazepam), often in steps, with administration of medication every 5 minutes until seizures subside.
- If cause is undetermined, acyclovir and ceftriaxone may be administered.
- If there is no response to the first 2 doses of anticonvulsants (refractory SE), rapid sequence intubation (RSI), which involves sedation and paralytic anesthesia, may be done while therapy continues. Combining phenobarbital and benzodiazepine can cause apnea, so intubation may be necessary.
- Antiepileptic medications are added.

Brain Tumors

Any type of **brain tumor** can occur in adults. Brain tumors may be primary, arising within the brain, or secondary as a result of metastasis:

- **Astrocytoma**: This arises from astrocytes, which are glial cells. It is the most common type of tumor, occurring throughout the brain. There are many types of astrocytomas, and most are slow growing. Some are operable while others are not. Radiation may be given after removal. Astrocytomas include glioblastomas, aggressively malignant tumors occurring most often in adults 45-70.
- **Glioblastoma**: This is the most common and most malignant adult brain tumor/astrocytoma. Treatment includes surgery, radiation, and chemotherapy, but survival rates are very low.
- **Brain stem glioma**: This may be fast or slow growing but is generally not operable because of location, although it may be treated with radiation or chemotherapy.
- **Craniopharyngioma**: This is a congenital, slow-growing, recurrent (especially if >5 cm) and benign cystic tumor that is difficult to resect and is treated with surgery and radiation.
- **Meningioma**: Slow growing recurrent tumors are usually benign and most often occur in women, ages 40 to 70; however, they can cause severe impairment/death, depending on size and location. Meningiomas are surgically removed if causing symptoms.
- **Ganglioglioma**: This can occur anywhere in the brain and is usually slow growing and benign.
- **Medulloblastoma**: There are many types of medulloblastoma, most arising in the cerebellum, malignant, and fast growing. Surgical excision is often followed by radiation and chemotherapy although recent studies show using just chemotherapy controls recurrence with less neurological damage.

- **Oligodendroglioma**: This tumor most often occurs in the cerebrum, primarily the frontal or temporal lobes, involving the myelin sheath of the neurons. It is slow growing and most common in those age 40-60.
- **Optical nerve glioma**: This slow growing tumor of the optic nerve is usually a form of astrocytoma. Optic nerve glioma is often associated with neurofibromatosis type I (NF1), occurring in 15%-40% of patients with NF1. Despite surgical, chemotherapy, or radiotherapy treatment, it is usually fatal.

STROKES

HEMORRHAGIC STROKES

Hemorrhagic strokes account for about 20% of all strokes and result from a ruptured cerebral artery, causing not only a lack of oxygen and nutrients but also edema that causes widespread pressure and damage:

- **Intracerebral** is bleeding into the substance of the brain from an artery in the central lobes, basal ganglia, pons, or cerebellum. Intracerebral hemorrhage usually results from atherosclerotic degenerative changes, hypertension, brain tumors, anticoagulation therapy, or use of illicit drugs, such as cocaine.
- **Intracranial aneurysm** occurs with ballooning cerebral artery ruptures, most commonly at the Circle of Willis.
- **Arteriovenous malformation**. Rupture of AVMs can cause brain attack in young adults.
- **Subarachnoid hemorrhage** is bleeding in the space between the meninges and brain, resulting from aneurysm, AVM, or trauma. This type of hemorrhage compresses brain tissue.

Treatment includes: The patient may need airway protection/artificial ventilation if neurologic compromise is severe. Blood pressure is lowered to control rate of bleeding but with caution to avoid hypotension and resulting cerebral ischemia (Goal – CPP >70). Sedation can lower ICP and blood pressure, and seizure prophylaxis will be indicated as blood irritates the cerebral cells. An intraventricular catheter may be used in ICP management; correct any clotting disorders if identified.

ISCHEMIA STROKES

Strokes (brain attacks, cerebrovascular accidents) result when there is interruption of the blood flow to an area of the brain. The two basic types are ischemic and hemorrhagic. About 80% are **ischemic**, resulting from blockage of an artery supplying the brain:

- **Thrombosis** in a large artery, usually resulting from atherosclerosis, may block circulation to a large area of the brain. It is most common in the elderly and may occur suddenly or after episodes of transient ischemic attacks.
- **Lacunar infarct** (a penetrating thrombosis in a small artery) is most common in those with diabetes mellitus and/or hypertension.
- **Embolism** travels through the arterial system and lodges in the brain, most commonly in the left middle cerebral artery. An embolism may be cardiogenic, resulting from cardiac arrhythmia or surgery. An embolism usually occurs rapidly with no warning signs.
- **Cryptogenic** has no identifiable cause.

Medical management of ischemic strokes with tissue plasminogen activator (tPA) (Activase®), the primary treatment, should be initiated within 3 hours (or up to 4.5 hours if inclusion criteria are met):

- **Thrombolytic,** such as tPA, which is produced by recombinant DNA and is used to dissolve fibrin clots. It is given intravenously (0.9 mg/kg up to 90 mg) with 10% injected as an initial bolus and the rest over the next hour.
- **Antihypertensives** if MAP >130 mmHg or systolic BP >220
- **Cooling** to reduce hyperthermia
- **Osmotic diuretics** (mannitol), hypertonic saline, loop diuretics (Lasix®), and/or corticosteroids (dexamethasone) to decrease cerebral edema and intracranial pressure
- **Aspirin/anticoagulation** may be used with embolism
- Monitor and treat hyperglycemia
- **Surgical Intervention:** Used when other treatment fails, may go in through artery and manually remove the clot

Symptoms of Brain Attacks in Relation to Area of Brain Affected

Brain attacks most commonly occur in the right or left hemisphere, but the exact location and the extent of brain damage from a **brain attack** affects the type of presenting symptoms. If the frontal area of either side is involved, there tends to be memory and learning deficits. Some symptoms are common to specific areas and help to identify the area involved:

- **Right hemisphere**: This results in left paralysis or paresis and a left visual field deficit that may cause spatial and perceptual disturbances, so people may have difficulty judging distance. Fine motor skills may be impacted, resulting in trouble dressing or handling tools. People may become impulsive and exhibit poor judgment, often denying impairment. Left-sided neglect (lack of perception of things on the left side) may occur. Depression is common as well as short-term memory loss and difficulty following directions. Language skills usually remain intact.
- **Left hemisphere**: Results in right paralysis or paresis and a right visual field defect. Depression is common and people often exhibit slow, cautious behavior, requiring repeated instruction and reinforcement for simple tasks. Short-term memory loss and difficulty learning new material or understanding generalizations is common. Difficulty with mathematics, reading, writing, and reasoning may occur. Aphasia (expressive, receptive, or global) is common.
- **Brain stem**: Because the brain stem controls respiration and cardiac function, a brain attack in the brain stem frequently causes death, but those who survive may have a number of problems, including respiratory and cardiac abnormalities. Strokes may involve motor or sensory impairment or both.
- **Cerebellum**: This area controls balance and coordination. Brain attacks in the cerebellum are rare but may result in ataxia, nausea and vomiting, and headaches and dizziness or vertigo.

TIA

Transient ischemic attacks (TIAs) from small clots cause similar but short-lived (minutes to hours) symptoms. Emergent treatment includes placing patient in semi-Fowlers or Fowler's position and administering oxygen. The patient may require oral suctioning if secretions pool. The patient's circulation, airway, and breathing should be assessed and IV access line placed. Thrombolytic therapy to dissolve blood clots should be administered within 1 to 3 hours. While a patient can recover fully from a TIA, they should be educated, because having a TIA increases an individual's risk for a stroke.

HEAD TRAUMA

BLUNT HEAD TRAUMA

Head trauma can occur as the result of intentional or unintentional blunt or penetrating trauma, such as from falls, automobile accidents, sports injuries, or violence. The degree of injury correlates with the impact force. The skull provides protection to the brain, but a severe blow can cause significant neurological damage. Blunt trauma can include:

- **Acceleration-deceleration injuries** are those in which a blow to the stationary head causes the elastic skull to change shape, pushing against the brain, which moves sharply backward in response, striking against the skull.
- **Bruising** can occur at the point of impact (*coup*) and the point where the brain hits the skull (*contrecoup*). So, a blow to the frontal area can cause damage to the occipital region.

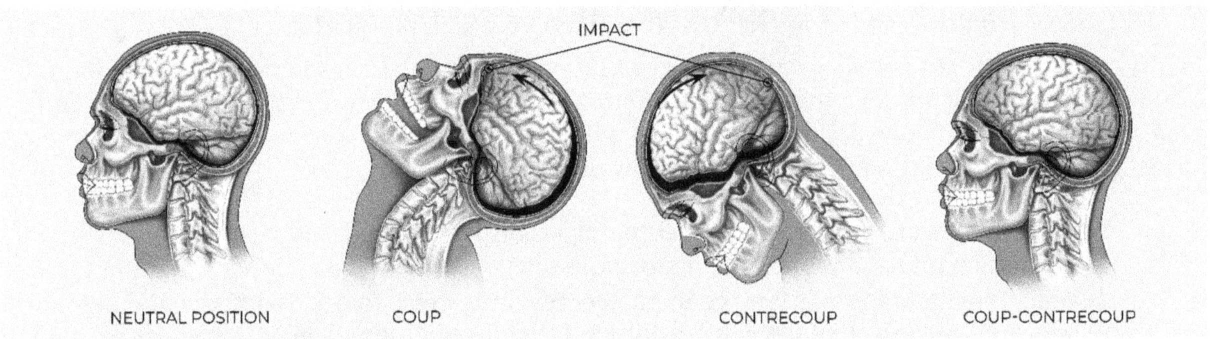

- **Shear injuries,** where vessels are torn, result from sudden movement of the brain.
- **Severe compression** may force the brain through the tentorial opening, damaging the brainstem.

CEREBRAL EDEMA AND INCREASED ICP SECONDARY TO HEAD TRAUMA

Head injuries that occur at the time of trauma include fractures, contusions, hematomas, and diffuse cerebral and vascular injury. These injuries may result in hypoxia, increased intracranial pressure, and cerebral edema. Open injuries may result in infection. Patients often suffer initial hypertension, which increases intracranial pressure, decreasing perfusion. Often the primary problem with head trauma is a significant increase in swelling, which also interferes with perfusion, causing hypoxia and hypercapnia, which trigger increased blood flow. This increased volume at a time when injury impairs auto-regulation increases cerebral edema, which increases intracranial pressure and results in a further decrease in perfusion with resultant ischemia. If pressure continues to rise, the brain may herniate. Concomitant hypotension may result in hypoventilation, further complicating treatment. Treatments include:

- Monitoring ICP and CCP
- Providing oxygen
- Elevating the head of the bed and maintaining proper body alignment
- Giving medications: Analgesics, anticonvulsants, and anesthetics
- Providing blood/fluids to stabilize hemodynamics

- Managing airway, providing mechanical ventilation if needed
- Providing osmotic agents, such as mannitol and hypertonic saline solution, to reduce cerebral edema

Concussions, Contusions, and Lacerations

A variety of different injuries can occur as a result of **head trauma**:

- **Concussions** are diffuse areas of bleeding in the brain and one of the most common injuries. They are usually relatively transient, causing no permanent neurological damage. They may result in confusion, disorientation, and mild amnesia, which last only minutes or hours.
- **Contusions/lacerations** are bruising and tears of cerebral tissue. There may be petechial areas at the impact site (coup) or larger bruising. Contrecoup injuries are less common in children than in adults. Areas most impacted by contusions and lacerations are the occipital, frontal, and temporal lobes. The degree of injury relates to the amount of vascular damage, but initial symptoms are similar to a concussion; however, symptoms persist and may progress, depending upon the degree of injury. Lacerations are often caused by fractures.

Skull Fractures

Skull fractures are a common mechanism of penetrating wounds causing cerebral lacerations. Open fractures are those in which the dura is torn, and closed fractures are those in which the dura remain intact. While fractures by themselves do not cause neurological damage, force is needed to fracture the skull, often causing damage to underlying structures. Meningeal arteries lie in groves on the underside of the skull, and a fracture can cause an arterial tear and hemorrhage. Skull fractures include:

- **Basilar**: Occurs in bones at the base of the brain and can cause severe brainstem damage. May see bruising around the ear ("Battles sign") and leaking of CSF from nose and ears ("Halo sign"—bloody fluid will develop a ring of clear fluid when placed on gauze or linens).
- **Comminuted**: Skull fractures into small pieces.
- **Compound**: Surface laceration extends to include a skull fracture.
- **Depressed**: Pieces of the skull are depressed inward on the brain tissue, often producing dural tears.
- **Linear/hairline:** Skull fracture forms a thin line without any splintering.

Traumatic Brain Injury

Traumatic brain injury (TBI) occurs when an external force damages the brain, thereby causing an alteration in its function. TBIs can be classified as mild, moderate or severe. Common causes of traumatic brain injury include falls, motor vehicle accidents, and assaults. Traumatic brain injuries are more common in males than females.

Signs and symptoms: Signs and symptoms of a traumatic brain injury may not be immediately present, depending on the severity of the injury. Symptoms may be subtle initially and then worsen. Symptoms include: loss of consciousness, headache, blurred vision, confusion, nausea, vomiting, fatigue, somnolence, dizziness, loss of balance or coordination, seizures, tinnitus, slurred speech, and photosensitivity.

Diagnosis: X-rays of the spine, CT and MRI of the head and angiography if penetrating injury occurred. The Glasgow coma scale is most commonly used to assess neurologic status in the TBI patient.

Treatment: Treatment of TBI includes frequent monitoring of vital signs, fluid balance and neurologic status. Intracranial pressure may also be monitored. Mannitol and hypertonic saline may be administered to decrease intracranial pressure and cerebral edema. Antiepileptic medications may be utilized to prevent or minimize seizure activity. In cases of severe injury, decompressive craniotomy and initiation of a hypothermia protocol may be used to reduce intracranial pressure, cerebral edema and cell death.

Brain Death

While each state has its own laws that describe the legal definition of **brain death,** most include some variation of this description:

- Brain death has occurred if the person has "sustained irreversible cessation of circulatory and respiratory functions; or has sustained irreversible cessation of all functions of the entire brain, including the brain stem."

Some states specify the number of physicians that must make the determination and others simply say the decision must be made in accordance with accepted medical practice. Criteria for determination of brain death include coma or lack of responsiveness, apnea (without ventilation), and absence of brainstem reflexes. In many states, findings must be confirmed by at least 2 physicians. **Tests used to confirm brain death** include:

- Cerebral angiograms: Delayed intracerebral filling or obstruction
- EEG: Lack of response to auditory, visual, or somatic stimuli
- Ultrasound (transcranial): Abnormal/lack of flow
- Cerebral scintigrams: Static images at preset time intervals
- Absence of oculocephalic reflex ("Doll's eyes"): patients eyes stay fixed when head is turned side to side
- Absence of oculovestibular reflex ("cold caloric"): When ice cold water is injected into the ear, the patient's eyes exhibit no response. The patient's HOB must be at least 20° for this test to be accurate

Delirium

Delirium is an *acute, sudden, and fluctuating change* in consciousness. Delirium occurs in 10-40% of hospitalized older adults and about 80% of patients who are terminally ill. Delirium may result from drugs, infections, hypoxia, trauma, dementia, depression, vision and hearing loss, surgery, alcoholism, untreated pain, fluid/electrolyte imbalance, and malnutrition. If left untreated, delirium greatly increases the risk of morbidity and death.

Signs/Symptoms: Reduced ability to focus/sustain attention, language and memory disturbances, disorientation, confusion, audiovisual hallucinations, sleep disturbance, and psychomotor activity disorder.

Diagnosis: Patient interview, history/chart/medication review, and possible blood tests to identify electrolyte imbalance/abnormalities.

Treatment includes:

- **Medications**: Trazodone, lorazepam, haloperidol—though these may make confusion worse in elderly patients
- **Procedures**: Provide a sitter to ensure safety, decreasing dosage of hypnotics and psychotropics, correct underlying cause

Prevention: Reorient patient frequently, ensure adequate rest/nutrition, monitor response to medications, and treat infections and dehydration/malnutrition early.

Agitation

Agitation is a common occurrence in the critically ill patient. Factors contributing to the development of agitation include drug or alcohol withdrawal, sleep deprivation, hypoxemia, electrolyte or metabolic imbalance, anxiety, pain, and adverse drug reactions. Delirium may also include agitation as a manifestation.

Diagnosis: The physiologic effects of agitation may include increases in heart rate, respiratory rate, blood pressure, intracranial pressure, and oxygen consumption. In addition, agitation can contribute to the self-removal of lines or tubes and combative behavior that may result in patient harm.

Treatment: Treatment of agitation involves the identification and correction of causative factors. The use of pharmacologic agents to manage pain, anxiety, and agitation are often utilized. Non-pharmacologic interventions including verbal de-escalation (when possible). The promotion of normal sleep patterns and relaxation techniques may also be effective. Early identification of signs and symptoms is also critical in the successful management of agitation.

Dementia

Dementia is a chronic condition in which there is progressive and irreversible loss of memory and function. There are many types of dementia a nurse may encounter:

1. **Creutzfeldt-Jakob disease**: Rapidly progressive dementia with impaired memory, behavioral changes, and incoordination
2. **Dementia with Lewy Bodies**: Similar to Alzheimer's, but symptoms may fluctuate frequently; may also include visual hallucinations, muscle rigidity, and tremors
3. **Frontotemporal dementia**: Causes marked changes in personality and behavior; characterized by difficulty using and understanding language
4. **Mixed dementia**: Combination of different types of dementia
5. **Normal pressure hydrocephalus**: Characterized by ataxia, memory loss, and urinary incontinence
6. **Parkinson's dementia**: Involves impaired decision making and difficulty concentrating, learning new material, understanding complex language, and sequencing
7. **Vascular dementia**: Memory loss less pronounced than that common to Alzheimer's, but symptoms are similar

Nursing considerations: Distraction is usually the best course of action to deter the patient with dementia. Reorient frequently, but do not argue with the patient. Avoid restraints or sedatives, which worsen confusion.

Endocrine Pathophysiology

Diabetes Mellitus Types 1 and 2

Diabetes mellitus is the most common metabolic disorder. Over 6% of adults have diabetes, but only two-thirds are diagnosed. Insulin resistance tends to increase in older adults, so there is less ability to handle glucose. Type II is more common in older adults, with incidence increasing with age.

- **Type I:** Immune-mediated form with insufficient insulin production because of destruction of pancreatic beta cells
  - **Symptoms** include pronounced polyuria and polydipsia, short onset, obesity or recent weight loss, and ketoacidosis present on diagnosis.
  - **Treatment** includes insulin as needed to control blood sugar, glucose monitoring 1–4 times daily, diet with carbohydrate control, and exercise.
- **Type II:** Insulin resistant form with defect in insulin secretion
  - **Symptoms** include long onset, obesity with no weight loss or significant weight loss, mild or absent polyuria and polydipsia, ketoacidosis or glycosuria without ketonuria, androgen-mediated problems such as hirsutism and acne (adolescents), and hypertension.
  - **Treatment** includes diet and exercise, glucose monitoring, and oral medications.

Diabetic Ketoacidosis

Diabetic ketoacidosis is a complication of type 1 diabetes mellitus, usually related to noncompliance with treatment, stress, illness, or lack of awareness of having diabetes (this event often being the first time that diabetes is diagnosed). Inadequate production of insulin results in glucose being unavailable for metabolism, so lipolysis (breakdown of fat) produces free fatty acids (FFAs) as an alternate fuel source. Glycerol is converted to ketone bodies which are used for cellular metabolism less efficiently than glucose. Excess ketone bodies are excreted in the urine (ketonuria) or exhalations. Acidosis of any type causes potassium in cells to shift to the serum. The ketone bodies lower serum pH, leading to ketoacidosis.

Symptoms include:

- Kussmaul respirations: "Ketone breath," or fruity smelling breath; progresses to CNS depression with loss of airway
- Fluid imbalance, including loss of potassium and other electrolytes from cellular death resulting in dehydration and diuresis with excess thirst
- Dangerous cardiac arrhythmias, related to potassium loss; hypotension, chest pain, tachycardia
- GI: Nausea/vomiting, abdominal pain, loss of appetite
- Neurological: malaise, confusion/lethargy progressing to coma

Diagnosis is based on:

- Labs: Blood glucose >250 mg/dL, lower Na and elevated K (switches after treatment), elevated beta-hydroxybutyrate (byproduct of ketones)
- ABG: pH <7.3, HCO_3 <18 mEq/L
- Urine: + glucose, ketones

Treatment and Potential Complications

Treatment of DKA:

- **Fluids**: Priority is fluid resuscitation with 1-2 liters of isotonic fluids given in the first hour, up to 8 liters in the first 24 hours. Potassium will be added to the fluids when levels begin to fall.
- **Insulin**: Continuous drip IV, with/without loading dose. Will usually begin at 0.1 unit/kg/ hour (5-7 units an hour generally), with a goal of decreasing blood glucose 50–75 mg/dL an hour. Blood glucose is checked every hour, and when levels are < 200 mg/dL, add dextrose to IV fluids to prevent rebound hypoglycemia.
- **Potassium**: Watch carefully, as fluids and insulin will cause rapid fall in serum levels. When K <5 mEq/L, it should be added to the IV fluids (Per liter: 20 mEq for K 4-5, 40 mEq for K 3–4). If potassium falls below 3, stop insulin drip and give 10–20 an hour until >3.5.
- **Sodium and Magnesium**: Na has an inverse relationship with potassium, and will increase as potassium falls. If sodium levels rise above 150 mEq, switch fluids to 0.45 NS. Low magnesium levels prevent potassium uptake, so replace as necessary.
- **Electrolytes**: Continue to monitor electrolytes and anion gap during ICU stay. When ABG and electrolytes normalized, transition to SQ insulin.

Potential complications include:

- Sudden electrolyte shifts (potassium) leading to catastrophic arrythmias, cerebral edema, and other complications
- Vomiting and decreased LOC leading to aspiration/ARDS
- Mechanical ventilation stops respiratory alkalosis and increases acidosis

HHNK

Hyperglycemic hyperosmolar nonketotic syndrome (HHNK) occurs in people without history of diabetes or with mild type 2 diabetes, resulting in persistent hyperglycemia leading to osmotic diuresis. Fluid shifts from intracellular to extracellular spaces to maintain osmotic equilibrium, but the increased glucosuria and dehydration results in hypernatremia and increased osmolarity. This condition is most common in those 50–70 years old and often is precipitated by an acute illness, such as a stroke, medications (thiazides), or dialysis treatments. HHNK differs from ketoacidosis because, while the insulin level is not adequate, it is high enough to prevent the breakdown of fat. Onset of symptoms often occurs over a few days. Glucose levels are often higher than those in DKA due to the gradual increase over time (often greater than 600), and the body living in a state of hyperglycemia, therefore the individual is not symptomatic until the blood glucose level is at an extreme high.

Symptoms: Polyuria, dehydration, hypotension, tachycardia, changes in mental status, seizures, hemiparesis.

Diagnosis: Increased glucose, Na, osmolality (urine and serum), BUN/Creatinine.

Treatment is similar to that for ketoacidosis:

- Insulin drip with frequent (hourly) blood sugar monitoring.
- Intravenous fluids and electrolytes.
- Correct blood glucose and other labs.

Acute Hypoglycemia

Acute hypoglycemia (hyperinsulinism) may result from pancreatic islet tumors or hyperplasia, increasing insulin production, or from the use of insulin to control diabetes mellitus. Hyperinsulinism can cause damage to the central nervous and cardiopulmonary systems, interfering with functioning of the brain and causing neurological impairment. Other causes may include: genetic defects (chromosome 11: short arm), severe infections, and toxic ingestion of alcohol or drugs (salicylates).

Symptoms include:

- Blood glucose <50-60 mg/dL
- Central nervous system: seizures, altered consciousness, lethargy, and poor feeding with vomiting, myoclonus, respiratory distress, diaphoresis, hypothermia, and cyanosis
- Adrenergic system: diaphoresis, tremor, tachycardia, palpitation, hunger, and anxiety

Diagnosis: Blood work, patient history, presentation.

Treatment depends on underlying cause:

- Glucose/Glucagon administration to elevate blood glucose levels
- Diazoxide (Hyperstat®) to inhibit release of insulin
- Somatostatin (Sandostatin®) to suppress insulin production
- Careful monitoring

Diabetes Insipidus

Diabetes insipidus (DI) is caused by a deficiency of the antidiuretic hormone (ADH), or vasopressin. DI may develop secondary to head trauma, primary brain tumor, meningitis, encephalitis, or surgical ablation or irradiation of the pituitary gland, or metastatic tumors. This is different from congenital nephrogenic diabetes insipidus, in which production of ADH is normal but the renal tubules do not respond.

Symptoms:

- Polydipsia—enormous quantities of fluid may be ingested (3-30 L/day)
- Polyuria—large volumes of very dilute urine is excreted (3-30 L/day); nocturia almost always occurs
- Dehydration and hypovolemia can develop quickly if urinary losses are not continuously replaced

Diagnosis: A water deprivation test is the most reliable diagnostic test, but should only be done while the patient is under constant supervision. The test measures urine production, blood electrolyte levels, and weight over about 12 hours, during which the person is not allowed to drink. At the end of the 12 hours, vasopressin is given and a diagnosis of DI is confirmed if the person's excessive urination stops, BP rises to normal, and HR is normal.

Treatment includes:

- **Hormonal drugs**—Desmopressin, a synthetic analog of vasopressin, has prolonged antidiuretic activity, lasting 12 to 24 hours in most patients, and may be given intranasally, SQ, IV, or orally. Overdosage can lead to water intoxication, so monitor neurological status.

- **Nonhormonal drugs**—Three groups of nonhormonal drugs can reduce polyuria:
  - Diuretics, primarily thiazides (hydrochlorothiazide)
  - Vasopressin-releasing drugs (chlorpropamide or carbamazepine)
  - Prostaglandin inhibitors (indomethacin)

SIADH

Syndrome of inappropriate secretion of antidiuretic hormone (SIADH) is related to hypersecretion of the posterior pituitary gland. This causes the kidneys to reabsorb fluids, resulting in fluid retention, and triggers a decrease in sodium levels (dilutional hyponatremia), resulting in production of only concentrated urine. This syndrome may result from central nervous system disorders, such as brain trauma, surgery, or tumors. It may also be triggered by other disorders, such as tumors of various organs, pneumothorax, acute pneumonia, and other lung disorders. Some medications (vincristine, phenothiazines, tricyclic antidepressants, and thiazide diuretics) may also trigger SIADH.

Symptoms: Edema, dyspnea, crackles on auscultation, anorexia with nausea and vomiting, irritability, stomach cramps, alterations of personality, stupor and seizures (related to progressive sodium depletion).

Diagnosis: Increased urine specific gravity, decreased Na and serum osmolality.

Treatment includes: (treat underlying cause)

- Correct fluid volume excess and electrolytes.
- Monitor urine output continuously: <0.5-1 mL/kg/hour is cause for concern.
- Seizure precautions.
- With SIADH expect low serum sodium and serum osmolality with high urine osmolality.

Chronic Adrenal Insufficiency (Addison's Disease)

Adrenal/Adrenocortical insufficiency (Addison's disease) is caused by damage to the adrenal cortex related to a variety of causes, such as autoimmune disease or genetic disorders, but it may relate to destructive lesions or neoplasms. Without treatment the condition is life threatening.

Symptoms may be vague and the condition undiagnosed until 80–90% of the adrenal cortex has been destroyed:

- Chronic weakness and fatigue
- Abdominal distress with nausea and vomiting
- Salt or licorice craving as a result of aldosterone deficiency
- Pigmentary changes in skin and mucous membranes, hyperpigmentation
- Hypotension
- Hypoglycemia
- Recurrent seizures (more common in children)

Treatment includes hormone replacement therapy with glucocorticoids (cortisol) and mineralocorticoids (aldosterone), which may be taken orally or by monthly parenteral injections. Androgen replacement is sometimes recommended for women.

Note: During times of stress or illness, the demand for glucocorticoids may increase, and dosages up to 3 times the normal dosage may be needed to prevent an acute crisis.

Acute Adrenal Insufficiency (Adrenal Crisis)

Acute adrenal insufficiency (adrenal crisis) is a sudden, life-threatening condition resulting from an exacerbation of primary chronic adrenal insufficiency (Addison's disease), often precipitated by sepsis, surgical stress, adrenal hemorrhage related to septicemia, anticoagulation complications, and cortisone withdrawal related to a decreased or inadequate dose to compensate for stress. Acute adrenal insufficiency may occur in those who do not have Addison's disease, such as those who have received cortisone for various reasons, usually a minimum of 20 mg daily for at least 5 days.

Symptoms:

- Fever
- Nausea and vomiting
- Abdominal pain
- Weakness and general fatigue
- Disorientation, confusion
- Hypotensive shock
- Dehydration
- Electrolyte imbalance with hyperkalemia, hypercalcemia, hypoglycemia and hyponatremia

Treatment:

- IV fluids in large volume
- Glucocorticoid
- 50% dextrose if indicated (hypoglycemia)
- Mineralocorticoid may be needed after intravenous solutions
- The precipitating cause must be identified and treated as well

Hyperthyroidism

Hyperthyroidism (thyrotoxicosis) usually results from excess production of thyroid hormones (Graves' disease) from immunoglobulins providing abnormal stimulation of the thyroid gland. Other causes include thyroiditis and excess thyroid medications.

Symptoms vary and may be non-specific, especially in the elderly:

- Hyperexcitability
- Tachycardia (100-160) and atrial fibrillation
- Increased systolic (but not diastolic) BP
- Poor heat tolerance, skin flushed and diaphoretic
- Dry skin and pruritis (especially in the elderly)
- Hand tremor, progressive muscular weakness
- Exophthalmos (bulging eyes)
- Increased appetite and intake but weight loss

Treatment includes:

- Radioactive iodine to destroy the thyroid gland. Propranolol may be used to prevent thyroid storm. Thyroid hormones are given for resultant hypothyroidism.
- Antithyroid medications, such as Propacil® or Tapazole® to block conversion of T4 to T3.

- Surgical removal of thyroid is used if patients cannot tolerate other treatments or in special circumstances, such as large goiter. Usually one-sixth of the thyroid is left in place and antithyroid medications are given before surgery.

Review Video: 7 Symptoms of Hyperthyroidism
Visit mometrix.com/academy and enter code: 923159

Review Video: Graves' Disease
Visit mometrix.com/academy and enter code: 516655

Review Video: Thyroid and Antithyroid
Visit mometrix.com/academy and enter code: 666133

THYROTOXIC STORM

Thyrotoxic storm is a severe type of hyperthyroidism with sudden onset, precipitated by stress such as injury or surgery, in those un-treated or inadequately treated for hyperthyroidism. If not promptly diagnosed and treated, it is fatal. Incidence has decreased with the use of antithyroid medications but can still occur with medical emergencies or pregnancy. Diagnostic findings are similar to hyperthyroidism and include increased T3 uptake and decreased TSH.

Symptoms:

- Increase in symptoms of hyperthyroidism
- Increased temperature >38.5 °C
- Tachycardia >130 with atrial fibrillation and heart failure
- Gastrointestinal disorders such as nausea, vomiting, diarrhea, and abdominal discomfort
- Altered mental status with delirium progressing to coma

Treatment:

- Controlling production of thyroid hormone through antithyroid medications such as propylthiouracil and methimazole
- Inhibiting release of thyroid hormone with iodine therapy (or lithium)
- Controlling peripheral activity of thyroid hormone with propranolol
- Fluid and electrolyte replacement
- Glucocorticoids, such as dexamethasone
- Cooling blankets
- Treatment of arrhythmias as needed with antiarrhythmics and anticoagulation

HYPOTHYROIDISM

Hypothyroidism occurs when the thyroid produces inadequate levels of thyroid hormones. Conditions may range from mild to severe myxedema. There are a number of causes:

- Chronic lymphocytic thyroiditis (Hashimoto's thyroiditis)
- Excessive treatment for hyperthyroidism
- Atrophy of thyroid
- Medications such as lithium and iodine compounds
- Radiation to the area of the thyroid
- Diseases that affect the thyroid such as scleroderma
- Iodine imbalances

Symptoms may include chronic fatigue, menstrual disturbances, hoarseness, subnormal temperature, low pulse rate, weight gain, thinning hair, thickening skin. Some dementia may occur with advanced conditions. Clinical findings may include increased cholesterol with associated atherosclerosis and coronary artery disease. Myxedema may be characterized by changes in respiration with hypoventilation and CO_2 retention resulting in coma.

Treatment involves hormone replacement with synthetic levothyroxine (Synthroid®) based on TSH levels, but this increases the oxygen demand of the body, so careful monitoring of cardiac status must be done during early treatment to avoid myocardial infarction while reaching euthyroid (normal) level.

Pheochromocytoma

Pheochromocytoma is a rare tumor of chromaffin tissue. Ninety percent of these occur in the adrenal medulla, 10% are bilateral, and 10% are malignant. These tumors produce epinephrine and norepinephrine, leading to episodic symptoms of headaches, chest pain, palpitations, diaphoresis, tremor, nausea, vomiting, weight loss, and constipation. Initial diagnosis requires a 24-hour urine test to check for metanephrine, VMA, and catecholamines. These are always elevated with pheochromocytoma. If associated with a multiple endocrine neoplasia (MEN) syndrome, then one must check serum free metanephrine. Then one should begin imaging with CT or MRI scanning of the adrenals. If the adrenals appear normal, a radiolabeled iodine (called MIBG-metaiodobenzylguanidine scintigraphy) scan can localize extra-adrenal pheochromocytoma tissue or metastases. This scan uses a compound that concentrates in the adrenals to highlight the pheochromocytoma tissue. Treatment is surgical. But first, phenoxybenzamines are used to block the catecholamines, and then beta-blockers are used to control heart rate. Surgery has a 90% cure rate. Urinary catecholamines should be followed for at least 10 years.

Hyperaldosteronism

Hyperaldosteronism leads to hypokalemia and hypernatremia (and often resulting hypertension). In fact, patients with untreated hypertension and potassium <2.8meq/dL often have primary hyperaldosteronism:

- **Aldosterone-producing adenoma** (Conn's syndrome) accounts for most primary hyperaldosteronism and affects women more often than men.
- **Idiopathic hyperaldosteronism** accounts for about 30% of primary hyperaldosteronism and has no identifiable changes on imaging.
- **Glucocorticoid suppressible hyperaldosteronism** is familial and rare.
- **Aldosterone-producing adrenocortical carcinoma** is another rare cause and presents with hyperandrogenism.

Diagnosis of hyperaldosteronism requires diastolic hypertension without edema, low renin levels that do not respond to volume depletion, and high aldosterone levels that fail to drop with saline boluses. An adrenal CT scan is performed to distinguish between Conn's syndrome and idiopathic hyperaldosteronism. Treatment includes spironolactone or eplerenone to block the mineralocorticoid receptor, normalizing potassium and improving blood pressure. Adrenalectomy is indicated for unilateral hyperplasia or Conn's syndrome.

Cushing Syndrome and Cushing's Disease

Cushing syndrome results when **cortisol levels** are increased. Most commonly, this is due to steroid treatment with **prednisone**. Endogenous causes include a pituitary adenoma producing excess amounts of adrenocorticotropic hormone (ACTH) which leads to elevated cortisol (termed

Cushing's disease) or a primary tumor of the adrenal gland causing increased cortisol secretion. Forms of cancer (e.g., lung, carcinoid) can present with ectopic sources of ACTH secretion. Patients will develop proximal muscle weakness, muscular atrophy, truncal obesity with thin arms and legs, round facies, buffalo hump, and purple striae usually across the abdomen. Patients may bruise easily, have non-healing sores, and women may be affected with hirsutism and oligomenorrhea/amenorrhea. Osteoporosis can occur as can glucose intolerance. For diagnosis a patient should be screened with one of the following: 24-hour urine free cortisol x3, low dose (1 mg) dexamethasone suppression test, midnight serum or salivary cortisol. Once Cushing syndrome is established, determine the cause using an ACTH and simultaneous cortisol measurement (elevated = adrenal adenoma or carcinoma) or a high-dose (8 mg overnight, or 2-day) dexamethasone suppression test (differentiates between pituitary cause and ectopic ACTH cause). Patients should be weaned off prednisone if possible. Removal of a pituitary adenoma can decrease ACTH production. Removal of an adrenal adenoma or other ectopic source of hormone secretion can decrease cortisol levels. Complications include hypertension, CV disease, DM, osteoporosis, risk of adrenal crisis, and psychosis.

Hyperparathyroidism

Hyperparathyroidism occurs when there is **overproduction of parathyroid hormone (PTH)**. Normal range is 10-55 pg/mL. This occurs more often in women and those over 50 years old. Hypercalcemia (total Ca^{++} >10.4 mg/dL) is the most common finding in hyperparathyroidism. Patients may complain signs of hypercalcemia which can be easily remembered with *bones, stones, groans, and moans.* This includes **bone pain** due to demineralization, **kidney stones**, **abdominal groans** (nausea, vomiting, constipation, loss of appetite), and **psychiatric moans** (nervous system issues: muscle weakness, fatigue, lethargy, depression, confusion). Polyuria can occur with renal failure. Cardiac arrhythmias, hypertension, and even coma can occur. Ca^{++} levels >12 mg/dL may be due to cancer, and therefore cancer must be ruled out, especially if Ca^{++} levels rise rapidly. Hyperparathyroidism is treated with parathyroidectomy of affected glands.

Hypoparathyroidism

Hypoparathyroidism is the **deficiency of PTH**. This is more common in women and is usually due to accidental damage during thyroid/neck surgery, radioactive iodine treatment for hyperthyroidism, radiation, or due to autoimmune causes. As Ca^{++} levels drop, patients may complain of paresthesia of the fingers, toes, and perioral area. Patients will show other signs of neuromuscular irritability with muscle aches, hyperreflexia, carpopedal spasm (tetany), laryngospasm, and facial grimacing. A positive Chvostek sign (unilateral spasm of the facial muscles when the facial nerve is tapped) and a positive Trousseau sign (carpal spasm when upper arm is compressed with a blood pressure cuff) may be present. Irritability, confusion, fatigue, seizures, brittle hair and nails, and personality changes may occur. Diagnose with an ionized Ca^{++} level (<4.7 mg/dL), reduced PTH, and elevated phosphate. Treat with Ca^{++} and vitamin D supplements. Patients with renal failure must also reduce the amount of phosphate in their diet. Patients with tetany are treated with IV calcium gluconate.

Paget's Disease

Paget's disease is a disease of high bone turnover and disorganized osteoid formation. It is most prevalent in patients in the northeast US or of European descent and in older patients. The disease is usually asymptomatic, being detected on radiographs. However, it may present with bone pain, fractures, and bony deformities. Commonly involved bones include the skull, femur, tibia, pelvis, and humerus. Specifically, with skull involvement, the patient may note frequent headaches and increasing hat size, sometimes associated with deafness. Examination findings include frontal bossing, bowed legs, and superficial erythema and warmth, due to the increased vascularity of the bones. This disease is diagnosed with increased alkaline phosphatase, and elevated urinary hydroxyproline. Calcium and phosphorous are often normal. Imaging reveals hyperdense and enlarged bones in some regions and erosions in others. Bone scanning reveals increased uptake in certain areas. Treatment includes bisphosphonate and management of complications, including CHF, spinal cord compression, or nerve entrapment.

Immunologic and Oncologic Pathophysiology

Immune Deficiencies

There are multiple disorders that fall into the category of **primary immunodeficiency diseases.** These disorders are genetic or inherited disorders in which the body's immune system does not function properly. These disorders may involve low levels of antibodies, defects in the antibodies, or defects in cells that make up the immune system (T-cells, B-cells). Common variable immune deficiency is a common immune deficiency diagnosed in adulthood. This disorder is characterized by low levels of serum immunoglobins and antibodies, which substantially increases the risk of infection.

- **Signs and symptoms**: Recurrent infections are the hallmark sign of immune deficiency disorders. Recurrent infections most often involve the ears, sinuses, bronchi, and lungs. Lymphadenopathy may occur as well as splenomegaly. GI symptoms may include abdominal pain, nausea, vomiting, diarrhea and weight loss. Some patients may experience polyarthritis. Granulomas are also common and may occur in the lungs, lymph nodes, liver, and skin.
- **Diagnosis**: A physical assessment and patient history are used to diagnose immune deficiency disorders. Since immune deficiency disorders are genetic or inherited, family history should also be evaluated. Lab tests such as serum antibodies, serum immunoglobin levels and a complete blood count may also be used to assist in the diagnosis of immune deficiency disorders.
- **Treatment**: Patients with immune deficiency disorders often receive immunoglobulin replacement. Long term antibiotics may also be administered for recurrent infections. Educate patients to frequently wash hands, cook foods thoroughly, avoid large crowds, and other infection prevention techniques.

Congenital Immunodeficiencies

Congenital immunodeficiencies include:

- **Common variable immunodeficiency** is primarily an IgG deficiency due to absent plasma cells and B cell differentiation. These patients have increased susceptibility to encapsulated organisms and are more likely to develop bronchiectasis from the recurrent damage. They are also at higher risk for B cell neoplasms, GI malignancy, and autoimmune disease. Test is with functional antibody response and treatment with IVIG.
- **Congenital Agammaglobulinemia** (Bruton's, x-linked) usually leads to a susceptibility to recurrent pyogenic infections and low IgG and no IgA, IgM, IgE, IgD, or B cells.

- **Selective IgA deficiency** is the most common Ig deficiency and leads to recurrent sinopulmonary infections. It has association with recurrent giardiasis, GI malignancy, and autoimmune disorders, including celiac sprue. One should withhold IVIG due to possible anaphylactic reaction to IgA.
- **Wiskott-Aldrich syndrome** is the combination of thrombocytopenia, eczema, and immunodeficiency. It has associated low IgM and elevated IgA and IgE. BMT treats this successfully.

Complement Deficiencies

There are **deficiencies of all parts of the complement pathway**, including the following:

- **Classical deficiency** may include C1 (q, r, s), C2, and C4. This leads to immune complex syndromes and pyogenic infection, such as recurrent sinopulmonary infections with encapsulated bacteria. There is an association with SLE and other rheumatoid diseases. C2 is the most common deficiency in Caucasians in the US.
- **C3 and Alternative complement deficiency** may lead to immune complex syndromes and recurrent infections, such as severe pyogenic infections. It may also be associated with HUS.
- **Membrane attack complex (MAC) deficiency** is also known as terminal complement deficiency. This is associated with recurrent Neisseria infections (which can cause meningitis and sepsis) and immune complex diseases. The CH50 assay must be checked to determine the activity of the classical pathway. CH50 may also be used to follow disease activity in SLE.

Autoimmune System Disorders

Allergic interstitial/tubulointerstitial nephritis is inflammation and edema of the interstitial areas of the kidneys. Up to 92% of cases caused by allergic reaction to medications, such as antibiotics (B-lactams, fluoroquinolones, macrolides, and anti-tuberculin drugs), antivirals, NSAIDs, PPIs, antiepileptics, diuretics, chemotherapy, and allopurinol. **Symptoms** include fever, rash, and renal enlargement as well as fatigue, nausea, vomiting, and weight loss. **Diagnosis** is by renal biopsy. Urine tests may show eosinophils, blood, RBC casts and sterile pyuria. Increased protein may be seen in response to NSAIDs. **Treatment** is primarily supportive but requires stopping the triggering medication.

Eosinophilic esophagitis is the accumulation of eosinophils in the esophagus, resulting in chronic inflammation. Damage from proteins produced in esophageal tissue causes scarring and narrowing, resulting in dysphagia, vomiting, choking, GERD, upper abdominal pain, heartburn, and regurgitation. **Causes** include allergic reaction to pollens or foods. **Risk factors** include cold/dry climate, male gender, family history, allergies, and asthma. **Diagnosis** is per endoscopy with biopsy. Blood tests may help confirm allergic reactions. **Treatment** may include dietary limitations, PPIs, and topical steroids. Some may require dilation of the esophagus.

Churg-Strauss syndrome (AKA **eosinophilic granulomatosis with polyangiitis**) is an idiopathic form of pulmonary vasculitis that can affect multiple systems (skin and lungs most often) as well as affecting small- and medium-sized arteries in those with asthma. **Symptoms** include dyspnea, chest pain, skin rash, myopathy, arthropathy, rhinitis, sinusitis, abdominal pain, blood in stools, and paresthesia (from the involvement of nerves). The syndrome is characterized by eosinophilia >1500 cells/mcL or >10% of peripheral total WBC count. X-rays or CTs may show transient opacities or multiple nodules. Tissue biopsies typically show allergic granulomas. **Treatment** usually begins with corticosteroids but other immunosuppressive drugs (cyclophosphamide, methotrexate, azathioprine) may be used, especially if critical organs are involved. The goal of treatment is remission, but patients usually need to take drugs at least 2 years before they are tapered off of the drugs. Up to 50% of patients have relapses.

NEUTROPENIA

Neutropenia is identified as a **polymorphonuclear neutrophil count** equal to or less than 500/mL. **Chronic neutropenia** is a sustained condition of minimal neutrophils lasting 3 or more months. Neutropenia may occur from a decreased production of **white blood cells** (e.g., from chemotherapy or radiation therapy). It may also occur from a loss of white blood cells from autoimmune disease processes. Neutropenia is silent but dangerous. It leaves essentially no neutrophils to fight any threat of infection. Neutrophils make up as much as 70% of the white blood cells circulating in the blood. Neutropenia can be the cause of a septic situation, which can be life-threatening. Up to 70% of patients experiencing a fever while in a neutropenic state will die within 48 hours if not treated aggressively.

LEUKOPENIA

Leukopenia is defined as a decrease in white blood cells. Neutropenia is defined as a low number of neutrophils and is often used interchangeably with the term leukopenia. With a decrease in the number of circulating white blood cells, the patient is at an increased risk for the development of an infection. Leukopenia and neutropenia can occur from either a decrease in the production of white blood cells or an increase in their destruction. Infections, malignancy, autoimmune disorders, medications (including chemotherapy) and a history of radiation therapy may contribute to the development of leukopenia/neutropenia.

Signs and symptoms: Malaise, fever, chills, night sweats, shortness of breath, headache, cough, abdominal pain, tachycardia, and hypotension. A patient with neutropenia/leukopenia is at risk for the development of infections including pneumonia, skin infections, urinary tract infections and gastrointestinal infections. In addition, the patient is at an increased risk for sepsis.

Diagnosis: Complete blood count including an absolute neutrophil count. In addition, a bone marrow biopsy may be performed to determine the cause of the decrease in neutrophils.

Treatment: Supportive therapy is used in the treatment of leukopenia including the aggressive treatment of infections that may develop. Precautions should be taken to protect the patient from additional infections, including strict adherence to sterile technique and infection control procedures. Hematopoietic growth factors may also be given to stimulate the production of neutrophils.

LYMPHEDEMA

Lymphedema results from untreated or incurable **edema**. It is a chronic condition marked by swelling and accumulated fluids within the tissue. This accumulation is a result of lymphatic drainage failure, inadequate lymph transport capacity, an increased lymph production, or a combination of these. Primary disease is a result of **inadequately developed lymphatic pathways**, while the secondary disease process is due to **damage outside of the pathways**. The process is worsened and complicated as **macrophages** are released to control inflammation caused by the increased release of fibroblasts and keratinocytes. There is a gradual increase in adipose tissue and leakage of lymph through the skin. The skin and tissues gradually thicken and change in color, texture, tone, and temperature. It begins to blister and produce hyperkeratosis, warts, papillomatosis, and elephantiasis. There is an ever-increasing risk of infection and further complications.

HIV/AIDS

AIDS is a progression of infection with **human immunodeficiency virus** (HIV). AIDS is diagnosed when the following criteria are met:

- HIV infection
- CD4 count less than 200 cells/mm^3
- AIDS defining condition, such as opportunistic infections (cytomegalovirus, tuberculosis), wasting syndrome, neoplasms (Kaposi sarcoma), or AIDS dementia complex

Because there is such a wide range of AIDS defining conditions, the patient may present with many types of **symptoms**, depending upon the diagnosis, but more than half of AIDS patients exhibit:

- Fever
- Lymphadenopathy
- Pharyngitis
- Rash
- Myalgia/arthralgia
- It is important to review the following:
  - CD4 counts to determine immune status
  - WBC and differential for signs of infection
  - Cultures to help identify any infective agents
  - CBC to evaluate for signs of bleeding or thrombocytopenia

Treatment aims to cure or manage opportunistic conditions and control underlying HIV infection through highly active anti-retroviral therapy (HAART), 3 or more drugs used concurrently.

Hodgkin's Disease

Hodgkin's disease (HD) (lymphoma) is cancer originating in the lymphatic system, resulting in impairment of the immune system. The cancer eventually spreads outside the lymphatic system to other organs. With HD, the lymphatic system produces large abnormal B cells (Reed-Sternberg cells), impairing the ability of the body to produce antibodies. Diagnosis may include biopsy of enlarged nodes, CBC, radiographs, CT scan, MRI, gallium scan to show spread of HD, PET scan, and bone marrow biopsy.

Symptoms:

- Painless, enlarged lymph nodes (neck, axillary, clavicular, and femoral areas), sometimes to greater than 1 inch in diameter, with enlargement progressing from one nodal group to another
- Fever with chills and night sweats
- Anorexia
- Pruritus, weakness and fatigue, opportunistic infections
- Other symptoms relate to the area affected by the lymphoma, such as chest pain, cough and dyspnea, or abdominal pain and swelling

Treatment:

- Stabilizing patient
- Treating opportunistic infections
- Referral to oncology/radio-therapy for radiation and chemotherapy

LEUKEMIA

Leukemia is a condition in which the proliferating cells compete with normal cells for nutrition. Leukemia affects all cells because the abnormal cells in the bone marrow depress the formation of all elements, resulting in several consequences, regardless of the type of leukemia:

- Decrease in production of **erythrocytes** (RBCs), resulting in anemia
- Decrease in **neutrophils**, resulting in increased risk of infection
- Decrease in **platelets**, with subsequent decrease in clotting factors and increased bleeding
- Increased risk of **physiological fractures** because of invasion of bone marrow that weakens the periosteum
- Infiltration of **liver, spleen, and lymph glands**, resulting in enlargement and fibrosis
- Infiltration of the **CNS**, resulting in increased intracranial pressure, ventricular dilation, and meningeal irritation with headaches, vomiting, papilledema, nuchal rigidity, and coma progressing to death
- **Hypermetabolism** that deprives cells of nutrients, resulting in anorexia, weight loss, muscle atrophy, and fatigue

Review Video: Leukemia
Visit mometrix.com/academy and enter code: 940024

LUNG CANCER

SCLC

Small cell lung cancer (SCLC) is a rapidly-growing variant of lung cancer found in about 15% of new cases. Its origin is in the bronchi and this type of lung cancer occurs predominantly in smokers. At the time of diagnosis, the disease is usually symptomatic and metastases have generally already occurred. There are 3 subtypes of SCLC: oat cell or small-cell carcinoma, intermediate cell, and small cell combined with squamous cell carcinoma or adenocarcinoma. Differential diagnosis includes tests to distinguish it from slower-growing non-small cell lung cancer, lymphoma, sarcoidosis, metastases due to other primary tumors, or infectious processes. In addition to routine procedures like history, physical examination, and laboratory tests, SCLC is generally staged using imaging tests. In particular, a CT scan with contrast is done to assess the involvement in the lung and other sites, and an MRI of the brain and/or a bone scan may also be done to look for metastases. A bone marrow biopsy may also be indicated.

NSCLC

Non-small cell lung cancer (NSCLC) is a blanket term for several histological types of lung cancer not classified as SCLC. The major histological variants are adenocarcinoma, squamous cell carcinoma, and large cell. The large cell type is anaplastic, which means the cells are relatively undifferentiated. Diagnosis of NSCLCs includes exclusion of small cell lung carcinoma, metastatic lung lesions from other primary sources, sarcoidosis, and infections. The clinician generally stages the disease through use of history, physical examination, and laboratory tests. Imaging studies usually include not only CT scans but also positron emission tomography (PET) and, if metastases are suspected, a brain MRI and possibly a bone scan. Mediastinal node biopsies are generally performed if the PET scan indicates later stage disease; various types of incisions can be made, such as those into the sternum or mediastinum.

LUNG CANCER TREATMENT

Since **SCLC** is an aggressive disease, surgical procedures are not useful and not generally performed. If the cancer is relatively limited, chemotherapy and irradiation of both the chest and brain (to prevent brain metastases) are done. Otherwise, several cycles of combination or multi-agent chemotherapy are tried but the prognosis is poor.

For **NSCLC**, surgical resection is usually effective for the early stages I and II. For stages IIIA and IIIB, indicating metastatic involvement, chemotherapy possibly combined with radiation is generally used either before surgery (IIIA) or as the treatment modality. If the latter patients also have a malignant pleural effusion, they are treated as stage IV. Stage IV patients are given combination chemotherapy, mainly to improve their quality of life. Individuals with recurrent NSCLC are also treated with combination chemotherapy.

Breast Cancer

Staging

The American Joint Committee on Cancer **TNM Staging** has recently developed a complex staging classification for breast cancer. In general, however, early invasive breast cancer would be Stage I or II (IIA or IIB). In these stages, there is either no lymph node involvement or only same-side axillary region lymph node involvement with no distant metastases. Nevertheless, diagnostic tests should include bilateral mammography (and possibly other imaging techniques), blood profiles, hepatic and renal function tests, serum alkaline phosphatase levels, and lymph node biopsy or mapping. Assays for prognostic factors like high levels of HER2 or hormone receptors may also be done. Management is surgery that either conserves the breast or a modified radical mastectomy in which the pectoral muscles are not removed. If there is nodal involvement or other factors exist (such as positive hormone receptors or large tumor size), adjuvant chemotherapy or endocrine treatment is added.

Locally Advanced or Recurrent Breast Cancer or Distant Metastases

Locally advanced stage III breast cancer is a comprehensive term for a highly heterogeneous grouping. All Stage III patients have either some sort of nodal involvement and/or their tumor has extended into the chest wall or skin. They do not have distant metastases. Once the disease has reached this stage, multiple treatment strategies are needed, including chemotherapy (and endocrine therapy in receptor-positive women), surgery, and radiation. Locally recurrent breast cancer, on the other hand, is generally due to insufficient removal of the primary lesion (such as with breast conservation surgery); it can often be managed with further surgery, although other modalities may be needed if there has been nodal or metastatic spread. Once there is metastatic involvement, therapies are merely palliative and the prognosis is poor.

Prostate Cancer

At present, about one out of nine men will develop **prostate cancer** at some point, and approximately 2-3% of those will die of the disease. There are familial groupings of prostate cancer; for example, mutations in the RNASEL and MSR1 loci coding for host response to infection appear to predispose a man to prostate cancer. Diet affects susceptibility to prostate cancer; in particular, consumption of red meat cooked at high temperature to release aromatic compounds is highly correlated to development of the cancer. Ethnicity may play a role, as African Americans in the U. S. have an especially high rate of prostate cancer, but this may be due in part to diet.

Mechanisms That Contribute to Development of Prostate Cancer

Germline mutations in the RNASEL and MSR1 genes have been associated with an increased risk of developing **prostate cancer**. There is some evidence that inflammation and infection may play a role in the progression of the disease, and development of lesions termed proliferate inflammatory atrophy (PIA) may predispose a man to later prostate intraepithelial neoplasia and prostate cancer. Molecular changes have also been closely associated with disease progression. These include somatic inactivation of the GSTP1 gene, which fosters susceptibility to oxidant and electron-accepting carcinogens and depression of various functions caused by gene mutations, such as the PTEN tumor-suppressor gene, NKA3.1, and CDKN1B. As discussed previously, screening tests include serum prostate-specific antigen (PSA) levels and digital rectal examination. Diagnosis is generally confirmed by core needle biopsy.

Colon Cancer

The factor most closely associated with development of **colon cancer** is age, with about 9 out 10 cases identified after age 50. The vast majority of cases have not been correlated to any heritable gene mutation. However, there is a several-fold increase in risk of development of the disease when a close relative is affected, and there are several familial syndromes related to colon cancer (most notably familial adenomatous polyposis or FAP and HNPCC or hereditary nonpolyposis colon cancer). Risk of colon cancer has been associated with certain dietary practices, including high intake of low fiber and high fat foods. It has also been associated with environmental influences, such as exposure to tobacco. The disease often develops through mutations attributable to either chromosomal instability or to a lesser extent microsatellite (repetitive DNA sequence) instability. The genetic change most often found in patients with both precursor adenomatous polyps or actual colon cancer is a defective APC tumor suppressor locus.

Procedures for Prevention, Diagnosis, and Staging of Colon Cancer

Identification of individuals with familial syndromes or known genetic changes associated with colon cancer is theoretically a means of preventing colon cancer. Realistically, at present this is rarely done. COX-2 inhibitors, which are basically anti-inflammatory agents, are sometimes used as chemo preventive drugs. Patients usually present with symptoms like anemia, fatigue, weight loss, or changes in bowel habits. A small portion of them have other cancers and up to 40% have polyps in addition to the primary tumor. Colonoscopy is suggested as a diagnostic procedure every 10 years beginning at age 50, and it involves inspection of the entire large intestine using a flexible fiberoptic endoscope. Benign polyps, possible cancer precursors, can be immediately excised. Other diagnostic probes include sigmoidoscopy and virtual colonoscopy. Staging is usually done utilizing imaging techniques like CT scans, MRIs, or PET scans. Liver metastases, common in conjunction with colorectal cancers, can be best visualized using intraoperative ultrasound.

Staging

There are several classification systems for **staging colorectal cancers**. The most common scheme utilized is the Astler-Coller modified Duke's system. The emphasis of this classification scheme is the depth of tumor invasion into the colon wall. The modified Astler-Coller (MAC), the traditional Duke, and the American Joint Committee on Cancer or AJCC (based on TMN) classification schemes are interrelated. According to Astler-Coller, MAC A is comprised of lesions limited to the mucosa or sub mucosa; MAC B1 and B2 involve extension into or through the muscularis propria; MAC C1, 2, or 3 imply nodal involvement along with extension into or through the bowel wall; MAC D means evidence of distant metastases. These correspond roughly to Duke's A, B, C and D. The AJCC or TMN classification defines stages 0 (carcinoma in situ) through IV.

Tumor Lysis Syndrome

Tumor lysis syndrome occurs when intracellular contents are released from tumor cells, leading to electrolyte imbalances (hyperkalemia, hyperphosphatemia, hypocalcemia and hyperuricemia) when the kidneys are unable to excrete the large volume of metabolites. Tumor lysis syndrome is most common after treatment of hematologic malignancies but can occur due to any type of tumor that is sensitive to chemotherapy. The primary goals of therapy for tumor lysis syndrome are to increase urine production through IV hydration in order to prevent renal failure and to decrease uric acid concentration, usually with administration of allopurinol. The urine pH should be maintained at 7 or higher. Electrolyte levels should be closely monitored, as hyperkalemia is a risk. Patients at moderate risk (intermediate grade lymphomas, acute leukemias) should begin prophylactic allopurinol before chemotherapy, and those at higher risk (high grade lymphomas or acute leukemias with WBC count >50,000) should begin rasburicase.

Hematologic Pathophysiology

Anemia

Anemia occurs when there is an insufficient number of red blood cells to sufficiently oxygenate the body. As a result of the decreased level of oxygen being supplied to the organs, the body will attempt to compensate by increasing cardiac output and redistributing blood to the brain and heart. In return, the blood supply to the skin, abdominal organs, and kidneys is decreased. Anemia can occur from blood loss, increased destruction of red blood cells (hemolytic anemia), or as a result of a decreased production in red blood cells.

Signs and symptoms: Pallor, fatigue, hypotension, weakness and mental status changes. As perfusion decreases and the body attempts to compensate for the lack of oxygenation, tachycardia, chest pain, and shortness of breath may occur. In hemolytic anemias, jaundice and splenomegaly may occur as the result of the breakdown of red blood cells and the excretion of bilirubin.

Diagnosis: A complete blood count, reticulocyte count, and iron studies may be used to diagnose anemia.

Treatment: The treatment of anemia is focused on treating the underlying cause. Parenteral iron may be given for patients with iron deficiency anemias caused from chronic blood loss, or inadequate iron intake or absorption. Blood transfusions are used to treat patients with active bleeding as well as those patients who are displaying significant clinical symptoms. Erythropoietin stimulating proteins may also be utilized to decrease the need for a transfusion.

Sickle Cell Disease

Sickle cell disease is a recessive genetic disorder of chromosome 11, causing hemoglobin to be defective so that red blood cells (RBCs) are sickle-shaped and inflexible, resulting in their accumulating in small vessels and causing painful blockage. While normal RBCs survive 120 days, sickled cells may survive only 10 to 20 days, stressing the bone marrow that cannot produce fast enough and resulting in severe anemia. There are 5 variations of sickle cell disease, with sickle cell anemia the most severe. Different types of crises occur (aplastic, hemolytic, vaso-occlusive, and sequestrating), which can cause infarctions in organs, severe pain, damage to organs, and rapid enlargement of liver and spleen. Complications include anemia, acute chest syndrome, congestive heart failure, strokes, delayed growth, infections, pulmonary hypertension, liver and kidney disorders, retinopathy, seizures, and osteonecrosis. Sickle cell disease occurs almost exclusively in African Americans in the United States, with 8% to 10% carriers.

Review Video: Sickle Cell Disease
Visit mometrix.com/academy and enter code: 603869

Treatment

Treatment for **sickle cell disease** includes:

- **Prophylactic penicillin** for children from 2 months to 5 years to prevent pneumonia
- **IV fluids** to prevent dehydration
- **Analgesics** (morphine) during painful crises
- **Folic acid** for anemia
- **Oxygen** for congestive heart failure or pulmonary disease
- **Blood transfusions** with chelation therapy to remove excess iron OR erythropheresis, in which red cells are removed and replaced with healthy cells, either autologous or from a donor
- **Hematopoietic stem cells transplantation** is the only curative treatment, but immunosuppressive drugs must be used and success rates are only about 85%, so the procedure is only used on those at high risk. It requires ablation of bone marrow, placing the patient at increased risk.
- **Partial chimerism** uses a mixture of the donor and the recipient's bone marrow stem cells and does not require ablation of bone marrow. It is showing good success.

Polycythemia Vera

Polycythemia vera is a condition in which there is abnormal production of blood cells in the bone marrow. Erythrocytes (red blood cells) are primarily affected. The disease is more common in men older than 40 years. Polycythemia may be primary or secondary, related to conditions causing hypoxia. The blood increases in viscosity, resulting in a number of **symptoms**:

- Dizziness, headache, weakness, and fatigue
- Dyspnea, especially when supine
- Flushing of skin, blue-tinged skin discoloration, and red lesions
- Itching after warm bath
- Left upper abdominal fullness and splenomegaly
- Phlebitis from blood clots
- Vision disturbances
- Complications include stroke, hemorrhage, and heart failure

Diagnosis includes CBC with differential, chemistry panel, bone marrow biopsy, and Vitamin B12 level. Red cell mass will be more than 25% above normal.

Treatment includes:

- **Phlebotomy** to remove 500 mL (lesser amounts for children) of blood to decrease blood viscosity, repeated weekly until hematocrit stable (less than 45%)
- Referral for **chemotherapy** (hydroxyurea) to suppress marrow production
- **Interferon** to decrease need for phlebotomy

Von Willebrand Disease

Von Willebrand disease is a group of congenital bleeding disorders (inherited from either parent) affecting 1-2% of the population, associated with deficiency or lack of von Willebrand factor (vWF), a glycoprotein that is synthesized, stored, and secreted by vascular endothelial cells. This protein interacts with thrombocytes to create a clot and prevent hemorrhage; however, with von Willebrand disease, this clotting mechanism is impaired. There are 3 types:

- **Type I**: Low levels of vWF and also sometimes factor VIII (dominant inheritance)
- **Type II**: Abnormal vWF (subtypes a, b) may increase or decrease clotting (dominant inheritance)
- **Type III**: Absence of vWF and less than 10% factor VIII (recessive inheritance)

Symptoms vary in severity and include bruising, menorrhagia, recurrent epistaxis, and hemorrhage.

Treatment includes:

- **Desmopressin acetate** parenterally or nasally to stimulate production of clotting factor (mild cases)
- **Severe bleeding**: factor VIII concentrates with vWF, such as Humate-P

Hemophilia

Hemophilia is an inherited disorder in which the person lacks adequate clotting factors. There are 3 types:

- **Type A**: lack of clotting factor VIII (90% of cases)
- **Type B**: lack of clotting factor IX
- **Type C**: lack of clotting factor XI (affects both sexes, rarely occurs in the United States)

Both Type A and B are usually X-linked disorders, affecting only males. The severity of the disease depends on the amount of clotting factor in the blood.

Symptoms:

- Bleeding with severe trauma or stress (mild cases)
- Unexplained bruises, bleeding, swelling, joint pain
- Spontaneous hemorrhage (severe cases), often in the joints but can be anywhere in the body
- Epistaxis, mucosal bleeding
- First symptoms often occur during infancy when the child becomes active, resulting in frequent bruises

Treatment:

- Desmopressin acetate parenterally or nasally to stimulate production of clotting factor (mild cases)
- Infusions of clotting factor from donated blood or recombinant clotting factors (genetically engineered), utilizing guidelines for dosing
- Infusions of plasma (Type C)

Disseminated Intravascular Coagulation

Pathology

Disseminated intravascular coagulation (DIC) (consumption coagulopathy) is a secondary disorder that is triggered by another disorder such as trauma, congenital heart disease, necrotizing enterocolitis, sepsis, and severe viral infections. DIC triggers both coagulation and hemorrhage through a complex series of events. Trauma causes tissue factor (transmembrane glycoprotein) to enter the circulation and bind with coagulation factors, triggering the coagulation cascade. This stimulates thrombin to convert fibrinogen to fibrin, causing aggregation and destruction of platelets and forming clots that can be disseminated throughout the intravascular system. These clots increase in size as platelets adhere to the clots, causing blockage of both the microvascular systems and larger vessels, which can result in ischemia and necrosis. Clot formation triggers fibrinolysis and plasmin to breakdown fibrin and fibrinogen, causing the destruction of clotting factors and resulting in hemorrhage. Both processes, clotting and hemorrhage, continue at the same time, placing the patient at high risk for death, even with treatment.

Symptoms and Treatment

The onset of **symptoms of DIC** may be very rapid or be a slower chronic progression from a disease. Those who develop the chronic manifestation of the disease usually have fewer acute symptoms and may slowly develop ecchymosis or bleeding wounds.

Symptoms include:

- Bleeding from surgical or venous puncture sites
- Evidence of GI bleeding with distention, bloody diarrhea
- Hypotension and acute symptoms of shock
- Petechiae and purpura with extensive bleeding into the tissues
- Laboratory abnormalities:
  - Prolonged prothrombin and partial prothrombin times
  - Decreased platelet counts and fragmented RBCs
  - Decreased fibrinogen

Treatment includes:

- Identifying and treating underlying cause
- Massive blood transfusion protocol; replacement of blood products, such as platelets and fresh frozen plasma
- Anticoagulation therapy (heparin) to increase clotting time
- Cryoprecipitate to increase fibrinogen levels
- Coagulation inhibitors and coagulation factors

Thrombocytopenia

Thrombocytopenia is a deficiency of circulating platelets in the blood. It can be caused by a decrease in the production of platelets from the bone marrow or an increase in destruction of platelets. Thrombocytopenia may also be caused from the use of heparin. Heparin induced thrombocytopenia can occur after heparin therapy (average 4-14 days post therapy) and is characterized by a decrease in platelet count to less than 50% of baseline or the occurrence of an unexplained thrombolytic event. A decreased production of platelets within the bone marrow can occur as a result of malignancy, bone marrow failure, infection, alcohol abuse, or a nutritional deficiency. An increase in the destruction of platelets may occur in disseminated intravascular coagulation, vasculitis, thrombotic thrombocytopenic purpura, sepsis, or idiopathic thrombocytopenic purpura.

Signs and symptoms: Signs and symptoms may include petechiae, ecchymosis, bleeding from the mouth or gums, epistaxis, pallor, weakness, fatigue, splenomegaly, blood in the urine or stool, and jaundice.

Diagnosis: Physical exam and lab studies including complete blood count, partial thromboplastin time and prothrombin time may be used to diagnosis thrombocytopenia. A bone marrow biopsy may be indicated to determine the cause of the decreased production of platelets.

Treatment: Treatment of thrombocytopenia involves identifying and treating the underlying cause. Medications that decrease the platelet count should be held. Platelet transfusions may be administered to patients with extremely low counts (less than 50,000) or if spontaneous bleeding occurs. Platelet transfusions are contraindicated in patients with thrombotic thrombocytopenia purpura.

ITP

The autoimmune disorder **idiopathic thrombocytopenic purpura (ITP)** causes an immune response to platelets, resulting in decreased platelet counts. ITP affects primarily children and young women although it can occur at any age. The acute form primarily occurs in children, but the chronic form affects primarily adults. Platelet counts are usually 150,000–400,000 per mcL. With ITP, platelet levels are less than 100,000. Maintaining a platelet count of at least 30,000 is necessary to prevent intracranial hemorrhage, the primary concern. The cause of ITP is unclear and may be precipitated by viral infection, sulfa drugs, and conditions, such as lupus erythematosus. ITP is usually not life threatening and can be controlled. **Symptoms** include:

- Bruising and petechiae with hematoma in some cases
- Epistaxis
- Increased menstrual flow in post-puberty females

Treatment includes:

- Corticosteroids to depress immune response and increase platelet count
- Splenectomy may be indicated for chronic conditions
- Platelet transfusions
- Avoiding aspirin, ibuprofen, or other NSAIDs

HITTS

Heparin-induced thrombocytopenia and thrombosis syndrome (HITTS) occurs in patients receiving heparin for anticoagulation. There are two types:

- **Type I** is a transient condition occurring within a few days and causing depletion of platelets (<100,000 mm^3), but heparin may be continued as the condition usually resolves without intervention.
- **Type II** is an autoimmune reaction to heparin that occurs in 3–5% of those receiving unfractionated heparin and also occurs with low-molecular-weight heparin. It is characterized by low platelets (<50,000 mm^3) that are ≥50% below baseline. Onset is 5–14 days but can occur within hours of heparinization. Death rates are <30%. Heparin-antibody complexes form and release platelet factor 4 (PF4), which attracts heparin molecules and adheres to platelets and endothelial lining, stimulating thrombin and platelet clumping. This puts the patient at risk for thrombosis and vessel occlusion rather than hemorrhage, causing stroke, myocardial infarction, and limb ischemia with symptoms associated with the site of thrombosis.

Treatment includes:

- Discontinuation of heparin
- Direct thrombin inhibitors (lepirudin, argatroban)
- Monitor for signs/symptoms of thrombus/embolus

ReoPro-Induced Coagulopathy

ReoPro® (abciximab) is used to prevent cardiac ischemia for those undergoing percutaneous cardiac intervention by inhibiting the aggregation of platelets. It is used with aspirin and/or weight-adjusted low dose heparin and potentiates the action of anticoagulants. However, its use with non-weight adjusted, longer acting heparin can cause thrombocytopenia with increased risk of hemorrhage, especially with readministration of the drug, which can induce the formation of antibodies and an allergic reaction that is characterized by anaphylaxis and thrombocytopenia, referred to as **ReoPro-induced coagulopathy**. Because of the danger of hemorrhage, ReoPro® is contraindicated if there is active bleeding or a history of bleeding or CVA within the 2 years prior, history of a CVA, platelet count <100,000 mm^3, or recent history of oral anticoagulation. Careful monitoring of platelet counts prior to administration and the use of weight-adjusted low dose heparin is important to prevent bleeding. Heparin should be discontinued after the PCI.

Gastrointestinal Pathophysiology

Abdominal Trauma

Splenic Injuries

The **spleen** is the most frequently injured solid organ in blunt trauma. Injuries to the spleen are the most common because the spleen is not well protected by the rib cage and is very vascular. Symptoms may be very non-specific. Kehr sign (radiating pain in left shoulder) indicates intra-abdominal bleeding and Cullen sign (ecchymosis around umbilicus) indicates hemorrhage from ruptured spleen. Some may have right upper abdominal pain although diffuse abdominal pain often occurs with blood loss, associated with hypotension. Splenic injuries are **classified** according to the degree of injury:

- I: Tear in splenic capsules or hematoma
- II: Laceration of parenchyma (<3 cm)
- III: Laceration of parenchyma (≥3cm)
- IV: Multiple lacerations of parenchyma or burst-type injury

Treatment: Because removing the spleen increases the risk of life-threatening infections, every effort (bed rest, transfusion, reduced activity for at least 8 weeks) is done to avoid surgery (argon gas, fibrin "glue", or therapeutic ultrasound). Lab testing for the absence of Howell-Jolly bodies indicates the spleen in functioning properly. If conservative efforts fail (usually occurs in first 72 hours), a splenectomy is performed. After surgery, the patient has an increased risk for infection and thrombosis. Lifetime anticoagulation therapy and vaccinations (combo of pneumonia/meningitis/influenza B vaccine) should be administered.

Hepatic Injuries

Hepatic injury is the most common cause of death from abdominal trauma. It is particularly dangerous as hematoma rupture can occur hours to 6 weeks after the time of injury. Because hepatic injury is often associated with multiple organ damage, symptoms may be non-specific and difficult to diagnose. Therefore, elevation in liver transaminase levels or elevation of right hemidiaphragm on x-ray in trauma patients indicates damage that may require further examination. Liver injuries are classified according to the **degree of injury**:

- I: Tears in capsule with hematoma
- II: Laceration(s) of parenchyma (<3 cm)
- III: Laceration(s) of parenchyma (≥3 cm)
- IV: Destruction of 25-75% of lobe from burst injury
- V: Destruction of >75% of lobe from burst injury
- VI: Avulsion [tearing away]

Hemodynamically stable patients are managed medically, but surgical repair may be necessary if the patient is unstable or bleeding. Hemorrhage is a common complication of hepatic injury and may require ligation of hepatic arteries or veins. Treatment often includes intravenous fluids for fluid volume deficit as well as blood products (plasma, platelets) for coagulopathies. Surgical or angiographic embolization of the tear may be indicated in severe injury.

Abdominal Compartment Syndrome

Abdominal trauma with pronounced shock increases risk of **compartment syndrome**, in which the pressure in the abdomen increases to the point of acute ischemia and anoxia of the tissues. Causes include edema of the intestines (trauma/surgical manipulation), reduced expansion of abdominal cavity (burns), hemorrhage, and capillary leakage after excessive fluid resuscitation.

Signs/Symptoms: Increased airway pressures and acute respiratory distress syndrome, decreased U/O, and cerebral edema.

Diagnosis: Increased intra-abdominal pressure (>20 cmH_2O), measured by a Foley catheter or NG tube with a pressure transducer or water-column manometry; elevated CVP and ICP, decreased CO and GFR.

Treatment includes:

- Medications: Sudden release of pressure and reperfusion may cause acidosis, hyperkalemia, vasodilation, and cardiac arrest. The patient should be given crystalloid solutions before decompression. Treatment may also include milrinone, dopamine, and mannitol.
- Surgical decompression.

Prevention: If risk for compartment syndrome exists, the wound should not be closed, but left open and covered with a sterile dressing. Negative-pressure wound therapy may be used to decrease risk.

Peritonitis

Peritonitis (inflammation of the peritoneum) may be primary (from infection of blood or lymph) or, more commonly, secondary, related to perforation or trauma of the gastrointestinal tract. Common causes include perforated bowel, ruptured appendix, abdominal trauma, abdominal surgery, peritoneal dialysis or chemotherapy, or leakage of sterile fluids, such as blood, into the peritoneum.

Symptoms: Diffuse abdominal pain with rebound tenderness (Blumberg's sign), abdominal rigidity, paralytic ileus, fever (with infection), nausea and vomiting, and sinus tachycardia.

Diagnosis: Increased WBC (>15,000), abdominal Xray/CT, paracentesis, blood and peritoneal fluid culture.

Treatment includes:

- Intravenous fluids and electrolytes
- Broad-spectrum antibiotics
- Laparoscopy as indicated to determine cause of peritonitis and effect repair

Appendicitis

Appendicitis is inflammation of the appendix often caused by luminal obstruction and pressure within the lumen; secretions build up and can eventually perforate the appendix. Diagnosis can be made difficult by the fact that there is some variation in the exact location of the appendix in some patients. Appendicitis can occur in all ages, but children younger than 2 years usually present with peritonitis or sepsis because of difficulty in early diagnosis. **Symptoms** include:

- Acute abdominal pain, which may be epigastric, periumbilical, right lower quadrant, or right flank with rebound tenderness
- Anorexia
- Nausea and vomiting
- Positive psoas and obturator signs
- Fever may develop after 24 hours
- Malaise
- Bowel irregularity and flatulence

Diagnosis is based on clinical presentation, CBC (although leukocytosis may not be present), urinalysis, and imaging studies (usually an abdominal CT with contrast).

Cholecystitis

Cholecystitis can result in obstruction of the bile duct related to calculi as well as pancreatitis from obstruction of the pancreatic duct. In **acute cholecystitis**, there is fever, leukocytosis, right upper quadrant abdominal pain, and inflammation of the gallbladder. The disease is most common in overweight women 20-40 years of age, but can occur in pregnant women and people of all ages, especially those who are diabetic or elderly. Cholecystitis may develop secondary to cystic fibrosis, obesity, or total parenteral nutrition. Many times, cholecystitis may resolve in about 7-10 days on its own, but acute cholecystitis may need surgical intervention to prevent complications such as gangrene in the gallbladder or perforation. Diagnosis is confirmed by ultrasound of gallbladder showing thickening of gallbladder walls or positive Murphy's sign, or a HIDA scan showing failure to fill.

Symptoms:

- Severe right upper quadrant or epigastric pain (ranging from 2-6 hours per episode)
- Nausea and vomiting
- Jaundice
- Altered mental status
- Positive Murphy's sign

Treatment:

- Antibiotics for sepsis/ascending cholangitis
- Antispasmodic agents (glycopyrrolate) for biliary colic and vomiting
- Analgesics (note that opioids result in increased sphincter of Oddi pressure)
- Antiemetics
- Surgical consultation for possible laparoscopic or open cholecystectomy

Erosive vs. Nonerosive Gastritis

Gastritis is inflammation of the epithelium or endothelium of the stomach. Types include:

- **Erosive**: Typically caused by alcohol, NSAIDs, illness, portal hypertension, and/or stress. Risk factors include severe illness, mechanical ventilation, trauma, sepsis, organ failure, and burns. Patients may be essentially asymptomatic but may have hematemesis or "coffee ground" emesis. Treatment depends on cause and severity but often includes a proton pump inhibitor (such as omeprazole 20-40 mg per day). Some may receive an H2-rceptor (such as ranitidine or famotidine). Those with portal hypertension may respond to propranolol or nadolol or portal decompression.
- **Nonerosive**: Typically caused by Helicobacter pylori infection or pernicious anemia. H. pylori infection can lead to gastric and duodenal ulcers. Treatment for H. pylori is per antibiotics and proton pump inhibitors with standard triple or standard quadruple therapy. Pernicious anemia is treated with vitamin B-12. Gastritis may also be caused by a wide range of pathogens, including parasites, so treatment depends on the causative agent.

Gastroenteritis

Viral Gastroenteritis

Viral gastroenteritis (commonly referred to as stomach flu) is characterized by nausea, vomiting, abdominal cramping, watery (may become bloody) diarrhea, headache, muscle aches, and fever. Viral gastroenteritis is spread through the fecal-oral route. Common causes include:

- **Norovirus**: Symptoms generally include diarrhea and vomiting with symptoms persisting for 1-3 days. Most people do not require treatment, but if diarrhea or vomiting is severe, an antiemetic or antidiarrheal may be prescribed if the patient is younger than 65. If severe dehydration occurs, the patient may require intravenous fluids until she is able to resume adequate oral intake.
- **Rotavirus**: Symptoms include watery diarrhea, nausea, vomiting, abdominal pain and cramping, lack of appetite and fever. Patients may become easily dehydrated and require rehydration with Pedialyte or Rice-Lyte or IV fluids. Medications are usually not needed but the rotavirus vaccine prevents severe rotavirus-related diarrhea and is given in 3 doses (2 months, 4 months, and 6 months).

Bacterial Gastroenteritis

Bacterial gastroenteritis generally results in cramping, nausea, and severe diarrhea. Some bacteria cause gastroenteritis because of enterotoxins that adhere to the mucosa of the intestines and others because of exotoxins that remain in contaminated food. Some bacteria directly invade the intestinal mucosa. Bacterial gastroenteritis is commonly caused by:

- ***Salmonella***: Sudden onset of bloody diarrhea, abdominal cramping, nausea, and vomiting, leading to dehydration. Infection may become systemic and life-threatening. Treatment is supportive although antibiotics may be administered to those at risk.

- ***Campylobacter***: Bloody diarrhea, cramping, fever, for up to 7 days that usually resolves but may become systemic in those who are immunocompromised. Treatment is primarily supportive with antibiotics only for those at risk.
- ***Shigella* spp.**: Most common in children <5 and presents with fever, abdominal cramping, and bloody diarrhea, persisting 5-7 days. Treatment is primarily supportive (rehydration) although those at risk (very young, old, immunocompromised) may receive antibiotics because the disease may become systemic.
- ***Escherichia coli***: Different strains are associated with traveler's diarrhea and food-borne illnesses, and severity varies. Most result in diarrhea, nausea, vomiting, and cramping, but some strains (0157) may develop into life-threatening hemolytic uremic syndrome (HUS). Treatment is supportive. Antibiotics increase risk of developing HUS.

Parasitic Gastroenteritis

Parasitic gastroenteritis is generally caused by infection with protozoa (one-celled pathogens):

- ***Giardia intestinalis***: Common cause of waterborne (drinking and recreational) disease and non-bacterial diarrhea, resulting from fecal contamination. Symptoms include diarrhea, abdominal cramping, flatulence, greasy floating stools, nausea and vomiting as well as weight loss. Symptoms usually persist for up to 3 weeks although some develop chronic disease. Metronidazole is the drug of choice: Adults, 250 mg TID for 5-7 days. Pediatrics, 15 mg/kg/day in 3 doses for 5-7 days.
- ***Cryptosporidium parvum***: About 10,000 cases occur in the US each year, usually from contact with fecal-contaminated water. Symptoms include watery diarrhea, abdominal pain, nausea, vomiting, weight loss, and fever and persist for up to 2 weeks although a severe chronic infection may occur in those who are immunocompromised. Treatment for non-HIV-infected patients (medications ineffective for HIV patients): Adults and children >11, Nitazoxanide 500 mg BID for 3 days. Pediatrics, 1-3 years 100 mg BID for 3 days; 4-11 years 200 mg BID for 3 days.

Constipation and Impaction

Constipation is a condition with bowel movements less frequent than normal for a person, or hard, small stool that is evacuated fewer than 3 times weekly. Food moves through the GI from the small intestine to the colon in semi-liquid form. Constipation results from the colon, where fluid is absorbed. If too much fluid is absorbed, the stool can become too dry. People may have abdominal distention and cramps and need to strain for defecation.

Fecal impaction occurs when the hard stool moves into the rectum and becomes a large, dense, immovable mass that cannot be evacuated even with straining, usually as a result of chronic constipation. In addition to abdominal cramps and distention, the person may feel intense rectal pressure and pain accompanied by a sense of urgency to defecate. Nausea and vomiting may also occur. Hemorrhoids will often become engorged. Fecal incontinence, with liquid stool leaking about the impaction, is common.

Medical Procedures to Evaluate Causes of Constipation

Medical procedures to evaluate causes of **constipation** should be preceded by a careful history as this may help to define the type and guide the choice of diagnostic procedures. Most tests are necessary only for severe constipation that does not respond to treatment. Medical diagnostic procedures may include the following:

- **Physical exam** should include rectal exam and abdominal palpation to assess for obvious hard stool or impaction.
- **Blood tests** can identify hypothyroidism and excess parathyroid hormone.
- **Abdominal x-ray** may show large amounts of stool in the colon.
- **Barium enema** can indicate tumors or strictures causing obstruction.
- **Colonic transit studies** can show defects of the neuromuscular system.
- **Defecography** shows the defecation process and abnormalities of anatomy.
- **Anorectal manometry studies** show malfunction of anorectal muscles.
- **Colonic motility studies** measure the pattern of colonic pressure.
- **Colonoscope** allows direct visualization of the lumen of the rectum and colon.

Bowel Obstructions

Bowel obstruction occurs when there is a mechanical obstruction of the passage of intestinal contents because of constriction of the lumen, occlusion of the lumen, adhesion formation, or lack of muscular contractions (paralytic ileus). Symptoms include abdominal pain, rigidity, and distention, n/v, dehydration, constipation, and respiratory distress from the diaphragm pushing against the pleural cavity, sepsis and shock. Treatment includes strict NPO, insertion of naso/orogastric tube, IV fluids and careful monitoring; may correct spontaneously, severe obstruction requires surgery.

Bowel Infarctions

Bowel infarction is ischemia of the intestines related to severely restricted blood supply. It can be the result of a number of different conditions, such as strangulated bowel or occlusion of arteries of the mesentery, and may follow untreated bowel obstruction. Patients present with acute abdomen and shock, and mortality rates are very high even with resection of infarcted bowel. Treatment includes replacing volume, correcting the underlying issue, improving blood flow to the mesentery, insertion of NGT, and/or surgery.

Intestinal Perforation

Intestinal perforation is a partial or complete tear in the intestinal wall, leaking intestinal contents into the peritoneum. Causes include trauma, NSAIDs (elderly, patients with diverticulitis), acute appendicitis, PUD, iatrogenic (laparoscopy, endoscopy, colonoscopy, radiotherapy), bacterial infections, IBS, and ingestion of toxic substances (acids) or foreign bodies (toothpicks). The danger posed by infection after perforation varies depending upon the site. The stomach and proximal portions of the small intestine have little bacteria, but the distal portion of the small intestine contains aerobic bacteria, such as *E. coli,* as well as anaerobic bacteria.

Signs/Symptoms: (appear within 24-48 hours): Abdominal pain and distention and rigidity, fever, guarding and rebound tenderness, tachycardia, dyspnea, absent bowel sounds/paralytic ileus with nausea and vomiting; Sepsis and abscess or fistula formation can occur.

Diagnosis: Labs: elevated WBC; lactic acid and pH change as late signs. X-ray and CT will show free air in abdominal cavity.

Treatment includes:

- Prompt antibiotic therapy and surgical repair with peritoneal lavage
- The abdominal wound may be left open to heal by secondary intention and to prevent compartment syndrome

Gastroesophageal Reflux

Gastroesophageal reflux (GER) occurs when the lower esophageal sphincter fails to remain closed, allowing the contents of the stomach to back into the esophagus. This reflux of the acid containing contents of the stomach may cause irritation of the lining of the esophagus. Over time, damage to the lining of the esophagus can occur. In some patients, this may lead to the formation of Barrett's esophagus. In Barrett's esophagus, the lining of the esophagus begins to resemble the tissue lining the intestine. Patients with Barrett's esophagus have an increased risk of developing esophageal adenocarcinoma.

Signs and symptoms: Heartburn, dysphagia, belching, water brash, sore throat, hoarseness, and chest pain.

Diagnosis: Clinical signs/symptoms, ambulatory esophageal reflux monitoring (this test uses a thin pH probe that is placed in the esophagus). Data is collected on the amount of acid entering the esophagus along with the presence of clinical symptoms. Endoscopy may be used in the diagnosis of GERD in patients with persistent or progressive symptoms.

Treatment: GER is often treated with proton pump inhibitors (inhibit gastric acid secretion). Surgical therapy may be utilized if medical management is unsuccessful. Patients are taught to eliminate foods that trigger symptoms (chocolate, caffeine, alcohol, and highly acidic foods). In addition, patients with GERD should avoid meals 2-3 hours before bed and may find it helpful to sleep with the head of the bed elevated to alleviate symptoms.

Peptic Ulcer Disease

Peptic ulcer disease (PUD) includes both ulcerations of the duodenum and stomach. They may be primary (usually duodenal) or secondary (usually gastric). Gastric ulcers are commonly associated with ***H. pylori*** infections (80%) but may be caused by aspirin and NSAIDs. *H. pylori* are spread in the fecal-oral route from person to person or contaminated water and cause a chronic inflammation and ulcerations of the gastric mucosa. PUD is 2 to 3 times more common in males and is associated with poor economic status that results in a crowded, unhygienic environment, although it can occur in others. Usually other family members have a history of ulcers as well.

Symptoms include abdominal pain, nausea, vomiting, and GI bleeding in children younger than 6 years with epigastric and postprandial pain and indigestion in older children and adults.

Treatment includes:

- Antibiotics for *H. pylori*: amoxicillin, clarithromycin, metronidazole
- Proton pump inhibitors: lansoprazole or omeprazole
- Bismuth
- Histamine-receptor antagonists: cimetidine, ranitidine, famotidine

Review Video: Peptic Ulcers
Visit mometrix.com/academy and enter code: 184332

Inflammatory Bowel Disease

Ulcerative Colitis

Ulcerative colitis is superficial inflammation of the mucosa of the colon and rectum, causing ulcerations in the areas where inflammation has destroyed cells. These ulcerations, ranging from pinpoint to extensive, may bleed and produce purulent material. The mucosa of the bowel becomes swollen, erythematous, and granular. Patients may present emergently with **severe ulcerative colitis** (having >6 blood stools a day, fever, tachycardia, anemia) or with **fulminant colitis** (>10 blood stools per day, severe bleeding, and toxic symptoms) These patients are at high risk for megacolon and perforation. For patients with severe and fulminant ulcerative colitis:

Symptoms:

- Abdominal pain
- Anemia
- F&E depletion
- Bloody diarrhea/rectal bleeding
- Diarrhea
- Fecal urgency
- Tenesmus
- Anorexia
- Weight loss
- Fatigue
- Systemic disorders: Eye inflammation, arthritis, liver disease, and osteoporosis as immune system triggers generalized inflammation

Treatment:

- Glucocorticoids
- Aminosalicylates
- Antibiotics if signs/symptoms of toxicity
- D/C anticholinergics, NSAIDS, and antidiarrheals
- If fulminant: Admitted & monitored for deterioration. Kept NPO, and given IV F&E replacement. NGT for decompression if intestinal dilation is present. Knee-elbow position to reposition gas in bowel. Colectomy for those with megacolon or who are unresponsive to therapy.

Crohn's Disease

Crohn's disease manifests with inflammation of the GI system. Inflammation is transmural (often leading to intestinal stenosis and fistulas), focal, and discontinuous with aphthous ulcerations progressing to linear and irregular-shaped ulcerations. Granulomas may be present. Common sites of inflammation are the terminal ileum and cecum. The condition is chronic, but patients with severe or fulminant disease (fevers, persistent vomiting, abscess, obstruction) often present emergently for treatment.

Symptoms:

- Perirectal abscess/fistula in advanced disease
- Diarrhea
- Watery stools
- Rectal hemorrhage

- Anemia
- Abdominal pain (commonly RLQ)
- Cramping
- Weight loss
- Nausea and vomiting
- Fever
- Night sweats

Treatment:

- Triamcinolone for oral lesions, aminosalicylates, glucocorticoids, antidiarrheals, probiotics, avoid lactose, and identify and eliminate food triggers.
- For patients who present with toxic symptoms: hospitalization for careful monitoring, IV glucocorticoids, aminosalicylates, antibiotics, and bowel rest. Parenteral nutrition for the malnourished.
- For repeated relapses (refractory):
  - Immunomodulatory agents (azathioprine, mercaptopurine, methotrexate) or Biologic therapies (infliximab). Bowel resection if unresponsive to all treatment or with ischemic bowel.

Diverticular Disease

Diverticular disease is a condition in which diverticula (saclike pouchings of the bowel lining that extend through a defect in the muscle layer) occur anywhere within the GI tract. About 20% of patients with diverticular disease will develop **acute diverticulitis**, which occurs as diverticula become inflamed when food or bacteria are retained within the diverticula. This may result in abscess, obstruction, perforation, bleeding, or fistula. Diagnosis is best confirmed by abdominal CT with contrast (showing a localized thickening of the bowel wall, increased density of soft tissue, and diverticula in the colon). Many patients have normal lab studies, but some present with leukocytosis, elevated serum amylase, and pyuria on urinalysis.

Symptoms (similar to appendicitis):

- Steady pain in left lower quadrant
- Change in bowel habits
- Tenesmus
- Dysuria from irritation
- Recurrent urinary infections from fistula
- Paralytic ileus from peritonitis or intra-abdominal irritation
- Toxic reactions: fever, severe pain, leukocytosis

Treatment:

- Rehydration and electrolytes per IV fluids
- Nothing by mouth initially
- Antibiotics, broad spectrum (IV if toxic reactions)
- NG suction if necessary, for obstruction
- Careful observation for signs of perforation or obstruction

Acute Gastrointestinal Hemorrhage

Gastrointestinal (GI) hemorrhage may occur in the upper or lower gastrointestinal track. The primary cause (50-70%) of GI hemorrhage is gastric and duodenal ulcers, generally caused by stress, NSAIDs or infection with *Helicobacter pylori.*

Symptoms: Abdominal pain and distention, coffee-ground emesis/hematemesis, bloody or tarry stools, hypotension with tachycardia.

Diagnosis: Stool occult blood (Guaiac test), EGD, colonoscopy, GI Bleed scan.

Treatment includes:

- Medications: Fluid replacement with blood transfusions if necessary, antibiotic therapy for *Helicobacter pylori,* continuous pantoprazole IV to prevent further irritation
- Endoscopic thermal therapy to cauterize or injection therapy (hypertonic saline, epinephrine, ethanol) to cause vasoconstriction
- Arteriography with intra-arterial infusion of vasopressin and/or embolizing agents, such as stainless-steel coils, platinum microcoils, or Gelfoam pledgets
- Vagotomy and pyloroplasty if bleeding persists

Prevention: Prophylactic medications (pantoprazole [Protonix] IV is common).

Hernias

Hernias are protrusions into or through the abdominal wall and may occur in children and adults. Hernias may contain fat, tissue, or bowel. There are a number of types:

- **Direct inguinal hernias** occur primarily in adults and rarely incarcerate.
- **Indirect inguinal hernias** related to congenital defect is most common on the right in males and can incarcerate, especially during the first year and in females.
- **Femoral hernias** occur primarily in women and may incarcerate.
- **Umbilical hernias** occur in children, especially those of African-American descent, and rarely incarcerate. They may also occur in adults, primarily women, and may incarcerate.
- **Incisional hernias** are usually related to obesity or wound infections, and may incarcerate.

Hernias are evident on clinical examination.

Symptoms of incarceration include:

- Severe pain
- Nausea and vomiting
- Soft mass at hernia site
- Tachycardia
- Temperature

Treatment for hernias includes:

- Reduction if incarceration is very recent with patient in Trendelenburg position and gentle compression
- Surgical excision and fixation
- Broad-spectrum antibiotics

HEPATIC CIRRHOSIS

COMPENSATED

Cirrhosis is a chronic hepatic disease in which normal liver tissue is replaced by the fibrotic tissue that impairs liver function. There are 3 types:

- **Alcoholic** (from chronic alcoholism) is the most common type and results in fibrosis about the portal areas. The liver cells become necrotic, replaced by fibrotic tissue, with areas of normal tissue projecting in between, giving the liver a hobnail appearance.
- **Post-necrotic** with broad bands of fibrotic tissue is the result of acute viral hepatitis.
- **Biliary**, the least common type, is caused by chronic biliary obstruction and cholangitis, with resulting fibrotic tissue about the bile ducts.

Cirrhosis may be either compensated or decompensated. **Compensated cirrhosis** usually involves non-specific symptoms, such as intermittent fever, epistaxis, ankle edema, indigestion, abdominal pain, and palmar erythema. Hepatomegaly and splenomegaly may also be present.

DECOMPENSATED

Decompensated cirrhosis occurs when the liver can no longer adequately synthesize proteins, clotting factors, and other substances so that portal hypertension occurs.

Symptoms:

- Hepatomegaly
- Chronic elevated temperature
- Clubbing of fingers
- Purpura resulting from thrombocytopenia, with bruising and epistaxis
- Portal obstruction resulting in jaundice and ascites
- Bacterial peritonitis with ascites
- Esophageal varices
- Edema of extremities and presacral area resulting from reduced albumin in the plasma. Vitamin deficiency from interference with formation, use, and storage of vitamins, such as A, C, and K
- Anemia from chronic gastritis and decreased dietary intake
- Hepatic encephalopathy with alterations in mentation
- Hypotension
- Atrophy of gonads

Treatment varies according to the symptoms and is supportive rather than curative as the fibrotic changes in the liver cannot be reversed:

- Dietary supplements and vitamins
- Diuretics (potassium sparing), such as Aldactone® and Dyrenium®, to decrease ascites
- Colchicine to reduce fibrotic changes
- Liver transplant (the definitive treatment)

FULMINANT HEPATITIS

Fulminant hepatitis is a severe acute infection of the liver that can result in hepatic necrosis, encephalopathy, and death within 1 to 2 weeks. Most hepatitis is caused by infection with hepatitis viruses A, B, C, D, or E, but it can also be caused by numerous viruses, toxic chemicals (carbon tetrachloride), metabolic diseases (Wilson disease), and drugs, such as acetaminophen. Fulminant hepatitis can result from any of these factors. Fulminant hepatitis can be divided into 3 stages according to the duration from jaundice to encephalopathy:

0 to 7 days = Hyperacute liver failure
7 to 28 days = Acute liver failure
28 to 72 days = Subacute liver failure

Symptoms:

- Poor feeding/anorexia
- Increased intracranial pressure with cerebral edema and encephalopathy
- Coagulopathies
- Renal failure
- Electrolyte imbalances

Treatment:

- Identify and treat underlying cause
- Intracranial pressure monitoring and treatment
- Diuresis; liver transplantation may be necessary
- Survival rates vary from 50% to 85%

Portal Hypertension

Portal hypertension occurs when obstructed blood flow increases blood pressure throughout the portal venous system, preventing the liver from filtering blood and causing the development of collateral blood vessels that return unfiltered blood to the systemic circulation. Increasing serum aldosterone levels cause sodium and fluid retention in the kidneys, resulting in hypervolemia, ascites and esophageal varices. Portal hypertension can be caused by any liver disease, especially cirrhosis and inherited or acquired coagulopathies that cause thrombosis of the portal vein.

Symptoms: Ascites with distended abdomen, esophageal varices with bleeding, dyspnea, abdominal discomfort, fluid/electrolyte imbalances.

Diagnosis: Labs (CBC, BMP, liver panel, Hep B &C), abdominal ultrasound or CT/MRI, EGD, Hemodynamic measurement of the hepatic venous pressure gradient (HVPG)

Treatment includes:

- Restricted sodium intake & use diuretics as needed
- Endoscopic treatment of obstruction
- Portal vein shunting redirecting blood from the portal vein to the vena cava
- Liver transplant in severe cases
- These patients are at high risk for esophageal varices, which, if they rupture, can cause instantaneous hemorrhage and death

Esophageal Varices

Esophageal varices are torturous, dilated veins in the submucosa of the esophagus (usually the distal portion). They are a complication of cirrhosis of the liver, in which obstruction of the portal vein causes an increase in collateral vessels and resulting decrease in circulation to the liver, increasing the pressure in the collateral vessels. This causes the vessels to dilate. Because they tend to be fragile and inelastic, they tear easily, causing sudden, massive esophageal hemorrhage.

Signs/Symptoms: Usually asymptomatic until rupture; projectile vomiting bright red blood, dark stools, and shock.

Diagnosis: EGD, capsule endoscopy, CT, and MRI.

Treatment (in the case of rupture) includes:

- Emergent fluid and blood replacement
- IV vasopressin, somatostatin, and octreotide to decrease venous pressure and provide vasoconstriction/clotting
- Endoscopic injection with sclerosing agents and band ligation
- Esophagogastric balloon tamponade using Sengstaken-Blakemore and Minnesota tubes (Note—always inflate gastric balloon first, keep scissors nearby in case of balloon migration, do not use longer than 24 hrs as there is increased risk of ulceration from pressure.)
- Transjugular intrahepatic portosystemic shunting (TIPS) creates a channel between systemic and portal venous systems to reduce portal hypertension

Hepatic Coma

Hepatic coma or **hepatic encephalopathy** occurs when the liver's inability to remove ammonia and other toxins from the bloodstream causes a decrease in neurologic function. Hepatic encephalopathy often occurs in patients with severe liver disease, most commonly in patients diagnosed with cirrhosis of the liver. The fibrous tissue that forms in cirrhosis affects the liver structure and impedes the blood flow to the liver, ultimately causing the liver to fail. There are four stages of hepatic encephalopathy ranging from grade 0 to grade 4. Grade 4 encephalopathy is defined as hepatic coma. Neurologic alterations may progress slowly and if left untreated may result in irreversible neurologic damage.

Signs and symptoms: Altered mental status, personality or mood changes, poor judgment, and poor concentration. As symptoms progress, patients may experience agitation, disorientation, drowsiness, increasing confusion, lethargy, slurred speech, tremors, and seizures. In grade 4 encephalopathy, patients become unresponsive and ultimately comatose.

Diagnosis: Physical assessment, lab tests including a complete blood count, liver function tests, serum ammonia levels, BUN, creatinine and electrolyte levels, CT or MRI of the brain, and electroencephalogram may be used to diagnose hepatic encephalopathy.

Treatment: Address precipitating factors such as infection, gastrointestinal bleeding, dehydration, hypotension, or alcohol use. Other treatment options may include limiting protein intake, administration of lactulose to prevent the absorption of ammonia, and the administration of an antibiotic such as neomycin, rifaximin, or Flagyl to reduce the serum ammonia level.

Biliary Atresia

Biliary atresia is a rare life-threatening condition that occurs in infancy of unknown cause. Bile ducts are tubes that transport bile from the liver to the gallbladder (where it is stored) and the small intestine (where it aids in digestion). Biliary atresia occurs when the bile ducts (either inside or outside of the liver) become inflamed, causing damage to the ducts and an impedance of bile flow. Without treatment, the trapped bile causes damage to the liver eventually causing it to fail. The life expectancy for infants with untreated biliary atresia is approximately 2 years.

Signs and symptoms: Early identification is key in successfully treating biliary atresia. Signs and symptoms include dark urine, gray or white stools, slow weight gain and delayed growth, jaundice, abdominal swelling and itching.

Diagnosis: Physical assessment, abdominal films, ultrasound, lab tests including bilirubin levels, and liver biopsy.

Treatment: The only treatment options for biliary atresia are liver transplant or the Kasai procedure. Named after the surgeon who invented it, the Kasai procedure involves using a loop of intestine to act as a new bile duct and removing the damaged ducts. Flow of bile is then restored to the small intestine. The Kasai procedure is most successful when performed on younger infants (less than 3 months old).

Acute Pancreatitis

Acute pancreatitis is related to chronic alcoholism or cholelithiasis in 90% of patients, but may have unknown etiology. It may also be triggered by a variety of drugs (tetracycline, thiazides, acetaminophen, and oral contraceptives). Complications may include shock, acute respiratory distress syndrome, and MODs.

Signs/Symptoms: acute pain (mid-epigastric, LUQ, or generalized), nausea and vomiting, abdominal distention.

Diagnosis: Serum lipase (>2x normal), amylase (less accurate), CT with contrast, abdominal U/S, MRI cholangiopancreatography, ERCP.

Treatment (supportive) includes:

- **Medications**: IV fluids, antiemetics, antibiotics (if necrosis is secondary to infection), and analgesia. NOTE: do not give morphine, can cause spasms in sphincter of Oddi, making pain worse.
- **TPN, NPO, or restricted to clear liquids** may help manage vomiting, ileus, and aspiration.
- **Surgical**: may remove gallbladder and biliary duct obstructions if cause of recurrent pancreatitis.

Prevention: Avoid smoking and alcohol consumption; limit fat intake and increase fresh fruits/vegetables and water.

Malnutrition and Malabsorption in Critically Ill Patients

Malabsorption occurs when an abnormality or alteration in the gastrointestinal tract affects the absorption of nutrients through the small intestine. It can also occur with damage to the small intestine due to infection, trauma, surgery, or radiation therapy; patients in ICU's are at an increased risk due to multiple illnesses, intubation/prolonged NPO status, vasopressors decreasing blood flow to the bowel, and other factors that make receiving adequate nutrition difficult. Malabsorption often leads to **malnutrition**. Hospitalized malnourished patients are at a higher risk for infection, respiratory failure, heart failure, arrhythmias and delayed or decreased wound healing.

Signs and symptoms: Bloating, cramping, gas, chronic diarrhea, failure to thrive, muscle wasting, weight loss, steatorrhea, anemia, electrolyte imbalance and vitamin/mineral deficiencies.

Diagnosis: Serum electrolytes, complete blood count, ferritin, vitamin B12, folate, albumin, and protein. Stool fat testing may be performed to assess for the presence of fat in the stool that occurs in certain disorders that affect fat absorption. Endoscopy may be used to diagnose an abnormality in the mucosa lining of the bowel.

Treatment: Replacement of nutrients that have been lost as a result of malabsorption as well as treatment for the cause of the malabsorption. Supplemental treatment with enzymes found to be deficient may also be incorporated into the treatment plan.

Prevention: Ensure patients with prolonged "NPO" status have alternative means of nutrition (TPN, tube feeds, etc.).

Genitourinary Pathophysiology

Incontinence

Urinary incontinence occurs more commonly in women than men and can range from an intermittent leaking of urine to a full loss of bladder control. Causes of urinary incontinence may include neurologic injury (including cerebral vascular accidents), infections, weakness of the muscles of the bladder and certain medications including diuretics, antihistamines and antidepressants. **Stress incontinence** is defined as an involuntary leakage of urine with sneezing, coughing, laughing, lifting, or exercising. **Urge incontinence** is defined as an uncontrollable need to urinate on a frequent basis. **Total incontinence** is the full loss of bladder control.

Signs and symptoms: Urinary frequency and urgency may accompany the inability to control urine. If urinary incontinence is severe, incontinence associated dermatitis may occur, predisposing the patient to skin breakdown and the development of pressure ulcers.

Diagnosis: Physical assessment and presence of symptoms. Ultrasound, urinalysis, urodynamic testing and cystoscopy may be used to determine the underlying cause.

Treatment: Treatment options are dependent on the type of urinary incontinence and the severity. Bladder training and pelvic muscle exercises may be utilized to strengthen muscles to control leakage of urine. In female patients with stress incontinence, a vaginal pessary may be inserted into the vagina to help support the bladder. Suburethral slings may also be surgically implanted to support the urethra. Anticholinergics, antispasmodics and tricyclic antidepressants may also be used in the treatment of urinary incontinence.

Hydronephrosis

Hydronephrosis is a symptom of a disease involving swelling of the kidney pelvises and calyces because of an obstruction that causes urine to be retained in the kidney. In chronic conditions, symptoms may be delayed until severe kidney damage has occurred. Over time, the kidney begins to atrophy. The primary conditions that predispose to hydronephrosis include:

- Vesicoureteral reflux
- Obstruction at the ureteropelvic junction
- Renal edema (non-obstructive)
- Any condition that impairs drainage of the ureters can cause backup of the urine

Symptoms vary widely depending upon cause and whether the condition is acute or chronic.

- Acute episodes are usually characterized by flank pain, abnormal creatinine and electrolyte levels, and increased pH.
- The enlarged kidney may be palpable as a soft mass.

Treatment includes:

- Identifying the cause of obstruction and correcting it to ensure adequate drainage.
- A nephrostomy tube, ureteral stent or pyeloplasty may be done surgically in some cases.
- A urinary catheter may be inserted if there is outflow obstruction from the bladder.

Renal and Ureteral Calculi

Renal and urinary calculi occur frequently, more commonly in males, and can relate to diseases (hyperparathyroidism, renal tubular acidosis, gout) and lifestyle factors, such as sedentary work. Calculi can form at any age, most composed of calcium, and can range in size from very tiny to larger than 6 mm. Those smaller than 4 mm can usually pass in the urine easily.

Diagnostic studies include clinical findings, UA, pregnancy test to rule out ectopic pregnancy, BUN and creatinine if indicated, ultrasound (for pregnant women and children), IV urography. Helical CT (non-contrast) is diagnostic.

Symptoms occur with obstruction and are usually of sudden onset and acute:

- Severe flank pain radiating to abdomen and ipsilateral testicle or labium majus, abdominal or pelvic pain (young children)
- Nausea and vomiting
- Diaphoresis
- Hematuria

Treatment includes:

- Instructions and equipment for straining urine
- Antibiotics if concurrent infection
- Extracorporeal shock-wave lithotripsy
- Surgical removal: percutaneous/standard nephrolithotomy
- Analgesia: opiates and NSAIDs

Acute Tubular Necrosis

Acute tubular necrosis (ATN) occurs when a hypoxic condition causes renal ischemia that damages tubular cells of the glomeruli so they are unable to adequately filter the urine, leading to acute renal failure. Causes include hypotension, hyperbilirubinemia, sepsis, surgery (especially cardiac or vascular), and birth complications. ATN may result from nephrotoxic injury related to obstruction or drugs, such as chemotherapy, acyclovir, and antibiotics, such as sulfonamides and streptomycin. Symptoms may be non-specific initially and can include life-threatening complications.

Symptoms include:

- Lethargy
- Nausea and vomiting
- Hypovolemia with low cardiac output and generalized vasodilation
- Fluid and electrolyte imbalance leading to hypertension, CNS abnormalities, metabolic acidosis, arrhythmias, edema, and congestive heart failure
- Uremia leading to destruction of platelets and bleeding, neurological deficits, and disseminated intravascular coagulopathy (DIC)
- Infections, including pericarditis and sepsis

Treatment includes:

- Identifying and treating underlying cause, discontinuing nephrotoxic agents
- Supportive care
- Loop diuretics (in some cases), such as Lasix®
- Antibiotics for infection (can include pericarditis and sepsis)
- Kidney dialysis

Acute Kidney Injury

Acute kidney injury (AKI), previously known as acute renal failure, is an acute disruption of kidney function that results in decreased renal perfusion, a decrease in glomerular filtration rate and a buildup of metabolic waste products (azotemia). Azotemia is the accumulation of urea, creatinine and other nitrogen containing end products into the bloodstream. The regulation of fluid volume, electrolyte balance and acid base balance is also affected. The causes of acute kidney injury are divided into pre-renal (caused by a decrease in perfusion), intrarenal or intrinsic (occurring within the kidney) and post-renal (caused by the inadequate drainage of urine). Acute kidney injury is common in hospitalized patients and even more common in critically ill patients, carrying a mortality rate of 50-80%. Risk factors for acute kidney injury include advanced age, the presence of co-morbid conditions, pre-existing kidney disease and a diagnosis of sepsis.

Signs and symptoms: Malaise, fatigue, lethargy, confusion, weakness, change in urine color, change in urine volume and flank pain.

Diagnosis: Urinalysis, serum BUN and creatinine levels, renal ultrasound, CT or MRI and renal biopsy.

Treatment: The treatment of acute kidney injury is based on the underlying cause. Treatment options may include fluid and electrolyte replacement, diuretic therapy, fluid restriction, renal diet, and low dose dopamine to increase renal perfusion. Hemodialysis may also be necessary in patients with acute kidney injury.

Chronic Kidney Disease

Chronic kidney disease (CKD) occurs when the kidneys are unable to filter and excrete wastes, concentrate urine, and maintain electrolyte balance because of hypoxic conditions, kidney disease, or obstruction in the urinary tract. It results first in azotemia (increase in nitrogenous waste in the blood) and then in uremia (nitrogenous wastes cause toxic symptoms.) When >50% of the functional renal capacity is destroyed, the kidneys can no longer carry out necessary functions and progressive deterioration begins over months or years. Symptoms are often non-specific in the beginning with loss of appetite and energy.

Symptoms and complications are as follows:

- Weight loss
- Headaches, muscle cramping, general malaise
- Increased bruising and dry or itchy skin
- Increased BUN and creatinine
- Sodium and fluid retention with edema
- Hyperkalemia
- Metabolic acidosis

- Calcium and phosphorus depletion, resulting in altered bone metabolism, pain, and retarded growth
- Anemia with decreased production on RBCs. Increased risk of infection
- Uremic syndrome

Treatment includes:

- Supportive/symptomatic therapy
- Dialysis and transplantation
- Diet control: Low protein, salt, potassium, and phosphorus
- Fluid limitations
- Calcium and vitamin supplementation
- Phosphate binders

Uremic Syndrome

Uremic syndrome is a number of disorders that can occur with end-stage renal disease and renal failure, usually after multiple metabolic failures and decrease in creatinine clearance to <10 mL/min. There is compromise of all normal functions of the kidney: fluid balance, electrolyte balance, acid-base homeostasis, hormone production, and elimination of wastes. Metabolic abnormalities related to uremia include:

- **Decreased RBC production:** The kidney is unable to produce adequate erythropoietin in the peritubular cells, resulting in anemia, which is usually normocytic and normochromic. Parathyroid hormone levels may increase, causing calcification of the bone marrow, causing hypoproliferative anemia as RBC production is suppressed.
- **Platelet abnormalities:** Decreased platelet count, increased turnover, and reduced adhesion leads to bleeding disorders.
- **Metabolic acidosis:** The tubular cells are unable to regulate acid-base metabolism, and phosphate, sulfuric, hippuric, and lactic acids increase, leading to congestive heart failure and weakness.
- **Hyperkalemia:** The nephrons cannot excrete adequate amounts of potassium. Some drugs, such as diuretics that spare potassium may aggravate the condition.
- **Renal bone disease:** ↓ Calcium, ↑ phosphate, ↑ parathyroid hormone, ↓ utilization of vitamin D lead to demineralization. In some cases, calcium and phosphate are deposited in other tissues (metastatic calcification).
- **Multiple endocrine disorders:** Thyroid hormone production is decreased and abnormalities in reproductive hormones may result in infertility/impotence. Males have ↓ testosterone but ↑ estrogen and LH. Females experience irregular cycles, lack of ovulation and menses. Insulin production may increase but with decreased clearance, resulting in episodes of hypoglycemia or decreased hyperglycemia in those who are diabetic.
- **Cardiovascular disorders:** Left ventricular hypertrophy is most common, but fluid retention may cause congestive heart failure and electrolyte imbalances, dysrhythmias. Pericarditis, exacerbation of valvular disorders, and pericardial effusions may occur.
- **Anorexia and malnutrition:** Nausea and poor appetite contribute to hypoalbuminemia, sometimes exacerbated by restrictive diets.

Pyelonephritis

Pyelonephritis is a potentially organ-damaging bacterial infection of the parenchyma of the kidney. Pyelonephritis can result in abscess formation, sepsis, and kidney failure. Pyelonephritis is especially dangerous for those who are immunocompromised, pregnant, or diabetic. Most infections are caused by *Escherichia coli.* **Diagnostic studies** include urinalysis, blood and urine cultures. Patients may require hospitalization or careful follow-up.

Symptoms vary widely but can include:

- Dysuria and frequency, hematuria, flank and/or low back pain
- Fever and chills
- Costovertebral angle tenderness
- Change in feeding habits (infants)
- Change in mental status (geriatric)
- Young women often exhibit symptoms more associated with lower urinary infection, so the condition may be overlooked.

Treatment includes:

- Analgesia
- Antipyretics
- Intravenous fluids
- Antibiotics: started but may be changed based on cultures
    - IV ceftriaxone with fluoroquinolone orally for 14 days
    - Monitor BUN. Normal 7-8 mg/dL (8-20 mg/dL >age 60). Increase indicates impaired renal function, as urea is end product of protein metabolism.

Cystitis

Cystitis is a common and often-chronic low-grade kidney infection that develops over time, so observing for symptoms of urinary infections and treating promptly are very important.

Changes in **character of urine**:

- **Appearance**: The urine may become cloudy from mucus or purulent material. Hematuria may be present.
- **Color**: Urine usually becomes concentrated and may be dark yellow/orange or brownish in color.
- **Odor**: Urine may have a very strong or foul odor.
- **Output**: Urinary output may decrease markedly.

Pain: There may be lower back or flank pain from inflammation of the kidneys.

Systemic: Fever, chills, headache, and general malaise often accompany urine infections. Some people suffer a lack of appetite as well as nausea and vomiting. Fever usually indicates that the infection has affected the kidneys. Children may develop incontinence or loose stools and cry excessively.

Treatment:

- Increased fluid intake
- Antibiotics

Nephrotoxic Agents

Medications are a common cause of renal damage, especially among older patients. The **nephrotoxic effects** may be reversible if the drug is discontinued before permanent damage occurs. Those at increased risk include patients who are older than 60, have a history of renal insufficiency, suffer from volume depletion, or have diabetes mellitus, sepsis, or heart failure. Initial signs may be quite subtle. Preventive measures include baseline renal function tests and monitoring of renal function and vital signs during treatment. The following are some common effects, and the drugs that may cause them:

- **Chronic interstitial nephritis**: Acetaminophen, lithium, carmustine, cisplatin, cyclosporine.
- **Acute interstitial nephritis**: NSAIDs, acyclovir, beta-lactams, rifampin, quinolones, sulfonamides, vancomycin, indinavir, loop/thiazide diuretics, lansoprazole, allopurinol, phenytoin, ranitidine.
- **Rhabdomyolysis**: Amitriptyline, diphenhydramine, doxylamine, benzodiazepines, haloperidol, lithium, ketamine, methadone, methamphetamine, statins.
- **Crystal nephropathy**: Acyclovir, foscarnet, ganciclovir, quinolones, sulfonamides, indinavir, methotrexate, triamterene.
- **Tubular cell toxicity**: Aminoglycosides, amphotericin B, pentamidine, adefovir, tenofovir, contrast dye, zoledronate.
- **Thrombotic microangiopathy**: Cyclosporine, clopidogrel, mitomycin-C, quinine.
- **Impaired intraglomerular hemodynamics**: NSAIDs, cyclosporine, tacrolimus, ACE inhibitors.
- **Glomerulonephritis**: NSAIDs, lithium, beta-lactams, interferon-alpha, gold therapy, pamidronate.

Phimosis and Paraphimosis

Phimosis and paraphimosis are both restrictive disorders of the penis that occur in males who are uncircumcised or incorrectly circumcised. **Phimosis** is the inability to retract the foreskin proximal to the glans penis, sometimes resulting in urinary retention or hematuria. **Treatments** include:

- Dilating the foreskin with a hemostat (temporary solution)
- Circumcision
- Application of topical steroids (triamcinolone 0.025% twice daily) from end of foreskin to glans corona for 4 to 6 weeks

Paraphimosis occurs when the foreskin tightens above the glans penis and cannot be extended to normal positioning. This results in edema of the foreskin and circulatory impairment of the glans penis, sometimes progressing to gangrene, so immediate treatment is critical. Symptoms include pain, swelling, and inability to urinate. **Treatments** include:

- Compression of the glans to reduce edema (wrapping tightly with 2-inch elastic bandage for 5 minutes)
- Reducing edema by making several puncture wounds with 22 to 25-gauge needle
- Local anesthetic and dorsal incision to relieve pressure

Testicular Torsion

Testicular torsion is a twisting of the spermatic cord within or below the inguinal canal, causing constriction of blood supply to the testis. Testicular torsion is most common at puberty but can occur at any age, sometimes precipitated by strenuous athletic participation or trauma, but it can also occur during sleep.

Symptoms include acute onset of severe testicular pain and edema, although children may present with nonspecific abdominal discomfort initially.

Diagnosis is based on clinical examination that demonstrates a firm scrotal mass. Color-flow duplex Doppler ultrasound may be helpful if diagnosis is not clear.

Treatment includes:

- **Manual detorsion** (usually 1.5 rotations) with elective surgical repair. Right testicle is usually rotated counterclockwise and left, clockwise. Reduction of pain should occur. If pain increases with rotation, then rotation should be done in the opposite direction.
- **Emergency surgical repair** (if manual detorsion not successful)

Epididymitis and Orchitis

Epididymitis, infection of the epididymis, is often associated with infection in a testis (epididymo-orchitis). In children, infection may be related to congenital anomalies that allow reflux of urine. In sexually active males 35 years or younger, it is usually related to STDs. In men older than 40, it is often related to urinary infections or benign prostatic hypertrophy with urethral obstruction.

Symptoms include progressive pain in lower abdomen, scrotum, and/or testicle. Late symptoms include large tender scrotal mass.

Diagnosis includes: Clinical examination. Pyuria. Urethral culture for STDs. Sonography.

Orchitis alone is rare but occurs with mumps, other viral infections, and epididymitis. Ultrasound may be needed to rule out testicular torsion.

Treatment for both conditions depends upon the cause, but epididymitis usually resolves with antibiotics:

- Younger than 40, associated with STDs:
  - Ceftriaxone 250 mg IM and doxycycline 100 mg twice daily for 10 days
- Older than 35, associated with other bacteria:
  - Ciprofloxacin 500 mg twice daily for 10-14 days
  - Levofloxacin 250 mg daily for 10-14 days
  - TMP/SMS DS twice daily for 10-14 days

Prostatitis

Prostatitis is an acute infection of the prostate gland, commonly caused by *Escherichia coli, Pseudomonas aeruginosa, Staphylococcus aureus,* or other bacteria. *Symptoms* include fever, chills, lower back pain, urinary frequency, dysuria, painful ejaculation, and perineal discomfort. PSA will often be elevated in this patient population, unrelated to prostate cancer. *Diagnosis* is based on clinical findings of perineal tenderness and spasm of rectal sphincter. *Treatments* include Ciprofloxacin 500 mg orally twice daily for 1 month **or** TMP/SMX DS twice daily for 1 month. Most patients also have a urethral culture to check for STDs. Patients with suspected bacteremia should be admitted for monitoring.

Benign Prostatic Hypertrophy

Benign prostatic hypertrophy/hyperplasia usually develops after age 40. The prostate may slowly enlarge, but the surrounding tissue restrains outward growth, so the gland compresses the urethra. The bladder wall also goes through changes, becoming thicker and irritated, so that it begins to spasm, causing frequent urinations. The bladder muscle eventually weakens and the bladder fails to empty completely.

Symptoms include urgency, dribbling, frequency, nocturia, incontinence, retention, and bladder distention.

Diagnosis may include IVP, cystogram, and PSA.

Treatment includes: Catheterization for urinary retention/bladder distention. Surgical excision. Avoid fluids close to bedtime, double void, avoid caffeine and alcohol, alpha-adrenergic antagonists, and 5-alpha-reductase inhibitors.

PID

Pelvic inflammatory disease (PID) comprises infections of the upper reproductive system, often ascending from vagina and cervix, and includes salpingitis, endometritis, tubo-ovarian abscess, peritonitis, and perihepatitis. *Neisseria gonorrhoeae* and *Chlamydia trachomatis* are implicated in most cases but some infections are polymicrobial. Complications include increase in ectopic pregnancy and tubal factor infertility. *Symptoms* include lower abdominal pain, vaginal pain, discharge, or bleeding, dyspareunia, dysuria, fever, and nausea and vomiting.

Diagnostic studies include:

- Pregnancy test
- Vaginal secretion testing, endocervical culture
- CBC
- Syphilis, HIV, and hepatitis testing
- Transvaginal pelvic ultrasound
- Endometrial biopsy
- Laparoscopy for definitive diagnosis

Treatments include:

- Broad spectrum antibiotics:
  - (Inpatient) Cefotetan 2 g IV every 12 hours or every 6 hours with doxycycline 100 mg every 12 hours
  - (Outpatient) Ceftriaxone 250 mg IM x 1 dose with doxycycline 100 mg orally every 12 hours for 14 days with metronidazole 500 mg twice daily for 2 weeks for patients who had gynecological procedures recently
- Laparoscopy to drain abscesses if symptoms do not improve in 72 hours or less
- Treatment specific to associated disorders (such as HIV or hepatitis)

Vulvovaginitis

Vulvovaginitis is inflammation of vulvar and vaginal tissues:

- **Bacterial vaginosis** (Gardnerella vaginalis or other bacteria)
- **Fungal infections** (usually Candida albicans)

- **Parasitic infections** (Trichomonas vaginalis)
- **Allergic contact vaginitis** (from soaps or other irritants)
- **Atrophic vaginitis** (postmenopause)

Symptoms include vaginal odor, swelling, discharge, or bleeding, pain and discomfort, or severe itching (common with *C. albicans).*

Diagnostic studies include:

- Physical exam and culture of discharge, pH testing with nitrazine paper: Greater than 4.5 is typical of bacterial and trichomonas infections. Less than 4.5 is typical of fungal infections.

Treatment includes:

- **Bacterial infections**: Metronidazole 500 mg orally twice daily for 7 days AND Metronidazole 0.75% gel intravaginally twice daily for 5 days AND Clindamycin 2% cream intravaginally at bedtime for 7 days
- **Fungal infections**: Fluconazole 150 mg tablet in 1 dose OR vaginal creams, tablets, or suppositories, such as butoconazole 2% cream for 3 days or tioconazole 6.5% ointment for 1 dose
- **Parasitic (trichomonas):** Metronidazole 2 g orally in 1 dose

Ovarian Cysts

Ovarian cysts can grow within or on the ovaries. When a normal monthly follicle continues to grow, this is known as a functional cyst, of which there are two types:

- A follicular cyst begins when the follicle doesn't rupture or release its egg, but continues to grow.
- A corpus luteum cyst develops when fluid accumulates inside the follicle after it releases its egg.

Functional cysts are usually harmless, rarely cause pain, and often resolve on their own within 2-3 months. Other types of ovarian cyst include the following:

- **Cystadenomas** form on the exterior of an ovary and may enlarge and cause pain.
- **Endometriomas** develop as a result of endometriosis, where some of the tissue attaches to the ovary and causes pain during menses and sexual activity.
- **Dermoid cysts**, also called teratomas, can contain tissue, such as skin or teeth, because they from embryonic cells. They may enlarge and cause pain but are rarely cancerous.

Polycystic ovaries have multiple cysts. Ovarian cysts may cause problems if they rupture or hemorrhage and if they twist or become infected. Presenting symptoms include **hypotension** and **hypovolemia** if hemorrhage occurs, pain (often acute) and tenderness in the lower abdomen on the affected side, lower back pain, dysuria, and weight gain.

Diagnostic studies include a pregnancy test to rule out ectopic pregnancy, ultrasound with Doppler flow.

Treatment depends upon the type of cyst and complications:

- Emergency surgery for torsion
- Antibiotics for infection
- Hormone therapy may be useful for endometrioma

Bartholin Cysts

The Bartholin glands are small glands located on both sides of the vagina in the lips of the *labia minora*. The glands help to lubricate the vulvar area. A **Bartholin cyst** occurs when a duct to one gland becomes obstructed, usually because of infection or trauma, resulting in swelling and formation of a cyst (usually 1 to 3 cm but may be much larger with infection). Bartholin cyst is most common in women in their 20s. Blockage may result from tumors as well, but usually in women older than 40.

Symptoms of a Bartholin cyst include:

- Palpable mass on one side of the vagina (usually painless)
- Pain and tenderness and increasing size of lesion if infection and abscess occurs

Treatment includes:

- Warm, moist compresses or sitz baths
- Antibiotics for infection
- Surgical incision and drainage may be necessary in some cases

Integumentary Pathophysiology

Cellulitis

Cellulitis occurs when an area of the skin becomes infected, usually following injury or trauma to the skin. Cellulitis is most likely to be caused by staphylococcus or streptococcus bacteria. Patients with peripheral vascular disease, diabetes mellitus, and immunosuppression are at a higher risk for the development of cellulitis. Signs and symptoms include: pain, erythema, and warmth at the affected site that progresses rapidly. In addition, the patient may experience fever, chills, fatigue and malaise. Diagnosis is made by physical exam. Labs include complete blood count, culture of the involved area and blood. Treatment for cellulitis is the administration of antibiotics. Surgical irrigation and debridement may be indicated in severe cases.

Septic Arthritis

Septic arthritis is defined as an invasion of the joint space by bacteria, virus or fungi. Elderly patients, immunosuppressed patients, and those with prosthetic joints are at an increased risk for septic arthritis. The most commonly affected joints include the knee, hip, shoulder, ankle and wrist. Signs and symptoms include joint pain, fever, impaired range of motion, chills, edema, erythema, warmth and the abnormal presence of fluid (effusion) surrounding the joint. Diagnosis is made by aspiration of the fluid with stain and culture, x-ray, and blood tests including CBC and cultures. Treatment is the administration of antibiotics. Surgical irrigation and debridement may also be indicated. The patient will likely undergo physical therapy as part of their recovery to improve and restore mobility and range of motion.

Extravasation

Extravasation occurs when an intravenously infused vesicant medication or fluid leaks from the vein and into the subcutaneous space. Vesicant medications are those that cause tissue injury if extravasated and that may ultimately lead to tissue necrosis. Extravasation and infiltration are similar in nature, with infiltration occurring when the infusate is a non-vesicant solution or medication. Extravasation occurs more commonly in peripheral IVs; however, it can also occur with central venous catheters. Common vesicant agents include several chemotherapeutic agents, vancomycin, electrolytes, dobutamine, norepinephrine, phenytoin, promethazine, propofol, and vasopressin.

Signs and symptoms: Pain, burning, erythema, and edema at the site of the extravasation. Oftentimes, a blood return from the peripheral IV or central venous catheter is not present. Long term complications include complex regional pain syndrome, tissue necrosis, and nerve or tendon damage.

Diagnosis: Physical assessment and review of patient symptoms and medications/infusions administered.

Treatment: Early recognition is key to the successful treatment of an extravasation. When an extravasation is suspected, the IV infusion should be immediately stopped and the infusion site assessed. For some medications, antidotes may be available to minimize the damage caused by the extravasation. Heat or cold therapy may also be utilized depending on the medication. In cases of severe damage, debridement, skin grafting, and even amputation may result.

Tissue Damage Related to Allergic Contact Dermatitis

Contact dermatitis is a localized response to contact with an allergen, resulting in a rash that may blister and itch. Common allergens include poison oak, poison ivy, latex, benzocaine, nickel, and preservatives, but there is a wide range of items, preparations, and products to which people may react.

Treatment includes:

- Identifying the causative agent through evaluating the area of the body affected, careful history, or skin patch testing to determine allergic responses
- Corticosteroids to control inflammation and itching
- Soothing oatmeal baths
- Pramoxine lotion to relieve itching
- Antihistamines to reduce allergic response
- Lesions should be gently cleansed and observed for signs of secondary infection
- Antibiotics are used only for secondary infections as indicated
- Rash is usually left open to dry
- Avoidance of allergen to prevent recurrence

Pressure Ulcers

Pressure ulcers occur when pressure from the weight of the body causes a decrease in perfusion, affecting arterial and capillary blood flow and resulting ischemia. Ulcers may then develop from pressure, shearing and friction. Common pressure points include the occiput, scapula, sacrum, buttocks, ischium and heels. Patients with a decreased level of consciousness, brain/spinal cord injuries, peripheral neuropathies, malnutrition, dehydration, PVD, or impaired mobility are at a higher risk for pressure ulcers. Critically ill patients are at an increased risk due to prolonged immobility, sedation, and often incontinence of urine and stool. In addition, patients on vasopressors are at a higher risk due to the constriction of the peripheral circulation.

Signs and symptoms: Early stages include redness, tenderness and firmness at the site of the ulcer. Once the ulcer progresses to severe tissue injury, bone, muscle, or tendons may be exposed, and there may be a yellow or black wound base in addition to pain and drainage at the site.

Diagnostics: Skin and wound assessment including staging of the ulcer.

Treatment: Wet-to-Dry dressings, Wound VAC® therapy, and hyperbaric oxygen may be used; a wound care consult is often advised.

Prevention: Begins with a risk assessment; the Braden scale is a commonly used scale. A score of 16 or below indicates that the patient is at risk. At-risk patients or patients with active ulcers should be placed on a turning and positioning schedule or on a specialty bed to relieve pressure. Moisture barriers and skin protectants may also be utilized.

National Pressure Ulcer Advisory Panel Staging

Pressure ulcers result from pressure or pressure with shear and/or friction over bony prominences. The **National Pressure Ulcer Advisory Panel (NPUAP) stages** include:

- **Suspected deep tissue injury**: Skin discolored, intact or blood blister
- **Stage I**: Intact skin with non-blanching reddened area
- **Stage II**: Abrasion or blistered area without slough but with partial-thickness skin loss
- **Stage III**: Deep ulcer with exposed subcutaneous tissue; tunneling or undermining may be evident with or without slough
- **Stage IV**: Deep ulcer, full thickness, with necrosis into muscle, bone, tendons, and/or joints
- **Unstageable**: Eschar and/or slough prevents staging prior to debridement

Patients should be placed on pressure reducing support surfaces and turned at least every two hours, avoiding the area(s) with a pressure ulcer. Wound care depends on the stage of the wound and the amount of drainage, but includes irrigation, debridement when necessary, antibiotics for infection, and appropriate dressing. Patients should be encouraged to have adequate protein and iron in their diets to promote healing and to maintain adequate hydration.

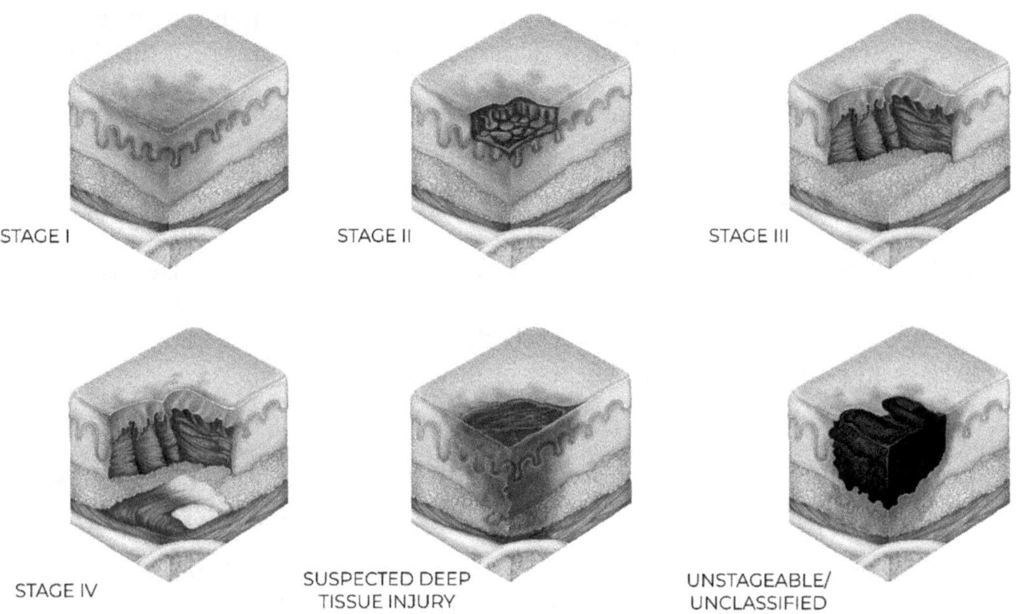

Infectious Wounds

All types of wounds have the potential to become infected. **Infectious wounds** are commonly health care acquired. Wound infections increase a patient's risk of sepsis, multisystem organ failure and death. Trauma patients are at an increased risk of developing an infected wound due to exposure to various contaminants that they may have encountered during their injury (e.g., dirt from a motor vehicle accident).

Signs and symptoms: Erythema, edema, induration, drainage, increasing pain and tenderness, fever, leukocytosis, and lymphangitis.

Diagnosis: Wound infections are diagnosed by wound cultures (anaerobic and aerobic). Fluid or tissue biopsy may also be performed.

Treatment: Wound infections are treated with antibiotics and a wound care regimen that includes routine cleaning and dressing of the wound. Wound care treatment is based on the type and severity of the wound. Surgical irrigation and debridement may also be indicated. For deep, complex wounds, a wound-care consult is often indicated.

Necrotizing Fasciitis

Necrotizing fasciitis is an infection that develops deep within the fascia, causing a rapidly developing tissue necrosis resulting in destruction and death of the soft tissue and nerves. Complications of necrotizing fasciitis may include the loss of the affected limb, sepsis, and death. Group A Streptococcus, Klebsiella, Clostridium, Escherichia coli, Staphylococcus aureus, and Aeromonas hydrophila are organisms that have the potential to cause necrotizing fasciitis.

Signs and symptoms: Edema, erythema, and pain at the affected site. Nausea, vomiting, fatigue, malaise, fever, and chills may also occur.

Diagnosis: Diagnosis is based on physical assessment and patient history. In addition, excisional deep skin biopsy and gram staining may be performed to determine the causative organism. CT/MRI may also be utilized to assess the extent of the infection.

Treatment: Treatment options for necrotizing fasciitis include antibiotics and fasciotomy with radical debridement. Hyperbaric oxygen therapy may also be utilized.

Surgical Wounds

Surgical wounds or incisions are made during a surgical procedure in a sterile, controlled environment. The American College of Surgeons has defined four classes of surgical wound types. This classification can help to predict how the wound will heal and the risk of infection.

- **Class I** is defined as clean (e.g., laparoscopic surgeries and biopsies).
- **Class II** is defined as clean contaminated (e.g., GI and GU surgeries).
- **Class III** is defined as contaminated (e.g., traumatic wounds such as a gunshot wound).
- **Class IV** is defined as dirty (e.g., traumatic wound from a dirty source).

Surgical wounds should be assessed for signs and symptoms of infection including erythema, edema, fever, increasing pain, and drainage. Surgical drains are commonly placed near the surgical incision to promote drainage—inspect drains for patency, amount and characteristics of drainage. Patients are often treated with antibiotics prophylactically to help prevent a surgical site infection. Wound vacuum assisted closure devices may also be utilized to remove blood or serous fluid from the surgical wound/incision site.

Tissue Damage

Abrasion is damage to superficial layers of skin, such as with road burn or ligature marks.

Contusion occurs when friction or pressure causes damage to underlying vessels, resulting in bruising. Contusions that are bright red/purple with clear margins have occurred within 48 hours and those with receding edges or yellow-brown discoloration are older than 48 hours.

Laceration is a tear in the skin resulting from blunt force, often from falls on protuberances, such as elbows, or other blunt trauma. Lacerations may be partial to full-thickness.

Avulsion is tissue that is separated from its base and lost or without adequate base for attachment.

Treatments include:

- Local anesthetic if needed
- Low pressure, high volume irrigation with 35-50 mL syringe of open wound with normal saline, water, or non-antiseptic nonionic surfactants, and mechanical scrubbing of surrounding tissue with disinfectant
- Topical antibiotics as indicated
- Prophylactic antibiotics or antibiotic irrigation if wound contaminated
- Suturing/debridement as needed
- Hydrocolloids, Steri-Strips, and transparent dressings to stabilize flaps

Musculoskeletal Pathophysiology

Immobility

Critical care patients are often **immobile** for extended periods of time, thereby increasing their risk of skin breakdown and the development of pressure ulcers, deep vein thrombosis, functional decline, decreased muscle mass, impaired coordination and gait, cardiovascular deconditioning, depression and constipation. Immobility leads to impaired physical functioning in which muscle mass is lost and weakness develops. Intensive care unit acquired weakness can develop during hospitalization and is associated with an increased hospital length of stay as well as an increased mortality rate. ICU acquired weakness may last years after discharge with residual effects often affecting the patient's quality of life. Progressive mobility is defined as the gradual progression of positioning and mobility techniques and should be utilized to improve muscle strength and provide the patient a greater ability to resume activities of daily living. Patients should be assessed daily for their readiness to progress in their mobility goals in order to prevent the adverse effects of immobility.

Gait Disorders

Functional movement disorders are defined as an involuntary, abnormal movement of part of the body in which pathophysiology is not fully understood. Functional tremors are the most frequent type of functional movement disorder. Dystonia, myoclonus and Parkinsonism are other types of functional movement disorders. Functional gait disorders are another type of functional movement disorder and are common in the elderly. Gait disorders can manifest as a dragging gait, knee buckling, small slow steps or "walking on ice," swaying gait, fluctuating gait, hesitant gait, and hyperkinetic gait in which there is excessive movement of the arms, trunk, and legs when ambulating. Patients with gait disorders are at an increased risk of falling. Gait disorders are diagnosed by a thorough clinical examination (including a neurologic assessment) and health history. Treatment for functional gait disorders includes strength and balance training. Assistive devices such as walkers and canes may also be utilized.

Falls

Falls are the most commonly occurring adverse event in the hospital setting. Confusion and agitation are factors that contribute to an increased risk for falling. In addition, impaired balance or gait, orthostatic hypotension, altered mobility, a history of falling, advanced age and the use of certain medications are additional risk factors. Approximately 30% of patient falls result in injury, some of which can significantly contribute to an increase in morbidity and mortality including fractures and subdural hematomas. Both physical and environmental factors contribute to patient falls, some of which are preventable. Fall prevention strategies include utilization of a standardized fall risk assessment to determine the patient's level of risk and subsequent care planning and interventions individualized to the patient. Fall prevention should also be balanced with progressive mobility. Many falls are related to toileting needs, and nurses often utilize scheduled rounding to address such needs.

Carpal Tunnel Syndrome

Carpal tunnel syndrome is a type of entrapment neuropathy in which the median nerve is compressed by thickening of the flexor tendon sheath, skeletal encroachment, or mass in the soft tissue. Carpal tunnel syndrome is often associated with repetitive hand activities, arthritis, hypothyroidism, diabetes, and pregnancy. Patients complain of pain in wrist, radiating to forearm, and numbness and tingling in the first 2 to 3 fingers, especially during the night.

Diagnosis is based on symptoms and tests such as:

- **Positive Tinel test**: Gentle percussion over medial nerve in inner aspect of wrist elicits numbness and pain.
- **Positive Phalen test**: The backs of the hands are pressed together and the wrists sharply flexed for 1 minute to elicit pain and numbness.

Treatment includes identifying and treating the underlying cause:

- Steroid injection may relieve symptoms
- Splint during the night or during repetitive activities
- Modification of activities
- Referral for decompression surgery in recalcitrant cases or those with severe loss of sensation

Infectious Arthritis

Infectious arthritis may be bacterial, viral (rubella, parvovirus, and hepatitis B), parasitic, or fungal, with **bacterial arthritis** causing the most rapid destruction to the joint. *Neisseria gonorrhoeae* (most common), *Staphylococcus*, *Streptococcus*, and *Escherichia coli* are the most common bacterial agents. The infection may be bloodborne or spread from an infection near the joint or from direct implantation or postoperative contamination of the wound. Usually the infection involves just one joint.

Symptoms include acute edema, erythema, and pain in a joint. Systemic reactions, such as fever and polyarthralgia, may occur, especially with gonorrhea.

Diagnosis requires a complete history and physical examination, arthrocentesis and synovial fluid culture, and WBC.

Treatment includes:

- Antibiotics as indicated by organism
- Arthrocentesis to drain fluid accumulation in joint (may need to be repeated)
- Analgesia

Bursitis and Tendinitis

Bursitis is inflammation of the bursa, fluid-filled spaces or sacs that form in tissues to reduce friction, causing thickening of the lining of the bursal walls. This can be the result of infection, trauma, crystal deposits, or chronic friction from trauma.

Tendinitis is inflammation of the long, tubular tendons and tendon sheaths adjacent to the bursa. Causes of tendinitis are similar to bursitis but tendinitis may also be caused by quinolone antibiotics. Frequently, both bursa and tendons are inflamed. Common types of bursitis include shoulder, olecranon (elbow), trochanteric (hip), and prepatellar (front of knee). Common types of tendinitis include wrist, Achilles, patellar, and rotator cuff.

Symptoms include pain with movement, edema, dysfunction, and decreased range of motion.

Diagnosis is by clinical examination, although x-rays may rule out fractures. The bursa may be aspirated diagnostically to aid in ruling out other diagnosis, like gout or infection.

Treatment for bursitis and tendinitis includes:

- Rest and immobilization
- NSAIDs
- Application of cold packs to affected area
- Steroid injections

Joint Effusion and Arthrocentesis

Joint effusion is the accumulation of fluid (clear, bloody, or purulent) within a joint capsule. Joint effusion can cause pressure on the joint and severe pain. **Arthrocentesis** relieves the pressure and the fluid aspirated can be examined to aid in diagnosis. Arthrocentesis is usually contraindicated in the presence of overlying infection, prosthetic joint, and coagulopathy without referral to an orthopedic specialist.

Procedure:

1. Patient is **positioned** according to joint to be aspirated and encouraged to relax muscles.
2. **Overlying area** is cleansed with povidone-iodine solution, air-dried a few minutes, and cleansed of iodine with alcohol wipe.
3. **Local anesthetic** is given to the area (but not into the joint) with 25- to 30-gauge needle (lidocaine 1-2%) or a regional nerve block for severe pain.
4. The joint is **aspirated** with insertion in a straight line, using a 30-60 mL syringe (depending upon expected amount of fluid) and an 18- to 22-gauge needle or IV catheter.
5. The joint is completely **drained** of fluid.
6. Observe for **complications**: bleeding, infection, or allergic reaction.

Lumbosacral Pain

Lumbosacral (low back) pain may be related to strain, muscular weakness, osteoarthritis, spinal stenosis, herniated disks, vertebral fractures, bony metastasis, infection, or other musculoskeletal disorders. Disk herniation or other joint changes put pressure on nerves leaving the spinal cord, causing pain to radiate along the nerve. Pain may be acute or chronic (more than 3 months).

Symptoms include local or pain radiating down the leg (radiculopathy), impaired gait and reflexes, difference in leg lengths, decreased motor strength, and alteration of sensation, including numbness.

Diagnosis is by careful clinical examination and history as well as x-ray (fractures, scoliosis, dislocations), CT (identifies underlying problems), MRI (spinal pathology), and/or EMG and nerve conduction studies. Diagnostic studies may be deferred in many cases for 4-6 weeks as symptoms may resolve over time. **Treatments** for nonspecific back pain include:

- Analgesia: acetaminophen, NSAIDS, opiates
- Encourage activity to tolerance but not bed rest
- Muscle relaxants: diazepam 5-10 mg every 6-8 hours
- Cold and heat compresses

Strains and Sprains

A **strain** is an overstretching of a part of the musculature ("pulled muscle") that causes microscopic tears in the muscle, usually resulting from excess stress or overuse of the muscle. Onset of pain is usually sudden with local tenderness on use of the muscle. A **sprain** is damage to a joint, with a partial rupture of the supporting ligaments, usually caused by wrenching or twisting that may occur with a fall. The rupture can damage blood vessels, resulting in edema, tenderness at the joint, and pain on movement with pain increasing over 2-3 hours after injury. An avulsion fracture (bone fragment pulled away by a ligament) may occur with strain, so x-rays rule out fractures.

Treatment for both strains and sprains includes:

- **RICE protocol**: rest, ice, compression, and elevation
- **Ice compresses** (wet or dry) applied 20-30 minutes intermittently for 48 hours and then intermittent heat 15-20 minutes 3-4 times daily
- Monitor **neurovascular status** (especially for sprain)
- **Immobilization** as indicated for sprains for 1-3 weeks

High Energy Joint Injuries

Low energy injuries include those that occur as a result of a fall from standing position or less than one-meter height, but **high energy injuries** include those with greater impact, such as from an automobile accident, fall from greater height, and sports accidents (downhill skiing, ice hockey) as well as gunshot wounds, stab wounds, and blast injuries. High energy injuries are likely to be more severe and may include:

- Fractures, both open and closed
- Compression fractures
- Dislocations and fracture-dislocations
- Comminution
- Strains and sprains, injury to ligaments and tendons
- Lacerations, bleeding
- Soft tissue trauma, edema, and ecchymosis
- Shock

Patients typically have severe pain, and the affected joint may be very unstable with obvious misalignment if fractures or dislocations are present. Older adults are particularly at risk for fractures because of osteoporosis, and healing may be impaired because of chronic disease. With high energy injuries, patients also have greater risk of complications, such as fat embolism, hemorrhage, pulmonary embolism, compartment syndrome, infection, neurological damage, avascular necrosis, and mal-union, delayed union, or non-union.

Fractures and Dislocations

Types of Fractures

Fractures and **dislocations** usually occur as the result of trauma, such as from falls and auto accidents, but *pathologic* fractures can result from minor force to diseased bones such as those with osteoporosis or metastatic lesions. *Stress* fractures are caused by repetitive trauma, such as from forced marching. *Salter* fractures involve the cartilaginous epiphyseal plate near the ends of long bones in children who are growing. Damage to this area can impair bone growth. Orthopedic injuries that are of special concern include:

- **Open fractures** with soft tissue injury overlying the fracture, including puncture wounds from external forces or bone fragments, can result in osteomyelitis.
- **Subluxation, partial dislocation of a joint, and luxation** (complete dislocation) can cause neurovascular compromise, which can be permanent if reduction is delayed. Dislocation of the hip can result in avascular necrosis of the femoral head.

Diagnosis and Treatment

Fractures and **dislocations** are commonly **diagnosed** by clinical examination, history, and radiographs. Careful inspection and observation of range of motion, palpation, and observation of abnormalities is important because pain may be referred. Neurovascular assessment should be done immediately to prevent vascular compromise. Radiographs should usually precede reduction of dislocations to ensure there are no fractures and follow reduction to ensure the dislocation is reduced.

Treatment includes:

- Analgesia and sedation as indicated
- Application of cold compresses and elevation of fractured area to reduce edema
- Reduction of fracture: steady and gradual longitudinal traction to realign bone
- Immobilization with brace, cast, sling, or splint indicated
- Reduction of dislocation: Varies according to area of dislocation
- Open fracture: Wound irrigation with NS
- Tetanus prophylaxis
- Antibiotic prophylaxis
- Referral to orthopedic specialist for open fractures, irreducible dislocations, and complications such as compartment syndrome or circulatory impairment

Pelvic Fractures

Pelvic fractures may be fairly benign or seriously life threatening, depending on the degree and type of fracture. They most often result from high-speed trauma related to vehicular accidents or skiing accidents:

- **Open book**: Pelvis is pulled apart, usually from frontal injury (may cause severe hemorrhage)
- **Closed book**: Lateral compression occurs from side injury
- **Vertical shear**: Injury occurs from fall

Indications of pelvic fracture include localized edema, tenderness, obvious pelvic deformity, abnormal pelvic movement, and abdominal bruising. Associated intra-abdominal injuries and complications are common, including paralytic ileus, hemorrhage, urethral, colon, or bladder laceration. Patients may develop sepsis, peritonitis, fat embolism syndrome, or DVT. Displaced fractures may require open reduction and internal fixation. Treatment usually includes bedrest (up to 6 weeks) with care in handling to prevent further injury. Patients should be turned and moved in accordance with specific physician's orders. Ambulation using walker or crutches may be allowed for non-displaced fractures.

Acetabular Fractures

Acetabular (hip-socket) fractures occur primarily in young adults with motor vehicle accidents or falls from a height, resulting in impact pressure from the head of the femur to the joint and frequently associated (up to 50% of cases) with other severe injuries, including dislocation (which can lead to avascular necrosis if not promptly reduced). Up to 20% of those with acetabular fractures also have pelvic fractures. The degree of displacement that occurs depends on the amount of force as well as the position of the femur during impact. Acetabular fracture may be classified as posterior-wall, posterior-column, anterior-column, or transverse. Acetabular fractures in children less than 12 years may result in growth arrest. Complications may include sepsis, chondrolysis, and injury to vessels and/or nerves. Post-traumatic arthritis of the joint may develop. Diagnosis is per examination, radiograph, and/or CT with Doppler ultrasound with suspected DVT. Treatment includes emergent closed reduction if necessary, longitudinal skeletal traction, and open reduction and internal fixation (ORIF) for displaced fractures and serious injury (usually delayed for 2-3 days because of initial bleeding).

Closed Fractures and Open Fractures

Closed fractures are those in which the damage to the bone and tissue (bleeding, swelling) remains enclosed within intact skin and does not invade any internal cavity. The bone segments are more likely to be aligned, although some comminution may have occurred from splintering when the bone breaks. It may be difficult to differentiate a closed fracture from an open fracture if there are abrasions and lacerations over the area of the fractures, but it is closed if there is no continuity between the fracture and the external injury.

Open fractures, on the other hand, cause an external wound and may result from fragments of the fractured bone penetrating the skin or an external force penetrating the skin and bone. Open fractures may also appear closed on the surface but invade a body cavity. Open fractures carry a much higher risk of contamination and infection as well as severe bleeding. The external wounds associated with open fractures may vary in size, but even small wounds are considered emergent because of risk of infection.

Fat Embolism as Complication of Traumatic Fracture

In instances of **traumatic fracture**, the possibility of **fat embolism** should be considered; this is especially true in fractures involving the long bones (femur, humerus). When the bone is fractured, this allows for some of the fatty marrow contained within the bone to escape. Because the fracture and subsequent trauma to the area surrounding the fracture results in broken vessels, it is possible that the fatty marrow can be introduced into the bloodstream. When this happens, the events are similar to that of a deep venous thrombosis; the fat embolus dislodges from the lumen of the vessel and travels to the lung. When the embolus enters the pulmonary circulation, it eventually blocks blood flow as the caliber of the vessel through which it travels decreases, keeping blood from flowing to the lung tissue. The disruption in blood flow results in inflammation and necrosis of the lung, and eventually pulmonary failure ensues.

Osteomyelitis

Musculoskeletal infections encompass a variety of different disorders with differing pathologies. Osteomyelitis, cellulitis, and septic arthritis are examples of musculoskeletal infections that can be both serious and debilitating in nature.

Osteomyelitis is an infection of the bone that can occur from an open fracture or an infection that has occurred somewhere else in the body. Osteomyelitis can also be caused by wounds or soft tissue infections that have progressed and extended to the bone. Signs and symptoms of osteomyelitis include pain, swelling, erythema and possible drainage at the site. The patient may also experience fever and chills. Diagnosis includes lab work including a complete blood count, erythrocyte sedimentation rate (ESR), C-reactive protein (CRP), and blood cultures, as well as radiologic testing that may include CT, MRI, X-ray, bone scan, or a bone biopsy. Treatment includes the administration of IV antibiotics. A needle aspiration may be performed to determine the organism and drain the area. Surgical irrigation and debridement may also be indicated.

Compartment Syndrome

Compartment syndrome occurs when there is an increase in the amount of pressure within a grouping of muscles, nerves, and blood vessels resulting in compromised blood flow to muscles and nerves. This is a medical emergency. If left untreated, tissue ischemia and eventual tissue death will occur. Compartment syndrome most often occurs after a fracture, particularly a long bone fracture, but can also occur with crushing syndrome and rhabdomyolysis. Risk factors include lower extremity trauma, massive tissue injury, venous obstruction, the use of certain medications (anticoagulants), burns and compressive dressings or casts. Compartment syndrome can affect the hand, forearm, upper arm, abdomen and lower extremities. It can be acute or chronic in nature with acute compartment syndrome requiring immediate intervention.

Signs and symptoms: Intense pain, decreased sensation and paresthesia, firmness at the affected site, swelling and tightness at the affected site, pallor and pulselessness (late signs).

Diagnosis: Physical assessment and the measurement of intra-compartmental pressures.

Treatment: The goal of treatment in compartment syndrome is decompression and the restoration of perfusion to the affected area. Surgical fasciotomy is often indicated to relieve pressure and prevent tissue death. Fasciotomy involves the opening of the skin and muscle fascia to release the pressure within the compartment and restore blood flow to the area.

Prevention: Leave large abdominal wounds open to drain, delay casting on affected extremities, and use flexible casts. Watch circumferential burns closely and perform frequent neurovascular checks on those at risk.

Rhabdomyolysis

Rhabdomyolysis occurs when damage of the cells of the skeletal muscles causes the release of toxins from injured cells into the bloodstream. Rhabdomyolysis may be caused by trauma, tissue ischemia, infection, certain medications (statins, selective serotonin reuptake inhibitors, lithium and antihistamines), sepsis, immobilization, extraordinary physical exertion, myopathies and cocaine or alcohol abuse. Additionally, rhabdomyolysis may occur with exposure to certain toxins such as snake/insect venoms or mushroom poisoning. In rare circumstances, the identifiable cause cannot be determined. The most serious complication of rhabdomyolysis is renal failure. Rhabdomyolysis may be life threatening. Early recognition and treatment are critical to avoid serious complications and for patients to make a full recovery.

Signs and symptoms: Electrolyte imbalance, muscle pain and weakness, fever, tachycardia, dehydration, fatigue, lethargy, hypotension and metabolic acidosis. Dark, reddish-brown urine may occur due to the presence of myoglobin released from the muscles and excreted into the urine.

Diagnosis: Laboratory studies such as creatinine kinase (CK) level, metabolic panel, urinalysis and blood gases.

Treatment: The treatment of rhabdomyolysis includes fluid administration to eliminate toxins and prevent renal failure. Bicarbonate may be administered to correct metabolic acidosis. Mannitol or dopamine may be administered to increase renal perfusion. Electrolyte replacement may also be indicated. In severe cases, emergency dialysis may be necessary.

Ear, Nose, and Throat Pathophysiology

Peritonsillar Abscess

Peritonsillar abscess (PTA), which usually derives from tonsillitis, progresses from cellulitis to abscess between the palatine tonsil and capsule. It is often polymicrobial. It usually occurs bilaterally between the ages of 20 to 30. Complications include obstruction of airway, rupture with aspiration of purulent material, septicemia, endocarditis, and epiglottitis. The infection is often polymicrobial. Symptoms include fever, pain, hoarseness, muffling of voice, dysphagia, tonsillar edema, erythema, exudate, and edema of palate with displacement of uvula.

Diagnosis:

- Aspiration of purulent material (usually diagnostic).
- CT with contrast, ultrasound.
- On exam: Displacement of the uvula, with enlarged tonsils.

Treatments include:

- Needle aspirations (often multiple) with needle penetrating 1 cm or less to avoid carotid artery.
- Abscess incision and drainage if aspiration not successful.
- IV volume replacement.
- **Antibiotics**: IV ampicillin-sublactam or clindamycin until culture results come back and in areas with high rates of CA-MRSA vancomycin may be added. Once the patient shows signs of clinical improvement, they may switch to oral antibiotics (needing 14 days total).

Dental Avulsions

Dental avulsions are the complete displacement of a tooth from its socket. The tooth may be reimplanted if done within one to two hours after displacement, although only permanent teeth are reimplanted, not primary.

Procedure:

1. Tooth can be **transported** from accident site to the emergency department in Hank solution, saline, or milk.
2. **Cleanse** tooth with sterile NS or Hank solution, handling only the crown and avoiding any disruption of fibers.
3. If tooth has been dry for 20 to 60 minutes, **soak** tooth in Hank solution for 30 minutes before reimplantation.
4. If tooth has been dry for more than 60 minutes, **soak** tooth in citric acid for 5 minutes, stannous fluoride 2% for 5 minutes, and doxycycline solution for 5 minutes prior to reimplantation.
5. Remove **clot** in socket and gently irrigate with NS.
6. Place tooth into **socket** firmly, cover with gauze, and have patient bite firmly on gauze until splinting can be applied.
7. Apply **splinting material and mold packing** over implanted tooth and 2 adjacent teeth on both sides (encompasses 5 teeth).

Dental Fractures

Dental fractures, most commonly of the maxillary teeth, may occur in association with other oral injuries and may be overlooked unless a careful dental examination is carried out. Fractures are classified according to severity of fracture with treatment to prevent further damage and necrosis.

- **Ellis I**: Chipping of enamel.
  - Smoothen rough edges.
- **Ellis II**: Fracture of enamel and dentin with pain on pressure and air sensitivity.
  - Protect dentin with glass ionomer dental cement and refer to dentist within 24 hours.

- **Ellis III**: Fracture of enamel, dentin, and pulp with pain on movement, air and temperature sensitivity; blood may be evident
    - Protect dentin with ionomer dental cement or calcium hydroxide base and refer to dentist for prompt treatment.
    - Administer oral analgesics.
- **Alveolar/root fracture:** Loose tooth and malocclusion, sensitivity to percussion.
    - Prompt referral to dentist for splinting and/or root canal.

Review Video: Anatomical and Clinical Parts of Teeth
Visit mometrix.com/academy and enter code: 683627

Recurrent Epistaxis

Recurrent epistaxis is common in young children (2 to 10 years), especially boys, and is often related to nose picking, dry climate, or central heating in the winter. Incidence also increases between 50 to 80 years of age, and may be caused by NSAIDs and anticoagulants. Kiesselbach plexus in the anterior nares has plentiful vessels and bleeds easily. Bleeding in the posterior nares is more dangerous and can result in considerable blood loss. Bleeding from the anterior nares is usually confined to one nostril, but from the posterior nares, blood may flow through both nostrils or backward into the throat and the person may be observed swallowing. People abusing cocaine may suffer nosebleeds because of damage to the mucosa. Hematocrit and hemoglobin should be done to determine if blood loss is significant. Bleeding should stop within 20 minutes. Treatment:

- Upright position, leaning forward so blood does not flow down throat.
- Applying pressure below the nares or by pinching the nostrils firmly for 10 minutes.
- Severe bleeding: packing and/or topical vasoconstrictors.
- Humidifiers may decrease irritation.

Bell's Palsy

Bell's palsy is caused by inflammation of cranial nerve VII, usually from a herpes simplex I or II infection, and generally affects only one side of the paired nerves. Onset is generally sudden, and symptoms peak by 48 hours with a wide range of presentation. **Symptoms** usually subside within two to six months but may persist one year:

- Mild weakness on one side of face to complete paralysis with distortion of features.
- Drooping of eyelid and mouth.
- Tearing in affected eye.
- Taste impairment.

Diagnosis includes:

- Neurological, eye, parotid gland, and ear exam to rule out other cranial nerve involvement or conditions.

Treatment includes:

- Artificial tears during daytime with lubricating ophthalmic ointment and patch at night to protect eye.
- Prednisone 60 mg daily for 5 days with tapering over 5 days.
- For severe cases use prednisone AND acyclovir 400 mg 5 times daily for 7 days.

Temporal Arteritis

Temporal arteritis (TA), also called giant cell arteritis, is inflammation of the blood vessels of the head, especially the temporal artery, and the thoracic aorta and branches. TA is commonly associated with polymyalgia rheumatica (30% or less of patients) but can occur with other systemic disorders such as lupus erythematous, Sjögren syndrome, and rheumatoid arthritis. TA is a progressive disorder that can result in blindness and is most common in those older than 50. **Symptoms** include:

- New onset of headaches.
- Vision fluctuations, including decreased visual acuity and loss of vision.
- Intermittent claudicating pain in jaw, tongue, and upper extremities.
- Fever.

Diagnosis includes:

- Temporal artery biopsy (definitive).
- ESR greater than 50 mm/h (may be normal in about 20%).
- CRP greater than 2.45 mg/dL.

Treatment should begin immediately if the diagnosis is suspected to prevent blindness:

- Prednisone 60 mg daily.

Trigeminal Neuralgia

Trigeminal neuralgia (tic douloureux) is a neurological condition in which blood vessels press on the trigeminal nerve as it leaves the brainstem causing severe pain on one side of the face or jaw. The shock-like pains may involve a small area or half the face and in rare cases both sides of the face at different times. The pain lasts from seconds to two minutes and is extremely debilitating and may be precipitated by movement, vibration, or contact with the face or mouth. Trigeminal neuralgia is most common in women older than 50. Patients may go through periods of remission and recurrences. Diagnosis is by history and neurological exam.

Treatment includes:

- **Carbamazepine** is the drug of choice and usually controls pain initially, but the effects may decrease over time.
- **Phenytoin or oxcarbazepine** may be used in place of carbamazepine.
- **Baclofen** (muscle relaxant) potentiates other drugs.
- **Surgical procedures** may be done if no response to medications.

Foreign Bodies

Foreign Bodies in the Ear

Foreign bodies in the **ear** (most often in children) can be organic or inorganic materials or insects. Careful history should be done to determine the type of foreign body before attempting removal. Children may require conscious sedation or general anesthesia for deep insertions. Irrigations should not be done if tympanic membrane is ruptured or cannot be visualized. Procedure:

1. Examine ear to determine if tympanic membrane is intact.
2. Drown insects with lidocaine 2% solution and then suction.
3. Irrigate small nonorganic particles with pulsatile flow aimed at wall of the canal.
4. Use cerumen loops, right-angle hooks, and/or alligator forceps to grasp and remove item.

5. Carefully examine the ear canal after removal of the item for lacerations or abrasions.
6. Topical antibiotic if extensive cutaneous abrasion or laceration or for organic material.

Foreign Bodies in the Eye

Foreign bodies in the **eye** should be assessed carefully with slit lamp with corneal examination using optical sectioning before attempting removal of the foreign body. Foreign bodies that penetrate the cornea full-thickness should not be removed in the ED, but superficial foreign bodies can safely be removed. Procedure:

1. Apply topical anesthetic to both eyes (to suppress blinking in the unaffected eye).
2. Eye held open by hand or with wire eyelid speculum.
3. Foreign body is carefully removed with small gauge needle or moistened cotton swab.
4. Rust ring from metallic objects should be removed with ophthalmic burr (if not over pupil), and patient referred to ophthalmologist for further rust ring removal within 24 hours.
5. Eyelid everted and examined carefully for further foreign bodies.
6. Abrasions treated as indicated.

Foreign Bodies in the Nares

Children may insert various organic and inorganic **foreign bodies** in the **nose**. In most cases, this is observed, but persistent unilateral obstruction of nose, foul discharge, or epistaxis is suggestive of foreign body. Small or uncooperative children may need to be restrained with conscious sedation or papoose board.

Procedure:

1. Vasoconstrictor/topical anesthetic applied: 1 mL of phenylephrine with 3 mL of lidocaine 4%.
2. Aerosolized racemic epinephrine may be used for decongestion, to loosen foreign body.
3. Examine nares with speculum.

Removal techniques:

- Positive pressure: Blowing nose on command. For small children, block opposite nares and have caregiver blow puff of air in mouth, forcing item out of nares.
- Suction with catheter.
- Use alligator or bayonet forceps to grasp item.
- Pass a curette behind item, rotate, and the use to pull item out.
- Pass Fogarty vascular catheter past item, inflate balloon, pull catheter back out.

Ludwig Angina

Ludwig angina is cellulitis, usually caused by *Streptococcus* or *Staphylococcus,* of the submandibular spaces and lingual space that can result in obstruction of the airway as the swelling in the mouth floor pushes the tongue superior and posterior.

Symptoms include:

- Evidence of poor dental hygiene and odontogenic abscess (usually from lower third molars or surrounding gums) that has spread into soft tissue.
- Dysphagia.
- Odynophagia, trismus, edema of the upper neck (midline).

- Erythema, stridor and cyanosis (late signs of obstruction).
- Changes in mental status.

Diagnosis includes:

- Examination of the head and neck to observe for swelling of the upper neck, floor of mouth, and tongue.
- CT scan.
- Culture (treatment should, however, begin immediately).

Treatments include:

- Nasotracheal intubation (with fiberoptic tube if necessary) and ventilation if respiratory obstruction.
- IV antibiotics, such as penicillin or clindamycin.
- Referral to surgeon for incision and drainage as indicated.

Otitis Externa

Otitis externa is infection of the external ear canal, either bacterial or mycotic. Common pathogens include bacteria, *Pseudomonas aeruginosa*, *Staphylococcus aureus,* and fungi, *Aspergillus* and *Candida.* OE is often caused by chlorine in swimming pools killing normal flora and allowing other bacteria to multiply. Fungal infections may be associated with immune disorders, diabetes, and steroid use.

Symptoms include:

- Pain, swelling, and exudate.
- Itching (pronounced with fungal infections).
- Red pustular lesions.
- Black spots over tympanic membrane (fungus).

Diagnosis: On exam, tenderness when touched on tragus or when the auricle is pulled, erythema, and history.

Treatment includes:

- Irrigate ear with Burow's solution or saline to clean and remove debris or foreign objects.
- **Bacteria**: Antibiotic ear drops, such as ciprofloxacin and ofloxacin. If impetigo, flush with hydrogen peroxide 1:1 solution and apply mupirocin twice daily for 5 to 7 days. Lance pointed furuncles.

- **Fungus**: Solution of boric acid 5% in ethanol; clotrimazole-miconazole solution with/without steroid for 5 to 7 days.
- Analgesics as needed.

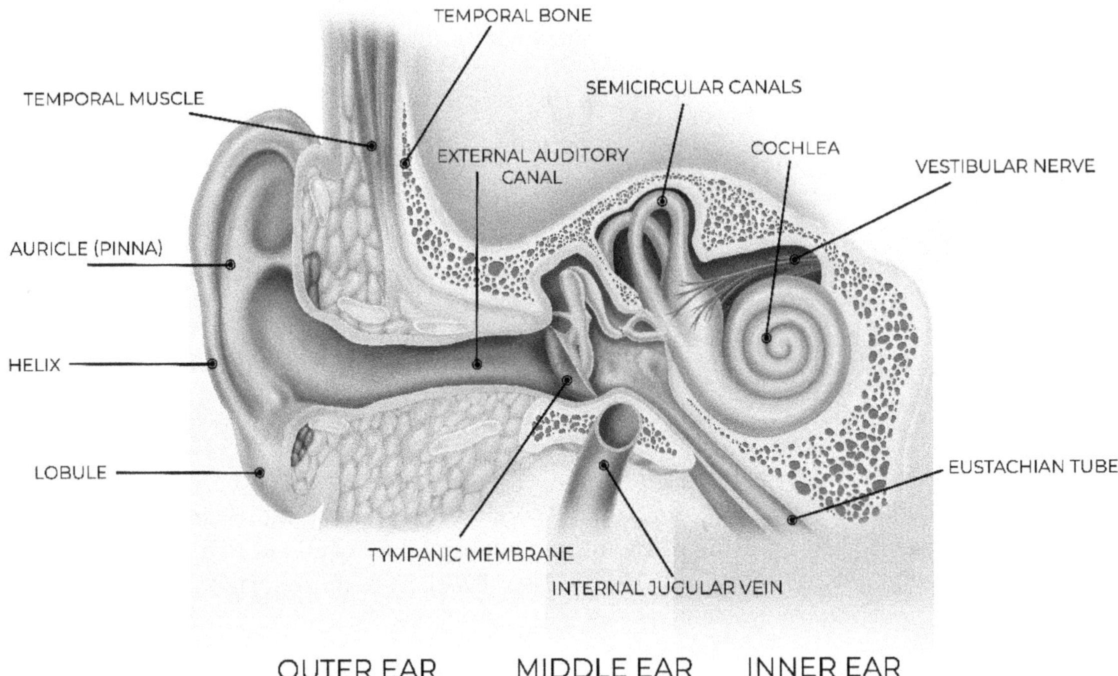

OTITIS MEDIA

Otitis media, inflammation of the middle ear, usually follows upper respiratory tract infections or allergic rhinitis. The eustachian tube swells and prevents the passage of air. Fluid from the mucous membrane pools in the middle ear, causing infection. Common pathogens include *Streptococcus pneumoniae, Haemophilus influenzae,* and *Moraxella catarrhalis.* Some genetic conditions, such as trisomy 21 and cleft palate, may include abnormalities of the eustachian tube, increasing risk. There are four forms:

- **Acute**: One to three weeks with swelling, redness, and possible rupture of the tympanic membrane, fever, pain (ear pulling), and hearing loss.
- **Recurrent**: Three episodes in six months or four to six in 12 months.
- **Bullous**: Acute infection with ear popping pressure in middle ear, pain, hearing loss, and bullae between layers of tympanic membrane, causing bulging.
- **Chronic**: Persists at least three months with thick retracted tympanic membrane, hearing loss, and drainage.

Diagnosis: Distinguishing features on assessment of acute otitis media include a bulging or perforated tympanic membrane, signs of inflammation, or purulent fluid present.

Treatment: 75% to 90% resolve spontaneously, so antibiotics are **withheld** for two to three days. Amoxicillin for 7 to 10 days. Referral for **tympanostomy and pressure-equalizing tubes** (PET) for severe chronic or recurrent infections.

Review Video: Otitis Media
Visit mometrix.com/academy and enter code: 328778

Mastoiditis

Mastoiditis usually results from extension of acute otitis media because the mucous membranes of the middle ear are continuous with the mastoid air cells in the temporal bone. All patients with otitis media should be considered at risk for mastoiditis. Patients with chronic otitis media also often develop chronic mastoiditis, which can result in formation of benign cholesteatoma. Signs and symptoms of mastoiditis include persistent fever, pain in or behind the ear (especially during the night), and hearing loss. Differential diagnoses may include Bell's palsy, otitis externa, and otitis media. Diagnosis is based on symptoms, CBC, audiometry, tympanocentesis or myringotomy with culture and sensitivities, and CT scan (definitive). **Acute mastoiditis** is treated with antibiotics, usually beginning with a 3rd generation cephalosporin or penicillin/aminoglycoside combination until culture and sensitivity results return. If spreading empyema or osteitis is present, then surgical mastoidectomy is required.

Sinusitis

Sinusitis is inflammation of the nasal sinuses, of which there are two maxillary, two frontal, and one sphenoidal, as ethmoidal air cells. Inflammation causes obstruction of drainage with resultant discomfort.

Symptoms include:

- Frontal and maxillary presents with pain over sinuses.
- Ethmoidal present with dull aching behind eye.
- Tenderness to palpation and percussion of sinuses.
- Mucosa of nasal cavity edematous and erythematous.
- Purulent exudate.

Diagnosis includes:

- Transillumination of sinus (diminished with inflammation).
- CT for those who are immunocompromised or if diagnosis is not clear.
- Careful examination to rule out spreading infection, especially with signs of fever, altered mental status, or unstable vital signs.

Treatment includes:

- Symptomatic relief with analgesia.
- Topical decongestants and nasal irrigation.
- Antimicrobial therapy if symptoms persist at least seven days or are severe (avoid routine use): Amoxicillin or TMP/SMX.
- Steroid nasal spray twice daily.

Meniere's Disease

Meniere's disease occurs when a blockage in the endolymphatic duct of the inner ear causes dilation of the endolymphatic space and abnormal fluid balance, which causes pressure or rupture of the inner ear membrane.

Symptoms include:

- Progressive fluctuating sensorineural hearing loss.
- Tinnitus.
- Pressure in the ear.

- Severe vertigo that lasts minutes to hours.
- Diaphoresis.
- Poor balance.
- Nausea and vomiting.

Diagnosis includes:

- Complete physical exam and evaluation of cranial nerves.
- Tuning fork sounds may lateralize to unaffected ear.
- Assessment of hearing loss.

Treatment:

- Low sodium diet.
- Vestibular suppressant (antihistamine): Meclizine.
- Benzodiazepine or SSRI for anxiety.
- Antiemetics, such as promethazine suppositories.
- Diuretics, such as hydrochlorothiazide.
- Referral for surgical repair for persistent vertigo, but this will not correct other symptoms.

Labyrinthitis

Labyrinthitis is a viral or bacterial inflammation of the inner ear, and it may occur secondary to bacterial otitis media. **Viral** labyrinthitis may be associated with mumps, rubella, rubeola, influenza, or other viral infections, such as upper respiratory tract infections. Because the labyrinth includes the vestibular system that is responsible for sensing head movement, labyrinthitis causes balance disorders. The condition often persists for 1 to 6 weeks with acute symptoms the first week and then decreasing symptoms. **Symptoms** include:

- Sudden onset of severe vertigo.
- Hearing loss and sometimes tinnitus.
- Nausea and vomiting.
- Panic attacks from severe anxiety related to symptoms.

Treatment includes:

- **Bacterial**: IV antibiotics.
- **Viral**: Symptomatic as for bacterial (except for antibiotics).
- Volume replacement.
- Antiemetics, such as promethazine suppositories.
- Vestibular suppressant (antihistamine): Meclizine.
- Benzodiazepine or SSRI for anxiety.
- Referral to surgeon for I&D if necessary.

TMD

Temporomandibular disorder (TMD) is jaw pain caused by dysfunction of the temporomandibular joint (TMJ) and the supporting muscles and ligaments. It may be precipitated by injury, such as whiplash, or grinding or clenching of the teeth, stress, or arthritis.

Symptoms include:

- Clicking or popping noises on jaw movement.
- Limited jaw movement or "locked" jaw.
- Acute pain on chewing or moving jaw.
- Headaches and dizziness.
- Toothaches.

Diagnosis includes:

- Complete dental exam with x-rays to rule out other disorders.
- MRI or CT may be needed.

Treatment usually begins conservatively:

- Ice pack to jaw area for 10 minutes followed by jaw stretching exercises and warm compress for 5 minutes 3 to 4 times daily.
- Avoidance of heavy chewing by eating soft foods and avoiding hard foods, such as raw carrots and nuts.
- NSAIDs to relieve pain and inflammation.
- Night mouthguard.
- Referral for dental treatments to improve bite as necessary.

Nasal Fracture

Nasal fracture can result from any type of blunt trauma to the face. Fracture may be overlooked because of edema, so careful examination of the nose with facial injuries is important. Common causes include altercations and sporting injuries. Septal cartilage is often fractured as well as nasal bones.

Symptoms include:

- Edema.
- Pain.
- Crepitation.
- Ecchymosis.
- Deformity.
- Nasal bleeding.

Diagnosis is based on clinical examination and otoscope. Radiographic studies are not indicated unless other facial fractures are suspected. Clear nasal discharge following injury to the face may indicate leaking of cerebrospinal fluid from torn meninges resulting from fracture of cribriform plate. A drop of clear drainage should be placed on filter paper and examined for a clear area around a central stain of blood. If CSF drainage is suspected, the patient should be placed upright, and have a CT scan and neurological consult.

Treatment for fracture includes:

- Realignment if necessary.
- Analgesia.
- Nasal decongestant.

- Protective covering.
- Packing only for persistent epistaxis.

Maxillary Fractures

Maxillary fractures of the face often are associated with significant other trauma because of the degree of force necessary to fracture the maxilla. Three primary types include:

- **Le Fort I**: Horizontal (low downward force)
- **Le Fort II**: Pyramidal (low or mid maxilla force)
- **Le Fort III**: Transverse (force to bridge of nose or upper maxilla)

However, many injuries are a combination with more than one type of fracture.

Symptoms may include:

- Malocclusion and open bite.
- Apparent lengthening of face.
- CSF rhinorrhea (clear nasal discharge).
- Periorbital ecchymosis.

Diagnosis: Grasping and moving the hard palate back and forth may shift the facial bones. Complete head, neck, ear, oral, and nasal examination with slit headlamp, suction as needed, nasal speculum, and otoscope. CT scans of face and brain.

Treatment:

- Stabilize patient and ensure patent airway.
- Disimpaction of displaced fragments manually.
- Obtain pre-injury photograph to guide surgical fixation.
- Referral to surgeon for fixation.

Fever and Fibromyalgia

Febrile Seizure

Febrile seizure is a generalized seizure associated with high fever (usually more than 38°C [100.4°F]) from any type of infection (upper respiratory tract, urinary) but without intracranial infection or other cause, occurring between six months and five years of age. Careful clinical examination must be conducted to rule out more serious disorders. Laboratory tests are conducted in relation to symptoms. Lumbar puncture is not usually indicated unless intracranial infection is suspected. Seizures usually last less than 15 minutes and are without subsequent neurological deficit.

Treatment includes:

- Fever control: Acetaminophen 10-15 mg/kg every 4-6 hours OR ibuprofen 10 mg/kg every 6-8 hours. Antipyretics are NOT recommended as prophylaxis for recurrent febrile seizures.
- Tepid water bath (NOT alcohol).
- Antiepileptic drugs (AEDs) are usually not advised unless seizures are complex or continuous, child is younger than 6 months, or there is a preexisting neurological disorder: IV diazepam 0.1-0.2 mg/kg or IV lorazepam 0.05-0.1 mg/kg. (May cause lethargy.)

Fibromyalgia

Fibromyalgia is a complex syndrome of disorders that include fatigue, chronic generalized muscle pain, and focal areas of tenderness persisting for at least three months. The cause of fibromyalgia is not clear and has only recently been recognized as a distinct disorder. Diagnosis is by clinical exam and ruling out joint and muscle inflammation that could be cause of the pain. On clinical exam there are specific points of tenderness, usually in multiple areas of the body.

Symptoms:

- Fatigue.
- Pain and stiffness unresponsive to treatment, persisting for months.
- Sleep disorders.
- Irritable bowel syndrome.
- Stiffness in neck and shoulders associated with headache and pain in face.
- Sensitivity to odor, noises, and lights.
- Mood disorders, such as depression, anxiety.
- Dysmenorrhea.
- Paresthesia in hands and feet.

Treatment:

- **Analgesia**: Acetaminophen, tramadol, or NSAIDs.
- **Antidepressants**, such as amitriptyline, nortriptyline, or fluoxetine. Duloxetine and venlafaxine have been shown to reduce pain.
- **Antiseizure medication**: Pregabalin is the first FDA-approved treatment for the pain of fibromyalgia.
- **Referral** for physical therapy and/or cognitive therapy.

Psychosocial Pathophysiology

Developmental Delays and Intellectual Disability

Developmental delays occur when a patient does not progress mentally at the same rate as the general population. **Intellectual disability** is a condition in which individuals may have difficulty adapting to changing environments, need guidance in decision-making, and have self-care or communication deficits. Behaviors range from shy and passive to hyperactive and aggressive. Intellectual disability may be inherited (Tay-Sachs), toxin-related (maternal alcohol consumption), perinatal (hypoxia), environmental (lack of stimulation/neglect), or acquired (encephalitis, brain injury). Diagnosis involves performance results from standardized tests with behavior analysis. Intellectual disability classifications are based on IQ:

- **55-69 (mild, 85% of cases):** Educable to about 6th grade level. May not be diagnosed until adolescence. Usually able to learn skills and be self-supporting but may need assistance and supervision.
- **40-54 (moderate, 10% of cases):** Trainable and may be able to work and live in sheltered environments or with supervision.
- **25-39 (severe, 3-4% of cases):** Language usually delayed and can learn only basic academic skills and perform simple tasks.
- **≤25 (profound, 1-2% of cases):** Usually associated with neurological disorder with sensorimotor dysfunction. Require constant care and supervision.

Nursing considerations: Always treat patients according to their developmental level, not their physical age. This is especially important when considering education and consent. People with developmental delays are at increased risk for injury and abuse.

Personality Disorder

A **personality disorder** is a fixed and enduring set pattern or traits of behavior that **deviate from expected behaviors within a culture**. These disorders inhibit the individual's ability to have meaningful interpersonal relationships, to be fulfilled, or to enjoy life. Onset usually occurs during adolescence or early adulthood. A personality disorder is an attitude directed toward the whole world including one's own self. This attitude is expressed through thoughts, feelings, and behaviors. Many times, the behaviors will become less extreme as the person gets older.

DSM Classification Groupings

The **DSM-5** lists 10 personality disorders grouped into three clusters: A, B, and C.

- **Cluster A** includes disorders that are characterized by odd or eccentric behaviors and a tendency for social awkwardness and withdrawal.
- **Cluster B** includes disorders that are characterized by erratic, highly emotional, dramatic, or impulsive behaviors.
- **Cluster C** includes disorders that are characterized predominantly by fearful or anxious symptoms.

Bipolar Disorder

Bipolar disorder causes severe mood swings between hyperactive states and depression, accompanied by impaired judgment because of distorted thoughts. The hypomanic stage may allow for creativity and good functioning in some people, but it can develop into more severe mania, which may be associated with psychosis and hallucinations with rapid speech and bizarre behavior, and then into periods of profound depression. While most cases are diagnosed in late adolescence, there is increasing evidence that some children present with symptoms earlier; especially at risk are children with a bipolar parent. Bipolar disorder is associated with high rates of suicide, so early diagnosis and treatment is critical.

Symptoms may be relatively mild or involve severe rapid cycling between mania and depression.

Treatment includes both medications (usually given continually) to prevent cycling and control depression and psychosocial therapy, such as cognitive therapy, to help control disordered thought patterns and behavior. Psychiatric referral should be made.

Depression

Depression is a mood disorder characterized by profound feelings of sadness and withdrawal. It may be acute (such as after a death) or chronic with recurring episodes over a lifetime. The cause appears to be a combination of genetic, biological, and environmental factors. A major depressive episode is a depressed mood, profound and constant sense of hopelessness and despair, or loss of interest in all or almost all activities for a period of at least two weeks. Some drugs may precipitate depression: diuretics, Parkinson's drugs, estrogen, corticosteroids, cimetidine, hydralazine, propranolol, digitalis, and indomethacin. Depression is associated with neurotransmitter dysregulation, especially serotonin and norepinephrine. Major depression can be mild, moderate, or severe.

Symptoms include changes in mood, sadness, loss of interest in usual activities, increased fatigue, changes in appetite and fluctuations in weight, anxiety, and sleep disturbance.

Treatment includes tricyclic antidepressants (TCAS) and SSRIs, but SSRIs have fewer side effects and are less likely to cause death with an overdose. Counselling, undergoing cognitive behavioral therapy, treating underlying cause, and instituting an exercise program may help reduce depression.

Anxiety and Depression Due to Intensive Care Stays

Anxiety and depression affect over half of patients who are treated in intensive care not only during the stay but also after discharge, especially if care is long-term or if their needs for moderate or high care continue. Additionally, studies have shown that those who suffer depression during and after ICU stays have increased risk of mortality over the next two years. Patients with anxiety may appear restless (thrashing about the bed), have difficulty concentrating, exhibit tachycardia and tachypnea, experience insomnia and feelings of dread, and complain of various ailments, such as stomach ache and headache. Symptoms of depression may overlap (and patients may have both anxiety and depression) and may also include fatigue, insomnia, withdrawal, appetite change, irritability, pessimistic outlooks, feelings of worthlessness, sadness, and suicidal ideation. Brief screening tools for anxiety and depression should be used with all ICU patients and interventions per psychological referral made as needed.

Anxiety Disorders

Anxiety is a human emotion and experience that everyone has at some point during their life. Feelings of uncertainty, helplessness, isolation, alienation, and insecurity can all be experienced during an **anxiety response**. Many times, anxiety occurs without a specific known object or source. It can occur because of the unknown. Anxiety occurs throughout the life cycle, and therefore anxiety disorders can affect people of all ages. Populations that are most commonly affected include women, smokers, people under the age of 45, individuals that are separated or divorced, victims of abuse, and people in the lower socioeconomic groups. An individual can have one single anxiety disorder, experience more than one anxiety disorder, or have other mental health disorders all occurring at the same time.

Generalized Anxiety Disorder

Generalized anxiety disorder can be very insidious and occurs when an individual consistently experiences **excessive anxiety and worry**. This anxiety and worry will be present almost every day and lasts for a period of at least six months. The worry and anxiety will be uncontrollable, intrusive, and not related to any medical disease process. It will pertain to real-life events, situations, or circumstances and may occur along with mild depression symptoms. The individual will also experience three or more of the following symptoms: fatigue, inability to concentrate, irritability, insomnia, restlessness, loosing thought processes or going blank, and muscle tension. The continued anxiety and worry will eventually affect daily functioning and cause social and occupational disturbances.

Comorbidities

Individuals with generalized anxiety disorder (GAD) will often have **other mental health disorders**. When a person has more than one psychological disorder occurring at the same time, these disorders are considered to be **comorbid**. Most patients suffering from GAD will have at least one more psychiatric diagnosis. The most common comorbid disorders can include major depressive disorder, social or specific phobias, panic disorder, and dysthymic disorder. It is also common for these individuals to have substance abuse problems, and they may look to alcohol or barbiturates to help control their symptoms of anxiety.

LEVELS OF ANXIETY

There are **four main levels of anxiety** that were named by **Peplau**. They are as follows:

1. **Mild anxiety** is associated with normal tensions of everyday life. It can increase awareness and motivate learning and creativity.
2. **Moderate anxiety** occurs when the individual narrows their field of perception and focuses on the immediate problem. This level decreases the perceptual field; however, the person can tend to other tasks if directed.
3. **Severe anxiety** leads to a markedly reduced field of perception and the person focuses only on the details of the problem. All energy is directed at relieving the anxiety and the person can only perform other tasks under significant persuasion.
4. **Panic** is the most extreme level of anxiety and associated with feelings of dread and terror. The individual is unable to perform any other tasks no matter how strongly they are persuaded to do so. This level can be life-threatening with complete disorganization of thought occurring.

PHYSICAL SYMPTOMS

Anxiety produces a very **physical response** and effects the largest body systems, such as cardiovascular, respiratory, GI, neuromuscular, urinary tract, and skin. Symptoms vary and can increase upon a continuum depending upon the level of anxiety the person is experiencing.

- **Cardiovascular symptoms** can include palpitation, tachycardia, hypertension, feeling faint or actually fainting, hypotension, or bradycardia.
- **Respiratory symptoms** can include tachypnea, shortness of breath, chest pressure, shallow respirations, or choking sensation.
- **GI symptoms** can include revulsion toward food, nausea, diarrhea, and abdominal pain or discomfort.

Even though anxiety occurs psychologically, it can produce extreme **physical responses** from the neuromuscular system, urinary tract, and skin. These symptoms can range from mild to severe depending upon the degree of anxiety the person is experiencing.

- **Neuromuscular symptoms** can include hyperreflexia, being easily startled, eyelid twitching, inability to sleep, shaking, fidgeting, pacing, wobbly legs, or clumsy movements.
- **Urinary tract symptoms** can include increased frequency and sensation of need to urinate.
- **Skin symptoms** can include flushed face, sweaty palms, itching, sensations of being hot and/or cold, pale facial coloring, or diaphoresis.

BEHAVIORAL AND AFFECTIVE RESPONSES

Behavioral and affective symptoms along with a multitude of physical symptoms are observable in anxious patients. The effects of these responses can affect the person experiencing the anxiety along with their relationships with others.

- Some **behavioral responses** can include restlessness and physical tension, hypervigilance, rapid speech, social or relationship withdrawal, decreased coordination, avoidance, or flight.

- **Affective responses** are the patient's emotional reactions and can be described subjectively by the individual. Patients may describe symptoms such as edginess, impatience, tension, nervousness, fear, frustration, jitteriness, or helplessness.

Cognitive Responses

Anxiety not only produces physical and emotional symptoms, but it can also greatly affect the individual's intellectual abilities. **Cognitive responses** to anxiety occur in three main categories. These include sensory-perceptual, thought difficulties, and conceptualization. Responses that affect the patient's **sensory-perceptual fields** can include feeling that their mind is unclear or clouded, seeing objects indistinctly, perceiving a surreal environment, increased self-consciousness, or hypervigilance. **Thinking difficulties** can include the inability to remember important information, confusion, inability to focus thoughts or attention, easily distracted, blocking thoughts, difficulty with reasoning, tunnel vision, or loss of objectivity. **Conceptual difficulties** can include the fear of loss of control, inability to cope, potential physical injury, developing a mental disorder, or receiving a negative evaluation. The patient may have cognitive distortion, protruding scary visual images, or uncontrollable repetition of fearful thoughts.

Panic Attacks

Panic attacks are short episodes (peaking in 5-10 minutes) of intense anxiety that can result in a wide variety of **symptoms** that include:

- Dyspnea
- Palpitations
- Hyperventilation
- Nausea and vomiting
- Intense fear or anxiety
- Pain and pressure in the chest
- Dizziness and fainting
- Tremors

Panic attacks may be associated with agoraphobia, depression, or intimate partner violence and abuse (IPVA), so a careful history is important. Typically, patients believe they are dying or having a heart attack and require reassurance and treatment, such as diazepam or lorazepam, in the ED for the acute episode. In severe cases, ASA may be given and EKG done to rule out cardiac abnormalities. Patients should be referred for psychiatric evaluation for ongoing medications such as SSRIs (sertraline, paroxetine, fluoxetine) to prevent recurrence. Panic attacks become chronic panic disorders if they are recurrent, with each attack each followed by at least a month of fear of another attack.

PTSD

Patients that experience a traumatic event may re-experience the trauma through distressing thoughts and recollections of the event. In addition, psychological effects of the trauma may include difficulty sleeping, emotional lability and problems with memory and concentration. Patients may also wish to avoid places or activities that remind them of their trauma. These are all characteristics of **post-traumatic stress disorder (PTSD)** and may cause patients extreme distress and significantly impact their quality of life.

Signs and symptoms: Nightmares, flashbacks, insomnia, symptoms of hyperarousal including irritability and anxiety, avoidance, and negative thoughts and feelings about oneself and others.

Diagnosis: PTSD is diagnosed through psychological assessment and criteria defined in the Diagnostic and Statistical Manual of Mental Disorders, Fifth Edition (DSM-5).

Treatment: Pharmacologic therapy may be utilized to help control the symptoms of PTSD. Non-pharmacologic therapy options include group and individual/family therapy, cognitive behavioral therapy, and anxiety management/relaxation techniques. Hypnosis may also be utilized.

STRESS

RELATIONSHIP BETWEEN STRESS AND DISEASE

Stress causes a number of physical and psychological changes within the body:

- Cortisol levels increase
- Digestion is hindered and the colon stimulated
- Heart rate increases
- Perspiration increases
- Anxiety and depression occur and can result in insomnia, anorexia or weight gain, and suicide
- Immune response decreases, making the person more vulnerable to infections
- Autoimmune reaction may increase, leading to autoimmune diseases

The body's **compensatory mechanisms** try to restore homeostasis. When these mechanisms are overwhelmed, pathophysiological injury to the cells of the body result. When this injury begins to interfere with the function of the organs or systems in the body, symptoms of dysfunction will occur. If the conditions are not corrected, the body changes the structure or function of the affected organs or systems.

ADAPTATION OF CELLS TO STRESS

The most common stressors to cells include the lack of oxygen, presence of toxins or chemicals, and infection. **Cells react to stress** by making the following changes:

- **Hypertrophy**: Cells swell, leading to an overall increase in the size of the affected organ.
- **Atrophy**: Cells shrivel and the overall organ size decreases in size.
- **Hyperplasia**: The cells divide and overgrowth and thickening of the tissue results.
- **Dysplasia**: The cells are changed in appearance as a result of irritation over an extended period of time, sometimes leading to malignancy.
- **Metaplasia**: Cells change type as a result of stress.

If the stress that caused the cells to change continues, the cells become injured and die. When enough cells die, organ and systemic failure occur.

PSYCHOLOGICAL RESPONSE TO STRESS

When stress is encountered, a person **responds** according to the threat perceived to compensate. The threat is evaluated as to the amount of harm or loss that has occurred or is possible. If the stress is benign (such as with marriage), then a challenge is present that demands change. Once the threat or challenge is defined, the person can gather information, resources, and support to make the changes needed to resolve the stress to the greatest degree possible. Immediate psychological response to stress may include shock, anger, fear, or excitement. Over time, people may develop chronic anxiety, depression, flashbacks, thought disturbances, and sleep disturbances. Changes may occur in emotions and thinking, in behavior, or in the person's environment. People may be more able to adapt to stress if they have many varied experiences, a good self-esteem, and a support network to help as needed. A healthy lifestyle and philosophical beliefs, including religion, may give a person more reserve to cope with stress.

Impact of Different Kinds of Stress

Everyone encounters **stress** in life and it **impacts** each person differently. There are the small daily "hassles," major traumatic events, and the periodic stressful events of marriage, birth, divorce, and death. Compounded stress experienced on a daily basis can impact health status over time. Stressors that occur suddenly are the hardest to overcome and result in the greatest tension. The length of time that a stressor is present affects the impact with long-term, relentless stress, such as that generated by poverty or disability, resulting in disease more often. If there is **ineffective coping**, a person will suffer greater changes resulting in even more stress. The nurse can help patients to recognize those things that induce stress in their lives, find ways to reduce stress when possible, and teach effective coping skills and problem-management.

Violence and Aggression

Violence and aggression are sometimes seen in critical care settings. The nurse must be aware of signs of impending violence or aggression in order to intervene and prevent injury to self or staff.

- **Violence** is a physical act perpetrated against an inanimate object, animal, or other person with the intent to cause harm. Violence often results from anger, frustration, or fear. It often occurs because the perpetrator believes that he is threatened in some way. Violence may occur suddenly without warning or following an escalating pattern of aggressive behavior.
- **Aggression** is the communication of a threat or intended act of violence that often occurs before the act of violence is carried out. This communication can occur verbally or nonverbally. Gestures, shouting, increasing volume of speech, invasion of personal space, and prolonged eye contact are all examples of aggression. The nurse should promptly recognize all forms of aggression and redirect or remove the patient from the situation to avoid an act of violence.

Management of Patients with Violent Behavior

Patients may exhibit **violent behavior** for a number of reasons, including metabolic disorders (hypoglycemia), neurological disorders (brain tumor), psychiatric disorders (schizophrenia), or substance abuse (drugs and alcohol). Patients who make threats or have a history of violent behavior should be approached with caution.

Diagnosis includes history, physical exam, CBC and chemistry panel, toxicology screening, ECG, and, in some cases, CT scans or lumbar punctures. Violent behavior tends to escalate from anxiety to defensiveness to aggression, so identifying these signs and providing support through information, setting limits, using restraints, and seclusion can avoid injuries. Handcuffs should not be removed in the ED, and patients who are so violent they must be restrained should not be allowed to leave the ED against medical advice.

Pharmacologic treatment includes:

- **Antipsychotic drugs**: Haloperidol 5 mg IM (1-2 mg for elderly patients)
- **Benzodiazepines**: Lorazepam 2-4 mg IM/IV (often in conjunction with antipsychotic drugs)
- **Hypnotics**: Droperidol 2.5 mg IM/IV

Homicidal Ideation

Homicidal ideation, the intention to kill another person, can occur for a variety of reasons:

- **Sociopathy/Psychopathy**: These patients usually appear quite normal and may even seem charming, but they can be very dangerous because they lack empathy for others. Some are involved in gangs in which violent behavior is expected and valued.
- **Psychosis**: Uncontrolled schizophrenia and paranoia may result in a patient behaving in a homicidal manner. In some cases, these changes may be brought about by pathology, such as TBI or brain tumor.
- **Medications**: Medications such as antidepressants, SSRIs, and antipsychotics as well as interferon have been associated with homicidal ideation in some patients. Patients on multiple medications may experience an involuntary intoxication that results in rage reactions and sometimes even the death of others.

Indications of homicidal ideation may include verbal threats, use of weapons, and violent behavior. Patients who express homicidal ideation or have attempted homicide require immediate psychiatric referral and may require restraint. The nurse should conduct a complete review of medications and notify security personnel if the patient poses a danger.

Suicidal Ideation

Patients may attempt **suicide** for many reasons, including severe depression, social isolation, situational crisis, bereavement, or psychotic disorder.

Suicidal indications are as follows:

- Depression or dysphoria
- Hostility to others
- Problems with peer relationships, and lack of close friends
- Post-crisis stress (divorce, death in family, graduation, college)
- Withdrawn personality; quiet or lonely appearance or behavior
- Change in behavior (dropping grades, unkempt appearance, change in sleeping patterns)
- A sudden increase in positive mood may indicate patient has a plan
- Co-morbid psychiatric problems (bipolar, schizophrenia)
- Substance abuse

The following are indicators of **high risk for repeated suicide attempt**:

- Violent suicide attempt (knives, gunshots)
- Suicide attempt with low chance of rescue
- Ongoing psychosis or disordered thinking
- Ongoing severe depression and feeling of helplessness
- History of previous suicide attempts
- Lack of social support system

Nursing considerations: Take all suicidal ideations seriously; do not minimize them. Suicidal patients should be watched continuously, given plastic utensils, break-away wall rails/shower heads, no cords/sharp instruments.

Psychosis

Psychosis is a severe reaction to stressors (psychological, physical) that results in alterations in affect and impaired psychomotor and behavioral functions, including the onset of hallucinations and/or delusions. Psychosis is not a diagnosis but is a symptom that may be caused by a mental disorder (such as schizophrenia or bipolar disease) or a physical disorder (such as a brain tumor or Alzheimer's disease). Psychosis may also be induced by some prescription drugs (muscle relaxants, antihistamines, anticonvulsants, corticosteroids, antiparkinson drugs), illicit drugs (cocaine, PCP, amphetamines, cannabis, LSD), and alcohol. Treatment depends on identifying the underlying cause of the psychosis and initiating treatment. For example, if caused by schizophrenia, then antipsychotic drugs and hospitalization in a mental health facility may be indicated. In most cases of drug-induced psychosis, stopping the drug alleviates the symptoms although some may benefit from the addition of a benzodiazepine or antipsychotic drug until symptoms subside.

Substance Abuse

Substance abuse is the abuse of drugs, medicines, or alcohol that causes mental and physical problems for the abuser and family. Abusers use substances out of boredom, to hide negative self-esteem, to dampen emotional pain, and to cope with daily stress. As the abuse continues, abusers become unable to take care of daily needs and duties. They lack effective coping mechanisms and the ability to make healthy choices. They can't identify and prioritize stress or choose positive behavior to resolve the stress in a healthy way. Some family members may act as codependents because of their desire to feel needed by the abuser, to control the person, and to stay with him or her. The nurse can help the family to confront an individual with their concerns about the person and their proposals for treatment. Family members can enforce consequences if treatment is not sought. Family members may also need counseling to learn new behaviors to stop enabling the abuser to continue substance abuse.

Pathophysiology of Addiction

Genetic, social, and personality factors may all play a role in the development of **addictive tendencies**. However, the main factor of the development of substance addiction is the pharmacological activation of the **reward system** located in the central nervous system (CNS). This reward systems pathway involves **dopaminergic neurons**. Dopamine is found in the CNS and is one of many neurotransmitters that play a role in an individual's mood. The mesolimbic pathway seems to play a primary role in the reward and motivational process involved with addiction. This pathway begins in the ventral tegmental area of the brain (VTA) and then moves forward into the nucleus accumbens located in the middle forebrain bundle (MFB). Some drugs enhance mesolimbic dopamine activity, therefore producing very potent effects on mood and behavior.

Indicators of Substance Abuse

Many people with **substance abuse** (alcohol or drugs) are reluctant to disclose this information, but there are a number of indicators that are suggestive of substance abuse:

Physical signs include:

- Burns on fingers or lips
- Pupils abnormally dilated or constricted, eyes watery
- Slurring of speech, slow speech
- Lack of coordination, instability of gait, tremors
- Sniffing repeatedly, nasal irritation, persistent cough
- Weight loss
- Dysrhythmias

- Pallor, puffiness of face
- Needle tracks on arms or legs
- Odor of alcohol/marijuana on clothing or breath

Behavioral signs include:

- Labile emotions, including mood swings, agitation, and anger
- Inappropriate, impulsive, or risky behavior
- Lying
- Missing appointments
- Difficulty concentrating, short term memory loss, blackouts
- Insomnia or excessive sleeping; disoriented, confused
- Lack of personal hygiene

Alcohol Withdrawal

Chronic abuse of ethanol (alcoholism) can lead to physical dependency. Sudden cessation of drinking, which often happens in the inpatient setting, is associated with **alcohol withdrawal syndrome.** It may be precipitated by trauma or infection and has a high mortality rate, 5-15% with treatment and 35% without treatment.

Signs/Symptoms: Anxiety, tachycardia, headache, diaphoresis, progressing to severe agitation, hallucinations, auditory/tactile disturbances, and psychotic behavior (delirium tremens).

Diagnosis: Physical assessment, blood alcohol levels (on admission).

Treatment includes:

- Medication: IV benzodiazepines to manage symptoms; electrolyte and nutritional replacement, especially magnesium and thiamine.
- Use the CIWA scale to measure symptoms of withdrawal; treat as indicated.
- Provide an environment with minimal sensory stimulus (lower lights, close blinds) & implement fall and seizure precautions.
- Prevention: Screen all patients for alcohol/substance abuse, using CAGE or other assessment tool. Remember to express support and comfort to patient; wait until withdrawal symptoms are subsiding to educate about alcohol use and moderation.

Multisystem Pathophysiology

Range of Severe Infection

There are a number of terms used to refer to **severe infections** which are often used interchangeably. It is important to know these terms to properly perform the continuum of care.

- **Bacteremia** is the presence of bacteria in the blood without systemic infection.
- **Septicemia** is a systemic infection caused by pathogens (usually bacteria or fungi) present in the blood.

- **Systemic inflammatory response syndrome** (SIRS) is a generalized inflammatory response affecting many organ systems. It may be caused by infectious or non-infectious agents, such as trauma, burns, adrenal insufficiency, pulmonary embolism, and drug overdose. If an infectious agent is identified or suspected, SIRS is an aspect of sepsis. Infective agents include a wide range of bacteria and fungi, including *Streptococcus pneumoniae* and *Staphylococcus aureus*. SIRS includes 2 of the following:
  - Elevated (>38 °C) or subnormal rectal temperature (<36 °C)
  - Tachypnea or $PaCO_2$ <32 mmHg
  - Tachycardia
  - Leukocytosis (>12,000) or leukopenia (<4000)
- **Sepsis** is the presence of infection either locally or systemically in which there is a generalized life-threatening inflammatory response (SIRS). It includes all the indications for SIRS as well as one of the following:
  - Changes in mental status
  - Hypoxemia without preexisting pulmonary disease
  - Elevation in plasma lactate
  - Decreased urinary output <5 mL/kg/hr for ≥1 hour
- **Severe sepsis** includes both indications of SIRS and sepsis as well as indications of increasing organ dysfunction with inadequate perfusion and/or hypotension.
- **Septic shock** is a progression from severe sepsis in which refractory hypotension occurs despite treatment. There may be indications of lactic acidosis.
- **Multi-organ dysfunction syndrome** (MODS) is the most common cause of sepsis-related death. Cardiac function becomes depressed, acute respiratory distress syndrome (ARDS) may develop, and renal failure may follow acute tubular necrosis or cortical necrosis. Thrombocytopenia appears in about 30% of those affected and may result in disseminated intravascular coagulation (DIC). Liver damage and bowel necrosis may occur.

SHOCK

There are a number of different types of **shock**, but there are general characteristics that they have in common. In all types of shock, there is a marked decrease in tissue perfusion related to hypotension, so that there is insufficient oxygen delivered to the tissues and inadequate removal of cellular waste products, causing injury to tissue:

- Hypotension (systolic below 90 mmHg); this may be somewhat higher (110 mmHg) in those who are initially hypertensive
- Decreased urinary output (<0.5 mL/kg/hr), especially marked in hypovolemic shock
- Metabolic acidosis
- Peripheral/cutaneous vasoconstriction/vasodilation resulting in cool, clammy skin
- Alterations in level of consciousness

Types of shock are as follows:

- **Distributive:** Preload decreased, CO increased, SVR decreased
- **Cardiogenic:** Preload increased, CO decreased, SVR increased
- **Hypovolemic:** Preload decreased, CO decreased, SVR increased

Septic Shock

Septic shock is caused by toxins produced by bacteria and cytokines that the body produces in response to severe infection, resulting in a complex syndrome of disorders. **Symptoms** are wide-ranging:

- **Initial**: Hyper- or hypothermia, increased temperature (>38 °C) with chills, tachycardia with increased pulse pressure, tachypnea, alterations in mental status (dullness), hypotension, hyperventilation with respiratory alkalosis ($PaCO_2$ ≤30 mmHg), increased lactic acid, unstable BP, and dehydration with increased urinary output
- **Cardiovascular**: Myocardial depression and dysrhythmias
- **Respiratory**: Acute respiratory distress syndrome (ARDS)
- **Renal**: Acute kidney injury (AKI) with decreased urinary output and increased BUN
- **Hepatic**: Jaundice and liver dysfunction with an increase in transaminase, alkaline phosphatase, and bilirubin
- **Hematologic**: Mild or severe blood loss (from mucosal ulcerations), neutropenia or neutrophilia, decreased platelets, and DIC
- **Endocrine**: Hyperglycemia, hypoglycemia (rare)
- **Skin**: Cellulitis, erysipelas, and fasciitis, acrocyanotic and necrotic peripheral lesions

Diagnosis and Treatment

Septic shock is most common in newborns, those >50, and those who are immunocompromised. There is no specific test to confirm a diagnosis of septic shock, so **diagnosis** is based on clinical findings and tests that evaluate hematologic, infectious, and metabolic states: Lactic acid, CBC, DIC panel, electrolytes, liver function tests, BUN, creatinine, blood glucose, ABGs, urinalysis, ECG, radiographs, blood and urine cultures.

Treatment must be aggressive and includes:

- Oxygen and endotracheal intubation as necessary
- IV access with 2-large bore catheters and central venous line
- Rapid fluid administration at 0.5L NS or isotonic crystalloid every 5-10 minutes as needed (to 4-6 L)
- Monitoring urinary output to optimal >30 mL/hr (>0.5-1 mL/kg/hr)
- Inotropic or vasoconstrictive agents (dopamine, dobutamine, norepinephrine) if no response to fluids or fluid overload
- Empiric IV antibiotic therapy (usually with 2 broad spectrum antibiotics for both gram-positive and gram-negative bacteria) until cultures return and antibiotics may be changed
- Hemodynamic and laboratory monitoring
- Removing source of infection (abscess, catheter)

Distributive Shock

Distributive shock occurs with adequate blood volume but inadequate intravascular volume because of arterial/venous dilation that results in decreased vascular tone and hypoperfusion of internal organs. Cardiac output may be normal or blood may pool, decreasing cardiac output. Distributive shock may result from anaphylactic shock, septic shock, neurogenic shock, and drug ingestions.

Symptoms include:

- Hypotension (systolic <90 mmHg or <40 mmHg below normal), tachypnea, tachycardia (>90) (may be lower if patient receiving β-blockers)
- Hypoxemia
- Skin initially warm, later hypoperfused
- Hyper- or hypothermia (>38 °C or <36 °C)
- Alterations in mentation
- Decreased urinary output
- Symptoms related to underlying cause

Treatment includes:

- Treating underlying cause while stabilizing hemodynamics
- Oxygen with endotracheal intubation if necessary
- Rapid fluid administration at 0.25-0.5 L NS or isotonic crystalloid every 5-10 minutes as needed to 2-3 L
- Vasoconstrictive and inotropic agents (dopamine, dobutamine, norepinephrine) if necessary, for patients with profound hypotension

Neurogenic Shock

Neurogenic shock is a type of distributive shock that occurs when injury to the CNS from trauma resulting in acute spinal cord injury (from both blunt and penetrating injuries), neurological diseases, drugs, or anesthesia, impairs the autonomic nervous system that controls the cardiovascular system. The degree of symptoms relates to the level of injury with injuries above T1 capable of causing disruption of the entire sympathetic nervous system and lower injuries causing various degrees of disruption. Even incomplete spinal cord injury can cause neurogenic shock.

Symptoms include:

- Hypotension and warm dry skin related to lack of vascular tone that results in hypothermia from loss of cutaneous heat
- Bradycardia (common but not universal)

Treatment includes:

- ABCDE (airway, breathing, circulation, disability evaluation, exposure)
- Rapid fluid administration with crystalloid to keep mean arterial pressure at 85-90 mmHg
- Placement of pulmonary artery catheter to monitor fluid overload
- Inotropic agents (dopamine, dobutamine) if fluids don't correct hypotension
- Atropine for persistent bradycardia

Anaphylactic Shock

Anaphylactic reaction or **anaphylactic shock** may present with a few symptoms or a wide range of potentially lethal effects.

Symptoms may recur after the initial treatment (biphasic anaphylaxis), so careful monitoring is essential:

- Sudden onset of weakness, dizziness, confusion
- Severe generalized edema and angioedema; lips and tongue may swell

- Urticaria
- Increased permeability of vascular system and loss of vascular tone leading to severe hypotension and shock
- Laryngospasm/bronchospasm with obstruction of airway causing dyspnea and wheezing
- Nausea, vomiting, and diarrhea
- Seizures, coma, and death

Treatments:

- Establish patent airway and intubate if necessary, for ventilation
- Provide oxygen at 100% high flow
- Monitor VS
- Administer epinephrine (Epi-pen® or solution)
- Albuterol per nebulizer for bronchospasm
- Intravenous fluids to provide bolus of fluids for hypotension
- Diphenhydramine if shock persists
- Methylprednisolone if no response to other drugs

Hypovolemic Shock/Volume Deficit

Hypovolemic shock occurs when there is inadequate intravascular fluid. The loss may be *absolute* because of an internal shifting of fluid or an external loss of fluid, as occurs with massive hemorrhage, thermal injuries, severe vomiting or diarrhea, and internal injuries (such as ruptured spleen or dissecting arteries) that interfere with intravascular integrity. Hypovolemia may also be *relative* and related to vasodilation, increased capillary membrane permeability from sepsis or injuries, and decreased colloidal osmotic pressure that may occur with loss of sodium and some disorders, such as hypopituitarism and cirrhosis.

Hypovolemic shock is **classified** according to the degree of fluid loss:

- **Class I:** <750 mL or ≤15% of total circulating volume (TCV)
- **Class II:** 750-1500 mL or 15-30% of TCV
- **Class III:** 1500-2000 mL or 30-40% of TCV
- **Class IV:** >2000 mL or >40% of TCV

Symptoms and Treatment

Hypovolemic shock occurs when the total circulating volume of fluid decreases, leading to a fall in venous return that in turn causes a decrease in ventricular filling and preload, indicated by ↓ in right atrial pressure (RAP) and pulmonary artery occlusion pressure (PAOP). This results in a decrease in stroke volume and cardiac output. This in turn causes generalized arterial vasoconstriction, increasing afterload (↑ systemic vascular resistance), causing decreased tissue perfusion.

Symptoms: Anxiety, pallor, cool and clammy skin, delayed capillary refill, cyanosis, hypotension, increasing respirations, weak, thready pulse.

Treatment is aimed at identifying and treating the cause:

- Administration of blood, blood products, autotransfusion, colloids (such as plasma protein fraction), and/or crystalloids (such as normal saline)
- Oxygen; intubation and ventilation may be necessary

- Medications may include vasopressors, such as dopamine. NOTE: Fluids must be given before starting vasopressors!

Post-Intensive Care Syndrome

Post-intensive care syndrome (PICS) refers to the disabilities that occur as the result of treatment in intensive care for critical illness, such as coronavirus patients with induced coma and weeks of mechanical ventilation. Impairments include:

- **Cognitive:** Difficulty speaking, impaired memory, difficulty concentrating, impaired executive function
- **Psychological:** Depression, anxiety, PTSD, delirium, lack of motivation. PICS can affect family members and caregivers as well because of the emotional stress they encounter, primarily exhibited with psychological problems (grief, anxiety, depression, insomnia, PTSD)
- **Physical**: Generalized weakness, dyspnea, insomnia, lethargy, fatigue, difficulty walking

These impairments may result from the critical illness or the interventions (medications, sedation, ventilation) that were included as part of treatment. Management includes early mobilization, orienting and interacting with the patient, minimizing medications and sedation, avoiding hypoxemia and hypoglycemia, assessing for delirium, and treating depression. Patients may need physical therapy to regain strength, respiratory and/or cardiac therapy, and psychological counseling. Some impairments may remain chronic.

Malignant Hyperthermia

Malignant hyperthermia is a life-threatening condition triggered by genetic susceptibility to inhalational anesthetics (except nitrous oxide and succinylcholine). Signs may occur within 10-20 minutes of induction or delayed >24 hours. Risk factors include large, strong muscles and a history of unexplained fevers or family history of death after surgery. Effects include:

- Increased cytoplasmic calcium, causing muscle contractions, including Masseter spasm (jaw clamps shut)
- Hypermetabolism with increasing temperature
- Cell leakage of potassium, myoglobin, and creatinine phosphokinase damages cells

Sympathetic nervous system compensation:

- Vasodilation and increased perspiration to combat rising temperature, increased circulating catecholamines cause tachycardia and subsequent vasoconstriction and increases vascular resistance
- Increased cardiac output outpaces oxygen demand with decreased mixed venous O_2 and arterial oxygen and development of lactic acidosis, hypotension, and increased ventilation

High temperature may be a late sign. Once temperature begins to increase, it may rise 1-2 °C every 5 minutes. Systemic manifestations may include cardiac dysrhythmias (ventricular), hemorrhage and/or DIC, increased ICP, kidney failure with oliguria, and cardiac arrest. Treatment includes stopping triggering agent, supportive treatment, and administration of dantrolene 1 mg/kg every five minutes until stabilized. Forced diuresis may be done to protect against renal failure. Internal and external cooling methods are used to reduce temperature.

Toxic Exposures

Carbon Monoxide Poisoning

Carbon monoxide (CO) poisoning occurs with inhalation of fossil fuel exhausts from engines, emission of gas or coal heaters, indoor use of charcoal, and smoke and fumes. The CO binds with hemoglobin, preventing oxygen carriage and impairing oxygen delivery to tissue.

Diagnosis includes history, on-site oximetry reports, neurological examination, and CO neuropsychological screening battery (CONSB) done with patient breathing room air, CBC, electrolytes, ABGs, ECG, chest radiograph (for dyspnea); *pulse oximetry is not accurate in these patients.*

Symptoms:

- Cardiac: chest pain, palpitations, decreased capillary refill, hypotension, and cardiac arrest
- CNS: malaise, nausea, vomiting, lethargy, stroke, coma, and seizure
- Secondary injuries: Rhabdomyolysis, AKI, non-cardiogenic pulmonary edema, multiple organ failure (MOF), DIC, and encephalopathy

Treatment includes:

- Immediate support of airway, breathing, and circulation
- Non-barometric oxygen (100%) by non-breathing mask with reservoir or ETT if necessary
- Mild: Continue oxygen for 4 hours with reassessment
- Severe: hyperbaric oxygen therapy (usually 3 treatments) to improve oxygen delivery

Cyanide Poisoning

Cyanide poisoning, from hydrogen cyanide (HCN) or cyanide salts, can result from sodium nitroprusside infusions, inhalation of burning plastics, intentional or accidental ingestion or dermal exposure, occupation exposure, ingestion of some plant products, and the manufacture of PCP. Inhalation of HCN causes immediate symptoms, and the ingestion of cyanide salts causes symptoms within minutes.

Diagnosis is by history, clinical examination, normal PaO_2 and metabolic acidosis.

Symptoms: Increase in severity and alter with the amount of exposure: tachycardia, hypertension, leading to bradycardia, hypotension, and cardiac arrest. Pink or cherry-colored skin because of oxygen remaining in the blood. Other symptoms include headaches, lethargy, seizures, coma, dyspnea, tachypnea, and respiratory arrest.

Treatment includes:

- Supportive care as indicated
- Removal of contaminated clothes
- Gastric decontamination
- Copious irrigation for topical exposure
- Antidotes:
    - Amyl nitrate ampule cracked and inhaled 30 seconds
    - Sodium nitrite (3%) 10 mL IV
    - Sodium thiosulfate (25%) 50 mL IV

Caustic Ingestions

Caustic ingestions of acids (pH <7) such as sulfuric, acetic, hydrochloric, and hydrofluoric found in many cleaning agents and alkalis (pH >7) such as sodium hydroxide, potassium hydroxide, sodium tripolyphosphate (in detergents) and sodium hypochlorite (bleach) can result in severe injury and death. Acids cause coagulation necrosis in the esophagus and stomach and may result in metabolic acidosis, hemolysis, and renal failure if systemically absorbed. Alkali injuries cause liquefaction necrosis, resulting in deeper ulcerations, often of the esophagus, but may involve perforation and abdominal necrosis with multi-organ damage.

Diagnosis is by detailed history, airway examination (oral intubation if possible), arterial blood gas, electrolytes, CBC, hepatic and coagulation tests, radiograph, and CT for perforations.

Symptoms may vary but can include pain, dyspnea, oral burns, dysphonia, and vomiting.

Treatment includes:

- Supportive and symptomatic therapy
- <u>NO</u> ipecac, charcoal, neutralization, or dilution
- NG tube for acids only to aspirate residual
- Endoscopy in first few hours to evaluate injury/perforations
- Sodium bicarbonate for pH <7.10
- Prednisolone (alkali injuries)

Allergic Reactions

Exposure to certain toxins, medications, illegal substances and allergens can cause life threatening effects in some patients. The physiologic response of the patient is dependent on the agent and the degree of exposure. Tissue hypoperfusion and lactic acidosis often occur as a result of the exposure. This can lead to metabolic acidosis, shock, organ failure, and death.

Signs and symptoms: In allergic type reactions, urticaria, pruritus, chest, back or abdominal pain, facial flushing, shortness of breath, wheezing and stridor may occur. Beta- and alpha-adrenergic responses may occur with exposure to amphetamines, cocaine, ephedrine, and pseudoephedrine. This response is manifested by diaphoresis, hypertension, tachycardia and mydriasis. Diarrhea, nausea and vomiting can occur with exposure to certain toxins.

Diagnosis: Physical assessment and testing to discover the toxin, drug or allergen the patient was exposed to. Labs—blood gases, BMP, complete blood count, toxicology screen, urinalysis, and allergy testing.

Treatment: Priority is to eliminate exposure to the drug/toxin/allergen. Antidotes (if available) may be administered in the case of toxin exposure. Activated charcoal may be administered in the case of medication/drug overdose. For allergic reactions, antihistamines and corticosteroids may be administered. Severe allergic reactions may need to be treated with epinephrine. Dialysis may be indicated in some patients. Sodium bicarbonate may be administered for the treatment of metabolic acidosis caused by many toxic reactions.

Acetaminophen Toxicity

Acetaminophen toxicity from accidental or intentional overdose has high rates of morbidity and mortality unless promptly treated. *Diagnosis* is by history and acetaminophen level, which should be completed within 8 hours of ingestion if possible. Toxicity occurs with dosage >140 mg/kg in one dose or >7.5g in 24 hours.

Symptoms occur in stages:

1. (Initial) Minor gastrointestinal upset
2. (Days 2-3) Hepatotoxicity with RUQ pain and increased AST, ALT, and bilirubin
3. (Days 3-4) Hepatic failure with metabolic acidosis, coagulopathy, renal failure, encephalopathy, nausea, vomiting, and possible death
4. (Days 5-12) Recovery period for survivors

Treatment includes:

- GI decontamination with activated charcoal (orally or NG) <24 hours
- Toxicity is plotted on the Rumack-Matthew nomogram with serum levels >150 requiring antidote. The antidote is most effective ≤8 hours of ingestion but decreases hepatotoxicity even >24 hours.
- Antidote: 72-hour N-acetylcysteine (NAC) protocol includes 140 mg/kg initially and 70 mg/kg every 4 hours for 17 more doses (orally or IV)
- Supportive therapy: Continuous dialysis, fluids, blood pressure medications

Amphetamine and Cocaine Toxicity

Amphetamine toxicity may be caused by IV, inhalation, or insufflation of various substances that include methamphetamine (MDA or "ecstasy"), methylphenidate (Ritalin®), methylenedioxymethamphetamine (MDMA), and ephedrine and phenylpropanolamine. **Cocaine** may be ingested orally, IV or by insufflation while **crack cocaine** may be smoked. Amphetamines and cocaine are CNS stimulants that can cause multi-system abnormalities.

Symptoms may include chest pain, dysrhythmias, myocardial ischemia, MI, seizures, intracranial infarctions, hypertension, dystonia, repetitive movements, unilateral blindness, lethargy, rhabdomyolysis with acute kidney failure, perforated nasal septum (cocaine), and paranoid psychosis (amphetamines). Crack cocaine may cause pulmonary hemorrhage, asthma, pulmonary edema, barotrauma, and pneumothorax. Swallowing packs of cocaine can cause intestinal ischemia, colitis, necrosis, and perforation. **Diagnosis** includes clinical findings, CBC, chemistry panel, toxicology screening, ECG, and radiography.

Treatment includes:

- Gastric emptying (<1 hour). Charcoal administration
- IV access. Supplemental oxygen
- Sedation for seizures: Lorazepam 2 mg, diazepam 5 mg IV titrated in repeated doses
- Agitation: Haloperidol
- Hypertension: Nitroprusside/nicardipine, phentolamine IV
- Cocaine quinidine-like effects: Sodium bicarbonate

Salicylate Toxicity

Salicylate toxicity may be acute or chronic and is caused by ingestion of OTC drugs containing salicylates, such as ASA, Pepto-Bismol®, and products used in hot inhalers.

Diagnosis is by ferric chloride or Ames Phenistix tests. Symptoms vary according to age and amount of ingestion. Co-ingestion of sedatives may alter symptoms.

Symptoms include:

- <150 mg/kg: Nausea and vomiting
- 150-300 mg/kg: Vomiting, hyperpnea, diaphoresis, tinnitus, and alterations in acid-base balance
- >300 mg/kg (usually intentional overdose): Nausea, vomiting, diaphoresis, tinnitus, hyperventilation, respiratory alkalosis, and metabolic acidosis
- Chronic toxicity results in hyperventilation, tremor, and papilledema, alterations in mental status, pulmonary edema, seizures, and coma

Treatment includes:

- Gastric decontamination with lavage (≤1 hour) and charcoal
- Volume replacement (D5W)
- Sodium bicarbonate 1-2 mEq/kg
- Monitoring of salicylate concentration, acid-base, and electrolytes every hour
- Whole-bowel irrigation (sustained release tablets)

Benzodiazepine Toxicity

Benzodiazepine toxicity may result from accidental or intentional overdose with such drugs as Xanax®, Librium®, Valium®, Ativan®, Serax®, Versed®, and Restoril®. Mortality is usually the result of co-ingestion of other drugs.

Diagnosis is based on history and clinical exam, as benzodiazepine level does not correlate well with toxicity.

Symptoms: Non-specific neurological changes: Lethargy, dizziness, alterations in consciousness, and ataxia. Respiratory depression and hypotension are rare complications. Coma and severe central nervous depression are usually caused by co-ingestions.

Treatment includes:

- Gastric emptying (<1 hour)
- Charcoal
- Concentrated dextrose, thiamine, and naloxone if co-ingestions suspected, especially with altered mental status
- Monitoring for CNS/respiratory depression
- Supportive care
- Flumazenil (antagonist) 0.2 mg each minute to total 3 mg may be used in some cases but not routinely advised because of complications related to benzodiazepine dependency or co-ingestion of cyclic antidepressants. Flumazenil is contraindicated in patients with increased ICP.

Ethanol Overdose

Ethanol overdose affects the central nervous system as well as other organs in the body. Alcohol is an inhibitory neurotransmitter that depresses the central nervous system. In most states, the legal intoxication blood alcohol level is defined as 100 mg/dL. Blood alcohol levels of **500 mg/dL or greater** are associated with a high mortality rate. The central nervous system depressant effect is further enhanced when alcohol is mixed with other agents.

Ethanol is absorbed through the mucosa of the mouth, stomach, and intestines, with concentrations peaking about 30-60 minutes after ingestion. If people are easily aroused, they can usually safely sleep off the effects of ingesting too much alcohol, but if the person is semi-conscious or unconscious, emergency medical treatment should be initiated.

Symptoms include:

- Altered mental status with slurred speech and stupor
- Nausea and vomiting
- Hypotension
- Bradycardia with arrhythmias
- Respiratory depression and hypoxia
- Cold, clammy skin or flushed skin (from vasodilation)
- Acute pancreatitis with abdominal pain
- Lack of consciousness
- Circulatory collapse

Treatment includes:

- Careful monitoring of arterial blood gases and oxygen saturation
- Ensure patent airway with intubation and ventilation if necessary
- Intravenous fluids
- Dextrose to correct hypoglycemia if indicated
- Maintain body temperature (warming blanket)
- Dialysis may be necessary in severe cases

Gastric Emptying for Toxic Substance Ingestion

Gastric emptying for toxic substance ingestion should be done ≤60 minutes of ingestion for large life-threatening amounts of poison. The patient requires IV access, oximetry, and cardiac monitoring. Sedation (1-2 mg IV midazolam) or rapid sequence induction and endotracheal intubation may be necessary. Patients should be positioned in left lateral decubitus position with head down at 20° to prevent passage of stomach contents into duodenum, although intubated patients may be lavaged in the supine position. With a bite block in place, an orogastric Y-tube (36-40 Fr. for adults) should be inserted after estimating length. Placement should be confirmed with injection of 50 mL of air confirmed under auscultation and aspiration of gastric contents, as well as abdominal x-ray (pH may not be reliable depending on substance ingested). Irrigation is done by gravity instillation of about 200-300 mL warmed (45 °C) tap water or NS. The instillation side is clamped and drainage side opened. This is repeated until fluid returns clear. A slurry of charcoal is then instilled, and the tube is clamped and removed when procedures completed.

Burn Injuries

Types and Classifications

Burn injuries may be chemical, electrical, or thermal, and are assessed by the area, percentage of the body burned, and depth:

- **First-degree burns** are superficial and affect the epidermis, causing erythema and pain.
- **Second-degree burns** extend through the dermis (partial thickness), resulting in blistering and sloughing of epidermis.
- **Third-degree burns** affect underlying tissue, including vasculature, muscles, and nerves (full thickness).

Burns are classified according to the **American Burn Association's criteria**:

- **Minor**: Less than 10% body surface area (BSA). 2% BSA with third degree without serious risk to face, hands, feet, or perineum.
- **Moderate**: 10-20% combined second- and third-degree burns (children younger than 10 years or adults older than 40 years). 10% or less full thickness without serious risk to face, hands, feet, or perineum.
- **Major**: 20% BSA; at least 10% third-degree burns. All burns to face, hands, feet, or perineum that will result in functional/cosmetic defect. Burns with inhalation or other major trauma.

Systemic Complications

Burn injuries begin with the skin but can affect all organs and body systems, especially with a major burn:

- **Cardiovascular**: Cardiac output may fall by 50% as capillary permeability increases with vasodilation and fluid leaks from the tissues.
- **Urinary**: Decreased blood flow causes kidneys to increase ADH, which increases oliguria. BUN and creatinine levels increase. Cell destruction may block tubules, and hematuria may result from hemolysis.
- **Pulmonary**: Injury may result from smoke inhalation or (rarely) aspiration of hot liquid. Pulmonary injury is a leading cause of death from burns and is classified according to the degree of damage:
  - *First*: Singed eyebrows and nasal hairs with possible soot in airways and slight edema
  - *Second*: (At 24 hours) Stridor, dyspnea, and tachypnea with edema and erythema of upper airway, including area of vocal cords and epiglottis
  - *Third*: (At 72 hours) Worsening symptoms if not intubated and if intubated, bronchorrhea and tachypnea with edematous, secreting tissue
- **Neurological**: Encephalopathy may develop from lack of oxygen, decreased blood volume and sepsis. Hallucinations, alterations in consciousness, seizures, and coma may result.
- **Gastrointestinal**: Ileus and ulcerations of mucosa often result from poor circulation. Ileus usually clears within 48-72 hours, but if it returns it is often indicative of sepsis.
- **Endocrine/Metabolic:** The sympathetic nervous system stimulates the adrenals to release epinephrine and norepinephrine to increase cardiac output and cortisol for wound healing. The metabolic rate increases markedly. Electrolyte loss occurs with fluid loss from exposed tissue, especially phosphorus, calcium and sodium, with an increase in potassium levels. Electrolyte imbalance can be life-threatening if burns cover >20% of BSA. Glycogen depletion occurs within 12-24 hours and protein breakdown and muscle wasting occurs without sufficient intake of protein.

Management

Management of burn injuries must include both wound care and systemic care to avoid complications that can be life threatening. Treatment includes:

- Establishment of airway and treatment for inhalation injury as indicated:
    - Supplemental oxygen, incentive spirometry, nasotracheal suctioning
    - Humidification
    - Bronchoscopy as needed to evaluate bronchospasm and edema
    - β-Agonists for bronchospasm, followed by aminophylline if ineffective
    - Intubation and ventilation if there are indications of respiratory failure (This should be done prior to failure. Tracheostomy may be done if ventilation >14 days.)
- Intravenous fluids and electrolytes, based on weight and extent of burn. Parkland formula: Fluid replacement (mL) in first 24 hours = (mass in kg) × (body % burned) × 400
- Enteral feedings, usually with small lumen feeding tube into the duodenum
- NG tube for gastric decompression to prevent aspiration
- Indwelling catheter to monitor urinary output. Urinary output should be 0.5-2 mL/kg/hr
- Analgesia for reduction of pain and anxiety
- Topical and systemic antibiotics
- Wound care with removal of eschar and dressings as indicated

Chemical Burns

Chemical burns may result from contact with acid or alkali substances. The pH ranges from 1 to 14 with 7 neutral and extremely acidic 1 and extremely alkaline 14. Alkali burns tend to be more severe because acid burns denature proteins, resulting in formation of eschar that prevents deeper penetration of the acid. Alkaline burns, however, both denature proteins and hydrolyze fats, allowing for deeper penetration and tissue damage because of liquefaction necrosis. Hydrofluoric acid is similar to alkaline substances in that it also causes liquefaction necrosis. Symptoms vary depending on the substance, strength, and site of injury but often includes severe pain, tissue blistering and sloughing, and bleeding. Initial treatment includes removal of contaminated clothing and copious wound irrigation with water. If substances contain Na, K, Mg, or metallic lithium, then the burn area should be covered with mineral oil rather than irrigated. If hydrofluoric acid, copious water irrigations and soft-tissue injection or IV infusion of calcium gluconate may help reduce pain and tissue destruction. Patients may need fluid resuscitation and skin grafting. Complications include disfigurement, infection, and electrolyte imbalance.

Electrical Burns

Electrical injuries result from electricity passing through the body from contact with live wires, lighting strikes, and short-circuiting equipment. Injuries may be high voltage (≥1000 volts) or low voltage (<1000 volts). Electrical injuries can result in extensive subdermal burns. The injury severity correlates with resistance of tissue and current amperage (AC usually causes more damage than DC). Tissue with the highest degree of resistance tends to suffer the most damage with low voltage injury, but high voltage injury can destroy all tissue. Tissue resistance (highest to lowest) include bone >fat >tendons >skin >muscles >vessels > nerves.

- **Low voltage** injuries may cause cardiac dysrhythmias (VF), external burns, tissue damage, fractures and dislocations from muscle contractions, respiratory arrest, or oral burns (children particularly). Treatment includes monitoring and cardiac care as needed, topical antimicrobials, and excision and grafting if necessary.

- **High voltage** injuries may result in additional symptoms of myonecrosis, thrombosis, compartment syndrome, nerve entrapment syndrome. Treatment may include fluid resuscitation, wound debridement, fasciotomy, and amputation, topical antibiotics, systemic antibiotics, and analgesia.

Thermal Burns

Thermal burns are caused by heat (hot iron, stove, sun exposure) or fire. Burn injuries begin with the skin but can affect all organs and body systems, especially with a major burn. **Management** of burn injuries must include both wound care and systemic care to avoid complications that can be life threatening. Patients may experience open blistering wounds and severe pain. **Treatment** varies according to severity and may include:

- Establishment of airway and treatment for inhalation injury if necessary
- Cleansing of burned areas, flushing
- Debridement of open blisters (no needle aspiration)
- Tetanus immunization if needed
- Intravenous fluids and electrolytes, based on weight and extent of burn
- Enteral feedings, usually with small lumen feeding tube into the duodenum
- NG tube for gastric decompression to prevent aspiration
- Indwelling catheter to monitor urinary output. Urinary output should be 0.5-2 mL/kg/hr
- Analgesia for reduction of pain and anxiety
- Topical (usually silver sulfadiazine) and systemic antibiotics
- Wound care with removal of eschar and dressings as indicated
- Skin grafting

Complications include scarring, disfigurement, contractures, and infection.

Radiation Injuries

Radiation injuries may be caused by direct radiation in which waves pass through the body (locally or to the entire body), which can result in acute radiation illness and genetic damage. **Contamination** usually occurs from radioactive dust or liquid contacting the skin. It can be absorbed into the tissues (eventually causing chronic illnesses, such as cancer) or contaminate others who contact it. Contaminated material may also be ingested. The lethal dose of 50% of those exposed within 60 days (LD50/60) is 4.5 Gy with immediate intensive treatment.

Diagnosis for direct radiation is symptomatic as there is no specific test; however, contamination can be measured by Geiger counter.

Syndromes of **acute radiation sickness** vary according to exposure:

- **Hematopoietic**: (at least 2 Gy exposure) affects blood cell production. 2-12 hours after exposure: anorexia, nausea, vomiting, lethargy. Symptom-free week during which blood cell production decreases causing decreased WBC and platelet count, resulting in infection and hemorrhage with weakness and dyspnea. Recovery begins in 4-5 weeks if patient survives.
- **GI**: (at least 4 Gy exposure)
    - 2-12 hours after exposure: nausea, vomiting, diarrhea, dehydration. 4-5 days, fewer symptoms but lining of GI tract sheds, leaving ulcerated tissue.
    - Severe diarrhea (bloody) and dehydration and systemic infections

- **Cerebrovascular**: (20-30 Gy exposure) always fatal
    - Alterations in mental status, nausea, vomiting, and diarrhea (bloody), progressing to shock, seizures, coma, and death

Treatment includes:

- Decontamination if contamination irradiation or if source of irradiation not clear
- Complete history of event, including source of radiation
- Protocol for decontamination and securing of area should be followed, including use of individual dosimeters and protective coverings
- **Localized**: burn care and analgesia
- **Internal**: gastric decontamination, collection of urine and feces for 4 days to monitor rate of radioisotopes excretion, and collection of body fluids for bioassay
- **Whole body irradiation**: supportive treatment and prophylactic measures to combat opportunistic infections, hematopoietic growth factor for bone marrow depression

Heat-Related Illness

Children and the elderly are particularly vulnerable to **heat-related illness**, especially when heat is combined with humidity. Heat-related illnesses occur when heat accumulation in the body outpaces dissipation, resulting in increased temperature and dehydration, which can then lead to thermoregulatory failure and multiple organ dysfunction syndromes. Each year in the United States, about 29 children die from heat stroke after being left in automobiles. At temperatures of 72-96 °F, the temperature in a car rises 3.2 °F every 5 minutes, with 80% of rise within 30 minutes. Temperatures can reach 117 °F even on cool days. There are 3 types of heat-related illness:

- **Heat stress**: Increased temperature causes dehydration. Patient may develop swelling of hands and feet, itching of skin, sunburn, heat syncope (pale moist skin, hypotension), heat cramps, and heat tetany (respiratory alkalosis). Treatment includes removing from heat, cooling, hydrating, and replacing sodium.
- **Heat exhaustion**: Involves water or sodium depletion, with sodium depletion common in patients who are not acclimated to heat. Heat exhaustion can result in flu-like aching, nausea and vomiting, headaches, dizziness, and hypotension with cold, clammy skin and diaphoresis. Temperature may be normal or elevated to less than 106 °F. Treatment to cool the body and replace sodium and fluids must be prompt in order to prevent heat stroke. Careful monitoring is important and reactions may be delayed.
- **Heat stroke**: Involves failure of the thermoregulatory system with temperatures that may be more than 106 °F and can result in seizures, neurological damage, multiple organ failures, and death. Exertional heat stroke often occurs in young athletes who engage in strenuous activities in high heat. Young children are susceptible to nonexertional heat stroke from exposure to high heat. Treatment includes evaporative cooling, rehydration, and supportive treatment according to organ involvement.

Hypothermia

Hypothermia occurs with exposure to low temperatures that cause the core body temperature to fall below 95 °F (35 °C). Hypothermia may be associated with immersion in cold water, exposure to cold temperature, metabolic disorders (hypothyroidism, hypoglycemia, hypoadrenalism), or CNS abnormalities (head trauma, Wernicke disease). Many patients with hypothermia are intoxicated with alcohol or drugs.

Symptoms of hypothermia include pallor, cold skin, drowsiness, alterations in mental status, confusion, and severe shivering. The patient can progress to shock, coma, dysrhythmias (T-wave inversion and prolongation of PR, QRS, and QT) including atrial fibrillation and AV block, and cardiac arrest.

Diagnosis requires low-reading thermometers to verify temperature.

Treatment includes:

- Passive rewarming if cardiac status stable
- Active rewarming (external) with immersion in warm water or heating blankets at 40 °C, radiant heat
- Active rewarming (internal) with warm humidified oxygen or air inhalation, heated IV fluids, and internal (bladder, peritoneal pleural, GI) lavage
- Warming with extracorporeal circuit, such as arteriovenous or venovenous shunt that warms the blood
- Supportive treatment as indicated

Localized Cold Injuries

Frostnip is a superficial freeze injury that is reversible. **Frostbite** is damage to tissue caused by exposure to freezing temperatures, most often affecting the nose, ears, and distal extremities. As frostbite develops, the affected part feels numb and aches or throbs, becoming hard and insensate as the tissue freezes, resulting in circulatory impairment, necrosis of tissue, and gangrene. There are **3 zones of injury:**

- **Coagulation** (usually distal): severe, irreversible cellular damage
- **Hyperemia** (usually proximal): minimal cellular damage
- **Stasis** (between other 2 zones): severe but sometimes reversible damage

Symptoms vary according to the degree of freezing:

- **Partial freezing** with erythema and mild edema, stinging, burning, throbbing pain
- **Full-thickness freezing** with increased edema in 3-4 hours, edema and clear blisters in 6-24 hours, desquamation with eschar formation, numbness, and then aching and throbbing pain
- Prognosis is very good for **first-degree** and good for **second-degree** frostbite
- Full-thickness and into **subdermal tissue** freezing with cyanosis, hemorrhagic blisters, skin necrosis, and "wooden" feeling, severe burning, throbbing, and shooting pains
- Freezing extends into **subcutaneous tissue**, including muscles, tendons, and bones with mottled appearance, non-blanching cyanosis, and eventual deep black eschar

Prognosis is poor for **third-degree** and **fourth-degree** freeze injuries. Determining the degree of injury can be difficult because some degree of thawing may have occurred prior to admission to the hospital.

Treatment includes:

- Rapid rewarming with warm water bath (40-42 °C [104-107.6 °F]) 10-30 minutes or until the frostbitten area is erythematous and pliable
- Treatment for generalized hypothermia

Treatment **after warming**:

- Debridement of clear blisters but not hemorrhagic blisters
- Aloe vera cream every 6 hours to blistered areas
- Dressings, separating digits
- Tetanus prophylaxis
- Ibuprofen 12 mg/kg daily in divided doses
- Antibiotic prophylaxis if indicated (penicillin G 500,000 units IV every 6 hours for 24 to 72 hours)

Electrolyte Imbalances

Sodium

Sodium (Na) regulates fluid volume, osmolality, acid-base balance, and activity in the muscles, nerves, and myocardium. It is the primary **cation** (positive ion) in extracellular fluid (ECF), necessary to maintain ECF levels that are needed for tissue perfusion:

- Normal range: 135-145 mEq/L
- Hyponatremia: <135 mEq/L
- Hypernatremia: >145 mEq/L

Hyponatremia may result from inadequate sodium intake, excess sodium loss through diarrhea, vomiting, or NG suctioning, or illness, such as severe burns, fever, SIADH, and ketoacidosis.

- **Symptoms**: Irritability to lethargy and alterations in consciousness, cerebral edema with seizures and coma, dyspnea to respiratory failure.
- **Treatment**: Identify and treat underlying cause and provide Na replacement.

Hypernatremia may result from renal disease, diabetes insipidus, and fluid depletion.

- **Symptoms**: Irritability to lethargy to confusion to coma; seizures; flushing; muscle weakness and spasms; thirst.
- **Treatment**: Identify and treat underlying cause, monitor Na levels carefully, and give IV fluid replacement.

Potassium

Potassium (K) is the primary **electrolyte** in intracellular fluid (ICF) with about 98% inside cells and only 2% in ECF, although this small amount is important for neuromuscular activity. Potassium influences activity of the skeletal and cardiac muscles. Its level is dependent upon adequate renal functioning because 80% is excreted through the kidneys and 20% through the bowels and sweat:

- Normal range: 3.5-5.5 mEq/L
- Hypokalemia: <3.5 mEq/L. Critical value: <2.5 mEq/L
- Hyperkalemia: >5.5 mEq/L. Critical value: >6.5 mEq/L

A healthy NPO patient will need about 40 mEq of K per day to maintain serum K levels. (expect alterations in renal disease and other disease processes).

Hypokalemia is caused by loss of potassium through diarrhea, vomiting, gastric suction, and diuresis, alkalosis, decreased intake with starvation, and nephritis.

- **Symptoms**: Lethargy and weakness; nausea and vomiting; paresthesia and tetany; muscle cramps with hyporeflexia; hypotension; dysrhythmias with EKG changes: PVCs or flattened T-waves.
- **Treatment**: Treatment involves identifying and treating the underlying cause and replacing K. When possible, oral replacement is preferable to IV, as it allows slower adjustment of K levels. When given IV, K should be given no faster than 20 mEq/hour via central line if possible. If given peripherally, 10 mEq/hour is preferable for patient comfort.

Hyperkalemia is caused by renal disease, adrenal insufficiency, metabolic acidosis, severe dehydration, burns, hemolysis, and trauma. It rarely occurs without renal disease but may be induced by treatment (such as NSAIDs and potassium-sparing diuretics). Untreated renal failure results in reduced excretion. Those with Addison's disease and deficient adrenal hormones suffer sodium loss that results in potassium retention.

- **Symptoms**: The primary symptoms relate to the effect on the cardiac muscle: ventricular arrhythmias with increasing changes in EKG lead to cardiac and respiratory arrest, weakness with ascending paralysis and hyperreflexia, diarrhea, and increasing confusion.
- **Treatment**: Treatment includes identifying the underlying cause and discontinuing sources of increased K. Calcium gluconate to decrease cardiac effects. Sodium bicarbonate shifts K into the cells temporarily. Insulin and hypertonic dextrose shift K into the cells temporarily. Cation exchange resin (Kayexalate®) to decrease K. Peritoneal dialysis or hemodialysis to remove excess K.

Note: When a tourniquet is on, a patient opening and closing their hand can lead to falsely elevated K levels.

Calcium

More than 99% of **calcium (Ca)** is in the skeletal system with 1% in serum, but it is important for transmitting nerve impulses and regulating muscle contraction and relaxation, including the myocardium. Calcium activates enzymes that stimulate chemical reactions and has a role in coagulation of blood:

- Normal range: 8.2 to 10.2 mg/dL
- Hypocalcemia: <8.2. Critical value: <7 mg/dL
- Hypercalcemia: >10.2 mg/dL. Critical value: >12 mg/dL

Hypercalcemia may be caused by acidosis, kidney disease, hyperparathyroidism, prolonged immobilization, and malignancies. Crisis carries a 50% mortality rate.

- **Symptoms**: Increasing muscle weakness with hypotonicity; anorexia; nausea and vomiting; constipation; bradycardia and cardiac arrest.
- **Treatment**: Identify and treat underlying cause, loop diuretics, IV fluids, phosphate.

Hypocalcemia may be caused by a damage to the parathyroid resulting in hypoparathyroidism (directly decreasing calcium production), vitamin D resistance or inadequacy, or liver/kidney disease.

- **Symptoms**: Muscle cramping or spasms; seizures; numbness or tingling of the feet, hands, or lips; tetany if severe.
- **Treatment**: Identify and treat underlying cause, replace calcium by administering IV calcium gluconate in acute circumstances or increasing oral Vitamin D and calcium in chronic cases.

Phosphorus

Phosphorus, or phosphate, (PO_4) is necessary for neuromuscular and red blood cell function, the maintenance of acid-base balance, and provides structure for teeth and bones. About 85% is in the bones, 14% in soft tissue, and <1% in ECF.

- Normal range: 2.4-4.5 mEq/L
- Hypophosphatemia: <2.4mEq/L
- Hyperphosphatemia: >4.5 mEq/L

Hypophosphatemia occurs with severe protein-calorie malnutrition, excess antacids with magnesium, calcium, or aluminum, hyperventilation, severe burns, and diabetic ketoacidosis.

- **Symptoms**: Irritability, tremors, seizures to coma; hemolytic anemia; decreased myocardial function; respiratory failure.
- **Treatment**: Identify and treat underlying cause and replace phosphorus.

Hyperphosphatemia occurs with renal failure, hypoparathyroidism, excessive intake, and neoplastic disease, diabetic ketoacidosis, muscle necrosis, and chemotherapy.

- **Symptoms**: Tachycardia; muscle cramping; hyperreflexia and tetany; nausea and diarrhea.
- **Treatment**: Identify and treat underlying cause, correct hypocalcemia, and provide antacids and dialysis.

Magnesium

Magnesium (Mg) is the second most common intracellular electrolyte (after potassium) and activates many intracellular enzyme systems. Mg is important for carbohydrate and protein metabolism, neuromuscular function, and cardiovascular function, producing vasodilation and directly affecting the peripheral arterial system:

- Normal range: 1.7-2.2 mg/dL
- Hypomagnesemia critical value: <1.2 mg/dL
- Hypermagnesemia critical value: >4.9 mg/dL

Hypomagnesemia occurs with chronic diarrhea, chronic renal disease, chronic pancreatitis, excess diuretic or laxative use, hyperthyroidism, hypoparathyroidism, severe burns, and diaphoresis.

- **Symptoms**: Neuromuscular excitability or tetany; confusion, headaches, dizziness; seizure and coma; tachycardia with ventricular arrhythmias; respiratory depression.
- **Treatment**: Identify and treat underlying cause, provide magnesium replacement. IV magnesium is a vasodilator, 2 g over 60 mins.

Hypermagnesemia occurs with renal failure or inadequate renal function, diabetic ketoacidosis, hypothyroidism, and Addison's disease.

- **Symptoms**: Muscle weakness, seizures, and dysphagia with decreased gag reflex; tachycardia with hypotension.
- **Treatment**: Identify and treat underlying cause, IV hydration with calcium, and dialysis.

Review Video: Fluid and Electrolytes
Visit mometrix.com/academy and enter code: 384389

Acid Base Imbalances

Invasive Blood Gas Monitoring

Invasive blood gas monitoring options include the following:

- **Arterial blood gas (ABG)** is the most informative measurement of blood gas status. If an arterial catheter is in place, it is easily obtained by aspirating 1-2 mL of blood.
- **Venous blood gas (VBG)** is easier to obtain if an arterial catheter is not in place. In order to compare the values in the VBG with an ABG, make the following calculations:
    - Add 0.05 to the pH of the VBG.
    - Subtract 5-10 mmHg from the PCO_2 of the VBG.
- **Capillary Blood Gas (CBG)** can be obtained with a heel stick, without a venous or arterial line, but the values obtained in a CBG are the least accurate and are rarely useful. This is used most often in neonates.

Components of a Blood Gas Reading

The following are **components of a blood gas reading**:

- **pH** measures the circulating acid and base levels. Neutral pH for humans is 7.4. A value below 7.35 indicates acidosis and a value greater than 7.45 indicates alkalosis.
- **pCO_2** is the partial pressure of carbon dioxide and it determines the respiratory component of pH. An elevated pCO_2 lowers the pH. A low pCO_2 raises the pH. The pCO_2 value is dependent on adequate pulmonary ventilation and respiration. Changes in respiratory status quickly alter this value. Normal value range for pCO_2 is 35-45 mmHg.
- **pO_2** is the partial pressure of oxygen, which indicates how well the individual is transporting oxygen from the lungs into the bloodstream. Normal value is 75-100 mmHg.
- **HCO_3^-** is bicarbonate, the metabolic component of pH. This value may slowly change in response to abnormal pH, or a disease process may cause an elevation or depression. Low values decrease the pH and high values raise the pH. Normal value for bicarbonate is 22-26 mEq/L.

Metabolic and Respiratory Acidosis

Pathophysiology

- Metabolic acidosis
    - Increase in fixed acid and inability to excrete acid, or loss of base, with compensatory increase of CO_2 excretion by lungs.

- Respiratory acidosis
    - Hypoventilation and CO_2 retention with renal compensatory retention of bicarbonate (HCO_3) and increased excretion of hydrogen.

Laboratory

- Metabolic acidosis
    - Decreased serum pH (<7.35) and PCO_2 normal if uncompensated and decreased if compensated.
    - Decreased HCO_3.
- Respiratory acidosis
    - Decreased serum pH (< 7.35) and increased PCO_2.
    - Increased HCO_3 if compensated and normal if uncompensated.

Causes

- Metabolic acidosis
    - DKA, lactic acidosis, diarrhea, starvation, renal failure, shock, renal tubular acidosis, starvation.
- Respiratory acidosis
    - COPD, overdose of sedative or barbiturate (leading to hypoventilation), obesity, severe pneumonia/atelectasis, muscle weakness (Guillain-Barré), mechanical hypoventilation.

Symptoms

- Metabolic acidosis
    - Neuro/muscular: Drowsiness, confusion, headache, coma.
    - Cardiac: Decreased BP, arrhythmias, flushed skin.
    - GI: Nausea, vomiting, abdominal pain, diarrhea.
    - Respiratory: Deep inspired tachypnea.
- Respiratory acidosis
    - Neuro/muscular: Drowsiness, dizziness, headache, coma, disorientation, seizures.
    - Cardiac: Flushed skin, VF, ↓BP.
    - GI: Absent.
    - Respiratory: Hypoventilation with hypoxia.

Metabolic and Respiratory Alkalosis

Pathophysiology

- Metabolic alkalosis
    - Decreased strong acid or increased base with possible compensatory CO_2 retention by lungs.
- Respiratory alkalosis
    - Hyperventilation and increased excretion of CO_2 with compensatory HCO_3 excretion by kidneys.

Laboratory

- Metabolic alkalosis
    - Increased serum pH (>7.45).
    - PCO_2 normal if uncompensated and increased if compensated.
    - Increased HCO_3.
- Respiratory alkalosis
    - Increased serum pH (>7.45).
    - Decreased PCO_2.
    - HCO_3 normal if uncompensated and decreased if compensated.

Causes

- Metabolic alkalosis
    - Excessive vomiting, gastric suctioning, diuretics, potassium deficit, excessive mineralocorticoids and $NaHCO_3$ intake.
- Respiratory alkalosis
    - Hyperventilation associated with hypoxia, pulmonary embolus, exercise, anxiety, pain, and fever.
    - Encephalopathy, septicemia, brain injury, salicylate overdose, and mechanical hyperventilation.

Symptoms

- Metabolic alkalosis
    - Neuromuscular: Dizziness, confusion, nervousness, anxiety, tremors, muscle cramping, tetany, tingling, seizures.
    - Cardiac: Tachycardia and arrhythmias.
    - GI: Nausea, vomiting, anorexia.
    - Respiratory: Compensatory hypoventilation.
- Respiratory alkalosis
    - Neuro/muscular: Light-headedness, confusion, lethargy.
    - Cardiac: Tachycardia and arrhythmias.
    - GI: Epigastric pain, nausea, and vomiting.
    - Respiratory: Hyperventilation.

Infectious Diseases

Viral Infections

Herpes Simplex Virus Infections

There are 2 types of the **herpes simplex virus (HSV),** human herpesvirus 1 and 2. **HSV-1** usually causes a **gingivostomatitis** (often referred to as "cold sores" or "fever blisters") and is transmitted through **close contact. HSV-2** usually causes painful **genital lesions** through **sexual contact.** Either may be found in other areas of the body.

- **Incubation** period is around 2-12 days.
- The primary infection is usually more severe (causes systemic **symptoms**) than the reactivated infection, but it may be asymptomatic. After the primary infection, the virus remains dormant in the nerve ganglia, and can be reactivated especially during times of stress, illness, immunosuppression, or sun exposure. While patients are most contagious during times of active lesions, the disease may be spread while asymptomatic. The frequency of the outbreaks usually decreases over time.
- HSV **lesions** are grouped vesicles with an erythematous base. They are usually painful, and a prodrome of tingling, pain, or burning sensations may be felt hours to a couple days before the eruption. Lesions last for approximately 2-3 weeks in primary infection (up to 4 weeks with genital HSV), and 1-2 weeks in recurrent infections.
- HSV is **diagnosed** clinically and confirmed with a + culture, PCR test, or HSV antibody tests (HSV-1 or HSV-2: IgM= active or recent infection; IgG= previous infection).
- Symptomatic **treatment**, proper wound care, and antivirals (acyclovir, valacyclovir, or famciclovir) may be given.
- **Complications** include perinatal infection, keratitis, herpetic whitlow, herpes gladiatorum, secondary infections, and encephalitis.

Epstein-Barr Infection

Epstein-Barr virus (**EBV**) is a **herpesvirus** (human herpesvirus 4) and is responsible for causing **infectious mononucleosis.** After the initial infection, it remains latent in B cells and epithelial cells. It has been linked to certain epithelial and lymphatic neoplasms (e.g., nasopharyngeal carcinoma, Burkitt lymphoma, Hodgkin lymphoma).

- EBV is **transmitted** through **body fluids** like saliva, so it is sometimes referred to as the kissing disease. It is most common in teenagers and college-age young adults
- **Incubation** period is typically 30-50 days.
- **Symptoms** of EBV infection range from being asymptomatic to swollen painful lymph nodes, pharyngitis (can mimic strep pharyngitis), extreme fatigue, fever, and possibly hepatosplenomegaly. The WBC count is elevated (~10,000-20,000 cells/mL) with 10-30% atypical lymphocytes in the differential.
- Confirm **diagnosis** with a Mono Spot test or EBV antibody serology tests.
- **Treatment** is supportive, and antibiotics are not helpful in treating this viral infection. Therefore, avoid unnecessary antibiotics in those with EBV, especially since administration of ampicillin or amoxicillin is often associated with a pruritic, maculopapular rash. Analgesics, warm salt water gargles, increased fluid intake, and rest will help to relieve some of the symptoms. Symptoms may last for several weeks and fatigue may last even longer. Patients should avoid contact sports for up to 2 months.
- **Complications** include hepatitis, cytopenias (e.g., thrombocytopenia), Guillain Barré syndrome, and splenic rupture.

Measles, Mumps, and Rubella

Measles (rubeola) virus is highly contagious, is spread through **respiratory secretions** (incubation is 7-14 days), and peaks in late winter to spring. It causes a prodrome of high fever (4-7 days), cough, congestion, conjunctivitis; then Koplik spots (pathognomonic), and finally a maculopapular rash (spreads cephalocaudally). Report suspected cases immediately to the health dept. **Diagnose** with a + IgM antibody test (collected after 3 days of rash), viral culture, or PCR. **Treatment** is supportive.

Mumps (parotitis) is a viral infection that is spread via **saliva** (incubation is 12-24 days), and often occurs during winter and spring. It causes painful swelling of the salivary glands (parotid). Report to health dept. Supportive **treatment**. Complications include orchitis (infertility), pancreatitis, and meningitis.

Rubella (German measles) is a virus that spreads via **respiratory droplets** (incubation is 2-3 weeks), and peaks in the spring. There is a mild prodrome (fever, aches, sore throat, conjunctivitis, swollen nodes [esp. suboccipital, postauricular, & posterior cervical]), then a maculopapular rash (face 1st then down). Report to health dept. Confirm with rubella antibodies IgM or IgG. Symptomatic care.

Influenza

Influenza is a highly contagious viral infection that affects the entire **respiratory system** from the nose to the lungs. There are 3 types of influenza virus: **A** (causes epidemics), **B** (only in humans), and **C**. Types A and B are seen most often and are the strains that the annual flu vaccine is most effective against; and type C is not as common and much less severe.

- Prevention is key and annual, age-appropriate influenza **vaccines** should be given to those ≥6 months; 2 vaccines are required in first-time vaccine patients if 6 mo. through 8-year-olds (separated by 28 days).
- **Incubation** period is 1-4 days and it is spread via respiratory droplets.
- Though **symptoms** can be very similar, the flu and the common cold differ in that the flu has a very sudden onset. Symptoms of influenza include a high fever (may last up to 5 days), headache, myalgias, dry cough, rhinorrhea, and fatigue. There may also be vomiting and diarrhea, although children are more prone to this.
- Clinical judgement, community patterns, and rapid influenza tests (high specificity, but lower sensitivity) aid in **diagnosis**, but RT-PCR or viral culture definitively confirm the diagnosis; pulse oximetry and CXR as needed for pulmonary issues.
- Antibiotic **treatment** is not effective unless there is a secondary bacterial infection (e.g., pneumonia). Look for signs of secondary infections (e.g., dyspnea, cyanosis, fever that goes away and returns, confusion/lethargy). Supportive treatment with rest, fluids, and analgesics. Antivirals should be considered in those who are at high risk (<5 years old, elderly, pregnant, chronic conditions). These are most effective if initiated within 24-48 hours of symptom onset. The neuraminidase inhibitors (oseltamivir, zanamivir) treat type A, type B, and avian H5N1. There is extensive resistance to the adamantanes (amantadine, rimantadine) so they are rarely used.
- **Complications** include pneumonia, ARDS, and death.

Coronavirus

A **coronavirus** is a common virus that causes cold-like symptoms, including a cough, runny nose, sore throat, and congestion. Most cases of coronavirus are not dangerous and are often given little attention or go entirely unnoticed. However, specific coronavirus strains have led to two worldwide pandemics. The first, **Severe Acute Respiratory Syndrome (SARS)**, appeared in China in 2002 and quickly spread worldwide. Presenting symptoms of SARS were fever, cough, dyspnea, and general malaise. It was extremely virulent, spreading easily from person to person through close contact by way of contaminated droplets produced by coughing or sneezing. SARS was also very deadly, with a case fatality rate of nearly 10%. High rates of infection occurred in health care workers and others in contact with infected patients, so prompt diagnosis and proper isolation were essential. By 2004, there were no longer any documented active cases of SARS.

The most recent coronavirus outbreak was the **COVID-19** strain, which first appeared in December of 2019, in the Chinese city of Wuhan, and quickly became a global pandemic. Presentation of COVID-19 was similar to that of SARS, with the notable additional symptom of acute loss of taste/smell as a unique identifier. Much is still unknown about this strain, including exact transmission methods (though droplet transmission is suspected), effective treatment protocols, and long-term effects.

Precautions to take when treating patients with pandemic coronavirus include the following:

- Contact and droplet precautions, including eye protection and appropriate personal protection equipment.
- Airborne precautions (recommended by the CDC), especially with aerosol-producing procedures (ventilators, nebulizers, intubation).
- Immediate notification of public health authorities and institution of contact tracing.
- Activity restrictions of exposed health care workers planned in coordination with public health officials.

Cytomegalovirus

Cytomegalovirus (CMV) is a herpes virus, occurring in most people by the time they are adults.

- **Transmission** can occur through secretions during personal contact and from mother to baby before, during or after birth.
- Most cases have no **symptoms**, although a few infants will have fetal damage, such as jaundice, hepatitis, brain damage, or growth retardation.
- **Treatment** for those with severe infections is with ganciclovir, an antiviral drug.

Respiratory Syncytial Virus

Respiratory syncytial virus (RSV) is a virus that infects the respiratory tract, causing symptoms of nasal congestion, cough, sore throat, and headache. Severe cases can lead to high fever, breathing difficulties, severe cough, and cyanosis.

- Respiratory syncytial virus may **manifest** as a cold in adults and older children; however, there are some children who are more at risk of developing complications.
- **Transmission** is through contact with droplets from an infected person's nose or throat, generally through coughing and sneezing.
- Infants born prematurely, children with chronic lung disease, children with cystic fibrosis, and children who are in an immunocompromised state because of surgery or illness are at **high risk** of breathing difficulties, poor oxygenation, and even death from RSV.

Bacterial Infections

Diphtheria

Diphtheria, caused by *Corynebacterium diphtheriae*, is most prevalent in fall and winter.

- The **incubation** period is 2-7 days, possibly longer, and transmission is through direct contact with nasal, eye, and oral secretions.
- The **symptoms** are slight fever, nasal discharge, sore throat, feeling unwell, poor appetite, and swelling of the airway.
- If the disease is severe, death can result. The patient requires isolation, bed rest, fluids, antibiotics, medication for fever, and an antitoxin. The patient may also require oxygen therapy and tracheostomy if the airway is obstructed.

Tetanus

Tetanus, caused by *Clostridium tetani*, occurs all over the world. The spores formed by the bacillus are present in soil, dust, and the GI tracts of animals and humans.

- The **incubation** period is 3-21 days.
- **Symptoms** start with headache, irritability, jaw muscle spasms, and inability to open the mouth. This is followed by severe back muscle spasms, seizures, incontinence, and fever.
- **Treatment** requires human tetanus immune globulin, penicillin G, Valium, and placement on a ventilator. The environment should be kept quiet because the spasms are initiated by stimuli.

Fungal Infections

Cryptococcosis

Cryptococcosis is an infection resulting from inhaling the **fungus** *Cryptococcus neoformans,* which is found worldwide in soil (can be associated with bird droppings), or *Cryptococcus gattii,* which is associated with certain trees in the Northwest.

- Cryptococcosis is most often due to *C. neoformans*. It is often found among those with compromised immune systems and is an **AIDS-defining opportunistic infection**.
- Healthy patients may be asymptomatic and the only finding may be pulmonary lesions on CXR that resolve spontaneously. The fungus can disseminate and cause meningitis, encephalitis, cutaneous lesions, and affect long bones and other tissues. **Symptoms** are based on the area of involvement. Patients may experience cough, pleuritic chest pain, weight loss, and fever if there is pulmonary involvement; headache, double vision, light sensitivity, N/V, and confusion if CNS involvement; cutaneous lesions (papules, pustules, nodules, ulcers) if the skin is involved.
- **Diagnosis** includes microscopic analysis, culture (gold standard), or an antigen test (highly sensitive; good for detecting early infection) for *Cryptococcus* using CSF, tissue, sputum, blood, or urine. Check CSF by India ink (limited sensitivity) or culture so meningitis can be ruled out. Confirm that no mass lesion is present by CT or MRI before LP is performed.
- Mild cases may only require monitoring to ensure that the infection does not spread. In more advanced cases, the infection is treated with different antifungal medications (e.g., fluconazole for pulmonary infections, amphotericin B ± flucytosine for meningitis). The patient should also be monitored for CNS infection and medication side effects. AIDS patients may need lifelong antifungals.
- **Complications** include cryptococcal meningitis, neural deficits, optic nerve damage, and hydrocephalus.

Histoplasmosis

Histoplasmosis is an infection caused by inhalation of **spores** from the fungus *Histoplasma capsulatum* that is found in soil and is associated with bird and bat droppings (e.g., chicken coops, caves).

- Healthy patients are usually asymptomatic and those with symptoms are typically immunocompromised or those who've had a heavy exposure to spores. The primary **pulmonary infection** occurs 3-17 days after exposure and can present with flu-like symptoms. It is typically self-limited but may become chronic. Histoplasmosis can also spread through the **blood** and can cause progressive disseminated disease in the immunocompromised (high mortality rate); this is an **AIDS-defining illness**.
- **Diagnose** through antigen tests (urine, serum), histopathology, or cultures; order a CXR. Mild and even moderate acute pulmonary histoplasmosis may resolve on its own.
- If needed, **treat** mild to moderate infections with itraconazole and severe illness with amphotericin B.

Pneumocystis

Pneumocystis jiroveci is a **fungus** (previously known as *Pneumocystis* carinii) that causes **pneumonia** (PJP, previously PCP) in the immunocompromised. Most people have been exposed to this by the age of 3 or 4.

- **Symptoms** of PJP include a dry nonproductive cough, fever, dyspnea, and weight loss.
- CXR may show diffuse bilateral infiltrates or it may be normal; and pulse oximetry may be low, especially on exertion. **Diagnosis** is confirmed with sputum histopathology using sputum induction or bronchoalveolar lavage.
- **Treat** immediately with TMP-SMX (trimethoprim/sulfamethoxazole) for 21 days if HIV + and for 14 days in other cases. Steroids may be added for HIV patients with severe PJP. HIV/AIDS patients with CD4 counts <200/μL should receive PJP prophylaxis with TMP-SMX. Dapsone and pentamidine are alternatives.
- **Complications** include ARDS and death.

Candidal Infections

Candida is a type of yeast that may cause a variety of infections:

- **Oral thrush** is commonly seen in diabetic patients and those who are immunosuppressed (HIV or underlying neoplasm). Patients often complain of burning on the tongue or in the mouth, associated with "curd-like" white patches that can be scraped away leaving reddish tissue underneath. Diagnosis is with KOH prep. Treatment is with oral or topical antifungals, including nystatin (swish and swallow or troches).
- **Candida esophagitis** also occurs in the immunosuppressed population, and patients may complain of dysphasia, odynophagia, and chest pain. This is diagnosed on EGD and may be treated with oral or IV antifungals (ketoconazole).
- **Candidal intertrigo**, or diaper rash, presents with beefy-red lesions at skin fold areas as well as satellite lesions. Treatment is with topical antifungals.
- **Candidemia** is diagnosed with fungal blood cultures and may lead to osteomyelitis, endocarditis, and other complications. Treatment is with IV antifungals.

RINGWORM

Ringworm is caused by an infection from the *Tinea* fungus, which produces patches on the skin that have normal centers, giving the appearance of a ring.

- The fungus can cause hair loss and patches of scaly skin that may develop blisters that ooze or crust.
- It is **transmitted** by touching the affected skin or through objects that have touched the affected skin.
- Ringworm may be **diagnosed** by viewing the skin section under a Wood's lamp. Skin cultures may also be taken for examination to identify the fungus. A potassium hydroxide (KOH) exam involves scraping the affected skin and placing the skin sample in KOH to test for the presence of the fungus.

VECTOR-BORNE AND PARASITIC INFECTIONS

MALARIA

Malaria is a **blood-borne disease** caused by a **parasite** from the genus *Plasmodium and* found in tropical areas. There are 4 known to cause disease in humans (*P. malariae*, *P. vivax*, *P. ovale*, and *P. falciparum*). These protozoa are transmitted by the **female *Anopheles* mosquito**. They travel to the **liver** where they multiply, are released, and then infect the RBCs, where they continue to multiply. Incubation time can be as little as 9 days or as much as multiple years depending on the species of the infecting parasite.

- **Signs and symptoms** include headache, high fever with shaking chills and sweating (rigors; occurs when merozoites, an immature form of the parasite, are released from RBCs), jaundice, anemia, and hepatosplenomegaly. Take a thorough history including recent travel.
- **Diagnose** with 3 thin and thick blood smears (gold standard) stained with Giemsa (preferred) and obtained 12-24 hours apart. Labs typically show elevated LDH, thrombocytopenia, and atypical lymphocytes. Rapid antigen tests are also available as well as PCR.
- **Treat** with chloroquine. If travelling, chemoprophylaxis depends on the area of travel due to species and resistance patterns, and may include chloroquine, primaquine, mefloquine, Malarone®, or doxycycline. Report infections to your local or state health department.
- **Complications** include severe anemia and hemolysis, organ failure (liver, spleen, kidneys), cerebral malaria, ARDS, and death.

LYME DISEASE

Lyme disease occurs from a bite from a **deer tick** (blacklegged tick) infected with the **spirochete bacterium** *Borrelia burgdorferi*. It is the most common tick-borne disease in the U.S. and is more prevalent in heavily wooded areas. Adult ticks are more active during colder times whereas the nymphs (<2 mm in size) are more active in the warm, spring or summer months. Once the tick bites, it stays attached; however, it takes about 36-48 hours for nymphs and about 48-72 hours for adult ticks before the spirochete is transmitted to the person. **Incubation** period is 3-30 days. There are 3 stages to this disease: early localized, early disseminated, and chronic disseminated.

- **Stage 1** 75% have the characteristic expanding red rash (erythema migrans; can be large, ~30cm) which can progress to have central clearing (bull's eye), headache, fever, chills, myalgias, and fatigue.

- **Stage 2** occurs weeks to months after initial infection and involves systemic symptoms (flu-like), neck stiffness, headaches, migrating pain in muscles and joints, rashes, paresthesias, Bell's palsy, confusion, fatigue, myocarditis, and heart palpitations.
- **Stage 3** occurs months to years after initial infection and involves neurologic (e.g., encephalitis) and rheumatologic issues, especially arthritis of large joints (e.g., knee).

DIAGNOSIS AND TREATMENT OF LYME DISEASE

Diagnose Lyme disease using 2-tiered testing: antibodies (IgM, IgG), then Western blot. Antibiotic treatment for localized Lyme disease involves 2-3 weeks of doxycycline, amoxicillin, or cefuroxime axetil is started immediately after diagnosis. IV antibiotics may be needed for severe disease (e.g., IV ceftriaxone). Prevention is key by wearing clothes covering the skin, using tick repellents, showering soon after being outdoors in tick-prone areas, and thoroughly checking for ticks (especially in hard to see areas by using a mirror). The Lyme vaccine is no longer available and previous vaccine recipients are still at risk of contracting the disease as protection decreases over time. Complications are prevalent with untreated Lyme disease and include chronic arthritis, fatigue, chronic musculoskeletal issues, acrodermatitis chronica atrophicans, and memory and concentration issues. Report cases to the local health dept.

ROCKY MOUNTAIN SPOTTED FEVER

Rocky Mountain spotted fever is a tick-borne illness caused by Rickettsia rickettsii. It tends to occur in spring and summer throughout the United States.

- **Incubation** period is about one week.
- **Symptoms** include headache, fever, nausea, vomiting, loss of appetite, muscle pain, and rash on the ankles and wrists.
- **Treatment** requires an antibiotic, usually Vibramycin.

HELMINTH INFESTATIONS

Helminth infestations (worms) include **roundworms** [nematodes: *Ascaris*, hookworms (cause anemia), **filariae** (cause elephantiasis)] and **flatworms** [tapeworms (cause weight loss); **flukes** (intestinal or liver)]. **Pinworms** are a type of roundworm that cause enterobiasis and is the most common helminth infestation. Pinworms are more prevalent in warmer areas of the country and infestations occur more frequently in children. The worms lay eggs within the digestive tract and then travel to the anal area where they are usually found. Pinworms are highly contagious. As a patient itches the anal area where the eggs are located, the eggs cling to the fingers and can easily be transmitted to other people either directly or through food or surfaces. The eggs can survive for 2-3 weeks on inanimate objects.

- Patients may be asymptomatic or have intense anal itching that is usually worse at night and can cause insomnia. Abdominal pain, nausea, and vomiting can also occur.
- **Diagnose** with the "tape test" which involves pressing cellophane tape over the perianal area to pick up eggs or worms and examine under the microscope. Most other helminth infestations can be diagnosed with a stool sample for ova and parasites; filariasis requires a blood smear or antigen test.
- Anthelmintic medications are given in a single dose and repeated in 2 weeks to kill the pinworms and their larvae (mebendazole, albendazole, or pyrantel pamoate). The entire family and close contacts should be treated simultaneously since pinworms are so contagious.

Giardia Lamblia

Giardia lamblia is a protozoan that infects water supplies and spreads to children through the fecal-oral route. It is the most common cause of non-bacterial diarrhea in the United States, causing about 20,000 cases of infection each year in all ages.

- Children often become infected after swallowing recreational waters (pools, lakes) while swimming or putting contaminated items into the mouth. *Giardia* live and multiply within the small intestine where cysts develop.
- **Symptoms** occur 7-14 days after ingestion of 1 or more cysts and include diarrhea with greasy floating stools (rarely bloody), stomach cramps, nausea, and flatulence, lasting 2-6 weeks. A chronic infection may develop that can last for months or years.
- **Treatment** includes Furazolidone 5-8 mg/kg/day in 4 doses for 7-10 days or Metronidazole 40 mg/kg/day in 3 doses for 7-10 days. Chronic infections are often very resistant to treatment.

Toxoplasmosis

Toxoplasmosis is an infection caused by the **parasite** *Toxoplasma gondii*, which is commonly found in soil. It is widespread and transmitted through cat feces; however, it also may be contracted by eating undercooked meat (especially pork, lamb, or venison) or poorly washed vegetables. Toxoplasmosis can cause serious disease and can affect various organs; and immunocompromised and pregnant women and their unborn babies are especially likely to have side effects of the disease (the "T" in congenital TORCH infections).

- Healthy patients are usually asymptomatic; however, once infected the parasite can remain latent until the patient becomes immunocompromised and the parasite is reactivated causing **symptoms**. The disease can cause a flu-like illness with fever, myalgias, and lymphadenopathy. More serious effects include retinochoroiditis, brain lesions, and encephalitis. Congenital toxoplasmosis may cause retinochoroiditis, microcephaly, hydrocephalus, intellectual disability, and possibly miscarriage or stillbirth.
- **Diagnose** with serology for *Toxoplasma* antibodies IgM and IgG. Also, PCR may be used to test amniotic fluid, CSF, or tissue.
- **Treat** with pyrimethamine (preferred) plus folinic acid or sulfadiazine plus folinic acid. Pregnant women should avoid high-risk practices like changing the cat litter and should avoid sand boxes.

Geriatric Pathophysiology

Geriatric Syndromes

Geriatric syndromes represent a category of illnesses that is comprised of the most common non-disease conditions that are seen amongst the geriatric community. It is the responsibility of the nurse to be competent in these critical areas:

- **Falls**: As individuals age, their senses dull, leaving them vulnerable to falls due to a combination of sensory decline and chronic disease. Patients and caregivers should be provided with recommendations for fall prevention, and health care providers should create safe inpatient environments with proper fall prevention protocols.
- **Frailty**: A syndrome characterized by decreased stamina, strength, weight, and speed. This combination of issues results from the natural decline of aging and presents specific risks (falls, confusion, and depression) that must be assessed amongst the geriatric population.

- **Incontinence**: Urinary incontinence is an especially common ailment amongst the elderly population due to neurological conditions, physical limitations, and cognitive decline. This particular ailment is not only physically limiting and introduces risks for skin breakdown and infection, but it is socially limiting and can lead to psychological issues as well.
- **Delirium**: Confusion is the most common manifestation of any physical ailment amongst the elderly, along with the prevalence of dementia amongst the elderly. Delirium should never be cast aside in an elderly individual. Though common, it may be an indication of other more serious issues.
- **Functional Decline**: Functional decline is the diminished ability of an individual to carry out the activities of daily living to sustain independence and perform self-care. With this, comes the consideration for additional support, be it live-in care, nursing homes, or assisted living communities.

Additional Health Issues for the Elderly

The following are **additional health issues** for the elderly:

- **Antibodies and Immunity**: An elderly patient can react to an infection with antibodies that have been created by the body before, but if the infection is new, it is more difficult for the body to respond appropriately. Cells in the immune system cannot proliferate as easily in an older patient as in a younger one. The number of T-cells is stable, but they do not work as well and can have less cytotoxicity. Additionally, there is not as much thymus-gained immunity because the thymus gland is smaller. This also means it is harder for an older patient to make antibodies.
- **Allergies**: Identify the type of allergic response the patient has and to what allergens, especially when getting the patient history. Determine if the response is actually an allergy to a medication or an adverse effect of it.
- **Driving**: An elderly patient senses change with age. A decreased ability to hear does not mean a patient cannot drive, but sight is very important, including binocular sight, ability to see color, and ability to see in the dark.
- **REM**: Rapid eye movement starts approximately 120 minutes after going to sleep, and happens again in 3–4 evenly spread out increments that last 10–15 minutes. It is linked to skeletal muscle atonia, rapid eye movements, and dreaming. REM sleep occurs less frequently as one gets older. With aging, the patient is more likely to wake up, which affects their sleep quality.

Urinary Incontinence

Urinary incontinence (UI) is the involuntary loss of urine. Incidence increases with age and is more common in women. There are several types of urinary incontinence:

- **Transient**: Adverse medication reaction, urinary tract infection, severe constipation, immobility, mental disorders.
- **Urge or Reflex**: Detrusor muscle spasms cause an urgent desire to urinate because of neurological impairment in Parkinson's, stroke, Alzheimer's, and sitting. Can be triggered by drinking, hearing or seeing running water.
- **Stress (SUI)**: Increased intra-abdominal pressure from sneezing, coughing, laughing, pregnancy, childbirth damage to the detrusor muscle and pelvic floor fascia, and menopausal hormone changes. Twice as common in women as men.
- **Enuresis**: Bedwetting while asleep.

Decreased bladder strength, diminished ability to concentrate urine, and decreased urethral closing pressure following menopause are common causes of incontinence in the elderly. Incontinence is also influenced by depression, less mobility, decreased vision, and less awareness of feeling a full bladder. Voiding routines are helpful in managing incontinence among the elderly. The typical voiding routine for a fully-grown adult patient is as follows: The initial urge to go to the bathroom happens at the point of the bladder having 200-300 mL in it. Grown patients generally void 4-6 times daily, and most will not need to go during the night except when there is a condition that makes it so or if the patient is using diuretic medication. The sensation of the bladder beginning to fill up begins at 90-150 mL, and the need to go starts at 200-300 mL. Usually an hour or two will go by from the first feeling of needing to go and the point where the bladder is at full capacity. Full, easy capacity is around 300-600 mL. There should not be any leaking if going to the bathroom has to be postponed.

Age-Related Changes in Respiratory System

As a patient ages, the **respiratory system changes** in the following ways:

- **Rib cage becomes more rigid**. There will be more width measured across the anteroposterior chest. When a patient gets old, the number of alveoli decreases. They get inflexible and can no longer draw back. This means that the patient cannot breathe out as well, leading to more residual volume. There is less basilar inflation and the patient cannot get foreign bodies out as well. This condition also happens to someone who has kyphosis.
- **Decreased ability for the chest wall to work** so that it is harder to take a deep inhalation.
- **Trachea and bronchi increase in measurement** so that there is more unused area and lessened air volume that gets to the alveoli. Small airway shutting means there is less vital capacity and more residual volume.
- **Lung parenchyma is not as elastic** so that the alveoli do not function as effectively.
- **Breaths are not as deep and coughs are not as forceful** because the muscles are not as strong.

Chronic Diarrhea

Chronic diarrhea is more than three bowel movements per day, with watery stools lasting more than two weeks. It is more common and potentially more serious for the elderly population. The most common cause is infectious, but chronic diarrhea in the elderly population can also be caused by inflammatory bowel disease, diverticulitis, colon cancer, medication side effects, and irritable bowel syndrome. Take a careful history, including a list of travel destinations. Look for these signs and **symptoms of dehydration** in the physical exam:

- Flushed, dry skin
- Dark, scanty urine
- Fast pulse and respiration
- Fever
- Vomiting or nausea
- Head rushes
- Thirst
- Dry mouth
- Anorexia
- Chills
- Tingling
- Cramps

- Exhaustion
- Confusion
- Seizures
- Unconsciousness

Send stools to the lab for culture, ova and parasites, occult blood, fecal leukocytes, and *C. difficile* toxin, especially if the patient was recently hospitalized. Collect blood for a CBC and electrolytes. Order an abdominal x-ray, and follow up with a barium enema or colonoscopy, if indicated. Treat the underlying cause. Significantly dehydrated patients require hospital admission for IV therapy.

Muscle Wasting or Atrophy

Sarcopenia describes the process of progressive **muscle wasting** that is seen in the elderly population. Muscle protein production decreases with age, resulting in a loss of muscle mass, and eventually a loss of physical functional ability. Decreased activity and a lack of exercise contribute to the process of muscle wasting. As sarcopenia progresses, it leads to decreased mobility and puts patients at higher risk for developing other health problems. The process of muscle wasting can be slowed, halted, or reversed with treatment. The most effective treatment is exercise, specifically resistance training. Adequate nutrition, including sufficient amounts of Vitamin B_{12}, protein, and calcium is an important part of the treatment regimen. Use of growth hormone, estrogen or testosterone is controversial. Sarcopenia differs from **cachexia**, which is wasting from a chronic disease, most often cancer.

Fractures

Fractures are a common cause of disability in the elderly population. The elderly population is at higher risk for sustaining fractures due to decreased bone mass and strength, and increased risk for falls due to poor vision and balance. The most common locations for fractures in the elderly are the distal radius, proximal humerus, proximal femur and tibia, vertebrae, hip and pubic ramus. Most fractures are the result of minor trauma. Fractures are slightly more common in women. Make the diagnosis based on the history, physical exam, and x-ray results. Immobilize the fracture above and below the break. Administer analgesics. Refer the patient to a physiotherapist, an orthopedic surgeon, and a PSW. The goal of treatment is as rapid a return to normal activity as is possible. The elderly population is more vulnerable to complications, such as permanent functional impairment, bedsores and pulmonary embolism. The aide, nurse, or caregiver must turn the patient every two hours to minimize complications.

Lens and Age-Related Cataracts

The **lens** is the clear part of the eye behind the pupil that focuses light on the retina. **Cataracts** are categorized by gradual clouding or opacification of the lens. One or both eyes can be affected, and cataracts can be congenital. Incidence increases with age and affects 70% of people over the age of 75. Risk factors include trauma, radiation, diabetes, family history, smoking, alcoholism, sun exposure, steroid use and previous eye surgery. Signs and symptoms for cataracts include gradual lens clouding; blurry vision; decreased night vision; brown tint or color fading; halo or glare around lights; diplopia (double vision); trouble distinguishing blue and purple. An ophthalmologist makes the diagnosis by slit lamp exam and retinal exam. Cataracts are followed until they cause significant visual loss and then are treated by surgical removal of the clouded lens and replacement with a permanent intraocular or removable external lens.

Hearing Loss

Approximately 25% of adults over the age of 65 have varying degrees of **hearing loss**. Risk factors for hearing loss include:

- A positive family history
- Chronic exposure to loud noises, especially if hearing protection was not worn
- Use of ototoxic drugs, like Gentamicin, NSAIDs, loop diuretics, or cancer chemotherapy

Hearing loss can be either peripheral or central. **Peripheral hearing loss** results when the ear canal is obstructed by impacted wax, a foreign object, or damage to the middle or inner ear. **Central hearing loss** is the result of damage to the portions of the brain that are needed for hearing: Vestibulocochlear nerve, brain stem, contralateral inferior colliculus, superior olivary nucleus, inferior colliculi, ipsilateral medial geniculate nucleus of the thalamus, and primary auditory cortex below the superior temporal gyrus in the temporal lobe.

Sinusitis

Elderly individuals are at higher risk for the development of **sinusitis**. Causes include the drying out of the nasal passages, weakened nasal cartilage leading to obstruction, and a weakened immune system. The elderly population is also at increased risk for more severe infections and complications. Sinusitis can be acute or chronic. It is considered acute if symptoms have been present for less than four weeks. Patients usually present with fever, cough, facial pain, headache, mouth breathing, and nasal discharge. The diagnosis is generally made clinically; however, occasionally a CT scan and nasal swab for culture and sensitivity can be helpful. Treatment includes antibiotics and decongestants. Chronic sinusitis requires a referral to an ENT specialist (otorhinolaryngologist).

Hypogonadism

Male **hypogonadism** means that the testes do not produce sufficient quantities of testosterone. The patient will be impotent, infertile, and have little or no sex drive. Male hypogonadism can be present at birth from Klinefelter or Kallmann syndromes, and may present also with a micropenis and/or undescended testicles. Hypogonadism can occur later in life from pituitary or testicular tumors, especially if the man must be castrated (orchiectomy) to slow advancing prostate cancer. Hypogonadism results from aging in 30% of men over the age of 50 as **andropause**. Patients present with beard and body hair loss, decreased muscle mass, osteoporosis, gynecomastia (female pattern breast growth), and complain of erectile dysfunction (ED), emotional lability, fatigue, inability to concentrate, and decreased libido. Patients may also have hot flashes. The diagnosis is made based on the clinical picture and the serum testosterone level. Treatment is testosterone replacement therapy, but it can cause polycythemia. A good serum testosterone target level for seniors is 250-1,000 ng/dL.

Menopause

Menopause is cessation of menstrual cycles and childbearing. It is diagnosed after a woman has no periods for 12 *consecutive* months. Perimenopausal women skip periods for months but are not infertile. Menopause is usually a natural process of normal ageing. However, many women experience instant menopause through complete hysterectomy (TAHBSO), cancer chemotherapy, radiation exposure, early ovarian failure, or another pathological condition. The average age of menopause is 51; normal age range is 45-55. Late menopause is 60 and is a risk for uterine cancer. Symptoms of impending menopause include irregular periods, hot flashes, emotional lability and difficulty sleeping because of night sweats. Diagnosis is made clinically, and confirmed with blood tests for LH, FSH, estrogen, and thyroid panel. The onset of menopause produces an elevated follicle-stimulating hormone level and a decreased estradiol level. Treatment is combined estrogen and progesterone replacement therapy, antidepressants, gabapentin, and clonidine. Do not use estrogen alone if the woman still has her uterus, because it predisposes her to cancer.

Common Comorbidities Seen Amongst the Elderly Population

Geriatric comorbidities are combinations of chronic or acute illnesses that significantly increase the mortality rate amongst this population and are also associated with faster rates of disability exacerbation and functional decline. Understanding these comorbidities not only help the nurse manage these specific comorbidities, but also aid in the guidance of health promotion and disease prevention efforts to decrease the rates of comorbidity amongst their elderly patients. A 2010 study clustered comorbidities most commonly found in the elderly population into 3 groups (Ross, 2010). The three most common comorbidity patterns amongst the geriatric population include:

- **Cardiovascular/Metabolic Disorders**: Heart disease, MI, coronary artery disease and congestive heart failure often coincide with metabolic issues such as hypertension, diabetes, obesity, and gout.
- **Anxiety/Depression/Somatoform Disorders and Pain**: Pain (systemic, localized, or joint related) often coincide with psychological conditions such as anxiety, depression and cognitive decline. Gastrointestinal issues also seem to coincide with these psychological conditions.
- **Neuropsychiatric Disorders**: Psychiatric conditions such as Parkinson's and dementia, are often tied to neurological issues such as incontinence, vascular issues, and/or nerve pain.

Common Psychological Responses to Chronic Illness

Chronic illness not only effects the physical health of individuals, but often has many **psychological manifestations** as well. This psychological stress is tied to the most basic needs that are engrained in individuals as children, and therefore can cause the regression of the patient to adapt more childlike responses to chronic illness over time. Often these psychological responses to chronic illnesses are based on general concepts of fear, self-esteem, and loss of control.

- **Fear**: Chronic illness, when debilitating with possibly severe consequences, forces patients to face common fears of death, loss and pain. Remaining in a constant state of fear (stress) can lead to depression, anxiety and anger.
- **Self Esteem**: While in the early stages of chronic illness many patients find strength and determination to conquer the disease. But, after time, the inability to do so wears on the individual's sense of strength and capability. With a loss of self-esteem, can come feelings of despair and hopelessness, which often result in an increasing rate of decline. Patients with strong support systems and positive outlooks often fare better with chronic disease.
- **Loss of Control**: When chronic disease dictates an individual's life and abilities, the patient loses a sense of control over their own life. Losing one's independence can be extremely difficult mentally and emotionally, especially when the patient was previously active and healthy. By providing the patient with treatment options and educating the patient on self-care the nurse can attempt to return some elements of control to the patient, which can motivate them to own their fight against disease and find a new normal in their life that is manageable and fulfilling.

Core Competencies: Advanced Pharmacology

Principles of Pharmacology

Principles of Pharmacokinetics

Pharmacokinetics relates to the route of administration, the absorption, the dosage, the frequency of administration, the distribution, and the serum levels achieved over time.

- The **drug's rate of clearance (elimination)** and **doses needed** to ensure therapeutic benefit are considered. Most drugs are cleared through the kidneys, with water-soluble compounds excreted more readily than protein-soluble compounds.
- **Volume of distribution** (IV drug dose divided by plasma concentration) determines the rate at which the drug passes into tissue. Drug distribution depends on the degree of protein binding and ion trapping that takes place.
- **Elimination half-life** is the time needed for the concentration of a particular drug to decrease to half of its starting dose in the body. Approximately five half-lives are needed to achieve steady-state plasma concentrations if giving doses intermittently.
- **Context-sensitive half-life** is the time needed to reach 50% concentration after withdrawal of a continuously-administered drug.
- **Recovery time** is the length of time it takes for plasma levels to decrease to the point that the effect is eliminated. This is affected by plasma concentration.
- **Effect-site equilibrium** is the time between administration of a drug and clinical effect (the point at which the drug reaches the appropriate receptors) and must be considered when determining dose, time, and frequency of medications.
- The **bioavailability** of drugs may vary, depending upon the degree of metabolism that takes place before the drug reaches its site of action.

Principles of Pharmacodynamics

Pharmacodynamics relates to biological effects (therapeutic or adverse) of drug administration over time. Drug transport, absorption, means of elimination, and half-life must all be considered when determining effects. Responses may include continuous responses, such as blood pressure variations, or dichotomous response in which an event either occurs or does not (such as death). Information from pharmacodynamics provides feedback to modify medication dosage (pharmacokinetics). Drugs provide biological effects primarily by interacting with receptor sites (specific protein molecules) in the cell membrane. Receptors include voltage-sensitive ion channels (sodium, chloride, potassium, and calcium channels), ligand-gated ion channels, and transmembrane receptors. Agonist drugs exert effects after binding with a receptor while antagonist drugs bind with a receptor but have no effects, so they can block agonists from binding. The total number of receptors may vary, upregulating or downregulating in response to stimuli (such as drug administration). Dose-response curves show the relationship between the amount of drug given and the resultant plasma concentration and biological effects.

First Pass Metabolism and Drug Clearance

First pass metabolism is the phenomenon that occurs to ingested drugs that are absorbed through the gastrointestinal tract and enter the hepatic portal system. Drugs metabolized on the first pass travel to the liver, where they are broken down, some to the extent that only a small fraction of the active drug circulates to the rest of the body. This first pass through the liver greatly reduces the bioavailability of some drugs. Routes of administration that avoid first pass metabolism include intravenous, intramuscular, and sublingual.

Drug Clearance refers to the ability to remove a drug from the body. The two main organs responsible for clearance are the liver and the kidneys. The liver eliminates drugs by metabolizing, or biotransforming the substance, or excreting the drug in the bile. The kidneys eliminate drugs by filtration or active excretion in the urine. Drugs use either renal or hepatic methods of clearance. Kidney and liver dysfunction inhibit the clearance of drugs that rely on that organ for removal. Toxicity results from poor clearance.

Enterohepatic Recirculation of Drugs and Renally-Excreted Drugs

Enterohepatic recirculation refers to the process whereby a drug is effectively removed from circulation and then reabsorbed. The drug is secreted in bile, which is collected in the gall bladder and emptied into the small intestine, from which part of it is reabsorbed and part excreted in the feces. This reabsorption reduces the clearance of these drugs and increases their duration of action. Generally, drugs susceptible to enterohepatic recirculation are those with a molecular weight greater than 300 g/mol and those that are amphipathic (have both a lipophilic portion and a polar portion).

Renally-excreted drugs are metabolized (biotransformed) by the liver to a form that can be excreted by the kidneys. Others are excreted by the kidneys unchanged. Infants with decreased renal function demonstrate decreased urine output or elevated levels of BUN and creatinine. The nurse should avoid using drugs that depend on the kidneys for clearance if the infant has renal impairment as overdose may result.

Absorpation in Relation to Routes of Medication Administration

The absorption rate of a drug depends on its transfer from its site of administration to the circulatory system. Different **routes of administration** have different absorption characteristics:

- **Oral**: Ingested medications pass from the gastrointestinal tract into the blood stream. Most absorption occurs in the small intestine and is affected by gastric motility and emptying rate, drug solubility in gastrointestinal fluids, and food presence. Orally administered drugs are susceptible to first pass metabolism by the liver.
- **Intravenous**: Medications directly administered to the blood stream have 100% absorption. Peak serum levels are rapidly achieved. Some drugs are not tolerated intravenously, due to vein irritation or toxicity, and others must be given as an infusion.
- **Intramuscular**: Medications injected into a muscle are absorbed fairly rapidly because muscle tissue is highly vascularized. Drugs in lipid vehicles absorb more slowly than those in aqueous vehicles.
- **Subcutaneous**: Medications injected beneath the skin absorb more slowly because the dermis is less vascularized than muscle. Hypoperfusion and edema decrease absorption further.

Blood Drug Levels

Plasma drug levels are used for **therapeutic drug monitoring** because, although plasma is often not the site of action, plasma levels correlate well with therapeutic (effective) and toxic (dose-related adverse effects) responses to most drugs. The therapeutic range of a drug is that between the minimum effective concentration (level at which there is no therapeutic benefit) and the toxic concentration (level at which toxic effects occur). To achieve drug plateau (steady state), the drug half-life (time needed to decrease drug concentration by 50%) must be considered. Most drugs reach plateau with administration equal to four half-lives and completely eliminate a drug in 5 half-lives. Because drug levels fluctuate, peak (highest drug concentration) and trough (lowest drug concentration) levels may be monitored. Samples for trough levels are taken immediately prior to administration of another dose while peak samples are taken at various times, depending on the average peak time of the specific drug, which may vary from 30 minutes to 2 hours or so after administration.

Side Effects of Medications

All drugs can have **side effects**, and some are toxic at certain levels or in combination with other drugs. Some side effects will be minor and may go away after a week or two. Others can be severe or life threatening, such as anaphylaxis. Common side effects include nausea, vomiting, diarrhea, and rashes. Side effects may vary with individuals according to age, gender, and condition and may be related to non-compliance with treatment, incorrect dosage, polypharmacy, or drug interactions. Drug compendiums will list all possible side effects according to system or incidence. Pharmacologically similar medications usually have some common side effects among the drugs in that class. Nursing actions include:

- Always question the patient about allergies or previous drug reactions before administering medication.
- Educate the patient about possible side effects of all medications.
- Watch out for drug/drug or food/drug combinations that are dangerous.

Drug Interactions

Drug interactions occur when one drug interferes with the activity of another in either the pharmacodynamics or pharmacokinetics:

- With **pharmacodynamic interaction,** both drugs may interact at receptor sites causing a change that results in an adverse effect or that interferes with a positive effect.
- With **pharmacokinetic interaction**, the ability of the drug to be absorbed and cleared is altered, so there may be delayed effects, changes in effects, or toxicity. Interactions may include problems in a number of areas:
  - **Absorption** may be increased or (more commonly) decreased, usually related to the effects within the gastrointestinal system.
  - **Distribution** of drugs may be affected, often because of changes in protein binding.
  - **Metabolism** may be altered, often causing changes in drug concentration.
  - **Biotransformation** of the drug must take place, usually in the liver and gastrointestinal system, but drug interactions can impair this process.
  - **Clearance interactions** may interfere with the body's ability to eliminate a drug, usually resulting in increased concentration of the drug.

Specific Interactions

Some drugs will either increase or inhibit the actions of other drugs. They may interfere with receptor-site binding or the way in which the drug is metabolized or excreted. Certain drugs may cause drowsiness when taken together or with alcohol. Some foods will inhibit drug action, such as the inhibition of warfarin by vitamin K-containing foods. Other foods may cause toxic levels of a drug to accumulate. Grapefruit juice, for example, is metabolized by the same enzyme that metabolizes about 50 drugs, including digoxin and statins, and this can prevent the liver from breaking down drugs and lead to severe reactions. The nurse should always obtain a complete medication list from the patient, including prescription and over-the-counter medications, herbals, vitamins, minerals, and dietary supplements that are taken regularly and occasionally. All medications taken should be checked for **potential interactions with drugs or foods.**

Principles of Adult Medication Administration

Drug Classification

The following are different ways to classify drugs:

- **Therapeutic classification**: The common uses for the drug will place it in a certain therapeutic classification.
- **Pharmacological classification**: The action of the drug determines which pharmacological category a drug will be in.

All drugs have a **chemical name** and a **generic name,** which is simpler. A company making the drug can give it a **trade or brand name**. The generic form of a drug is generally cheaper but may differ in efficacy from a brand name drug due to a difference in the amount of drug that is absorbed for use in the body. The Controlled Substances Act restricts usage of certain drugs and classifies them according to schedules that include:

- **Schedule I**: Ecstasy, LSD, marijuana, peyote, Quaalude®, mescaline, psilocybin, heroin, and others
- **Schedule II**: Amphetamine, cocaine, codeine, fentanyl, Dilaudid®, Demerol®, Ritalin®, morphine, opium, and others
- **Schedule III**: Anabolic steroids, barbiturates, codeine, Vicodin®, and pentothal
- **Schedule IV**: Xanax®, Librium®, Klonopin®, Tranxene®, Redux®, Darvocet®, Valium®, Ativan®, Equagesic®, Versed®, phenobarbital, Restoril®, Sonata®, Ambien®
- **Schedule V**: Lomotil® and others

5 Rights of Medication Administration

The **5 rights of medication administration** are used to prevent/reduce medication errors in the hospital setting. Often these 5 rights are integrated into the scanning requirements of electronic documentation. The 5 rights of medication administration must also be incorporated into the prescriber's order:

- **Right Patient***:* Confirm the patient's identity using two identifiers, often being their full name and date of birth. Scanning will also confirm the patient's identity with their bar code and electronic health record.
- **Right Drug**: Check the name of the drug with the prescriber's order. By scanning the medication, the drug name will also be checked against the order.
- **Right Dose**: Check the dose of the drug with the prescriber's order. Some medications require a second nurse confirm any dosage calculations utilized before administration. Ensure the dosage is appropriate and contact the prescriber if there are any concerns.
- **Right route**: Routes include oral (PO), subcutaneous, intradermal, IV, or IM, amongst others. The route must also be confirmed with the prescriber's order.
- **Right time/frequency*:*** The drug may be administered as a one-time dose, PRN (as needed), or recurring administration (twice daily, every 8 hours, etc.).

Clinical Situations That Have Implications for Medication Administration

It is quite important to recognize clinical situations involving patients that may have **implications for the administration of medications**. For example, many patients have co-morbid conditions that will impact decisions about their medication administration. A patient with non-insulin-dependent diabetes and coronary artery disease who is being treated for a hip fracture would require oral hypoglycemic medications, cardiovascular medications, pain medication, and anti-coagulants. Another example would be an insulin-dependent diabetic patient with concomitant hypertension and renal failure. This patient would require insulin, anti-hypertensive medications, and dosing adjustments of medications secondary to renal failure. The nurse who is responsible for the patient must ensure that the correct dosages of each prescribed medication are administered on time. Potential negative side effects and drug-drug interactions should be avoided, and the patient should be monitored for adverse reactions to newly prescribed drugs.

Routes of Drug Administration

The **route of administration** is the manner by which a drug is introduced into the body. The most common routes of administration are:

- Enteral (oral, rectal, or by feeding tube)
- Topical (on the skin, in the eyes or nose, vaginal, or inhaled)
- Parenteral (IV, subcutaneous, intramuscular, intracardiac, intraosseous, intradermal, intrathecal, intraperitoneal, transdermal, transmucosal, intravitreal, and epidural)

There are many variations on these three basic routes of administration. The FDA acknowledges 111 different routes of administration. When deciding on the route of administration, the doctor and pharmacist consider:

- How fast the patient requires the drug
- How effective it will be by a given route
- The likelihood of toxicity
- The discomfort it will cause
- How likely the patient is to comply with the route
- How likely the route is to play into the patient's addictive habits

Injections

The three most common types of **injections** and the preferred injection sites are as follows:

- **Subcutaneous Injection**: Deliver the drug under the skin with a ½ inch, 24- or 25-gauge needle held at a 45° angle to reach the fat. Choose the upper arm, abdomen, thigh, or lower back as the site. The maximum amount of subcutaneous medication is 0.5 ml. An example is insulin for a patient with diabetes.
- **Intramuscular Injection**: Deliver the drug into the muscle with a 1 inch long, 20-gauge needle held at a 90° angle perpendicular to the muscle, to reach the deep tissue. For obese patients, use a 2-inch needle. Choose the vastus lateralis (thigh), ventrogluteal (hip), deltoid (upper arm), or dorsogluteal (buttocks) as the site. The maximum amount of IM medication is 5 ml. An example is Vitamin B12 for a patient with pernicious anemia.
- **Intravenous Injection**: Deliver the drug into a vein of the arm, hand, leg, foot, scalp, or neck with an Angiocath, butterfly, or Insyte Autoguard needle. Use a size from 14 gauge to 26 gauge, depending on the fluid and the patient. The nurse sets the drip rate per minute by adjusting the clamp and monitoring the drip chamber. An example of a drug requiring intravenous injection is Zoledronate, which is given yearly to prevent bone fractures for individuals with osteoporosis.

Two less frequently used forms of injection are: Intradermal (into the skin) for Mantoux TB test, and intraosseous access (IO) into the bone, which is used in emergency situations when other access sites are not available.

Herbal-Drug Contraindications

Patients on certain medications should not take some **herbals**. Some contraindications for common herbals include:

- **Echinacea**: Anti-anxiety meds, antifungals, heart medications, HIV medications, anabolic steroids, methotrexate, NSAIDs
- **Gingko Biloba**: Anticoagulants, NSAIDs, aspirin, acetaminophen
- **Garlic**: Anticoagulants, oral hypoglycemics, NSAIDs
- **Licorice**: Diuretics, digoxin, antihypertensives
- **St. John's Wort**: Antidepressants, anticoagulants, Tamoxifen, oral contraceptives, HIV medications, anesthetics. Action is similar to MAO inhibitor
- **Valerian**: Sedatives, anti-seizure meds, anesthetics, alcohol, opioids
- **Feverfew**: Anticoagulants, migraine meds, NSAIDs
- **Ginger**: Anticoagulants, NSAIDs
- **Ginseng**: Anticoagulants, antihypertensives, NSAIDs, opioids. Do not take when pregnant or lactating
- **Goldenseal**: Antihypertensives, diabetic medications, meds for kidney diseases. Do not take when pregnant or lactating
- **Kava-kava**: Alcohol, anti-seizure meds, antidepressants, sedatives, anesthetics, antipsychotics, NSAIDS, opioids
- **Saw Palmetto**: Hormone therapy
- **Hawthorn**: Digoxin

Clinical Practice

Health Promotion and Disease Prevention

Benefits of Knowing Epidemiological Practices

Epidemiology is important to nurses across all clinical settings, not just those in public health positions. Each and every nurse will treat a varied patient population during his or her career, and it is important for the nurse to create a plan of care that is tailored to the patient; the patient's age, race, career, and religion all represent different populations to which he or she belongs, and may affect clinical course, treatment, and outcome. Armed with **epidemiological knowledge** about his or her patients, the nurse can create a clinical decision-making framework, an effective care plan, and the means to share this information with his or her peers to aid in the care of other patients.

Health Promotion

Nurses **promote health** when they assist individuals to change behavior in ways that help them to attain and maintain the highest level of wellbeing possible. Health promotion is a very popular way to control healthcare costs and reduce illness and early death. Health is increasingly the topic of newscasts and literature. The public is demanding more information pertinent to the maintenance of health and to the ways in which the average person can act independently to do so. Health promotion is centered on ideal personal habits, lifestyles, and environmental control that decrease the risk for disease. The U.S. Public Health Service periodically identifies national health goals and most recently published a program called **Healthy People 2030**, with measurable goals to increase the general quality and years of life for all and to increase the health status of all groups to an equal level of wellness. Health promotion programs in the community are now offered by workplaces, clinics, schools, and churches, not just by hospitals as in the past.

Healthy People 2030

The **5 main goals of *Healthy People 2030*** are

1. Attaining healthy, thriving lives free of preventable disease, disability, injury and premature death.
2. Eliminating health disparities, achieving health equality, and increasing health literacy.
3. Creating environments conducive to health-promotion.
4. Improving health in all life stages.
5. Collaborating with leadership and key stakeholders in policy design that improves the health and well-being of all.

Healthy People 2030 has 62 topic areas with 355 total objectives divided across five sections:

- Health Conditions
- Health Behaviors
- Populations
- Settings and Systems
- Social Determinants of Health

Main Components of Health Promotion

Health promotion efforts are concentrated in four areas:

- Individuals must be educated to realize that their **lifestyle and choices** have a large impact on their health. They must then be motivated to choose to modify their personal risk factors and take the responsibility to do so.
- The emphasis on **good nutrition** as the biggest factor that impacts health and the length of life must be brought into general awareness. This is occurring via the media through numerous books and articles educating people about the essential nutrients needed to maintain health.
- **Stress** is a constant in a production-driven society. Individuals must learn ways to manage and decrease stress to achieve and maintain health and to decrease the effects of stress upon chronic illness, risk of infections, and trauma.
- **Physical fitness** helps cardiovascular status, relieves stress, controls weight, delays aging, promotes strength and endurance, and improves appearance and performance. Individuals must have programs that increase activity gradually to prevent injury and are designed to meet individual needs.

Health Self-Management

Health self-management includes health maintenance, disease prevention, and health promotion. Health maintenance is defined as strategies that help maintain and/or improve health over time. Health maintenance is dependent on three factors, which include health perception, motivation for behavioral change, and compliance to set goals. Disease prevention is an effort to limit the development or progression of lifestyle-related illness. **Disease prevention** can be categorized into primary, secondary, and tertiary prevention.

- **Primary prevention** measures are employed prior to disease onset and are used in health populations.
- **Secondary prevention** measures are used to screen, detect, and treat disease in earlier stages to prevent further progression or development of other complications.
- **Tertiary prevention** measures are used to prevent the onset of other complications or comorbid conditions.

Health promotion strategies include risk reduction strategies applied to the general population.

Influences on Decision to Modify Behavior to Achieve and Maintain Health

Many factors have an **influence on people's efforts to change behavior** in a way that improves and maintains their health status. These factors include age, ethnicity, gender, lifestyle, level of education, self-esteem, motivation, and self-image. The patient's support network and the availability of health promotion programs and healthcare systems also have an influence on healthcare behaviors. Some people may be prevented from accessing health promotion programs because of lack of medical insurance. Financial status and employment are important as well. The presence of addictions and diseases, the length of illness, and the severity of disabilities are all factors to be considered. The value placed on health, the threat of potential losses, and the perceived benefits of behavior modification are important motivating factors.

Strategies to Encourage Smoking Cessation

The **health impact associated with smoking** varies among smokers and can be affected by the number of cigarettes used daily, exposure to smoking-associated stimuli, and educational level. The presence of stress and depression, psychosocial problems, lack of coping mechanisms, low income, and long-term habitual behavior are problematic for the quitter. Nurses can promote smoking cessation by taking every opportunity to bring up the subject, educating about the dangers of smoking and benefits of quitting, and providing **resources** to help patients quit. Strategies include:

- Educating about the personal effects of smoking upon that individual
- Encouraging patients to set a quit date
- Referring to programs and smoking cessation information
- Educating about the use of nicotine replacements including nicotine gum, lozenges, inhalers, transdermal patches, and nasal sprays
- Educating about the use of medications such as Zyban®, Catapres®, and Chantix®
- Providing support via phone calls or office visits
- Discovering the reason for relapses
- Praising and rewarding any success in the quitting process

Healthy Nutrition Principles

Healthy nutrition principles include the following:

- Eating a range of different kinds of foods, and eating increased amounts fruits, vegetables, whole grains, poultry and fish.
- Diets should consist of 55-60% **carbohydrates**, less than 30% **fat**, and the rest should be **protein** (0.8-1.0 g/kg).
- Restrict **saturated fat** to <10%. Restrict **cholesterol** to 300 mg/day.
- Utilize moderate amounts of sugar, salt, and sodium.
- Take a **multivitamin** including folic acid if the patient is female and able to have children. Get 200-800 IU/day of vitamin D in order to absorb calcium.
- **Calcium** intake should be: 1300 mg/day for women age 13-18 or those who are pregnant/nursing; 1000 mg/day for women age 19-50 years; 1500 mg/day for age 51 years and older.
- Patients who are pregnant or having chemotherapy should not try to lose weight.
- **Weight loss** may improve diabetes, joint pain, inflammation, cardiovascular disease, hypothyroidism, or renal disease.

Disease Prevention for the Elderly

Although life spans are longer, **ongoing (chronic) diseases** are still the primary reason patients die. Elderly patients have more of an absolute chance of getting a disease, but they also react well to prevention. Keep good records of the elderly patient's history, including updating every year and following advice for patients over the age of 65 years. Evaluate nutrition, functional ability, alcoholic beverage intake (more than 2 alcoholic beverages a day constitutes abuse), smoking, illegal drugs, misuse of prescriptions, and exercise level.

- **Preventative measures** include a physical, screening assessments, and immunizations.
- Some **routine screenings** include: fasting glucose, papanicolaou smear, dipstick urinalysis, mammography, PPD, fecal occult blood/sigmoidoscopy, electrocardiogram, thyroid function, glaucoma and sight, hearing, and cholesterol.
- **Immunizations** include yearly flu shot, pneumococcal vaccine, and tetanus.

The following screens are controversial: depression for someone with no symptoms, dementia for someone with no symptoms, osteoporosis including bone densitometry for postmenopausal females (counsel females regarding hormone prophylaxis), colon and prostate cancer, and cholesterol for someone with no symptoms.

Health Screening

Young Adult Screenings

Health screening is encouraged for conditions that are very **likely to occur** and diseases that are **likely to kill** if they are not identified. The assessment should be trustworthy using proper techniques and proper follow-up.

Young adult (ages 20-39 years) screenings, according to the U.S. Preventive Services Task Force (USPSTF), should include:

- A full head-to-toe physical (every 5-6 years)
- Blood pressure screening (every 3-5 years if range is within normal: <130/85 mmHg)
- Cholesterol screening (every 5 years; more frequently when total cholesterol is higher than 200 mg/dL)
- PPD test for tuberculosis when patient has had known contact with TB or is at increased risk (health care workers, prisoners, homeless, or immunocompromised)
- Dental check-up (annually)
- Thyroid palpation (every 3 years)
- Depression screening (at every visit)
- Men perform self-testicular exam every month
- Women conduct a self-breast exam every month; should receive a clinical breast exam every 3 years
- Pap smear and pelvic assessments every 3-years (or up to 5 years in conjunction with HPV testing)
- Screening for gonorrhea and chlamydia for all sexually active individuals
- Health education and promotion (every time patient is seen)
- Influenza vaccination (annually)
- Td immunization every 10 years

Adult Screenings

Adults (age 40 and older) screenings, according to the USPSTF, should maintain the same schedule as young adults (unless indicated below) in addition to the following:

- A full head-to-toe physical (annually)
- Blood pressure screening (annually)
- ECG (over 40, annually; only when there are cardiac risks)
- Clinical breast exam (annually in women over 40)
- Mammogram (biennially in women over 50)
- General colorectal cancer screening for risks (annually), and colorectal cancer screening via colonoscopy (every 10 years for those over 50 until age 75)
- Prostate-specific antigen screening (men over 50 with average risk, or younger if higher risk; upon the patient's informed request only)

Diagnostic Testing and Procedures

Sources and Procedures for Obtaining Diagnostic Studies and Test Results

The advent of the electronic health record has somewhat simplified the **procedures for obtaining diagnostic studies and test results.**

- **Laboratory systems** are typically stand-alone systems that must be interfaced with the electronic health record. The laboratory component of the electronic health record often is utilized as a means to coordinate laboratory orders, laboratory results, and administrative details.
- **Radiology information systems** are typically utilized to enable unification of patient data such as orders, results, and actual images. Radiology information can be accessed using a picture archive and communication system (PACS). PACS can be used to obtain diagnostic medical scans from a variety of imaging devices.

Analyzing Normal and Abnormal Test Results and Diagnostic Studies

Knowledge of **normal and abnormal values for test results** and for diagnostic studies is a vital component of the nursing assessment. Nurses should have a basic knowledge of the purpose and procedures for typical laboratory tests, such as a blood test for complete blood count (CBC), and diagnostic practices, such as X-rays for bone fractures, as well as the specialized tests and studies relevant to their field of expertise. In addition, they should understand accepted standards or **norms**, and how normal values are defined by the facility where they are employed. These norms offer general guidelines for assessing any individual test results or diagnostic studies. Interpreting abnormal test results requires knowing what potential problems may be responsible and what mitigating factors in the patient's history, such as current medications or timing of the last meal, might be influencing these results. Often nurses are the first to review/receive critically abnormal lab results and must be sure to notify the physician immediately in case emergency interventions (such as electrolyte replacement or blood transfusions) must be ordered.

Medical Reasoning, Diagnostic Reasoning, Therapeutic Reasoning, and Therapeutic Uncertainty

Medical reasoning refers to the process by which clinicians gather data and information about a patient, and then use those data to arrive at a diagnosis and treatment plan. Diagnostic reasoning and therapeutic reasoning are subsets of medical reasoning. **Diagnostic reasoning** is the process that is used to determine the most likely diagnosis, while **therapeutic reasoning** is the process used to determine what the best treatment is for that particular patient suffering from that particular disease. While the patient is undergoing treatment, it is necessary for the clinician to evaluate the patient's response to treatment on a regular basis. If it is not clear whether the patient is improving, or whether another treatment might be more beneficial, a degree of **therapeutic uncertainty** is introduced. There is also therapeutic uncertainty when the clinician is trying to decide which treatment option to use if the first treatment fails.

Importance of Data Gathering to Diagnostic Reasoning

The **gathering and recording of data** are of utmost importance to the diagnostic evaluation process. The history and physical section of the patient chart contains a wealth of information (ideally) and should always be taken into consideration when developing a care plan for the patient. Because any number of clinicians can add information to the patient chart (and because all of these clinicians will be reading this information), it is important to record all information clearly and in an organized manner. This can be a daunting task when considering all of the different sources of information, including the patient interview, family member interviews, previous charts, and lab results. By keeping this information clear and concise, errors are minimized, and the differential diagnosis is comprehensive.

Sensitivity and Specificity in Relation to Diagnostic Testing

Some degree of error is inherent in almost all diagnostic testing. When ordering a diagnostic test for a patient, how confident can one be that the result will be accurate? The terms **sensitivity and specificity** are used to illustrate the accuracy of diagnostic tests. The sensitivity of a test refers to its ability to correctly identify patients who do have the disease. If a test is administered to 100 patients with diabetes, and all 100 patients test positive, the test is considered to have a sensitivity of 100%. If only 85 of those tested have a positive result, however, that means that the test has a false-negative rate of 15%, and a sensitivity of 85%. On the other hand, the specificity of a diagnostic test refers to its ability to identify patients who do not have the disease. If 100 nondiabetic patients are tested for diabetes, and 50 of them have a positive result, the test has a specificity of only 50%.

Differential Diagnosis Process

The **differential diagnosis** is an important tool that allows the clinician to familiarize him or herself with the patient's condition, understand the condition, create an effective treatment plan, and follow the progress of the patient. To start, thoroughly examine the patient's chart, making a list of all of the abnormal test results and laboratory values. Add to this list all of the patient's complaints. Once this list is complete, organize the test results, labs, and complaints by anatomic location or organ system. After breaking the list down by organ site, look for any relationships between symptoms and/or results. Create another list of those data that seem to be related, and list all of the diseases or conditions that explain the findings, eliminating any that do not fit.

Analytical Decision-Making

An **analytical decision** is one that is made after a systematic review and analysis of all factors involved in the decision. Concentration and awareness are important in the analytical decision-making process. In contrast with an intuitive decision, an analytical decision takes longer to make, because it is not automatic. The analysis involves an in-depth look at all factors and is based on scientific evidence (i.e., based on the outcomes of previous similar situations). Because an analytical decision is based on scientific evidence and facts, the outcome of the decision has a high predictive value; this means that by looking at previous outcomes, it is possible to predict the current outcome. Because the clinician has so carefully reviewed all factors, he or she will most likely not experience the emotional anxiety associated with an intuitive decision.

Intuitive Decision-Making

When a clinician makes an **intuitive decision**, he or she is making a decision not necessarily based on fact, but more so because it feels like the right decision. Of course, in most cases, one would not want a doctor making decisions this way, although in certain cases (say, a choice between 2 different types of treatment, each of which has the same general risks, or when all other options have been exhausted), it may be necessary. Although these decisions are not based on an analysis of the facts, there is something to be said about the so-called "gut instinct," which years of training and experience can hone. These decisions are made without spending a lot of time on the process of decision-making; though they are based on experience, the clinician may suffer some degree of anxiety about the decision and its outcome.

Influential Factors in Clinical Decision-Making Process

Although one would like to think that there isn't much variation in the clinical decision-making process, this simply is not true. The process, of course, will differ depending on the patient, the differential diagnosis, and the clinician. The first variable to consider is the clinician. The way that the clinician conducts the clinical decision-making process is influenced by the knowledge base of the clinician, as well as the level of his experience, the ability he possesses to think both critically and creatively, and the confidence that he has in his ability to make educated decisions. The acuity level of the patient is also a factor in the clinical decision-making process, as is the length of the differential. A time stressor is placed on the clinician when the condition of the patient is critical, and when there are more diseases that must be eliminated from the differential. An element of stress may also exist if the clinician has a high number of patients, especially if he has multiple high-acuity patients.

Questions to Consider When Dealing with Diagnostic and Therapeutic Uncertainty

Diagnosis and subsequent treatment are not easily arrived at for every patient because every patient is different. The clinical presentation of a heart attack, for example, may include severe chest pain, sweating, and nausea for one patient, and may have very mild, almost unnoticeable symptoms in another. **Diagnostic uncertainty** is especially prominent when dealing with diseases that have nonspecific symptoms; in these cases, it is important that the clinician recognize which of the possible diagnoses are life-threatening, and which are not. Ruling out the life-threatening possibilities should be higher on the clinician's list of priorities than the nonlife-threatening ones. Diagnostic testing, and subsequent treatment options, should also be evaluated according to the risks and benefits to the patient.

Degree of Clinical Uncertainty

Although the **degree of uncertainty** is somewhat dependent on the patient, the clinical setting can have an influence on the degree of uncertainty that the clinician is likely to encounter. For example, a clinic, such as a dermatology clinic, is a setting in which the degree of uncertainty is likely to be low; this is because the clinic is nonemergent, and because the clinic treats a specific, limited group of diseases with which the clinicians are very familiar. An urgent care clinic would fall somewhere in the middle because, although there is a wider range of diagnostic possibility, life-threatening emergencies are rarely encountered. An emergency room or a trauma center, on the other hand, sees a high degree of uncertainty because the clinicians see a wide range of diagnostic possibilities, and are expected to work at a fast pace.

Cardiovascular Diagnostics

Cardiac Enzymes

CK and CK-MB

Creatine kinase (CK) and CK-MB levels are evaluated every 6–8 hours in a suspected myocardial injury. Total CK and CK-MB (specific to cardiac cells) initially rise within the first 4–6 hours of an MI. A normal range would be 30 IU/L to 180 IU/L for CK and CK-MB totaling 0–5% of the CK level.

Assuming no further damage is sustained, peak levels (in excess of 6 times the normal range) are reached 12–24 hours after the injury. CK levels will return to normal within 3–4 days of the event. Small spikes in CK level might also occur following invasive cardiac procedures.

Troponin I and T

Troponin, which is found in cardiac and skeletal muscle, is a type of protein. Both troponin I and T (isolates of troponin) are found in the myocardium, but troponin T is also found in skeletal muscle, so it is less specific than troponin I. Troponin I, therefore, may be used to detect a myocardial infarction after non-cardiac surgery and to detect acute coronary syndrome. Troponin is released into the bloodstream when injury to the tissue (such as the myocardium) occurs and causes damage to the cell membranes, as occurs with myocardial injury.

- **Troponin I** (<0.05 ng/mL): Appears in 2-6 hours, peaks at 15-20 hours and returns to normal in 5-7 days. Exhibits a second but lower peak at 60-80 hours (biphasic).
- **Troponin T** (<0.2 ng/mL): Increases 2-6 hours after MI and stays elevated. Returns to normal in 7 days. (Less specific than troponin I)

Echocardiography

Echocardiography is a non-invasive ultrasound technology that is very useful for assessing and diagnosing anatomic heart abnormalities, blood flow, and valvular lesions:

- The **standard "2D Echo"** is used best for basic structural imaging, such as valvular lesions and assessment of pericardial disorders.
- The **transesophageal (TEE)** probe is an improved version of echocardiography, which allows better visualization of the left atrium and more precise evaluation of the valvular structure. TEE is also the best modality for evaluation of the thoracic aorta in the setting of suspected aortic dissection or aneurysm.
- **Doppler imaging** is used to measure blood flow, often in the context of velocity across a valve and a pressure gradient.
- **Bubble study** is an addition to echocardiography allowing the study to determine if there is right to left blood flow through a patent foramen ovale or a more distal intrapulmonary shunt of blood.

Stress Echocardiography

Basic **cardiac stress testing** consists of exercise EKG testing (EET) and exercise imaging testing. The exercise imaging testing may be broken down into exercise, or "stress" echocardiography, and exercise myocardial perfusion imaging.

Exercise imaging testing is usually performed with echocardiography. Stress echocardiography is performed similarly to exercise EKG testing and also requires that the patient meet at least 85% maximum heart rate in order to attain optimum sensitivity and specificity. (The maximum heart rate formula is 220 minus the person's age.) Of note, chemicals may substitute for exercise during the "stress" portion of the test. This may be performed with dobutamine (beta-1-agonist: cannot be used after beta-blocker administration) or adenosine (causes diffuse coronary dilatation, leading to decreased perfusion pressure and unmasking of defects, and cannot be used with asthma). Stress imaging allows the study to determine the actual area of ischemia and whether or not this is a reversible defect. Additional information obtained during echocardiography is cardiac output and measurement of viability.

Myocardial Perfusion Imaging Techniques

Stress perfusion studies are often interchanged with stress echocardiography, as they are both good at determining areas of ischemia and reversible wall motion defects. Myocardial perfusion imaging is often performed with the administration of adenosine to induce diffuse coronary dilatation, which unmasks perfusion defects. This test is performed using either thallium 201 or technetium 99. The use of these tracers allows for more exact determination of cardiac blood flow. Basically, the ischemic areas take up fewer tracers during peak "stress" than do normal areas. If these changes persist during rest, then this area is deemed infracted. Images may be repeated in 24 hours to determine if there is an increased area of viability.

Cardiovascular Procedures and Interventions

CARDIOVERSION

Cardioversion sends a timed electrical stimulation to the heart to convert a tachydysrhythmia (such as atrial fibrillation) to a normal sinus rhythm. Usually, anticoagulation therapy is done for at least 3 weeks prior to elective cardioversion to reduce the risk of emboli, and digoxin is discontinued for at least 48 hours prior. During the procedure, the patient is usually sedated and/or anesthetized. Electrodes in the form of gel-covered paddles or pads are placed in the anteroposterior position and then connected by leads to a computerized ECG and cardiac monitor with a defibrillator. The defibrillator is synchronized with the ECG so that the electrical current is delivered during ventricular depolarization (QRS). The timing must be precise in order to prevent ventricular tachycardia or ventricular fibrillation. Sometimes, drug therapy is used in conjunction with cardioversion; for example, antiarrhythmics (Cardizem®, Cordarone®) may be given before the procedure to slow the heart rate.

(**Arrhythmia**: Beginning Monophasic Shock, Beginning Biphasic Shock)

- **Atrial Fibrillation:** 50-100 J, 25 J.
- **Atrial Flutter**: 25-50 J, 15 J.
- **Ventricular Tachycardia** (monomorphic asymptomatic): 100-200 J, 50 J.

EMERGENCY DEFIBRILLATION

Emergency defibrillation delivers a non-synchronized shock that is given to treat acute ventricular fibrillation, pulseless ventricular tachycardia, or polymorphic ventricular tachycardia with a rapid rate and decompensating hemodynamics. Defibrillation can be given at any point in the cardiac cycle. It causes depolarization of myocardial cells, which can then repolarize to regain a normal sinus rhythm. Defibrillation delivers an electrical discharge through pads/paddles. In an acute care setting, the preferred position to place the pads is the anteroposterior position. In this position, one pad is placed to the right of the sternum about the second to third intercostal space, and the other pad is placed between the left scapula and the spinal column. This decreases the chances of damaging implanted devices, such as pacemakers, and this positioning has also been shown to be more effective for external cardioversion (if indicated at some point during resuscitation). There are two main types of defibrillator shock waveforms: monophasic and biphasic. Biphasic defibrillators deliver a shock in one direction for half of the shock, and then in the return direction for the other half, making them more effective and able to be used at lower energy levels. Monophasic defibrillation is given at 200-360 J and biphasic defibrillation is given at 100-200 J.

PERICARDIOCENTESIS

Pericardiocentesis is done with ultrasound guidance to diagnose pericardial effusion or with ECG and ultrasound guidance to relieve cardiac tamponade. Pericardiocentesis may be done as treatment for cardiac arrest or with presentation of PEA with increased jugular venous pressure. Non-hemorrhagic tamponade may be relieved in 60-90% of cases, but hemorrhagic tamponade requires thoracotomy, as blood will continue to accumulate until the cause of the hemorrhage is corrected. Resuscitation equipment must be available, including a defibrillator, intravenous line in place, and cardiac monitoring:

The **procedure** is as follows:

- Elevate the chest 45° to bring the heart closer to the chest wall, pre-medicate with atropine, and insert a nasogastric tube if indicated.
- Cleanse the skin with chlorhexidine or another appropriate cleanser.
- After insertion of the needle using ultrasound guidance, remove the obturator and attach a syringe for aspiration.
- The needle can often be replaced with a catheter after removal for drainage.
- A post-procedure chest x-ray should be done to check for pneumothorax.

Possible Complications: Pneumo/hemothorax, coronary artery rupture, hepatic injury, dysrhythmias, and false negative/positive aspiration.

PACEMAKERS

Pacemakers are used to stimulate the heart when the normal conduction system of the heart is defective. Pacemakers may be used temporarily or be permanently implanted. Temporary pacemakers for external cardiac pacing are commonly used in the emergency setting. Temporary pacemakers may be used prophylactically or therapeutically to treat a cardiac abnormality. Clinical uses include:

- To treat persistent **dysrhythmias** not responsive to medications
- To increase **cardiac output** with bradydysrhythmia by increasing rate
- To decrease **ventricular or supraventricular tachycardia** by "overdrive" stimulation of contractions
- To treat **secondary heart block** caused by myocardial infarction, ischemia, and drug toxicity
- To improve **cardiac output** after cardiac surgery
- To provide **diagnostic information** through electrophysiology studies, which induce dysrhythmias for purposes of evaluation
- To provide **pacing** when a permanent pacemaker malfunctions

Review Video: Pacemaker Care
Visit mometrix.com/academy and enter code: 979075

TRANSCUTANEOUS PACING

Transcutaneous pacing is used temporarily in an emergency situation to treat symptomatic bradydysrhythmias that don't respond to medications (atropine) and result in hemodynamic instability. Generally, the patient is provided oxygen and some sort of mild sedation before the pacing. The placement of pacing pads is usually one pacing pad (negative) on the left chest, inferior to the clavicle, and the other (positive) on the left back, inferior to the scapula, so the heart is sandwiched between the two. Lead wires attach the pads to the monitor. The rate of pacing is usually set around 80 bpm. The current is increased slowly until capture occurs—a spiking followed by QRS sequence—then the current is readjusted downward if possible just to maintain capture, keeping it 5-10 mA above the pacing threshold. Both demand and fixed modes are available, but demand mode is preferred. The patient should be warned that the shocks may induce pain.

Epicardial Pacing

Epicardial pacing wires may be attached directly to the exterior atria, ventricles, or both at the conclusion of surgery for CPB or valve repair in the event that postoperative pacing support is required or for those with risk of AV block because of medications used to control atrial fibrillation. Cold cardioplegia may precipitate the transient sinus node or AV node dysfunction. While some surgeons avoid placing epicardial pacing wires because of concerns about bleeding and cardiac tamponade on removal, recommendations include placing at least one ventricular pacing wire. A typical configuration for pacing wires is atrial pacing wires placed in a plastic disk that is sutured low on the right atrium. The two ventricular wires are attached over the right ventricular wall. Atrial pacing wires may be used to record atrial activity and, and with standard ECG, can help to distinguish atrial and junctional arrhythmias and ventricular arrhythmias. Pacing wires can also be used therapeutically to increase the heart rate to about 90 bpm in order to achieve optimal hemodynamics. The epicardial leads are intended for use of 7 days or less and may be less reliable if used for extended periods. The wires are removed by applying gentle traction.

Temporary Transvenous Pacemakers

Transvenous pacemakers, comprised of a catheter with a lead at the end, may be used prophylactically or therapeutically on a temporary basis to treat symptomatic bradycardias or heart blocks when other methods have failed. The catheter has a balloon tip that must be checked for leaks prior to insertion – this is usually done by inflating the catheter tip while submersed in normal saline and checking for bubbles. After the balloon's integrity is verified, the catheter is inserted through the femoral or jugular vein and the balloon is inflated. The catheter is then attached to an external pulse generator, and the settings are adjusted to achieve capture. The balloon is then deflated, and placement can be verified via ultrasound or chest x-ray.

Complications are similar to those of PCI and permanent pacemaker insertion, including infection, hemorrhage, catheter migration, perforation, embolism, thrombosis, and pacemaker syndrome.

Transvenous Pacer Settings

Temporary **transvenous pacing** utilizes bipolar leads with two tails, positive/proximal and negative/distal, and these must be connected properly to the pulse generator, with the distal end of the pacing lead to the negative terminal and the proximal end to the positive terminal. Once the transvenous pacing wire is inserted and the leads are connected to the pulse generator, it must be set to the patient's needs:

- **Rate**: The beats per minute are usually set between 70 and 80 (allowable range is generally 50-90), but this may vary according to individual needs.
- **Sensitivity**: The myocardial voltage needed for the pacing electrode to detect P or R waves. The sensitivity is usually set at 2 mV and then adjusted as needed to ensure capture. Most pacemakers can sense 0.3-10 mV from the atria and 0.8 to 29 mV from the ventricles, but setting it relatively low prevents oversensing.
- **Output**: The current or pulse produced by the pulse generator is usually set at 5 mA. The current is delivered rapidly, in about 0.6 ms.

Problems Related to Transvenous Pacing

With **transvenous pacing** (usually per a pulse generator connected to a pacing cable and a pacing wire, which is inserted into the right internal jugular to the right ventricle for ventricular pacing and right atrium for atrial pacing), sensing refers to the ability to detect electrical activity of the heart. Capture occurs when an artificial stimulus (the pulse generator) depolarizes the heart, indicated by a pacer spike followed by the QRS complex. **Problems** include:

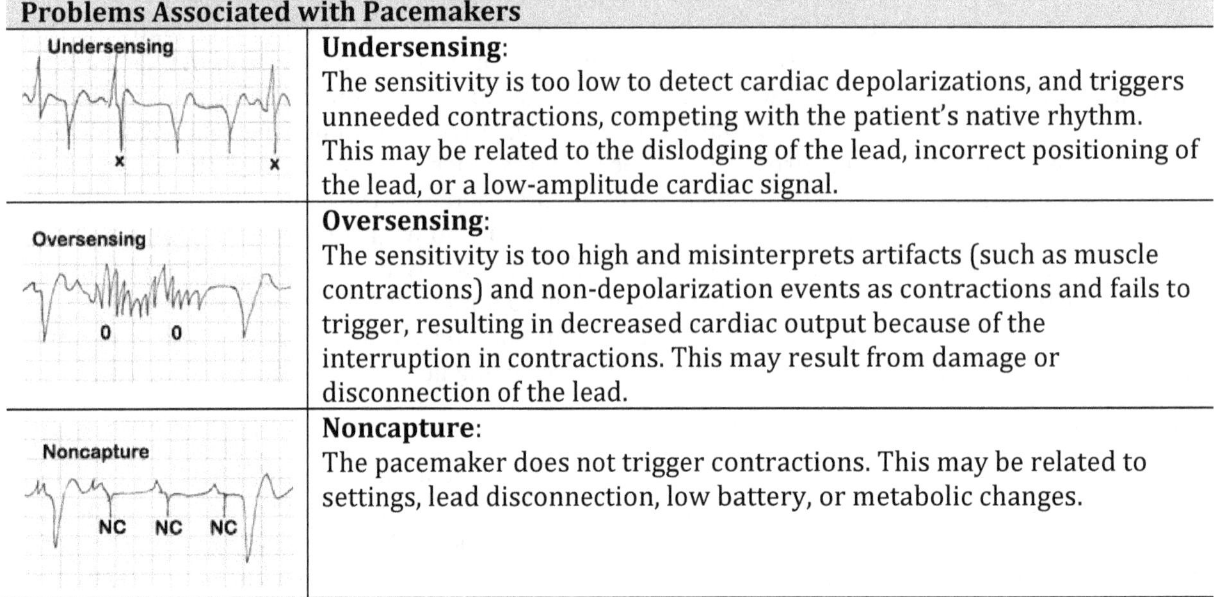

Problems Associated with Pacemakers	
Undersensing x x	**Undersensing**: The sensitivity is too low to detect cardiac depolarizations, and triggers unneeded contractions, competing with the patient's native rhythm. This may be related to the dislodging of the lead, incorrect positioning of the lead, or a low-amplitude cardiac signal.
Oversensing 0 0	**Oversensing**: The sensitivity is too high and misinterprets artifacts (such as muscle contractions) and non-depolarization events as contractions and fails to trigger, resulting in decreased cardiac output because of the interruption in contractions. This may result from damage or disconnection of the lead.
Noncapture NC NC NC	**Noncapture**: The pacemaker does not trigger contractions. This may be related to settings, lead disconnection, low battery, or metabolic changes.

Pacemaker Complications

Pacemakers, transvenous and permanent, are invasive foreign bodies and, as such, can cause a number of different **complications**:

- Infection, bleeding, or hematoma may occur at the entry site of leads for temporary pacemakers or at the subcutaneous area of implantation for permanent generators.
- Puncture of the subclavian vein or internal mammary artery may cause a hemothorax.
- The endocardial electrode may irritate the ventricular wall, causing ectopic beats or tachycardia.
- Dislodgement of the transvenous lead may lead to malfunction or perforation of the myocardium. This is one of the most common early complications.
- Dislocation of leads may result in phrenic nerve or muscle stimulation (which may be evidenced by hiccupping).
- Cardiac tamponade may result when the epicardial wires of temporary pacing are removed.
- General malfunctioning of the pacemaker may indicate dislodgement, dislocation, interference caused by electromagnetic fields, and the need for new batteries or a new generator.
- Pacemaker syndrome.

Pacemaker Syndrome

Pacemaker syndrome can occur with any type of pacemaker if there is inadequate synchronicity between the contractions of the atria and ventricles, resulting in a decrease in cardiac output and inadequate atrial contribution to the filling of the ventricles. Total peripheral vascular resistance may increase to maintain blood pressure, but hypotension occurs after decompensation.

- **Mild:**
    - Pulsations evident in the neck and abdomen
    - Cardiac palpitations
    - Headache and feeling of anxiety
    - General malaise and unexplained weakness
    - Pain or feeling of fullness in jaw and/or chest
- **Moderate:**
    - Increasing dyspnea on exertion with accompanying orthopnea
    - Dizziness, vertigo, and increasing confusion
    - Feeling of choking
- **Severe:**
    - Increasing pulmonary edema with dyspnea even at rest
    - Crackling rales
    - Syncope
    - Heart failure

Automatic ICD

The **automatic implantable cardioverter-defibrillator (AICD)** is similar to the pacemaker and is implanted in the same way, with one or more leads to the ventricular myocardium or the epicardium, but it is used to control tachycardia and/or fibrillation. Most AICDs consist of a pacing/sensing electrode, a pulse generator, and defibrillation electrodes. Severe tachycardia may be related to electrical disturbances, cardiomyopathy, or postoperative response to the repair of congenital disease. In some cases, it is not responsive to medications. When the pulse reaches a certain preset rate, then the device automatically provides a small electrical impulse to the atrial or ventricular myocardium to slow the heart. If fibrillation occurs, a higher energy shock is delivered. It takes 5 to 15 seconds for the device to detect abnormalities in the pulse rate, and more than one shock may be required so fainting can occur. Contemporary devices can function as both a pacemaker and an ICD, which is especially important for those who have episodes of both bradycardia and tachycardia. The use of adjunctive antiarrhythmics or ablation is important to prevent AICD shocks.

Closure Devices with PCI

Percutaneous catheter intervention (PCI) is often the treatment choice for patients with symptomatic coronary artery disease. Percutaneous transluminal coronary angioplasty (PTCA), arthrectomy, and stent insertion are common types of percutaneous catheter intervention procedures. While historically, manual compression has been utilized to achieve hemostasis after PCI, different types of devices exist to assist in achieving hemostasis post-procedure. Passive devices such as hemostasis pads and compression devices help to enhance hemostasis. Active devices are used at the femoral access site after the sheath used for the procedure is removed. There are different types of active devices, including percutaneous suture mediated devices, that use needles and sutures to suture the artery closed after the procedure. Collagen plugs are another type of closure, where collagen is injected into the supra-arterial space until hemostasis is achieved. These devices may be used independently or in combination. Clip devices such as implantable clips can be used to pull the edges of the arteriotomy together for closure. Active devices shorten the time to achieve hemostasis as well as the time the patient must remain hospitalized post-procedure.

Complications: Persistent coronary artery spasms, dissection of the coronary artery, thrombosis, bleeding, and hematoma formation. Other complications may arise depending on the type of closure device utilized. For example, the use of clip devices may result in arterial laceration, occlusion of the artery, or arterial stenosis.

PTCA and Stent Insertion

Percutaneous transluminal coronary angioplasty (PTCA) is a procedure done to reperfuse coronary arteries blocked by plaque or an embolus. Cardiac catheterization is done with a hollow catheter (sheath), usually inserted into the femoral vein or artery and fed through the vessels to the coronary arteries. When the atheroma is verified by fluoroscopy, a balloon-tipped catheter is fed over the sheath and the balloon is inflated with a contrast agent to a specified pressure to compress the atheroma. The balloon may be inflated a number of times to ensure that residual stenosis is <20%. Laser angioplasty using the excimer laser is also used to vaporize plaque. **Stents** may be inserted during the angioplasty to maintain patency. Stents may be flexible plastic or wire mesh and are typically placed over the catheter, which is inflated to expand the stent against the arterial wall. All patients with a stent must be discharged on aspirin, an antiplatelet, and a statin.

Complications include:

- **Intraoperative**: Perforation/dissection of the coronary artery, arrythmias, and vasospasm.
- **Postoperative**: Hemorrhage/hematoma at insertion site, thrombus/embolus, arteriovenous fistula/pseudoaneurysm, retroperitoneal bleed, and failure of angioplasty.

Intra-aortic Balloon Pump

The intra-aortic balloon pump (IABP) is a catheter with an inflatable balloon at the tip, which is inserted through the femoral artery and threaded into the descending thoracic aorta. The balloon inflates during diastole to increase circulation to the coronary arteries and then deflates during systole to decrease afterload. It is indicated in patients experiencing cardiogenic/septic shock, acute heart failure, unstable angina, and papillary or ventricular septal rupture.

Contraindications: Aortic valve stenosis and large aortic aneurysms.

Complications: Stroke, peripheral ischemia, renal injury, air embolus, and arrhythmias.

Nursing considerations are as follows:

- **Placement:**
  - Too high: occludes the left subclavian artery, which results in dizziness and decreased radial pulse.
  - Too low: occludes the renal artery, which results in flank pain and a sudden decrease in urine output.
  - Preventing displacement: the patient cannot bend his or her knees, sit up, or flex the hips more than 45°. Patient should remain in a supine position.
- **Timing**: In ECG mode, the balloon should inflate in the T-wave and deflate with the R. Do site checks, I&O, neuro-checks, and vascular checks every hour.
- If a **gas-leak alarm sounds** OR **blood is visible in the catheter**, this indicates balloon rupture/damage to the catheter. Immediately shut down the machine, place the patient in the Trendelenburg position, and notify the physician.

- **Weaning**: Decrease balloon volume/frequency to wean. Use the flutter function to prevent embolus while the catheter is still in place. After removal, the physician will allow bleeding for five seconds to eject clots.

Carotid Endarterectomy

A **carotid endarterectomy** involves clamping the carotids, opening the occluded artery, and removing the plaque that is occluding the artery. A shunt may be inserted during the procedure to ensure blood supply to the brain. Postoperative complications may include:

- **Hematoma:** May obstruct respiration; watch closely for increased respiratory effort and swelling near the airway.
- **Hypertension:** Especially in the first 48 postoperative hours, may increase risk of neurologic impairment and hematoma.
- **Hypotension:** Usually resolves in 24-48 hours, but may indicate myocardial infarction.
- **Hyperperfusion syndrome:** Caused by inadequate vasoconstriction of vessels dilated from long-term diminished blood flow. It can cause hemorrhage and edema, usually identified by severe unilateral headache relieved by raising the head.
- **Hemorrhage:** May be fatal or cause severe impairment.
- **Stroke:** Risk of plaque dislodging and forming an embolus; frequent neurological checks are crucial.

CABG

Coronary artery bypass graft (CABG) is a surgical procedure for the treatment of angina that does not respond to medical treatment, unstable angina, blockage of >60% in the left main coronary artery, blockage of multiple coronary arteries that include the proximal left anterior descending artery, left ventricular dysfunction, and previous unsuccessful PCIs. The surgery is performed through a midsternal incision that exposes the heart, which is chilled and placed on cardiopulmonary bypass with blood going from the right atrium to the machine and back to the body while the aorta is clamped to keep the surgical field free of blood. Bypass grafts are sutured into place to bypass areas of occluded coronary arteries. Grafts may be obtained from various sites: gastroepiploic artery, internal mammary artery, radial artery, or saphenous vein (commonly used, especially for emergency procedures).

Complications: Arrhythmias, infection, cardiac tamponade, cardiogenic shock, embolus/stroke, and renal or pulmonary dysfunction

MIDCAB and Port Access Coronary Artery Bypass Graft

Minimally-invasive direct coronary artery bypass (MIDCAB) applies a bypass graft through a 10 cm incision in the mid-chest without using cardiopulmonary bypass. Because the incision must be over the bypass area, this procedure is suitable only for bypass of one or two coronary arteries, usually on the left side of the heart. A small portion of rib is removed to allow access to the heart, and the internal mammary artery is used for grafting. Special instruments, such as a heart stabilizer, are used to limit movement of the heart during suturing. Surgery usually takes 2-3 hours and recovery time is decreased as patients have less pain. Because anastomosis is difficult on a beating heart, complications such as ischemia may occur during surgery, so a cardiopulmonary bypass machine must be available.

Port access coronary artery bypass graft is an alternative form of CABG that utilizes a number of small incisions (ports) along with cardiopulmonary bypass (CPB) and cardioplegia to do a video-assisted surgical repair. Usually, 3 or more incisions are required, with one in the femoral area to allow access to the femoral artery for a multipurpose catheter that is threaded through to the ascending aorta to return blood from the CPB, block the aorta with a balloon, provide a cardioplegic solution, and vent air. Another catheter is threaded through the femoral vein to the right atrium to carry blood to the CPB. An incision is also needed for access to the jugular vein for catheters to the pulmonary artery and the coronary sinus. One to three thoracotomy incisions are made for the insertion of video imaging equipment and instruments. While the midsternal incision is avoided, multiple incisions pose the potential for possible increased morbidity.

Cardiac Surgical Options for Repair of Cardiac Valves

There are a number of different surgical options for the **repair of cardiac valves**:

- **Valvotomy/Valvuloplasty** is usually done through cardiac catheterization. A valvotomy/valvuloplasty involves releasing valve leaflet adhesions or opening a stenosed valve. In balloon valvuloplasty, a catheter with an inflatable balloon is positioned in the stenotic valve and inflated and deflated a number of times to dilate the opening. Risks include stroke from a broken-off calcified valve and worsened valvular insufficiency/rupture.
- **Aortic valve replacement** is an open-heart procedure with cardiopulmonary bypass. Aortic valves are tricuspid (3 leaflets) and repair is usually not possible, so defective valves must be replaced with either mechanical (metal, plastic, or pyrolytic carbon) or biological (porcine or bovine) grafts.
- **Aortic homograft** uses part of a donor's aorta with the aortic valve attached to replace the recipient's faulty aortic valve and part of the ascending aorta.
- **Ross procedure** uses the patient's pulmonary artery with the pulmonary valve to replace the aortic valve and part of the aorta and then uses a donor graft to replace the pulmonary artery.

TAVR

Transcatheter aortic valve replacement (TAVR) is usually reserved for patients with advanced symptomatic stenosis of the aortic valve who are unable to tolerate open-heart surgery or are at high risk with the procedure. Symptoms of aortic stenosis include chest pain, peripheral edema, dyspnea, fainting, weakness, and heart failure. With a TAVR, patients generally receive a general anesthesia, and a catheter is inserted, usually transfemoral (most common), transaortic, or transapical. Two types of replacement valves are available in the US: a balloon-expandable valve (Sapien XT®) or a self-expanding valve (CoreValue®). Once the catheter with a balloon device and the replacement valve attached is in place in the aortic valve, the balloon is inflated to secure the replacement valve, then the balloon is deflated and the catheter is removed. With the self-expanding valve, the valve is attached to the catheter and expanded when it is in place in the stenotic valve and the catheter is removed.

Postoperative Care for Cardiac Surgery

The **recovery period** is discussed below:

- 2:1 nursing ratio; monitor hemodynamics closely (check vitals every 5-15 minutes).
- Warm patient according to policy; monitor ECG closely for arrhythmias during rewarming.
- Maintain MAP between 70-110 mmHg to prevent inadequate perfusion or graft rupture/hemorrhage; urine output should be >30 mL/hr.
- The patient will have multiple chest tubes; ensure output is not excessive (>200 mL/hr = hemorrhage) and does not suddenly stop/decrease.

- Auscultate heart sounds and evaluate extremities frequently to assess perfusion; hourly urine output should be 30 mL/hr OR 1 mL/kg/hr (gold standard).
- Monitor ABGS (every 2-4 hr during recovery) and adjust ventilator settings accordingly.
- Close blood sugar control (will probably be on insulin drip) and prophylactic cephalosporin to prevent infection.
- Monitor CMP and replace electrolyte imbalances as ordered.

Monitor for the following complications:

- Cardiac Tamponade: bleeding from graft sites into the pericardial sac
- Hypotension/shock: decreased cardiac output
- Arrhythmias: due to blood flow changes and cardioplegic solution – be prepared for epicardial pacing and defibrillation if needed
- Stroke (clots from grafts), infection (surgical site), etc.

Nursing considerations are as follows:

- Educate patient: recovery, possibility of Dressler's Syndrome and postoperative depression; adequate pain management and splinting.

Arterial Line Insertion

Indications for an **arterial line** include hemodynamic instability, frequent ABG monitoring, placement of IABP, monitoring arterial pressure, and medication administration when venous access cannot be obtained. Sterile technique is utilized for arterial line insertion. Insertions sites include radial (most common), femoral (second choice), brachial, or dorsalis pedis arteries.
Procedure:

- Verify adequate perfusion and position.
  - Radial: Perform modified Allen test and position wrist in dorsiflexion with an arm board.
  - Femoral: Place the patient in a supine position with the leg on the insertion side slightly abducted and extended.
- Prep and drape. Apply 1% lidocaine if the patient is conscious.
- Insert needle.
  - Over-the-needle catheter insertion: Needle is inserted at a 30-45° degree angle and decreased to a 10-15° angle when blood returns, catheter advanced into vessel, needle removed, and catheter connected to transducer.
  - Over-wire catheter insertion: Needle is inserted into the artery at a 30-45° angle until blood returns. A wire is then inserted and advanced through the needle, and needle removed, leaving the wire in place. A catheter is then advanced over the wire, wire removed, and catheter connected to transducer system.
- A small incision is made at insertion site and catheter sutured into place.

Complications include bleeding, coagulopathy, thrombosis (especially with larger catheters or smaller arteries), advanced atherosclerosis, and infection.

Review Video: Nursing Care of Arterial Lines
Visit mometrix.com/academy and enter code: 561047

Central Line Insertion

Central lines allow rapid administration of large volumes of fluid, blood testing, and CVP measuring. Central lines may be placed into the internal jugular vein (right preferred), subclavian vein, or femoral vein (usually avoided). The insertion site is located through an ultrasound. The patient is positioned, supine Trendelenburg (or legs elevated) for interior jugular, using sterile technique. Following skin prep, the CVC kit is placed on a sterile field and opened, the equipment is prepared, and the insertion site is again verified by a probe (covered with sterile cover). Topical anesthetic (lidocaine) is administered and the needle inserted with the triangulation or spear method, always pulling back on the plunger of the syringe so that blood returns when entering the vein. The syringe is removed and the guidewire inserted into needle ≤20 cm. The needle is then removed and the wire position verified with ultrasound. A small incision is made at the insertion site, and a dilator is applied over the wire and inserted about 2.5 to 3.5 cm. The catheter is placed over the wire and advanced into the vein (13 to 17 cm). The wire is then removed, the lines are flushed, and the catheter is sutured in place and dressing is applied. Long (24-inch) PICCs may be inserted in the basilic or cephalic veins and advanced into central circulation.

Intraosseous Infusion

Intraosseous (IO) infusion is an alternative to IV access for neonates, pediatric emergencies, and adult emergencies when rapid temporary access is necessary or when peripheral or vascular access can't be achieved. It is often used in pediatric cardiac arrest. Because yellow marrow replaces red marrow, access in those older than 5 is more difficult. Preferred sites include:

- 0-5: Proximal tibia (preferred)
- Older children and adults: Medial malleolus. The sternum can support higher infusion rates. Other sites include the distal femur, clavicle, humerus, and ileum.

IO infusion is used to administer fluids and anesthesia and to obtain blood samples. Equipment requires a special needle (13-20 gauge) as standard needles may bend. The bone injection gun (BIG) with a loaded spring facilitates insertion. The FAST needle is intended for use in the sternum of adults and prevents accidental puncture of the thoracic cavity. Knowledge of bony landmarks and correct insertion angle and site is important. The position is confirmed by aspiration of 5-10 mL of blood and marrow before infusion.

Vascular Interventions

Vascular interventions are required when a patient has a condition that is decreasing blood flow to the limbs, causing ischemia-related damage. Conditions that require a vascular intervention include acute occlusion (embolus), severe unresponsive vascular disease, ruptured/dissecting aneurysm, damaged vessels, or congenital defect.

- **Bypass grafts:** The MD uses a harvested vein from another part of the body (saphenous usually) or synthetic graft to bypass the occlusion. Because veins have valves, they must be reversed or stripped of valves prior to attachment; however, synthetic grafts have a higher failure rate. A common peripheral bypass is the femoropopliteal (Fem-pop) bypass, extending from the femoral artery around the blockage to the popliteal artery.
- **Embolectomy:** A catheter is inserted into the blocked artery and threaded through the thrombus. Then a balloon on the tip is inflated, and the physician removes the catheter, removing the clot with it.
- **Aortic Aneurysm Repair:** This is an intense procedure, requiring an open incision and the patient to be placed on cardiopulmonary bypass. The affected area is resected and replaced with a vascular or Dacron graft.

Nursing considerations: Monitor and control blood pressure carefully to protect the patency and integrity of the grafts. Neurologic and renal function should also be carefully monitored, as emboli could block the renal or cerebral artery. Frequent neuro, urine output, vascular, and dressing checks.

Possible Complications: Pulmonary infection, graft-site infection, renal dysfunction, occlusion, hemorrhage, and embolus/thrombus.

Fem-Pop Bypass

Femoropopliteal (Fem-Pop) bypass is used for femoral artery disease in order to bypass an occluded femoral artery above or below the knee. Either a man-made or a vein graft (such as the saphenous vein) is used and is sewn above the blocked area to the femoral artery and below to the popliteal artery, allowing the blood to bypass the occluded area. In addition to the incisions in the affected leg, if a vein graft is obtained from the other leg, the patient may also have a long incision where the vein was removed. Edema in the surgical sites is common and may persist for up to 3 months. Femoral popliteal bypass surgery is indicated for peripheral vascular insufficiency that does not respond to medical treatment, causes severe intermittent claudication and/or ischemic resting pain, and results in gangrene or other non-healing wounds, especially if the limb is at risk for amputation because of impaired oxygenation. The limb(s) must be monitored carefully in the postoperative period for color, sensation, warmth, and ability to move.

Peripheral Stents

Peripheral vascular stenting may be utilized as an intervention in the treatment of peripheral vascular insufficiency. Often performed in interventional radiology, the interventionalist uses balloon angioplasty to unblock the vessel under fluoroscopic guidance. A small balloon attached to a catheter is inserted into the occluded vessel and inflated to expand the arterial wall and compress the blockage. A small metal tube (stent) is then placed to support the vessel and maintain its patency. Stents are primarily made of stainless steel or a metal alloy. This intervention helps to restore circulation to the affected area and prevent restenosis of the vessel. There are different types of stents available based on the type of vessel affected and the type of lesion. Stenting may be used in both peripheral and coronary arteries.

- **Indications**: Stenting may be the initial choice of intervention in patients with iliac, renal, subclavian or carotid stenosis. Stenting may be indicated in patients with severe claudication, non-healing ulcers of the extremities, ischemic pain with rest, and in patients who have a high operative risk. Peripheral stenting often results in shorter hospital stays and shorter recovery times in comparison with surgical intervention.
- **Complications**: Complications that may occur in patients undergoing peripheral stenting include bleeding, infection, arterial spasm or rupture, dissection of the vessel, restenosis or thrombus formation within the vessel, and intravascular fracture of the stent.

Cardiovascular Pharmacology

Anti-Hypertensive Medications

The **classes of anti-hypertensive medications** are as follows: Diuretics, sympatholytics, vasodilators, calcium channel blockers, and angiotensin-converting enzyme inhibitors (ACE inhibitors).

- Diuretics include hydrochlorothiazide, chlorthalidone, chlorothiazide, indapamide, metolazone, amiloride, spironolactone, triamterene, furosemide, bumetanide, ethacrynic acid, and torsemide.
- Sympatholytics are clonidine, methyldopa, guanabenz, guanadrel, guanethidine, reserpine, labetalol, prazosin, and terazosin.
- Vasodilators include diazoxide, hydralazine, minoxidil, and nitroprusside sodium.
- Calcium channel blockers include amlodipine, nimodipine, isradipine, nicardipine, nifedipine, bepridil, diltiazem, and verapamil.
- ACE inhibitors include benazepril, captopril, enalapril, fosinopril, lisinopril, moexipril, quinapril, ramipril, and losartan.

Diuretics

Diuretics increase **renal perfusion and filtration**, thereby reducing preload and decreasing peripheral and pulmonary edema, hypertension, CHF, diabetes insipidus, and osteoporosis. There are different types of diuretics: loop, thiazide, and potassium sparing.

Loop Diuretics

Loop diuretics inhibit the reabsorption of sodium and chloride (primarily) in the ascending loop of Henle. They also cause increased secretion of other electrolytes, such as calcium, magnesium, and potassium, and this can result in imbalances that cause dysrhythmias. Other side effects include frequent urination, postural hypotension, and increased blood sugar and uric acid levels. They are short-acting so are less effective than other diuretics for control of hypertension.

- **Bumetanide** (Bumex®) is given intravenously after surgery to reduce preload or orally to treat heart failure.
- **Ethacrynic acid** (Edecrin®) is given intravenously after surgery to reduce preload.
- **Furosemide** (Lasix®) is used for the control of congestive heart failure as well as renal insufficiency. It is used after surgery to decrease preload and to reduce the inflammatory response caused by cardiopulmonary bypass (post-perfusion syndrome).

Review Video: Diuretics
Visit mometrix.com/academy and enter code: 373276

Thiazide Diuretics

Thiazide diuretics inhibit the **reabsorption of sodium and chloride** primarily in the early distal tubules, forcing more sodium and water to be excreted. Thiazide diuretics increase secretion of potassium and bicarbonate, so they are often given with supplementary potassium or in combination with potassium-sparing diuretics. Thiazide diuretics are the first line of drugs for treatment of **hypertension**. They have a long duration of action (12-72 hours, depending on the drug) so they are able to maintain control of hypertension better than short-acting drugs. They may be given daily or 3–5 days per week. There are numerous thiazide diuretics, including:

- Chlorothiazide (Diuril®)
- Bendroflumethiazide (Naturetin®)
- Chlorthalidone (Hygroton®)
- Trichlormethiazide (Naqua®)

Side effects include, dizziness, lightheadedness, postural hypotension, headache, blurred vision, and itching, especially during initial treatment. Thiazide diuretics cause sensitivity to sun exposure, so people should be counseled to use sunscreen.

Potassium-Sparing Diuretics

Potassium-sparing diuretics inhibit the **reabsorption of sodium** in the late distal tubule and collecting duct. They are weaker than thiazide or loop diuretics, but do not cause a reduction in potassium level; however, if used alone, they may cause an increase in potassium, which can cause weakness, irregular pulse, and cardiac arrest. Because potassium-sparing diuretics are less effective alone, they are often given in a combined form with a thiazide diuretic (usually chlorothiazide), which mitigates the potassium imbalance. Typical side effects include dehydration, blurred vision, nausea, insomnia, and nasal congestion, especially in the first few days of treatment.

- **Spironolactone** (Aldactone®) is a synthetic steroid diuretic that increases the secretion of both water and sodium and is used to treat congestive heart failure. It may be given orally or intravenously.
- **Eplerenone** is an antimineralocorticoid similar to spironolactone but with fewer side effects.

Antidysrhythmic Drugs

Antidysrhythmic drugs include a number of drugs that act on the conduction system, the ventricles and/or the atria to control dysrhythmias. There are 4 classes of drugs that are used as well as some that are unclassified:

- **Class I:** 3 subtypes of sodium channel blockers (quinidine, lidocaine, procainamide)
- **Class II:** β-receptor blockers (esmolol, propranolol)
- **Class III:** Slows repolarization (amiodarone, ibutilide)
- **Class IV**: Calcium channel blockers (diltiazem, verapamil)
- **Unclassified:** Miscellaneous drugs with proven efficacy in controlling arrhythmias (adenosine, electrolyte supplements)

Smooth Muscle Relaxants

Smooth muscle relaxants decrease peripheral vascular resistance, but may cause hypotension and headaches.

- Sodium nitroprusside (Nipride®) dilates both arteries and veins; rapid-acting and used for reduction of hypertension and afterload reduction for heart failure.
- Nitroglycerin (Tridil®) primarily dilates veins and is used sublingual or IV to reduce preload for acute heart failure, unstable angina, and acute MI. Nitroglycerin may also be used prophylactically after PCIs to prevent vasospasm.
- Hydralazine (Apresoline®) dilates arteries and is given intermittently to reduce hypertension.

CALCIUM CHANNEL BLOCKERS

Calcium channel blockers are primarily arterial vasodilators that may affect the peripheral and/or coronary arteries.

- Side effects: Lethargy, flushing, edema, ascites, and indigestion:
- Nifedipine (Procardia®) and nicardipine (Cardene®) are primarily arterial vasodilators, used to treat acute hypertension. Diltiazem (Cardizem®) and Verapamil (Calan®, Isoptin®) dilate primarily coronary arteries and slow the heart rate, thus are used for angina, atrial fibrillation, and SVT. *Note:* Nifedipine (Procardia®) should be avoided in older adults due to increased risk of hypotension and myocardial ischemia.

Review Video: Ca Channel Blockers
Visit mometrix.com/academy and enter code: 942825

ADDITIONAL VASODILATORS

B-type natriuretic peptide (BNP) (Nesiritide [Natrecor®]) is type of vasodilator (non-inotropic), which is a recombinant form of a peptide of the human brain. It decreases filling pressure, vascular resistance, and increases U/O.

- May cause hypotension, headache, bradycardia, and nausea. It is used short term for worsening decompensated CHF; contraindicated in SBP<90, cardiogenic shock, constrictive pericarditis, or valve stenosis.

Alpha-adrenergic blockers block alpha receptors in arteries and veins, causing vasodilation.

- May cause orthostatic hypotension and edema from fluid retention.
- Labetalol (Normodyne®) is a combination peripheral alpha-blocker and cardiac β-blocker that is used to treat acute hypertension, acute stroke, and acute aortic dissection.
- Phentolamine (Regitine®) is a peripheral arterial dilator that reduces afterload. It is used for HTN crisis in patients with pheochromocytoma, as well as a subcutaneous injection for extravasation of vessicants.

Selective specific dopamine DA-1-receptor agonists:

- Fenoldopam (Corlopam®) is a peripheral dilator affecting renal and mesenteric arteries and can be used for patients with renal dysfunction or those at risk of renal insufficiency.

INOTROPIC AGENTS

Inotropic agents are drugs used to increase cardiac output and improve contractibility. IV inotropic agents may increase the risk of death, but may be used when other drugs fail. Oral forms of these drugs are less effective than intravenous. Inotropic agents include:

- **β-Adrenergic agonists:**
  - **Dobutamine** improves cardiac output, treats cardiac decompensation, and increases blood pressure. It helps the body to utilize norepinephrine. Side effects include increased or labile blood pressure, increased heart rate, PVCs, N/V, and bronchospasm.
  - **Dopamine** improves cardiac output, blood pressure, and blood flow to the renal and mesenteric arteries. Side effects include tachycardia or bradycardia, palpitations, BP changes, dyspnea, nausea and vomiting, headache, and gangrene of extremities.

- **Phosphodiesterase III inhibitors:**
  - **Milrinone** (Primacor®) increases strength of contractions and cause vasodilation. Side effects include ventricular arrhythmias, hypotension, and headaches.
- **Digoxin (Lanoxin®):**
  - Increases contractibility and cardiac output and prevents arrhythmias.

Medications for Heart Failure

A patient with heart failure may be prescribed with one or multiple of the drugs below:

- **ACE inhibitors:** Captopril (Capoten®), enalapril (Vasotec®), and lisinopril (Prinivil®). Decrease afterload/preload and reverse ventricular remodeling; they also prevent neuropathy in DM. Contraindicated with renal insufficiency, renal artery stenosis, and pregnancy.
  - Side effects include cough (#1), hyperkalemia, hypotension, angioedema, dizziness, and weakness.
- **Angiotensin receptor blockers (ARBs):** Losartan (Cozaar®) and valsartan (Diovan®). Decrease afterload/preload and reverse ventricular remodeling, causing vasodilation and reducing blood pressure. They are used for those who cannot tolerate ACE inhibitors.
  - Side effects include cough (less common than with ACE inhibitors), hyperkalemia, hypotension, headache, dizziness, metallic taste, and rash.
- **β-Blockers:** Metoprolol (Lopressor®), carvedilol (Coreg®) and esmolol (Brevibloc®). Slow the heart rate, reduce hypertension, prevent dysrhythmias, and reverse ventricular remodeling. Contraindicated in bradyarrythmias, decompensated HF, uncontrolled hypoglycemia/diabetes mellitus, and airway disease.
  - Side effects: bradycardia, hypotension, bronchospasm, may mask signs of hypoglycemia.
- **Aldosterone agonist:** Spironolactone (Aldactone®). Decreases preload and myocardial hypertrophy and reduces edema and sodium retention but may increase serum potassium.
- **Furosemide (Lasix®)** is used for the control of congestive heart failure as well as renal insufficiency. It is used after surgery to decrease preload and to reduce the inflammatory response caused by cardiopulmonary bypass (post-perfusion syndrome).

Digoxin (Lanoxin®)

Digitalis drugs, most commonly administered in the form of digoxin (Lanoxin®), are derived from the foxglove plant and are used to increase myocardial contractility, left ventricular output, and slow conduction through the AV node, decreasing rapid heart rates and promoting diuresis. Digoxin does not affect mortality, but increases tolerance to activity and reduces hospitalizations for heart failure. Therapeutic levels (0.5-2.0 ng/mL) should be maintained to avoid digitalis toxicity, which can occur even if digoxin levels are within therapeutic range, so observation of symptoms is critical. Because patients with heart failure are often on diuretics which decrease potassium levels, they are at increased risk for toxicity.

Symptoms of toxicity are as follows:

- Early signs: Increasing fatigue, lethargy, depression, and nausea and vomiting; progress to severe diarrhea, blurred vision/yellow or green halos around lights, fatigue/weakness
- Arrythmias: SA or AV block, VT/VF, PVCs, and bradycardia

Treatment consists of the following:

- Monitor serum levels and symptoms.
- Digoxin immune FAB (Digibind®) may be used to bind to digoxin and inactivate it if necessary.

Glycoprotein IIB/IIIA Inhibitors

Glycoprotein IIB/IIIA Inhibitors are drugs that are used to inhibit platelet binding and prevent clots prior to and following invasive cardiac procedures, such as angioplasty and stent placement. These medications are used in combination with anticoagulant drugs, such as heparin and aspirin for the following:

- Acute coronary syndromes (ACS), such as unstable angina or myocardial infarctions
- Percutaneous coronary intervention (PCI), such as angioplasty and stent placement

These medications are contraindicated in those with a low platelet count or active bleeding:

- **Abciximab (ReoPro®)**: Used with both heparin and aspirin for ACS and PCI and affects platelet binding for 48 hours after administration.
- **Eptifibatide (Integrilin®)**: Used with both heparin and aspirin for ACS and PCI and affects platelet binding for 6-8 hours after administration. Should not be used in patients with renal problems.
- **Tirofiban (Aggrastat®)**: Used with heparin for PCI patients with reduced dosage for those with renal problems and affects platelet blinding for only 4-8 hours after administration.

Pharmacologic Measures to Maximize Perfusion

The primary focus of pharmacologic measures to **maximize perfusion** is to reduce the risk of **thromboses**:

- **Antiplatelet agents**, such as aspirin, Ticlid®, and Plavix®, which interfere with the function of the plasma membrane, interfering with clotting. These agents are ineffective to treat clots but prevent clot formation.
- **Vasodilators** may divert blood from ischemic areas, but some may be indicated, such as Pletal®, which dilates arteries and decreases clotting, and is used for control of intermittent claudication.
- **Antilipemic**, such as Zocor® and Questran®, slow progression of atherosclerosis.
- **Hemorheologic agents**, such as Trental®, reduce fibrinogen, reducing blood viscosity and rigidity of erythrocytes; however, clinical studies show limited benefit. It may be used for intermittent claudication.
- **Analgesics** may be necessary to improve quality of life. Opioids may be needed in some cases.
- **Thrombolytics** may be injected into a blocked artery under angiography to dissolve clots.
- **Anticoagulants**, such as Coumadin® and Lovenox®, prevent blood clots from forming.

Administration of Fibrinolytic (Thrombolytic) Infusions for MI

Fibrinolytic infusion is indicated for acute myocardial infarction under these conditions:

- Symptoms of MI, <6-12 hours since onset of symptoms
- ≥1 mm elevation of ST in ≥2 contiguous leads
- No contraindications and no cardiogenic shock

Fibrinolytic agents should be administered as soon as possible, within 30 minutes is best. All agents convert plasminogen to plasmin, which breaks down fibrin, dissolving clots:

- Streptokinase and anistreplase (1st generation)
- Alteplase or tissue plasminogen activator (tPA) (2nd generation)
- Reteplase and tenecteplase (3rd generation)

Contraindications

- Present or recent bleeding or history of severe bleeding
- History of intracranial hemorrhage
- History of stroke (<3 months unless within 3 hours)
- Aortic dissection or pericarditis
- Intracranial/intraspinal surgery or trauma within 3 months or neoplasm, aneurysm, or AVM

Relative contraindications

- Active peptic ulcer
- >10 minutes of CPR
- Advanced renal or hepatic disease
- Pregnancy
- Anticoagulation therapy
- Acute uncontrolled hypertension or chronic poorly controlled hypertension
- Recent (2–4 weeks) internal bleeding
- Non-compressible vascular punctures

Neurological Diagnostics

Lumbar Puncture

The **lumbar puncture** (spinal tap) is done between the 3rd and 4th or between the 4th and 5th lumbar vertebrae. The patient is in the lateral recumbent position with knees drawn toward the chest during the procedure. A local anesthetic is applied to prevent pain when the needle is inserted into the subarachnoid space to withdraw CSF and measure CSF pressure, which should be 70-200 mmH_2O.

Queckenstedt's test: Compress jugular veins on each side of the neck during the procedure. Note pressure and then release the veins and note pressure in 10-second intervals. Pressure should rise quickly with compression and fall quickly with release. Slower or no response indicates blockage of subarachnoid pathways.

Normal values (CSF analysis):

- Clear and colorless
- Protein: 15-45 mg/dL
- Glucose: 60-80 mg/dL
- Lactic acid: <25.2 mg/dL
- Culture: Negative
- RBCs: 0
- WBCs: 0.5/mL

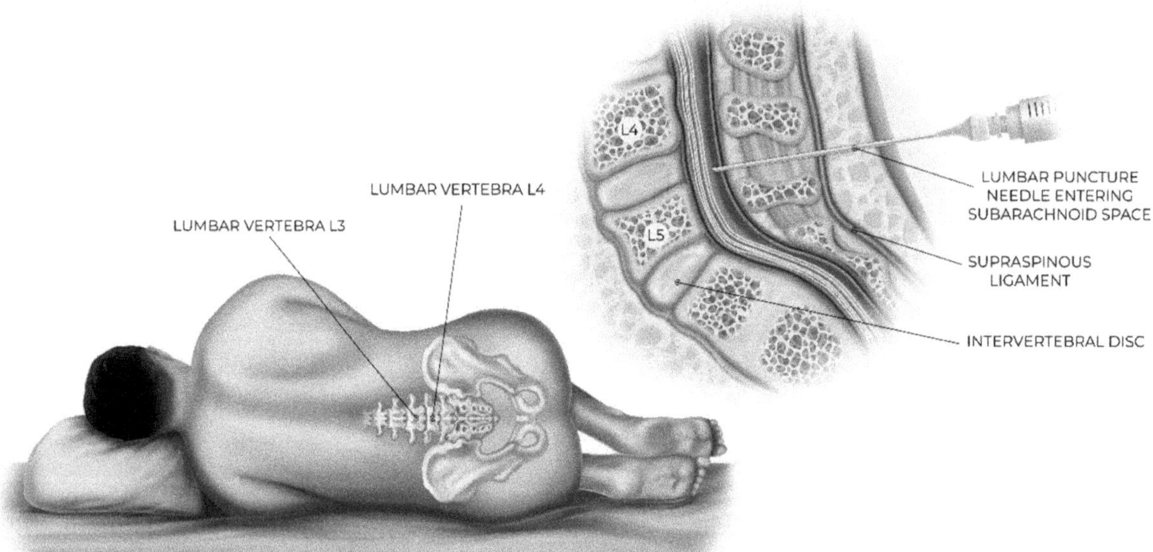

Avoiding Complications After Lumbar Puncture and Use of Epidural Blood Patch

After a **lumbar puncture**, the patient should remain in the prone position for at least 3 hours to ensure that the needle puncture sites through the dural and arachnoid areas remain separate in order to reduce the chance of CSF leakage. If >20 mL of CSF is removed, then the patient should remain prone for 2 hours, side-lying (flat) for 2-3 hours, and supine or prone for 6 additional hours. Relieving intracranial pressure by withdrawing CSF may cause herniation of the brain, so lumbar puncture should be done with care in the presence of increased ICP. The most common complaint is of spinal headache, which may occur within a few hours or several days of the procedure. Increased fluid intake may reduce risk of headache. If headache occurs, it may be treated with analgesics, fluids, and bed rest; however, if the headache is severe or persistent, an **epidural blood patch** may be done, with venous blood withdrawn and then injected into the epidural space at the site of the puncture to seal the leaking opening.

Neurological Procedures and Interventions

Clipping for Treatment of Aneurysm

Surgical clipping of a ruptured or large, unstable **aneurysm** is necessary because of the danger of rebleeding, 4% in the first 24 hours and 1-2% each day for the next month. Mortality rates with rebleeding are about 70%. Surgical repair is usually done within 48 hours. Clipping may be done prophylactically to prevent rupture. Clipping is done to secure the aneurysm without impairing circulation. Typically, a craniotomy is done and an incision is made into the brain to access the site of the aneurysm. When bleeding is controlled, a small spring-like clip (or sometimes multiple clips) is placed about the neck of the aneurysm. The bulging part of the aneurysm is drained with a needle to make sure that it does not refill and angiography may be done to ensure patency of the artery that feeds the aneurysm. It is possible during surgery for a clot to break away from the aneurysm with resultant extensive hemorrhage. Neurological damage may occur related to surgical manipulation, especially if access is difficult. Post-op monitoring includes frequent neurological checks—sometimes every hour, checking for signs and symptoms of stroke, hemorrhage or cerebral edema/increased ICP. An angiogram may be performed after surgery to confirm placement of clips and ensure there are no leaks.

Embolization for Treatment of Aneurysm or AVM

Embolization is a minimally-invasive method that is an alternative to clipping for some aneurysms and is also used for AVMs. There are different types of embolization, but all use percutaneous transfemoral catheterization and fluoroscopy. The catheter is fed through the femoral and carotid artery to the area requiring repair:

- AVM repair by introducing small silastic beads or glue into the feeder vessels, allowing blood flow to carry the material to the site. This may also be done prior to surgical repair.
- AVM or aneurysm repair by placing one or more detachable balloons into the aneurysm or an AVM and inflating it with a liquid polymerizing agent that solidifies.
- Aneurysm repair with endovascular coiling involves feeding very small platinum coils through the catheter to fill the aneurysm.

Results of endovascular coiling have been very positive, with risk of death or disability at one year over 22% lower than those treated with clipping, although distal ischemia related to emboli is a possible complication.

Surgical Excision of AVM

Surgical excision of AVM is the definitive treatment for AVMs as both embolization and radiotherapy treatment pose the risk that the abnormal vessels will recur. Sometimes, 2-3 different surgeries may be required for large AVMs. Usually nonfunctioning brain tissue surrounds the AVM, so it's possible to remove the AVM without damaging brain tissue. However, reperfusion bleeding may occur as blood is diverted to surrounding arterials that had dilated because of chronic ischemia. The sudden increase in blood flow and pressure may cause leakage of blood from the vessels. There may be extensive blood loss during surgery, so constant monitoring of arterial pressure and multiple IV cannulas are important. Embolization may be done prior to surgery to reduce bleeding. Hyperventilation and mannitol are often used, and β-blockers may be used to prevent hypertension and cerebral edema. Postoperatively, blood pressure is kept low to prevent reperfusion bleeding.

Evacuation of Hematomas

Evacuation of hematomas can be done in a number of different ways, including burr holes, needle aspiration, direct surgical craniotomy, or endoscopic craniotomy, but evacuation can pose considerable risks:

- **Epidural hematomas** are usually arterial but may be venous (20%) and are always medical emergencies and require craniotomy with evacuation before compression damage to the brain occurs. Prognosis is good if corrected early because underlying brain damage is rarely severe.
- **Subdural hematomas**, often from acceleration-deceleration accidents or abuse, involve damage to the brain tissue. Evacuation may be done if the hematoma is large and causing compression, but the brain tissue beneath hematomas is often extremely swollen. If the dura is opened, suddenly relieving the pressure may cause the brain to herniate through the opening, so aggressive therapy to reduce swelling preoperatively and careful surgical planning are necessary.

Craniotomies

Craniotomies for tumors or other surgical repair (AVMs, aneurysms) are increasingly done with micro-endoscopic equipment, but the surgical opening must be large enough to allow access and the use of necessary instruments. Procedures vary widely according to the reason for craniotomy, the type of tumor, and the age and condition of the patient. Direct craniotomies through the skull are needed in some instances, but newer approaches, including transnasal and transsphenoidal endoscopy are used when possible. Some areas of the brain are not accessible with craniotomy, but may be accessible through stereotactic radiosurgery with Gamma Knife® or CyberKnife®. Stereotactic radiosurgery is often used as a secondary treatment after primary removal of tumor for regrowth or residual tumor. Radiosurgery may be fractionated and given in a series of treatments. These non-invasive treatments are usually done while adults are awake.

Postoperative Care for Craniotomy Patients

In the post-operative period immediately following a **craniotomy**, the patient must be observed carefully for any **complications** or changes in condition:

- Monitor intracranial pressure
- Position the head in a midline, neutral position. HOB is elevated 30-45° for supratentorial surgery and is flat or only slightly elevated for infratentorial surgery
- Initiate anti-thromboembolism measures: Compression stockings or intermittent pneumatic compression device
- Monitor fluid balance (intake and output)
- Observe surgical wound for swelling and drainage; empty and measure drainage devices (usually bulb drains)
- Monitor oxygen saturation and ABGs to ensure proper oxygenation
- Monitor thermoregulation and prevent hyperthermia
- Administer analgesics and antiemetics routinely to maintain comfort and prevent stress or increased ICP from vomiting
- Administer corticosteroids to reduce postoperative swelling
- Administer anticoagulants (heparin) to prevent clotting

- Monitor laboratory status:
  - Complete blood count to observe for blood loss/infection
  - Electrolyte levels, especially observing for hyponatremia and/or hyperkalemia
  - Blood glucose level (may elevate with corticosteroids)

Burr Holes

Burr holes are small holes drilled through the skull, often as an emergent procedure to relieve increased intracranial pressure (such as from subdural, epidural hematoma, or hydrocephalus), to drain blood, or to remove foreign objects. Burr holes may also be used as access points for minimally-invasive surgeries on the brain, such as to remove a brain tumor. The burr holes are generally drilled with the patient under general anesthesia, and the opening may be closed or left open with a drain in place. The patient must be monitored for indications of bleeding or other surgical complications. Perioperative complications may include increased intracranial pressure from cerebral edema, seizures, intracranial bleeding, and coma. The patient's vital signs and neurological signs should be closely monitored. If a drain is in place, the amount and character of the drainage should be monitored. The patient may receive prophylactic antibiotics to reduce the risk of infection.

Ventricular Drains

Ventricular drains are inserted into one of the brain's lateral ventricles (usually on the right to prevent damage to the language center) to drain cerebrospinal fluid associated with hydrocephalus. The catheter is tunneled under the skin and sutured in place with an occlusive dressing covering the insertion site. The catheter drains into a collection chamber, which is separated from a drainage bag by a stopcock that can be opened or closed. A pressure scale (which should be leveled with zero at the tragus of the ear) is at the same level as the collection chamber. The target pressure should be determined by the neurosurgeon. The dressing should be changed only if soiled, and any indication of CSF leakage or blood in the CSF should be immediately reported. The CSF output should be measured and recorded hourly (after which the collection chamber is emptied into the drainage bag) and VS and neurological assessment at least every 4 hours. The catheter should be checked when the collection chamber is emptied to ensure it is patent and not kinked. During straining or activities that involve moving the patient, the drainage should be stopped, but for short periods only. Over drainage may result in headache.

Ventricular-peritoneal shunts may become occluded or disconnected, the catheter may be positioned incorrectly, and the valve pressure may not be adequate. If the shunt does not function properly, signs of hydrocephalus and increased intracranial pressure can occur. If there is a flush valve, this may relieve the obstruction, but obstruction may be difficult to assess with radiography, so a neurosurgical consult may be indicated for revision of the shunt.

Lumbar Drains

A **lumbar drain** is inserted in the lumbar region (usually L3-L4 or L4-L5) into the arachnoid space in order to drain cerebrospinal fluid. Indications for a lumbar drain include shunt infection, increased intracranial pressure, hydrocephalus, thoracoabdominal aortic aneurysm repair, and dural fistula (traumatic/postoperative). The patient should be positioned with the head of the bed elevated to 30 degrees and the transducer leveled to the phlebostatic axis or to the right atrium. The cerebrospinal fluid pressure should be monitored continuously and recorded at least every hour for the first 72 hours as well as the volume of drainage, which should be prescribed by the neurosurgeon. Over-drainage may cause a sudden decline in ICP and subarachnoid hemorrhage. Vital signs, neuromuscular and neurovascular checks should be carried out at least every hour for 24 hours. Systolic BP should be maintained ≥140 mmHg and fluid bolus administered for hypotension. After 24 hours, the patient may sit in a chair if stable, but CSF should not be drained while the patient is out of bed. Any sign of blood in CSF should be immediately reported to the neurosurgeon. Hemoglobin should be maintained at >9 mg/dL.

TRANSSPHENOIDAL HYPOPHYSECTOMY

The sella turcica is a depressed area that holds the pituitary gland (which extends down from the brain on a stalk) in the sphenoid bone at the base of the skull. Pituitary tumors < 10 mm diameter are removed in a **transsphenoidal hypophysectomy**. In addition to general anesthesia, supplemental infraorbital blocks may provide postoperative pain relief. Vasoconstrictors (such as epinephrine) with local anesthesia are usually administered intranasally to control bleeding. Microscopic surgery is done with an incision in the gingival mucosa beneath the upper lip then through the nasal septum and through the roof of the sphenoid cavity to access the base of the sella turcica and the pituitary tumor. Endoscopic surgery is done directly through the nares with removal of the mucosa but no incision. After microscopic surgery, stents are placed in the nasal septum and the nose packed. With both procedures, nasal discharge must be observed for CSF leakage ("Halo sign") and the patient cautioned not to blow the nose.

NEURO-ENDOVASCULAR INTERVENTIONS

COILING

Coiling is a minimally-invasive procedure used to treat cerebral aneurysm. A catheter is inserted in the femoral area and advanced to the aneurysm. Then a microcatheter with coil attached is fed through the catheter into the aneurysm until the coil fills the aneurysm. The coil is separated with an electrical current and the catheter is removed. In some cases, more than one coil may be needed. The coil is spring like and very thin. Blood enters the aneurysm about the coils and clots so that no further blood can enter, effectively sealing the aneurysm.

THROMBECTOMY

Thrombectomy is a procedure by which an endovascular clot is removed. Various techniques may be used, but a catheter is generally inserted into the femoral vein and advanced to the clot and then the clot may be suctioned, broken up mechanically and the pieces removed, or a helical thrombectomy device wrapped around the clot so that it can be removed. Thrombectomy is used as treatment for stroke to restore blood flow as well as for removal of clots in the arms or legs.

Neurologic Pharmacology

ANTICONVULSANTS

Carbamazepine (Tegretol®)

Use: Partial, tonic-clonic, and absence seizures; analgesia for trigeminal neuralgia

Side effects: Dizziness, drowsiness, nausea, and vomiting. Toxic reactions include severe skin rash, agranulocytosis, aplastic anemia, and hepatitis

Clonazepam (Klonopin®)

Use: Akinetic, absence, and myoclonic seizures; Lennox-Gastaut syndrome

Side effects: Behavioral changes, hirsutism or alopecia, headaches, and drowsiness. Toxic reactions include hepatotoxicity, thrombocytopenia, ataxia, and bone marrow failure.

Ethosuximide (Zarontin®)

Use: Absence seizures

Side effects: Headaches and gastrointestinal disorders. Toxic reactions include skin rash, blood dyscrasias (sometimes fatal), hepatitis, and lupus erythematosus.

Felbamate (Felbatol®)

Use: Lennox-Gastaut syndrome

Side effects: Headache, fatigue, insomnia, and cognitive impairment. Toxic reactions include aplastic anemia and hepatic failure. It is recommended only if other medications have failed.

Fosphenytoin (Cerebyx®)

Use: Status epilepticus prevention and treatment during neurosurgery

Side effects: CNS depression, hypotension, cardiovascular collapse, dizziness, nystagmus, and pruritus.

Gabapentin (Neurontin®)

Use: Partial seizures; post-herpetic neuralgia

Side effects: Dizziness, somnolence, drowsiness, ataxia, weight gain, and nausea. Toxic reactions include hepatotoxicity and leukopenia.

Lamotrigine (Lamictal®)

Use: Partial and primary generalized tonic-clonic seizures; Lennox-Gastaut syndrome

Side effects: Tremor, ataxia, weight gain, dizziness, headache, and drowsiness. Toxic reactions include severe rash, which may require hospitalization.

Levetiracetam (Keppra®)

Use: Partial onset, myoclonic, and generalized tonic-clonic seizures

Side effects: Idiopathic generalized epilepsy, dizziness, somnolence, irritability, alopecia, double vision, sore throat, and fatigue. Toxic reactions include bone marrow suppression and liver failure.

Oxcarbazepine (Trileptal®)

Use: Partial seizures

Side effects: Double or abnormal vision, tremor, abnormal gait, GI disorders, dizziness, and fatigue. A toxic reaction is hepatotoxicity.

Phenobarbital (Luminal®)

Use: Tonic-clonic and cortical local seizures; acute convulsive episodes; insomnia

Side effects: Sedation, double vision, agitation, and ataxia. Toxic reactions include anemia and skin rash.

Phenytoin (Dilantin®)

Use: Tonic-clonic and complex partial seizures

Side effects: Nystagmus, vision disorders, gingival hyperplasia, hirsutism, dysrhythmias, and dysarthria. Toxic reactions include collapse of cardiovascular system and CNS depression.

Primidone (Mysoline®)

Use: Grand mal, psychomotor, and focal seizures

Side effects: Double vision, ataxia, impotence, lethargy, and irritability. Toxic reactions include skin rash.

Tiagabine (Gabitril®)

Use: Partial seizures

Side effects: Concentration problems, weak knees, dysarthria, abdominal pain, tremor, dizziness, fatigue, and agitation.

Topiramate (Topamax®)

Use: Partial and tonic-clonic seizures; migraines

Side effects: Anorexia, weight loss, somnolence, confusion, ataxia, and confusion. Toxic reactions include kidney stones.

Valproate/Valproic acid (Depakote®, Depakene®)

Use: Complex partial, simple, and complex absence seizures; bipolar disorder

Side effects: Weight gain, alopecia, tremor, menstrual disorders, nausea, and vomiting. Toxic reactions include hepatotoxicity, severe pancreatitis, rash, blood dyscrasias, and nephritis.

Zonisamide (Zonegran®, Excegran®)

Use: Partial seizures

Side effects: Anorexia, nausea, agitation, rash, headache, dizziness, and somnolence. Toxic reactions include leukopenia and hepatotoxicity.

Hypertonic Saline Solution

Hypertonic saline solution (HSS) has a sodium concentration higher than 0.9% (NS) and is used to reduce intracranial pressure/cerebral edema and treat traumatic brain injury. Concentrations usually range from 2% to 23.4%. The hypertonic solution draws fluid from the tissue through osmosis. As edema decreases, circulation improves. HSS also expands plasma, increasing CPP, and counteracts hyponatremia that occurs in the brain after injury.

Administration:

- Peripheral lines: HSS <3% only
- Central lines: HSS ≥3%

HSS can be administered continuously at rates varying from 30-150 mL/hr. Rate must be carefully controlled. Fluid status must be monitored to prevent hypovolemia, which increases risk of renal failure. Boluses (typically 30 mL of 23.4%) may be administered over 15 minutes for acute increased ICP or transtentorial herniation.

Laboratory monitoring includes:

- Sodium (every 6 hours): Maintain at 145-155 mmol/L. Higher levels can cause heart/respiratory/renal failure.
- Serum osmolality (every 12 hours): Maintain at 320 mOsm/L. Higher levels can cause renal failure.

Mannitol

Mannitol is an osmotic diuretic that increases excretion of both sodium and water and reduces intracranial pressure and brain mass, especially after traumatic brain injury. Mannitol may also be used to shrink the cells of the blood-brain barrier in order to help other medications breach this barrier. Mannitol is administered per intravenous infusion:

- 2 g/kg in a 15-25% solution over 30-60 minutes

Cerebral spinal fluid pressure should show decrease within 15 minutes. Fluid and electrolyte balances must be carefully monitored as well as intake and output and body weight. Concentrations of 20-25% require a filter. Crystals may form if the mannitol solution is too cold and the mannitol container may require heating (in 80 °C water) and shaking to dissolve crystals, but the solution should be cooled to below body temperature prior to administration. Mannitol cannot be administered in polyvinylchloride bags as precipitates form. Side effects include fluid and electrolyte imbalance, nausea, vomiting, hypotension, tachycardia, fever, and urticaria.

Endocrine Diagnostics

Glucose Laboratory Test

Glucose is manufactured by the liver from ingested carbohydrates and is stored as glycogen for use by the cells. If intake is inadequate, glucose can be produced from muscle and fat tissue, leading to increased wasting. High levels of glucose are indicative of diabetes mellitus, which predisposes people to skin injuries, slow healing, and infection. Fasting blood glucose levels are used to diagnose and monitor this condition:

- Normal values: 70–99 mg/dL
- Impaired: 100–125 mg/dL
- Diabetes: ≥126 mg/dL

There are a number of different conditions that can increase glucose levels, including stress, renal failure, Cushing syndrome, hyperthyroidism, and pancreatic disorders. Medications, such as steroids, estrogens, lithium, phenytoin, diuretics, tricyclic antidepressants, may increase glucose levels. Other conditions, such as adrenal insufficiency, liver disease, hypothyroidism, and starvation can decrease glucose levels.

Hemoglobin A1C Laboratory Test

Hemoglobin A1C comprises hemoglobin A with a glucose molecule because hemoglobin holds onto excess blood glucose, so it shows the average blood glucose levels over a 3-month period and is used primarily to monitor long-term diabetic therapy:

- Normal value: <6%
- Elevation: >7%

Basic Thyroid Function Testing and Antibody Testing

Thyroid stimulating hormone (TSH) is produced by the pituitary as a result of thyrotropin releasing hormone (TRH) from the hypothalamus. TSH stimulates the thyroid to produce T4 (mostly) and T3. T4 is deiodinated to T3 (active hormone), and the free hormone is active while the majority is bound to albumin and thyroxine-binding globulin. The best testing of thyroid function is the free T4 (unbound). Free T4 and TSH testing allows appropriate screening for thyroid disease.

Additionally, certain antibodies are used to screen for thyroid disease. Thyroglobulin antibodies are found in 50% of patients with Graves' disease and about 90% of those with Hashimoto's thyroiditis. Thyroid peroxidase antibodies are detected in >90% of those with Hashimoto's thyroiditis. TSH receptor antibodies (TSHR) may be either thyroid stimulating immunoglobulin (TSI) which stimulate the receptor to produce thyroid hormone (found in Graves' disease), or TSHR-blocking antibodies, which may inhibit production of thyroid hormone.

Lab values to consider include:

- **Thyroid stimulating hormone (TSH)** (0.4-6.15 mIU/L). Increase in TSH indicates hypothyroidism and decrease indicates hyperthyroidism.
- **Free thyroxine**: (FT4) (0.9-2.4 ng/dL). FT4 is used to confirm TSH abnormalities. Serum T3 (80-180 ng/dL) and T4 (4.5-11.5 mcg/dL). These usually increase together, but T3 more accurately diagnoses hyperthyroidism. T3 resin uptake (25-35%). Increases with hyperthyroidism and decreases with hypothyroidism.

Additional Endocrine Function Studies

There is a wide range of **endocrine function studies**:

- **Pituitary:** Serum levels of pituitary hormones and hormones of target organs, dependent on stimulation by pituitary hormones, are measured to determine abnormalities.
- **Parathyroid:** Parathyroid hormone (PTH) level (10-65 ng/L) and serum calcium levels (8.5-10.2 mg/dL) both increase with hyperparathyroidism. Calcium levels decrease with hypoparathyroidism, and phosphate levels (2.5-4.5 mg/dL) increase.
- **Adrenal**: Catecholamine (urine and serum) levels: Epinephrine (<75 ng/L) and norepinephrine (<100-550 ng/mL) elevate with pheochromocytoma. Electrolyte and glucose levels.
- **ACTH** and **serum cortisol levels** and **ACTH stimulation test** to evaluate for Addison's. Dexamethasone suppression test for Cushing's disease.

Endocrine Pharmacology

Oral Hypoglycemic Agents

Oral hypoglycemic agents are **anti-diabetic treatments** generally used in the treatment of Type II Diabetes. There are five classic categories of oral hypoglycemic agents: sulfonylureas, biguanides, meglitinides, competitive inhibitors of alpha-glucosidases (located in the intestinal brush border), and thiazolidinediones. More recently, two additional novel classes of oral hypoglycemics, DPP-4 inhibitors and SGLT2 inhibitors, were introduced with proven effectiveness when in conjunction with changes in diet and exercise. Some examples of sulfonylurea oral hypoglycemic agents include the first-generation agents tolbutamide, tolazamide, chlorpropamide, and acetohexamide; and second-generation agents glyburide, glimepiride, and glipizide. The biguanide oral hypoglycemic agent is metformin. Metformin has the distinct advantage of not causing weight gain or hypoglycemic reactions. The meglitinide agent is repaglinide. Examples of alpha-glucosidase inhibitors are acarbose and miglitol. Alpha-glucosidase inhibitors bind tightly to intestinal alpha-glucosidases and decrease the post-prandial rise in glucose levels. The only available thiazolidinedione oral hypoglycemic agent is currently pioglitazone; troglitazone was removed from U.S. market in 2000 and rosiglitazone was removed from U.S. market in 2011. Examples of DPP-4 inhibitors include linagliptin, vildagliptin, sitagliptin and saxagliptin. Examples of SGLT2 inhibitors include canagliflozin, dapagliflozin and empagliflozin.

Insulin Used to Treat Glycemic Disorders

There are a number of different types of **insulin** with varying action times. Insulin is used to metabolize **glucose** for those whose pancreases do not produce insulin. People may need to take a combination of insulins (short and long-acting) to maintain glucose control. Duration of action may vary according to the individual's metabolism, intake, and level of activity:

- **Humalog** (Lispro H) is a fast acting, short acting insulin with onset in 5–15 minutes, peaking between 45–90 minutes and lasting 3–4 hours.
- **Regular** (R) is a relatively fast acting insulin with onset in 30 minutes, peaks in 2–5 hours, and lasts 5–8 hours.
- **NPH** (N) insulin is intermediate acting with onset in 1–3 hours, peaking at 6–12 hours, and lasting for 16–24 hours.
- **Insulin Glargine** (Lantus) is a long-acting insulin with onset in 3–6 hours, no peak, and lasting for 24 hours.
- **Combined NPH/Regular** (70/30 or 50/50) has an onset of 30 minutes, peaks at 7–12 hours, and lasts 16–24 hours.

Immunologic and Oncologic Diagnostics

Frozen Sections

Frozen sections are useful in the establishment and staging of a tumor when a decision as to the optimal type of surgical procedure is pending. They also provide information about the completeness of tumor removal post-surgery. They can elucidate the type of tissue involved so that it can be evaluated further, and they can aid in diagnosis through biopsy. However, the use of frozen sections is time-consuming and costly, so they should not be utilized when other options might be more complete or specific. Examination of the sections by a pathologist also has to be taken in context, because it is virtually impossible to examine every portion of the tissue. In addition, the use of freezing can damage tissue architecture and induce distortions.

Immunohistochemistry (IHC)

Immunohistochemistry (IHC) is a technique in which tissue antigens on frozen tissue sections are identified. The antigens are detected by the use of specific antibodies coupled to either fluorescent compounds or pigmented entities, allowing the pathologist to view these interactions on a fluoroscope or through a microscope. There are also various methods of amplifying the interactions, or enzymatically exposing masked antigens to aid in their visualization. IHC is used to distinguish between benign and malignant (antigen-positive) processes and to classify the type of tumor observed. It can also be a useful adjunct in determining the point of origin for the tumor and in identifying small areas that have metastasized. IHC can aid in the evaluation of the future aggressiveness of the tumor through the detection of characteristic nuclear antigens, and it can help predict therapeutic responses by identifying certain receptors, gene products, and proteins.

Fine Needle Aspiration (FNA)

In **fine needle aspiration (FNA),** a small gauge needle is used to extract cells from a tissue area that might be malignant and then the cells are observed microscopically. The procedure is usually done before surgery and is attempted in conjunction with other tools, such as X-rays and laboratory evaluations. FNA is relatively non-invasive and inexpensive. The utility of fine needle aspiration is dependent on the nature of the mass because FNA can only broadly classify it and identify types of cells involved. Other issues, such as the architecture of the mass and its precise classification, are difficult to predict with FNA alone.

Flow Cytometry

Flow cytometry is a method of analyzing populations of cells in suspension for various properties. The cells, such as tumor sample cells, are aspirated into the fluidic system of a machine called a flow cytometer. Here the cells are mixed with a fluid that places them in suspension and a unidirectional or laminar flow is created. As each cell flows past a laser sensor, photons emitted are picked up and intensified by photomultiplier tubes. Data is electronically converted into either histograms or dot plots that compare characteristics of the cells in the population. In addition, fluorochromes are usually injected into the mixture in order to further highlight and identify the cell populations. A fluorochrome is a fluorescent dye, i.e., a substance that absorbs light at a particular wavelength but can emit it at more than one wavelength such as fluorescein isothiocyanate (FITC).

Cytogenetic Analysis

Cytogenetic analysis combines the use of cultured tissues and various precise methodologies in the identification of chromosomal abnormalities. Tissue collection methods are designed to maximize the viability of the tumor cells ex vivo for analysis. Detailed patient information is sent to the laboratory along with the specimen, and the technician then chooses appropriate analysis techniques based upon this information. Usually a bone marrow aspirate (BMA) in sodium heparin is obtained for tumors of hematological origin; two to 3 milliliters of aspirate is generally sufficient. If it is impossible to obtain an adequate BMA (usually due to fibrotic tissue), peripheral blood samples or bone marrow biopsies may be taken instead. Other body fluids or tissues containing tumor cells may also be collected using sterile technique for cytogenetic analysis.

Molecular Diagnostics

Various **molecular diagnostic techniques** are utilized to scrutinize the nucleic acid content or protein gene products in samples from cancer patients. Specific gene mutations have been associated with the presence of many cancers or their presumptive development. The initial step in all these techniques is extraction of nucleic acids by cell disruption. A fresh blood sample is preferable, especially if RNA or DNA content is to be assessed. This decreases the risk of DNA degradation. The anti-coagulants of choice are either ethylenediaminetetraacetic acid (EDTA) or citrate, since heparin can attach to nucleic acids. Some studies further suggest EDTA to be superior to citrate for plasma DNA testing. If fresh samples cannot be promptly analyzed, proper storage conditions are critical. Refrigeration for a few days is generally acceptable, and frozen, liquid nitrogen-stored, or paraffin-embedded older samples can sometimes be used.

Tumor Marker Assays

Tumor marker assays quantify levels of certain molecules found in serum, other body fluids, cells, and tissues that have an association with the presence of malignancy. Most of the available assays are either radioimmunoassays (RIAs) or enzyme-linked immunosorbent assays (ELISAs), which respectively use radioisotopes or enzymes linked to various substances (often specific antibodies) as detection vehicles. The value of these immunoassays depends upon their specificity (i.e., their ability to accurately detect malignancy, versus normal tissue or benign growths) and sensitivity (the capacity for early detection during screening or preliminary diagnosis). The linearity of a test is important as well, as the concentration changes must be quantifiable and directly related to changes in tumor volume or response to treatment. At present, the measurement of cancer or tumor markers is generally more useful in the monitoring of disease, rather than in the initial diagnosis.

Tumor Markers Currently Used in the United States

In order for a tumor marker to be a good candidate for a screening assay, it should be both organ and cancer specific. Some markers—for example, carcinoembryonic antigen or CEA—are indicative of a malignant process, but they are not organ specific. In contrast, prostate specific antigen or total PSA is the ideal tumor marker for early detection or screening purposes because it is unique to the prostate. There is a range (4 to 10 ng/ml) where non-cancerous conditions, such as benign prostatic disease or BPH, can be picked up as well. When total PSA is combined with free PSA (which is lower in men with prostate cancer), the specificity of prostate cancer detection increases dramatically. Similarly, a carbohydrate marker called CA125 is a useful screening marker for ovarian cancer, if it is used in conjunction with other tests such as ultrasound. Thus, PSA and CA125 are valuable in screening settings, particularly if they show increases when measured sequentially. These screening assays are always serum or plasma-based.

Diagnostic and Prognostic Utility of Assays for Tumor Markers

Assays for tumor markers are generally more useful for **disease diagnosis** than screening, especially if they are used in conjunction with other types of tests, such as histology. Many of these markers are good adjuncts to tumor staging. Some of the more useful markers and their associated cancers follow:

- **CA125**: Useful for ovarian cancer diagnosis and monitoring in conjunction with other testing.
- **Alpha-Fetoprotein or AFP**: Informative for distinguishing between various types of germ cell tumors, especially when used together with measurement of *B*-Human chorionic gonadotrophin (*B*-hCG).
- **Carcinoembryonic antigen (CEA)**: Can be elevated in colorectal, breast, and lung carcinomas; however, elevated levels are not tumor specific but can still be of prognostic or monitoring value.
- **Tissue estrogen and progesterone receptors**: Have prognostic utility for the treatment of breast cancer, as test-positive individuals are responsive to antiestrogen therapies.
- **Tissue HER-2/neu**: Is useful in assessment of breast cancer patients for possible treatment with Herceptin.

Imaging Methods for Cancer Detection and Staging

There are advantages and disadvantages to the use of **imaging methods for cancer detection**. One advantage is that imaging methods are non-invasive. This can provide significant benefits in burdens, costs, and time. However, a key disadvantage is that tumor masses must be large enough for visualization by the imaging technique used. This is typically about 3 to 5 millimeters in diameter. Smaller lesions may well be missed. Other detection methods are theoretically much more sensitive. Cytology, for example, can detect a single cancerous cell. Realistically, however, laboratory methods usually only sample a small portion of the overall cancerous mass, whereas imaging techniques permit the technician to look at the entire tumor. Imaging techniques are also very useful in initial staging of the tumor and evaluation of changes after treatment.

Imaging Methods Used in Oncology

The following types of **imaging methods are currently used in oncology:**

- **Traditional radiographs**: Uses X-rays and development on films (or digital methods); useful for detection of bone tumors and lung cancer.
- **Mammography**: As above, but with specialized machinery to detect breast cancer.
- **Computed tomography or CT scans**: Uses a rotating source of X-rays and image digitalization for greater clarity and multiple views.
- **Angiography**: Uses a vascular introduction of iodinated contrast media while taking serial images (generally digital); similar injections can be done with CT scans.
- **Ultrasound**: Utilizes high-frequency sound waves to produce an image; it is most effective in detecting malignancies in the neck and pelvic region or in the gallbladder and liver areas.
- **Magnetic resonance imaging (MRI)**: Uses an electromagnetic field, which excites atomic nuclei, to produce a digitalized image; used primarily for detection of tumors in the brain, spinal cord, and musculoskeletal tissues.
- **Single-photon-emission computed tomography (SPECT):** Use the injection of long half-life radioisotopes (primarily ^{99m}Tc) tracers to look at perfusion into bone or thyroid areas.
- **Positron-emission tomography (PET)**: Uses the injection of positron emitter tracers, usually coupled with agents involved with glycolytic metabolism.

Immunologic and Oncologic Pharmacology

Immunosuppressant Drugs

Drugs	Actions	Side effects
Corticosteroids	Depress cell-mediated immune response, humoral immune response, and inflammation, reducing proliferation of T cells and B cells. Used with transplantations and to prevent GVHD disease.	Weight gain, edema, Cushing syndrome, hyperglycemia, bruising, and osteoporosis. Abruptly stopping drugs may trigger Addisonian crisis.
Ciclosporin	Inhibit activation of T cells. Used to prevent transplantation rejection and to treat autoimmune diseases and nephrotic syndrome.	Tremor, excessive facial hair, gingivitis, bone marrow suppression with increased risk of infection and cancer, especially skin cancer.
Intravenous immuno-globulin G (IVIG)	Used to combat immunosuppression by increasing antibodies to prevent infection or treat acute infection, such as Guillain-Barre. Used off-label for many different disorders and infections.	Dermatitis, headache, renal failure, and venous thrombosis. Infections can occur because IVIG is extracted from pooled plasma.

Review Video: Immunomodulators and Immunosuppressors
Visit mometrix.com/academy and enter code: 666131

Chemotherapy

Chemotherapy may be offered during palliative care to enhance patient comfort, wellbeing, and symptom control for **enhanced quality of life**. It is understood that the treatment is not expected to provide a cure and should not be given as a means to maintain a sense of false hope within the patient or family. It should be clear that the expectation of treatment is **prolonged survival** and **control of cancer-related symptoms**. Not all patients will benefit from palliative chemotherapy. The decision to provide chemotherapy is based on the clinical indicators and the patient's wishes. The benefit and cost ratios of treatment need to be considered. Tumor response to treatment, metastasis, and other disease specific factors will help define chemotherapy's usefulness for an individual patient. Patients also need to be aware that chemotherapy involves a commitment to repeated travel, hospitalizations, invasive procedures, and assessments in order to make an informed decision.

Chemotherapeutic Agents

The major chemotherapy agents are alkylating agents, antimetabolites, plant alkaloids, antitumor antibiotics, and steroid hormones.

- **Alkylating agents** work directly by attacking the DNA of cancers such as chronic leukemias, Hodgkin's disease, lymphomas, and lung, breast, prostate, and ovary cancers.
- **Nitrosoureas** inhibit repair in damaged DNA. They are able to cross the blood-brain barrier and are frequently used to treat brain tumors, lymphomas, multiple myeloma, and malignant melanoma.
- **Antimetabolites** block cell growth. This class of chemotherapeutic drugs is used to treat leukemias, choriocarcinoma, and gastrointestinal, breast, and ovary cancers.

- **Antitumor antibiotics** are a broad category of agents that bind to DNA and prevent RNA synthesis and are used with a wide variety of cancers.
- **Plant (vinca) alkaloids** are extracted from plants and block cell division. These are used to treat acute lymphoblastic leukemia, Hodgkin and non-Hodgkin lymphomas, neuroblastomas, Wilms tumor, and lung, breast, and testes cancers.
- **Steroid hormones** have an unclear action but may be useful in treating hormone-dependent cancers such as ovary and breast cancer.

Routes of Delivery

Chemotherapy treatments may be provided orally, intramuscularly, intravenously, intra-arterially, intralesionally (directly into the tumor), intraperitoneally, intrathecally, or topically. **Oral chemotherapy** is the easiest and often used in the home. **Intravenous delivery** is the most common chemotherapy route but **intramuscular delivery** may have more lasting effects. The goal of **intra-arterial chemotherapy** is to introduce the agent directly into the blood supply feeding the tumor or affected organ. Ovarian cancer with tumors greater than 2 cm in diameter may be treated with **intraperitoneal therapy**. Acute lymphocytic leukemia is primarily treated with **intrathecal administration. Intralesional treatments** are used for melanoma and Kaposi sarcoma. **Topical treatment** is most common with skin cancers.

Side Effects

Not every patient will experience every symptom, or in the same degree. **Side effects** can vary greatly; some can be easily controlled with additional medications. Many side effects are due to the effects of the chemotherapy on **cells**, such as bone marrow, hair, and gastrointestinal cells, which have a rapid mitotic rate and rapid turnover. Common side effects can include bone marrow suppression, hair loss (alopecia), mouth ulcers, sore throat and gums, heartburn, nausea, vomiting, loss of appetite, weight loss, anorexia and cachexia, anemia, nerve and muscle problems, dry or discolored skin, kidney and bladder irritation, fatigue, and increased bruising, bleeding, and infection. The patient's sexual function can also be affected, including possible infertility.

Risks

Infection is a common **concern of chemotherapy** because of the decreased number of **neutrophils** in the patient's system. **Neutropenia** is silent but dangerous, leaving no neutrophils to fight the threat of infections. Neutropenia can cause a septic situation, which can be life-threatening. Severe **anemia** may result in the need for blood transfusions. **Neurological damage** may include mild alterations in taste or smell, peripheral neuropathy, mental status changes, or seizures. Some anticancer drugs can cause **heart damage** if not monitored closely. Many anticancer drugs cause **kidney damage**, as well as increasing the risk of drug toxicity from decreased renal function. Anticancer drugs can also cause **cataracts** and **retina damage**.

Palliative Sedation

Palliative sedation is a treatment method focused on controlling and easing symptoms that have proven otherwise refractory or unendurable in nature. This process was originally named **terminal sedation**. It was changed to palliative sedation to emphasize the differences between symptom management and euthanasia. The purpose of palliative sedation is **symptom control**; it does not hasten or cause death. Through the monitored use of medications such as midazolam or propofol, relief can be provided through varying levels of unconsciousness. Among terminally ill patients, palliative sedation is most often used to calm persistent agitation and restlessness. The second most frequent need is for pain control, followed by confusion, shortness of breath, muscle twitching or seizures, and anguish.

Hematologic Diagnostics

Red Blood Cells

Red blood cells (RBCs or erythrocytes) are biconcave disks that contain **hemoglobin** (95% of mass), which carries oxygen throughout the body. The heme portion of the cell contains **iron**, which binds to the oxygen. RBCs live about 120 days, after which they are destroyed and their hemoglobin is recycled or excreted. Normal values of red blood cell count vary by gender:

- Males >18 years: 4.7-6.1 million per mm^3
- Females >18 years: 4.2-5.4 million per mm^3

The most common **disorders of RBCs** are those that interfere with production, leading to various types of **anemia**:

- Blood loss
- Hemolysis
- Bone marrow failure

The **morphology** of RBCs may vary depending upon the type of anemia:

- Size: Normocytes, microcytes, macrocytes
- Shape: Spherocytes (round), poikilocytes (irregular), drepanocytes (sickled)
- Color (reflecting concentration of hemoglobin): Normochromic, hypochromic

Laboratory Tests

A number of different tests are used to evaluate the condition and production of red blood cells in addition to the red blood cell count.

Hemoglobin: Carries oxygen and is decreased in anemia and increased in polycythemia. Normal values:

- Males >18 years: 14.0-17.46 g/dL
- Females >18 years: 12.0-16.0 g/dL

Hematocrit: Indicates the proportion of RBCs in a liter of blood (usually about 3 times the hemoglobin number). Normal values:

- Males >18 years: 40%-50%
- Females >18 years: 35%-45%

Mean corpuscular volume (MCV): Indicates the size of RBCs and can differentiate types of anemia. For adults, <80 is microcytic and >100 is macrocytic. Normal values:

- Males >18 years: 84-96 μm^3
- Females >18 years: 76-96 μm^3

Reticulocyte count: Measures marrow production and should rise with anemia. Normal values: 0.5%-1.5% of total RBCs.

WBC Count and Differential

White blood cell (leukocyte) count is used as an indicator of bacterial and viral infection. WBC count is reported as the total number of all white blood cells.

- Normal WBC for adults: 4,800-10,000
- Acute infection: 10,000+; 30,000 indicates a severe infection
- Viral infection: 4,000 and below

The **differential** provides the percentage of each different type of leukocyte. An increase in the white blood cell count is usually related to an increase in one type, and often an increase in immature neutrophils (bands), referred to as a "shift to the left," is an indication of an infectious process:

- Normal immature neutrophils (bands): 1%-3%, increases with infection
- Normal segmented neutrophils (segs) for adults: 50%-62%, increases with acute, localized, or systemic bacterial infections
- Normal eosinophils: 0%-3%, decreases with stress and acute infection
- Normal basophils: 0%-1%, decreases during acute stage of infection
- Normal lymphocytes: 25%-40%, increases in some viral and bacterial infections
- Normal monocytes: 3%-7%, increases during recovery stage of acute infection

C-Reactive Protein and Erythrocyte Sedimentation Rate

C-reactive protein is an acute-phase reactant produced by the liver in response to an inflammatory response that causes neutrophils, granulocytes, and macrophages to secrete cytokines. Thus, levels of C-reactive protein rise when there is inflammation or infection. It is helpful to measure the response to treatment for pyoderma gangrenosum ulcers:

- Normal values: 2.6-7.6 µg/dL

Erythrocyte sedimentation rate (sed rate) measures the distance erythrocytes fall in a vertical tube of anticoagulated blood in one hour. Because fibrinogen, which increases in response to infection, slows the fall, the sed rate can be used as a non-specific test for inflammation when infection is suspected. The sed rate is sensitive to osteomyelitis and may be used to monitor treatment response. Values vary according to gender and age:

- <50: Males 0-15 mm/hr; females 0-20 mm/hr
- >50: Males 0-20 mm/hr; females 0-30 mm/hr

Elements of the Coagulation Profile

The **coagulation profile** measures clotting mechanisms, identifies clotting disorders, screens preoperative patients, and diagnoses excessive bruising and bleeding. Values vary depending on lab:

- **Prothrombin time (PT)**: 10-14 seconds
    - Increases with anticoagulation therapy, vitamin K deficiency, decreased prothrombin, DIC, liver disease, and malignant neoplasm. Some drugs may shorten PT.

- **Partial thromboplastin time (PTT)**: 25-35 seconds
  - Increases with hemophilia A and B, von Willebrand disease, vitamin deficiency, lupus, DIC, and liver disease.
- **Activated partial thromboplastin time (aPTT)**: 21-35 seconds
  - Similar to PTT, but decreases in extensive cancer, early DIC, and after acute hemorrhage. Used to monitor heparin dosage.
- **Thrombin clotting time (TCT) or Thrombin time (TT)**: 7-12 seconds
  - Used most often to determine the dosage of heparin. Prolonged with multiple myeloma, abnormal fibrinogen, uremia, and liver disease.
- **Bleeding time**: 2-9.5 minutes
  - (Using the IVY method on the forearm) Increases with DIC, leukemia, renal failure, aplastic anemia, von Willebrand disease, some drugs, and alcohol.
- **Platelet count**: 150,000-400,000 per μL
  - Increased bleeding <50,000 (transfusion required) and increased clotting >750,000.

Hematologic Procedures and Interventions

Transfusion Components

Blood components that are commonly used for transfusions include:

- **Packed red blood cells:** RBCs (250-300 mL per unit) should be warmed >30 °C (optimal 37 °C) before administration to prevent hypothermia and may be reconstituted in 50-100 mL of normal saline to facilitate administration. RBCs are necessary if blood loss is about 30% (1,500-2,000 mL lost; Hgb ≤7). Above 30% blood loss, whole blood may be more effective. RBCs are most frequently used for transfusions.
- **Platelet concentrates:** Transfusions of platelets are used if the platelet count is <50,000 cells/mm^3. One unit increases the platelet count by 5,000-10,000 cells/mm^3. Platelet concentrates pose a risk for sensitization reactions and infectious diseases. Platelet concentrate is stored at a higher temperature (20-24 °C) than RBCs. This contributes to bacterial growth, so it is more prone to bacterial contamination than other blood products and may cause sepsis. Temperature increase within 6 hours should be considered an indication of possible sepsis. ABO compatibility should be observed but is not required.
- **Fresh frozen plasma** (FFP) (obtained from a unit of whole blood frozen ≤6 hours after collection) includes all clotting factors and plasma proteins, so each unit administered increases clotting factors by 2-3%. FFP may be used for deficiencies of isolated factors, excess warfarin therapy, and liver-disease-related coagulopathy. It may be used for patients who have received extensive blood transfusions but continue to hemorrhage. It is also helpful for those with antithrombin III deficiency. FFP should be warmed to 37 °C prior to administration to avoid hypothermia. ABO compatibility should be observed if possible, but it is not required. Some patients may become sensitized to plasma proteins.
- **Cryoprecipitate** is the precipitate that forms when FFP is thawed. It contains fibrinogen, factor VIII, von Willebrand, and factor XIII. This component may be used to treat hemophilia A and hypofibrinogenemia.

Autotransfusion

Autotransfusion (autologous blood transfusion) is collecting of the patient's blood and re-infusing it. This is life-saving if another donor's blood is not available. Blood in trauma cases is usually collected from a body cavity, such as pleural (hemothorax with ≥1,500 mL blood) or peritoneal space (rare). Autotransfusion is contraindicated if malignant lesions are present in the area of blood loss, contamination of pooled blood, or wounds >4-6 hours old. Commercial collection/transfusion kits (Pleur-Evac®, Thora-Klex®) are available, but blood can be collected through the chest tube into a sterile bottle, which is then disconnected and connected to IV tubing for infusion, or the blood in the bottle may be transferred to a blood collection bag for use. Commercial kits use either a chest tube or suction tube to withdraw blood and provide specific procedures. Blood is filtered. Heparin is not routinely used, but citrate phosphate dextrose (CPD) (25-70 mL per 500 mL blood) is often added to the aspirant to prevent clotting. Complications from autotransfusion are rare.

Plasmapheresis

With **plasmapheresis,** whole blood is removed from the body, anticoagulant is added, cellular components are separated from the plasma (which is removed), and cellular components are suspended in saline, albumin (most common), or another substitute for plasma. This is reinfused into the patient. The purpose is to remove harmful antibodies found in plasma. ACE inhibitors increase risk of hypotension and should be withheld for 24 hours before the procedure. Machine settings may vary. Typically, the patient's height and weight are entered into the automated system to aid in calculating the plasma volume. The patient must be carefully monitored during the procedure for signs of hypocalcemia (perioral/fingertip tingling, alterations in mental status, VT), which requires the administration of calcium; hypomagnesemia (confusion, headaches, dizziness, twitching), which requires administration of magnesium; and hypotension, which requires saline bolus. If the patient shows indications of transfusion reaction, the infusion must be discontinued and medications (diphenhydramine, corticosteroids) administered. The patient should be kept warm to avoid hypothermia. Post-procedure, the patient may experience thrombocytopenia and hypofibrinogenemia, so the patient must be observed for signs of bleeding.

Exchange Transfusion

Exchange transfusions replace a person's blood with donor blood to remove sickled blood for sickle cell anemia or to remove toxins. The exchange may be complete or partial. An automated machine is generally used, and the time on the machine ranges from 1 to 4 hours. (If done manually, removal and replacement are done in cycles with blood first removed followed by replacement.) A catheter is inserted (usually in the arm) to drain the blood and another, usually in the femoral area (under local or moderate sedation), to administer donor blood, plasma, or another substitute for plasma. During the exchange, the patient's VS must be carefully monitored. If the patient exhibits signs of hypocalcemia (perioral/finger tingling) then calcium is administered. Some may receive calcium routinely during administration. Blood may be taken from the femoral line for testing after the exchange. When the femoral catheter is removed, pressure must be applied to the area for at least 5 minutes and the patient instructed to lie flat for at least 30 minutes to prevent bleeding.

Leukocyte Depletion

Red blood cell and platelet transfusions typically contain some leukocytes, which are recognized as foreign by the immune system of a patient receiving the transfusion. This can lead to adverse reactions, especially in patients who are immunocompromised. **Leukocyte depletion** is carried out by various processes, including filtration. One disadvantage to leukodepletion of RBCs is that the process results in the loss of about 10% of the RBCs, and some hemolysis may occur. Leukocyte depleted RBCs are given in volumes of 200 to 250 mL within a 4-hour time period.

Transfusion Administration

Prior to the transfusion of any blood component, the nurse should obtain the patient's transfusion history along with a consent form. A type and crossmatch must be completed on the patient's blood and an IV in place for administration. An 18-gauge catheter is standard, but 22-gauge can also be used at a slower rate. Baseline vital signs need to be taken prior to starting the infusion, and then the patient should be under direct observation for at least the first 15 minutes. Vital signs should be monitored at 5 minutes, 15 minutes, and then at least every 30 minutes during the transfusion and one hour post-transfusion.

Blood Conservation

Blood conservation includes methods to:

- **Minimize the loss of blood during surgical procedures**: May include regional anesthesia instead of general, positioning to reduce blood loss, cell salvage, autotransfusion, non-invasive monitoring (BP, pulse oximetry), limited blood draws, normovolemic hemodilution, and medications to reduce bleeding (vitamin K, tranexamic acid, desmopressin, somatostatin, vasopressin, recombinant factor VIIa).
- **Lower the threshold for receiving transfusions**: Transfusion threshold lowered from 10 to 7 g/dL.
- **Maintain the hematocrit at acceptable levels**: Administration of oral or parenteral iron therapy to increase tolerance for blood loss. Erythropoietin alpha may also be administered perioperatively to stimulate the production of RBCs.
- **Ensure optimal oxygenation of tissue**: Hyperoxic ventilation during surgery, crystalloid/colloid volume replacement, and utilizing techniques to minimize consumption of oxygen.

Blood conservation includes a commitment to bloodless surgery as much as possible, especially through the utilization of minimally-invasive procedures.

Massive Transfusion Protocol

A massive transfusion protocol (MTP) is a proactive standardized protocol used during an uncontrolled hemorrhage, designed to ensure effective management of massive blood loss and to improve patient outcome.

Indications for activation of **massive transfusion protocol** (MTP) include:

- Uncontrolled hemorrhage.
- Actual/anticipated use of ≥4 units of RBCs in less than 4 hours or ≥10 units in 24 hours (some may need up to 30 units in 8 hours).
- Hemodynamic instability despite initial management of bleeding and resuscitation efforts that should include avoiding hypothermia and the use of excessive crystalloid.
- Allowing permissive hypotension to 80-100 systolic BP to help control bleeding. Autotransfusion may be used when appropriate.

Protocols may vary somewhat:

- MTPs are activated by a clinician in response to massive bleeding, generally after transfusion of 4-10 units.
- Obtain baseline laboratory tests (CBC, coagulation screen, blood gases, and chemistry panel) and repeat CBC, blood gases, coagulation screen, and ionized calcium test hourly.
- MTP packs have a predetermined ratio (e.g. 1:1:1 or 2:1:1 ratio) of RBCs, FFPs, and platelet units for transfusion, prepared by the blood bank for rapid and timely delivery.
- Targets of resuscitation include:
    - Mean arterial pressure (MAP) around 60 mmHg
    - Core temperature >35° C
    - Hemoglobin 7–9 g/dL
    - pH 7.35–7.45
    - Lactate <4 mmol/L
    - Calcium >1.1 mmol/L
    - Platelets >50,000
    - PT/aPTT <1.5 times normal
    - INR ≤1.5
    - Fibrinogen >1.5–2.0 g/L

Transfusion-Related Complications

There are a number of **transfusion-related complications**, which is the reason that transfusions are given only when necessary. Complications include:

- **Infection**: Bacterial contamination of blood, especially platelets, can result in severe sepsis. A number of infective agents (viral, bacterial, and parasitic) can be transmitted, although increased testing of blood has decreased rates of infection markedly. Infective agents include HIV, hepatitis C and B, human T-cell lymphotropic virus, CMV, WNV, malaria, Chagas' disease, and variant Creutzfeldt-Jacob disease (from contact with mad cow disease).
- **Transfusion-related acute lung injury (TRALI):** This respiratory distress syndrome occurs ≤6 hours after transfusion. The cause is believed to be antileukocytic or anti-HLA antibodies in the transfusion. It is characterized by non-cardiogenic pulmonary edema (high protein level) with severe dyspnea and arterial hypoxemia. Transfusion must be stopped immediately and the blood bank notified. TRALI may result in fatality but usually resolves in 12-48 hours with supportive care.
- **Graft vs. host disease:** Lymphocytes cause an immune response in immunocompromised individuals. Lymphocytes may be inactivated by irradiation, as leukocyte filters are not reliable.
- **Post-transfusion purpura:** Platelet antibodies develop and destroy the patient's platelets, so the platelet count decreases about 1 week after transfusion.
- **Transfusion-related immunosuppression:** Cell-mediated immunity is suppressed, so the patient is at increased risk of infection, and in cancer patients, transfusions may correlate with tumor recurrence. This condition relates to transfusions that include leukocytes. RBCs cause a less pronounced immunosuppression, suggesting a causative agent is in the plasma. Leukoreduction is becoming more common to reduce transmission of leukocyte-related viruses.
- **Hypothermia**: This may occur if blood products are not heated. Oxygen utilization is halved for each 10 °C decrease in normal body temperature.

Hematologic Pharmacology

ANTICOAGULANTS

Common **anticoagulants** used at home and in the hospital setting are discussed below, including possible complications and the antidotes for each:

- **Antithrombin activators**: Heparin (unfractionated) and derivatives, LWM (Dalteparin, Enoxaparin, tinzaparin), and Fondaparinux.
  - Possible complications: Thrombocytopenia, bleeding/hemorrhage, osteopenia, hypersensitivity.
  - Antidote: Protamine sulfate 1% solution—dosage varies according to drug and drug's dosage. (1 mg protamine neutralizes 100 units of heparin or 1 mg of enoxaparin.)
- **Direct thrombin inhibitors**: Hirudin analogs (bivalirudin, desirudin, lepirudin). Others: Apixaban, Argatroban, and dabigatran.
  - Possible complications: Bleeding/hemorrhage, GI upset, backpain, hypertension, headache.
  - No antidote is available.
- **Direct Xa inhibitor**: Rivaroxaban
  - Possible complications: Bleeding/hemorrhage.
  - No antidote is available.
- **Antithrombin (AT)**: Recombinant human AT, Plasma-derived AT
  - Possible complications: Bleeding/hemorrhage, hypersensitivity.
  - No antidote is available.
- **Warfarin**
  - Possible complications: Bleeding/hemorrhage. Drug interactions may cause thrombosis or increased risk of bleeding.
  - Antidote: Vitamin K_1 usually at 2.5 mg PO or 0.5–1.0 mg IV. If ineffective, FFP or fresh whole blood may be administered.

HEPARIN

PHARMACOLOGY

Heparin is an **anticoagulant** derived from the intestinal mucosa of the pig and the lung of the pig. The mechanism of action of heparin is to bind to the surface of the endothelial cell membrane. The activity of heparin depends upon plasma protease inhibitor antithrombin III. Antithrombin III inhibits thrombin and other anti-clotting proteases. In addition, heparin binding causes a change in antithrombin III inhibitor form, resulting in increased antithrombin-protease complex formation activity. After antithrombin-protease complex formation, heparin is subsequently released and is available to bind to more antithrombin molecules.

RISK FACTORS

The major **risk factor** of **heparin** use is hemorrhage. Predisposing factors for hemorrhage include advanced age and renal failure. Prolonged use of heparin can result in osteoporosis and fractures. Other risk factors of heparin use include transient thrombocytopenia, severe thrombocytopenia, paradoxical thromboembolism, and heparin-induced aggregation of platelets. These risks can be reduced by careful selection of patients who receive heparin therapy, careful control of the dosage of heparin, and meticulous monitoring of the partial thromboplastin time, or PTT. It is important to remember that thrombocytopenia or the development of a thrombus may be due to heparin itself.

CONTRAINDICATIONS

There are numerous **contraindications** to the use of **heparin**, including: hypersensitivity to heparin; diseases of the hematologic system (hemophilia, purpura, or thrombocytopenia); uncontrolled hypertension; intracranial bleed; infectious endocarditis; active tuberculosis; gastrointestinal ulcers; cancer of the gastrointestinal visceral organs; severe liver dysfunction; severe kidney dysfunction; and threatened miscarriage or abortion. Heparin is contraindicated in the following medical procedures: following brain surgery; following spinal cord surgery; following eye surgery; after a lumbar puncture; and after regional anesthesia blocks. The effects of heparin may be reversed by stopping heparin or by the use of a specific antagonist (protamine sulfate).

Review Video: Heparin - An Injectable Anti-Coagulant
Visit mometrix.com/academy and enter code: 127426

WARFARIN

PHARMACOLOGY

Warfarin causes a deficiency in prothrombin in the plasma and is used as an **anti-thrombotic agent** and to decrease the risk of embolism in humans. This agent causes the liver to manufacture less of the proteins necessary for blood coagulation. Since it is 99% bound to albumin in the plasma, warfarin has a high bio-availability. The mechanism of action of warfarin involves prothrombin, factor VII, factor IX, factor X, and protein C. Warfarin inhibits the g-carboxylation of the glutamate residues in the aforementioned factors. The mechanism of action of warfarin also involves vitamin K. Warfarin has a slow onset of action, usually 24 hours, and a typical duration of 2 to 5 days. Using increased dosages of warfarin as loading dosages will serve to speed up the onset of anti-coagulation. Patients on warfarin must discontinue this medication five days before planned surgery due to its longer duration.

DRUG-DRUG INTERACTIONS

Warfarin has many **drug-drug interactions**, the most serious of which increases the risk of bleeding. Sulfinpyrazone and phenylbutazone interact with warfarin to cause enhanced decrease in prothrombin, increased inhibition of platelets, and increased risk of peptic ulcer. The following drugs can have adverse effects when co-administered with warfarin: antibiotics such as metronidazole, azithromycin, clarithromycin, dirithromycin, erythromycin, roxithromycin, and telithromycin; broad-spectrum antibiotics such as amoxicillin, imipenem, levofloxacin; antifungal agents such as fluconazole, miconazole, and ketoconazole; barbiturates; and trimethoprim-sulfamethoxazole, amiodarone, cimetidine, and disulfiram. Aspirin inhibits metabolism of the warfarin and nonsteroidal anti-inflammatory drugs (NSAIDs) inhibit the clotting of platelets. The third-generation cephalosporins increase the risk of bleeding with warfarin because these drugs destroy the intestinal bacteria that produce vitamin K. Always check on possible drug-drug interactions when administering warfarin and monitor patients who might be at risk.

Review Video: Warfarin: Most Popular Anticoagulant?
Visit mometrix.com/academy and enter code: 844117

THROMBOLYTICS

Thrombolytics are drugs used to dissolve clots in myocardial infarction, ischemic stroke, DVT, and pulmonary embolism. Thrombolytics may be given in combination with heparin or low-weight heparin to increase anticoagulation effect. Thrombolytics should be administered within 90 minutes but may be given up to 6 hours after an event. They may increase the danger of hemorrhage and are contraindicated with hemorrhagic strokes, recent surgery, or bleeding. Thrombolytics include:

- **Alteplase tissue-type plasminogen activator** (t-PA) (Activase®) is an enzyme that converts plasminogen to plasmin, which is a fibrinolytic enzyme. t-PA is used for ischemic stroke, MI, and pulmonary embolism and must be given IV within 3–4.5 hours or by catheter directly to the site of occlusion within 6 hours.
- **Anistreplase** (Eminase®) is used for treatment of acute MI and is given intravenously in a 30-unit dose over 2–5 minutes.
- **Reteplase** (Retavase®) is a plasminogen activator used after MI to prevent CHF (contraindicated for ischemic strokes). It is given in 2 doses, a 10-unit bolus over 2 minutes and then repeated in 30 minutes.
- **Streptokinase** (Streptase®) is used for pulmonary emboli, acute MI, intracoronary thrombi, DVT, and arterial thromboembolism. It should be given within 4 hours but can be given after up to 24 hours. Intravenous infusion is usually 1,500,000 units in 60 minutes. Intracoronary infusion is done with an initial 20,000-unit bolus and then 2000 units per minute for 60 minutes.
- **Tenecteplase** (TNKase®) is used to treat acute MI with large ST elevation. It is administered in a one-time bolus over 5 seconds and should be administered within 30 minutes of the event.

Contraindications to thrombolytic therapy include:

- Evidence of cerebral or subarachnoid hemorrhage or other internal bleeding or history of intracranial hemorrhage, recent stroke, head trauma, or surgery (ruled out by CT scan before administration for ischemic stroke)
- Uncontrolled hypertension, seizures
- Intracranial AVM, neoplasm, or aneurysm
- Current anticoagulation therapy
- Low platelet count (<100,000 mm^3)

Gastrointestinal Diagnostics

Liver Function Studies

Liver function studies are described below:

- **Bilirubin:** Determines the ability of the liver to conjugate and excrete bilirubin: direct 0.0–0.3 mg/dL, total 0.0–0.9 mg/dL, and urine bilirubin which should be 0.
- **Total protein:** Normal: 6.0–8.0 g/dL (Albumin: 4.0–5.5 g/dL, Globulin: 1.7–3.3 g/dL). Normal albumin/globulin (A/G) ratio: 1.5:1 to 2.5:1, measured by serum protein electrophoresis.
- **Prothrombin time (PT):** 100% or clot detection in 10 to 14 seconds. PT increases with liver disease. International normalized ratio (INR) (PT result/normal average): <2 for those not receiving anticoagulation; 2.0–3.0 for those receiving anticoagulation; critical value >3 in patients receiving anticoagulation therapy.
- **Alkaline phosphatase:** 36–93 units/L in adults. (Normal values vary with method.) Indicates biliary tract obstruction if no bone disease.
- **AST (SGOT):** 10–40 units. (Increases with liver cell damage.)
- **ALT (SGPT):** 5–35 units. (Increases with liver cell damage.)

- **GGT, GGTP:** 5–55 μ/L females, 5–85 μ/L males. (Increases with alcohol abuse.)
- **LDH:** 100–200 units. (Increases with alcohol abuse.)
- **Serum ammonia:** 150–250 mg/dL (Increases with liver failure.)
- **Cholesterol:** Increases with bile duct obstruction and decrease with parenchymal disease.

Nutritional Lab Monitoring

Total Protein and Albumin

Total protein levels can be influenced by many factors, including stress and infection, but it may be monitored as part of an overall nutritional assessment. Protein is critical for general health and wound healing, and because metabolic rate increases in response to a wound, protein needs increase:

- Normal values: 6–8 g/dL
- Diet requirements for wound healing: 1.25–1.5 g/kg/day

Albumin is a protein that is produced by the liver and is a necessary component for cells and tissues. Levels decrease with renal disease, malnutrition, and severe burns. Albumin levels are the most common screening to determine protein levels. Albumin has a half-life of 18–20 days, so it is sensitive to long-term protein deficiencies more than short-term.

- Normal values: 3.5–5.5 g/dL
- Mild deficiency: 3.0–3.5 g/dL
- Moderate deficiency: 2.5–3.0 g/dL
- Severe deficiency: <2.5 g/dL

Levels below 3.2 correlate with increased morbidity and death. Dehydration (poor intake, diarrhea, or vomiting) elevates levels, so adequate hydration is important to ensure meaningful results.

Prealbumin

Prealbumin (transthyretin) is most commonly monitored for acute changes in nutritional status because it has a half-life of only 2–3 days. Prealbumin is a protein produced in the liver, so it is often decreased with liver disease. Oral contraceptives and estrogen can also decrease levels. Levels may rise with Hodgkin's disease or the use of steroids or NSAIDS. Prealbumin is necessary for transportation of both thyroxine and vitamin A throughout the body, so if prealbumin levels fall, both thyroxine and vitamin A utilization are also affected:

- Normal values: 16–40 mg/dL
- Mild deficiency: 10–15 mg/dL
- Moderate deficiency: 5–9 mg/dL
- Severe deficiency: <5 mg/dL

Prealbumin is a good measurement because it quickly decreases when nutrition is inadequate and rises quickly in response to increased protein intake. Protein intake must be adequate to maintain levels of prealbumin. Death rates increase with any decrease in prealbumin levels.

Transferrin

Transferrin, which transports about one-third of the body's iron, is a protein produced by the liver. It transports **iron** from the intestines to the bone marrow where it is used to produce **hemoglobin**. The half-life of transferrin is about 8–10 days. It is sometimes used as a measure of nutritional status; however, transferrin levels are sensitive to many factors. Levels rapidly decrease with protein malnutrition. Liver disease and anemia can also depress levels, but a decrease in iron, commonly found with inadequate protein, stimulates the liver to produce more transferrin, which increases transferrin levels but also decreases production of albumin and prealbumin. Transferrin levels may also increase with pregnancy, use of oral contraceptives, and polycythemia. Thus, transferrin levels alone are not always reliable measurements of nutritional status:

- Normal values: 200–400 mg/dL
- Mild deficiency: 150–200 mg/dL
- Moderate deficiency: 100–150 mg/dL
- Severe deficiency: <100 mg/dL

EGD

Esophagogastroduodenoscopy (EGD) with a flexible fiberscope equipped with a lighted fiberoptic lens allows direct inspection of the mucosa of the esophagus, stomach, and duodenum. The scope has a still or video camera attached to a monitor for viewing during the procedure. The scope may be used for biopsies or therapeutically to dilate strictures or treat gastric or esophageal bleeding. The patient is positioned on the left side (head supported) to allow saliva drainage. Conscious sedation (midazolam, propofol) is commonly used along with a topical anesthetic spray or gargle to facilitate placing the lubricated tube through the mouth into the esophagus. Atropine reduces secretions. A bite guard in the mouth prevents the patient from biting the scope. The airway must be carefully monitored through the procedure (which usually takes about 30 minutes), including oximeter to measure oxygen saturation. While perforation, bleeding, or infection may occur, most complications are cardiopulmonary in nature and relate to drugs (conscious sedation) used during the procedure, so reversal agents (flumazenil, naloxone) should be available.

Review Video: GI Diagnostic Procedures
Visit mometrix.com/academy and enter code: 645436

Gastrointestinal Procedures and Interventions

NG Tubes, Sump Tubes, and Levin Tubes

Nasogastric **(NG) tubes** are plastic or vinyl tubes inserted through the nose, down the esophagus, and into the stomach. **Sump tubes** are radiopaque with a vent lumen to prevent a vacuum from forming with high suction. **Levin tubes** have no vent lumen and are used only with low suction. NG tubes drain gastric secretions, allow sampling of secretions, or provide access to the stomach and upper GI tract. They are used for lavage after medication overdose, for decompression, and for instillation of medications or fluids. NG tubes are contraindicated with obstruction proximal to the stomach or gastric pathology, such as hemorrhage.

Tube-insertion length is estimated: earlobe to xiphoid + earlobe to nose tip + 15 cm.

The tube is inserted through the naris with the patient upright, if possible, and swallowing sips of water. Vasoconstrictors and topical anesthetic reduce gag reflex. Placement is checked with insufflation of air or aspiration of stomach contents and verified by x-ray. The NG is secured and drainage bag provided. Tubes attached to continuous low or intermittent high suction must be monitored frequently.

Levin Tube

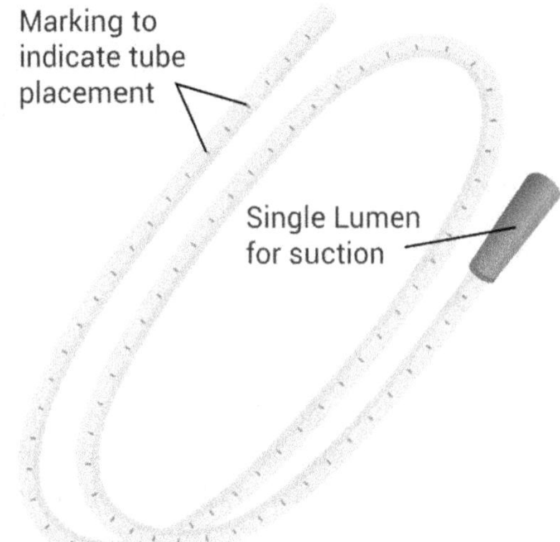

PEG Tube

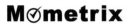

Percutaneous endoscopic gastrostomy (PEG), used for tube feedings, involves intubation of the esophagus with the endoscope and insertion of a sheathed needle with a guidewire through the abdomen and stomach wall so that a catheter can be fed down the esophagus, snared, and pulled out through the opening where the needle was inserted and secured. The PEG tube should not be secured to the abdomen until the PEG is fully healed, which usually takes 2 to 4 weeks, because tension caused by taping the tube against the abdomen may cause the tract to change shape and direction. The tract should be straight to facilitate insertion and removal of catheters. Once the tract has healed, the original PEG tube can generally be replaced with a balloon gastrostomy tube. External stabilizing devices can be applied to the skin to hold the tube in place but should be placed 1 to 2 cm above the skin surface to prevent excessive tension that may result in buried bumper syndrome (BBS) in which the internal fixation device becomes lodged in the mucosal lining of the gastric wall, resulting in ulceration.

DRAINS

The following are different **types of drains** a patient may have, including pertinent nursing considerations:

- **Simple drains** are latex or vinyl tubes of varying sizes/lengths. They are usually placed through a stab wound near the area of involvement.
- **Penrose drains** are flat, soft rubber/latex tubes placed in surgical wounds to drain fluid by gravity and capillary action.

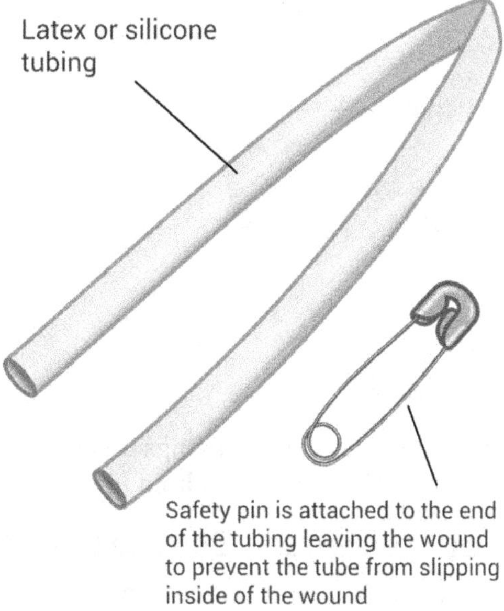
Latex or silicone tubing
Safety pin is attached to the end of the tubing leaving the wound to prevent the tube from slipping inside of the wound

- **Sump drains** are double-lumen or tri-lumen tubes (with a third lumen for infusions). The multiple lumens produce venting when air enters the inflow lumen and forces drainage out of the large lumen.
- **A percutaneous drainage catheter** is inserted into the wound to provide continuous drainage for infection/fluid collection. Irrigation of the catheter may be required to maintain patency. Skin barriers and pouching systems may also be necessary.

SAFE PERCUTANEOUS DRAINAGE KIT

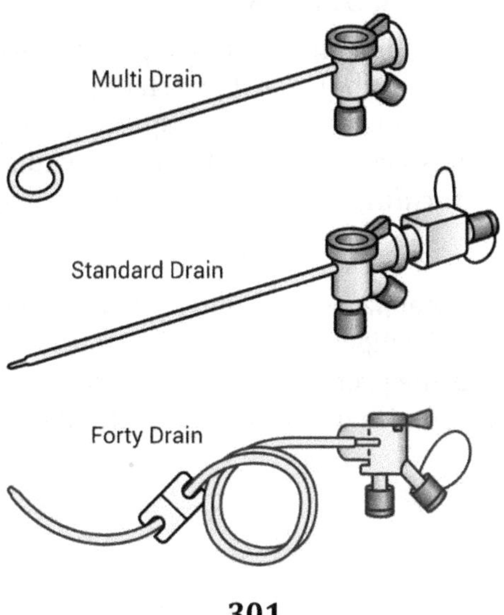
Multi Drain
Standard Drain
Forty Drain

- **Closed drainage systems** use low-pressure suction to provide continuous gravity drainage of wounds. Drains are attached to collapsible suction reservoirs that provide negative pressure. The nurse must remember to always re-establish negative pressure after emptying these drains. There are two types in frequent use:
    - *Jackson-Pratt® is* a bulb-type drain that is about the size of a lemon. A thin plastic drain from the wound extends to a squeeze bulb that can hold about 100 mL of drainage.

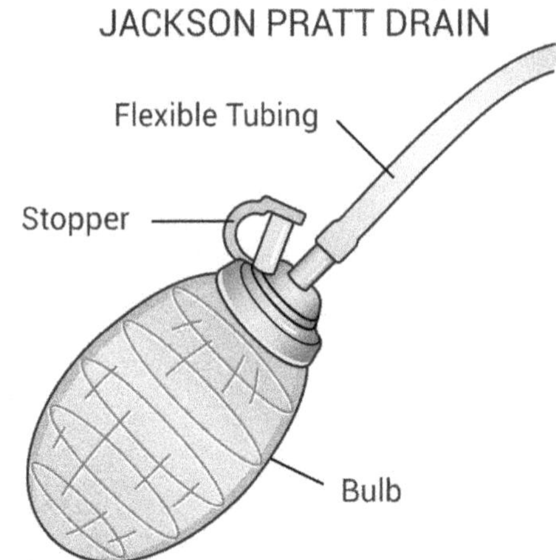

    - *Hemovac®* is a round drain with coiled springs inside that are compressed after emptying to create suction. The device can hold up to 500 mL of drainage.

Determining the Caloric Requirements of Critically Ill Patients

When an individual requires hospitalization for a critical illness, his or her **caloric requirements** must be determined so that normal body function is maintained, and so that recovery is as quick as possible. There are many factors that must be considered when attempting to determine the requirements of an ill patient. First, the **age** of the patient is important. If the patient is a growing child or adolescent, he or she will have very different nutritional requirements than an elderly individual would have. Also, to be considered is the **physical and nutritional status** of the patient, independent of the illness. A patient who is normally very active would have different requirements than an overweight, sedentary individual. Along the same lines, **comorbidities**, such as diabetes and atherosclerosis, need to be considered, as well as overall **stress levels** of the patient.

Enteral Support and Parenteral Support

Enteral nutrition is a method of providing nutrition to a patient through a tube; the tube may be placed in either the nose (a nasogastric tube), the stomach (a percutaneous endoscopic gastrostomy [PEG] tube), or the small bowel (a percutaneous endoscopic jejunal [J] tube). When the tube has been placed, nutrition can be administered through the tube and absorbed by the patient's digestive system. Various **enteric formulas** exist, and the choice is dependent on the nutritional requirements of the patient.

Parenteral nutrition (also called total parenteral nutrition [**TPN**]) is a method of providing nutrition that completely bypasses the digestive system by administering nutrition through an intravenous line. Enteral support is the preferred method of providing nutrition, although in patients suffering from some compromise of the gastrointestinal tract, parenteral nutrition is the only option.

Trouble-Shooting Problems Related to Enteral Feedings

Feeding tubes are commonly found in the critical care setting, as many patients are intubated and unable to take oral nutrition or medication. General maintenance involves checking placement before flushing anything into the tube (prevents aspiration), flushing the tubes with at least 30 mL of water before and after use, and every 4 hours. Never crush enteric-coated medications, and keep the HOB inclined at least 30° at all times during feeding. **Complications** include:

- **Vomiting/aspiration:** Caused by incorrect placement, gastric emptying, and/or formula intolerance.
    - Treatment: Confirm placement by checking pH (preferred to air bolus); delay feeding one hour and check residual volume before resuming. Refrigerate formula, check expiration, and use only for 24 hours.
- **Diarrhea:** Caused by rapid feeding, antibiotics/medications, intolerance of formula or hypertonic formula, and/or tube migration.
    - Treatment: Reduce rate of feeding, evaluate medications, avoid hanging feedings longer than 8 hours, and add fiber or decrease sodium in the feed.
- **Displacement of tube**:
    - Treatment: For NG tube, replace using the other nostril, only if not surgically placed. For G-tube or J-tube, cover the site and notify the physician.
    - Prevention: secure all tubes with the appropriate device and mark placement to identify migration.
- **Tube occlusion**:
    - Treatment: Check for kinks and obvious problems. Aspirate fluid, instill warm water, and aspirate to loosen occlusion. The physician may order an enzyme or sodium bicarb solution.

TPN

Total parenteral nutrition (TPN) is an intravenous hypertonic solution containing glucose, fat emulsion, protein, minerals, and vitamins. TPN is generally given through a central line (PICC if short-term), and used only when other methods of nutrition are not feasible.

Nursing Considerations:

- **Infection prevention**: Use aseptic technique for feedings and dressing changes; change solution, filter, and tubing every 24 hours, discard cloudy solutions, and monitor the site for signs of infection.
- **Risk of embolus/contamination**: Use micropore filter (TPN without fat emulsion) or 1.2-micron filter (TPN with fat emulsion); heparin can be added to the solution. Never infuse any medication or product in the same line as the TPN; blood cannot be drawn from this line either.
- **Malnutrition and Electrolytes**: Check daily weight and check BMP and CBC 3x a week until stable, then weekly. Check the label and ingredients before administration and watch for signs of fluid overload. A cloudy blood specimen could indicate hyperlipidemia. Patients on TPN are also at risk for hyperammonemia (demonstrated by asterixis and altered mental status) and azotemia (demonstrated by dehydration and elevated BUN).

- **Hyper/Hypoglycemia**: Initiate slowly, increasing rate over 24-48 hours. NEVER try to "catch-up" at a higher rate if there is a delay/pause in feeding; only administer with a pump and do not change the rate without order. If the bag runs out, hang a bag of D10W until a new bag can be obtained. Monitor BG every 4-6 hours; sliding scale insulin may be used.

Gastrointestinal Surgery

Whipple

The **Whipple** (pancreaticoduodenectomy) procedure is used to surgically remove the head of the pancreas, the gallbladder, part of the bile duct, the duodenum, and sometimes the distal portion of the stomach. After excision, the remaining pancreas, bile duct, and intestinal stump are sutured to the intestine so that secretions empty into the intestine. The Whipple procedure may be done as an open procedure or laparoscopically. This procedure is used primarily for malignant or benign tumors of the head of the pancreas but can also be used for chronic pancreatitis, duodenal cancer, cancer of the ampulla, and cholangiocarcinoma. Whipple is recommended only if the cancer has not spread beyond the pancreas and has not invaded major vessels. Usually, the pancreas is still able to produce adequate insulin, but the production of pancreatic enzymes may be impaired. A pylorus-preserving variation preserves the stomach and part of the pylorus to decrease nutritional deficiencies and weight loss associated with the standard Whipple.

Post-op treatment includes monitoring fluid/electrolyte balance and monitoring drains. These patients have a very high risk of developing numerous complications, including peritonitis, bowel obstruction, sepsis, and acute abdomen, along with others.

Esophagectomy and Esophagogastrectomy

Esophageal cancer starts in the inner layer of the esophagus and spreads. It may develop after long-term reflux because of cell changes brought about by gastric acid. Symptoms include throat or epigastric discomfort, increasing dysphagia and inability to swallow solids, unexplained weight loss, hoarseness, hiccups, hematemesis, and the feeling of something in the throat. *Treatment* for esophageal cancer involves surgical removal of the affected portion of the esophagus. Two common procedures include:

- **Esophagectomy** is the removal of all or part of the esophagus with the distal end resutured to the stomach or an intestinal graft used to replace the excised portion of the esophagus.
- **Esophagogastrectomy** is the removal of the distal portion of the esophagus, lymph nodes, and the upper portion of the stomach, after which the remaining esophagus and stomach are reattached.

Postoperative Management

Postoperative management for esophagectomy/gastrectomy includes the following:

- Monitor intubation and ventilation (increased risk for ARDS), encourage pulmonary hygiene, and monitor chest tubes (change in color or sudden increase in drainage could indicate leak; notify physician).
- Subcutaneous emphysema in the chest/neck could indicate a leak in the anastomosis and should be reported immediately.
- Manage pain, which is often severe; a PCA or epidural may be used initially.
- Hemodynamics: IV fluids, 100-200 mL/hr, bolus PRN; however, be cautious as there is an increased risk of pulmonary edema.
- Monitor the NG tube; **NEVER replace or irrigate the NG tube**, as it could damage the anastomosis. Notify MD if complications arise.

- Maintain NPO for 5-7 days; nutrition should be provided via J-tube or TPN.
- Drains: Penrose, Jackson-Pratt, possible drainage collection bag at the base of the cervical incision for saliva if >250 mL in 8 hr.
  NOTE: Patients often have history of alcohol abuse; observe for signs of DTs/withdrawal.
- Prior to initiating oral intake, a fluoroscopic examination with water-soluble contrast will be done to check for leaks. If no leaks, patients begin with clear liquids and progress to 6 to 8 small meals per day.

Bariatric Gastrointestinal Surgery

Bariatric surgery is used to promote weight loss in the morbidly obese (100 pounds over normal weight or BMI of 35-40). Surgery is done to restrict intake and/or prevent the absorption of calories. Procedures are open surgical or laparoscopic and include:

- **Banding** places a band around the upper portion of the stomach, creating a small pouch with a small distal opening to slow gastric emptying.
- **Sleeve gastrectomy** removes about 2/3 of the stomach, and a distal part of the small intestine is attached, bypassing part of the small intestine, reducing absorption.
- **Roux-en-Y** uses staples and a vertical band to decrease the size of the stomach, creating a small pouch. Then, a section of the small intestine is attached to the pouch, bypassing the first and second segments of the intestine to reduce absorption.
- **Gastric ballooning** places a balloon in the stomach and fills it with liquid to decrease stomach capacity; this is used primarily in Europe.

Nursing considerations: Use extreme caution with post-bariatric NG/PEG tubes – generally do not check placement/irrigate with normal amounts (risk of rupturing stomach); ensure patient maintains strict NPO. There is an increased risk of respiratory complications post-surgery.

Monitoring Devices for Abdominal Compartment Syndrome

Measurement of **intra-abdominal pressure** is obtained by attaching a pressure transducer or water-column manometer to a Foley catheter in the bladder, because bladder pressure correlates with abdominal pressure. The patient should be in the supine position if possible. The bladder must be empty for accurate measurement. The catheter should be clamped and transducer zeroed at the iliac crest along the midaxillary line. Then, 2-25 mL (usually about 10 mL for critically ill) of fluid is injected into the bladder and left in place for 30-60 seconds before the reading pressure following a patient expiration. Compartment pressures should be <30 mmHg and the difference between diastolic BP and compartment pressure should be >30 mmHg. Intraabdominal pressure may also be checked with an indwelling NG tube. If the risk for compartment syndrome exists, the wound should not be closed. Sudden release of pressure and reperfusion may cause acidosis, vasodilation, and cardiac arrest, so the patient should be given crystalloid solutions before decompression.

Indwelling Fecal Management Systems

Indwelling fecal management systems are used for incontinent clients with loose or watery stools in order to prevent skin breakdown, discomfort, odor, and contamination of wounds, and to control the spread of organisms, such as *Clostridium difficile,* in bedridden or immobile clients. A number of different devices, such as the Flexi-Seal® FMS, are available and work similarly. A typical management system includes:

- A silicone catheter
- A silicone retention balloon at end of the catheter
- A 45-mL syringe
- Charcoal filter collection bags

The application of the fecal management system is relatively simple: The catheter is inserted into the rectum and the balloon is inflated with water or saline (using the 45-mL syringe) to hold it in place and to block fecal leakage. Some systems, such as Flexi-Seal® FMS, have a pop-up button to indicate when the balloon is adequately filled for the size of the rectum. The catheter contains an irrigation port so that irrigating fluid can be instilled if necessary. The charcoal filter collection bag is attached to the end of the silicone catheter to contain fecal material.

Gastrointestinal Pharmacology

Histamine Receptor Antagonists

Histamine (H) receptor antagonists (actually reverse agonists) are used to treat conditions in which excessive **stomach acid** causes heartburn and GERD. They block histamine 2 (H_2) (parietal) cell receptors in the stomach, thereby decreasing acid production. These drugs are used less commonly now than proton-pump inhibitors. Common H_2 antagonists include:

- **Cimetidine (Tagamet®)**: The first H_2 antagonist, it is used less frequently than others because of inhibition of enzymes that results in drug interactions, especially with contraceptive agents and estrogen.
- **Ranitidine (Zantac®)**: This was developed to decrease drug interactions and improve patient tolerance. Its activity is about 10 times that of cimetidine. It may be used in combination with other drugs to treat ulcers.
- **Famotidine (Pepcid®)**: This may be combined with an antacid to increase the speed of effects as it has a slow onset. It may be used pre-surgically to reduce post-operative nausea.
- **Nizatidine (Axid®)**: The last H_2 antagonist developed, it is about equal in potency and action to ranitidine.

Antacids

Antacids are medications used to reduce **stomach acids** by raising the pH and neutralizing the acids present. They are commonly used to treat heartburn or indigestion. Adverse reactions are relatively rare unless taken to excess or with renal impairment. Drugs include:

- **Aluminum hydroxide** (Amphojel®) may cause constipation and with renal impairment, hypophosphatemia and osteomalacia.
- **Magnesium hydroxide** (Milk of Magnesia®) may cause diarrhea and with renal impairment can cause hypermagnesemia.
- **Aluminum hydroxide with magnesium hydroxide** (Maalox®, Mylanta®) may cause nausea, vomiting and diarrhea, yeast infection (thrush), or hypophosphatemia.
- **Calcium carbonate** (TUMS®, Rolaids®, Titralac®) may cause gastric distention. Excess calcium intake may cause toxic reactions, including kidney stones and renal failure, so excess intake should be avoided.
- **Alka-Seltzer®** combines sodium bicarbonate with aspirin and citric acid so this compound may cause gastric irritation, nausea and vomiting, and tarry stools.

- **Bismuth subsalicylate** (Pepto-Bismol®). Pepto-Bismol® may react with sulfur in the body to create a black tongue and black stools, but this is temporary. Pepto-Bismol® has been associated with Reye's syndrome in children with influenza or chickenpox.

Proton Pump Inhibitors

Proton pump inhibitors (PPIs) are now used more frequently than histamine receptor antagonists. PPIs interfere with an **acid-producing enzyme** in the stomach wall, reducing stomach acid. PPIs are used to treat GERD, stomach ulcers, and *H. pylori* (with antibiotics). PPIs are similar in action and include:

- Esomeprazole (Nexium®)
- Lansoprazole (Prevacid®)
- Omeprazole (Prilosec®)
- Pantoprazole (Protonix®)
- Rabeprazole (Aciphex®)
- Omeprazole/sodium bicarbonate (Zegerid®) (Long-acting form of omeprazole)

Common side effects include gastrointestinal upset (nausea, diarrhea, and constipation), headache, and rash. In rare instances, PPIs may cause severe muscle pain; however, they are usually well-tolerated with few adverse effects. PPIs may interfere with the absorption of some drugs, such as those that are affected by stomach acid. Absorption of ketoconazole is impaired, and absorption of digoxin is increased, sometimes leading to toxicity. Omeprazole impacts the hepatic breakdown of drugs more than other PPIs and may cause increased levels of diazepam, phenytoin, and warfarin.

Review Video: Gastroenterological Drugs
Visit mometrix.com/academy and enter code: 455152

Genitourinary Diagnostics

Renal Function Studies

Renal function studies are described below:

- **Osmolality (urine):** Normal: 350-900 mOsm/kg/day. Shows early changes when the kidney has difficulty concentrating urine.
- **Osmolality (serum):** Normal: 275-295 mOsm/kg. Gives a picture of the amount of solute in the blood.
- **Uric acid:** Normal: 3.0-7.2 mg/dL. Increases with renal failure.
- **Creatinine clearance (24-hour):** Normal: 75-125 mL/min. Evaluates the amount of blood cleared of creatinine in 1 minute. Approximates the GFR.
- **Serum creatinine:** Normal: 0.6-1.2 mg/dL. Increase with decreased renal function, urinary tract obstruction, and nephritis.
- **Urine creatinine:** Normal: 11-26 mg/kg/day. Product of muscle breakdown. Increase with decreased renal function.
- **Blood urea nitrogen (BUN):** Normal: 7-8 mg/dL (8-20 mg/dL if age >60). An increase indicates impaired renal function, as urea is the end product of protein metabolism.
- **BUN/creatinine ratio:** Normal: 10:1. Increases with hypovolemia. With intrinsic kidney disease, the ratio is increased.
- **Urinalysis:** Tests various qualities of a urine sample that are reflective of kidney function and other disease processes.

Urinalysis

Urinalysis components and normal findings are described below:

- **Color:** Pale yellow/amber and darkens when urine is concentrated or other substances (such as blood or bile) are present.
- **Appearance:** Clear but may be slightly cloudy.
- **Odor:** Slight. Bacteria may give urine a foul smell, depending upon the organism. Some foods, such as asparagus, change the odor.
- **Specific gravity:** Normal: 1.005 to 1.025. May increase if protein levels increase or if there is fever, vomiting, or dehydration.
- **pH:** Usually ranges from 4.5-8 with an average of 5-6.
- **Sediment:** Red cell casts from acute infections, broad casts from kidney disorders, and white cell casts from pyelonephritis. Leukocytes >10 per mL^3 are present with urinary tract infections.
- **Glucose, ketones, protein, blood, bilirubin, and nitrate:** Negative. Urine glucose may increase with infection (with normal blood glucose). Frank blood may be caused by some parasites and diseases but also by drugs, smoking, excessive exercise, and menstrual fluids. Increased red blood cells may result from lower urinary tract infections.
- **Urobilinogen:** 0.1-1.0 units.

IVP and Radionucleotide Renal Scan

Intravenous pyelogram (IVP) is done to identify structural defects and tumors and to observe urinary structures. The patient is administered an IV contrast medium and may be administered antihistamine or corticosteroid before the test to minimize allergic response. Serum creatinine and BUN are done prior to the IVP to ensure that the contrast medium can be excreted. During the procedure, radiographs are taken once every minute for five minutes and then again after 15 minutes (giving the contrast medium time to pass into the bladder). A post-voiding radiograph shows how efficiently the bladder is able to empty. Fluid intake should be increased post-procedure to flush contrast.

Radionucleotide renal scan with dimercaptosuccinic acid (DMSA) requires IV administration of a radioactive element followed by a series of CT scans taken over 20 minutes to 4 hours. The scan is used to assess function and perfusion of the kidney and can detect lesions, atrophy, and scars and differentiate among different causes for hydronephrosis. The patient must be well-hydrated and may need to be catheterized to measure the output of urine.

Renal Biopsy

Renal biopsy to remove a small segment of cortical tissue helps to identify the extent of **kidney disease** with acute renal failure, transplant rejection, glomerulopathies, and persistent hematuria or proteinuria. Preoperative coagulation studies determine the risk of bleeding. The biopsy is done percutaneously per needle biopsy (guided by fluoroscopy or ultrasound) or surgically through a small flank incision. A urine specimen must be obtained so it can be compared with a post-procedure specimen. **Post-procedure**:

- Maintain the patient in a supine position immediately after the procedure for 4-6 hours and on bed rest overnight.
- Monitor urine for hematuria and compare it with the preop specimen.
- Monitor VS every 5-15 minutes for the first hour and then less frequently. To minimize bleeding, maintain blood pressure <140/90.
- Note anorexia, vomiting, and abdominal discomfort that may suggest bleeding.

- Note pain: Severe colicky pain may indicate a clot in the ureter.
- Monitor urinalysis and CBC post-procedure.
- Maintain fluid intake at 3,000 mL/day in absence of renal insufficiency.
- Provide blood component therapy and surgical repair if bleeding occurs.

Renal Ultrasound

Renal ultrasound is a non-invasive method of viewing the **urinary structures**. Most patients that present with kidney disease of unknown origin should undergo a renal ultrasound to assess for possible obstruction. An ultrasound uses ultrasonic sound waves transmitted by a transducer, which picks up reflected sound waves that a computer converts to electronic images. An ultrasound can show fluid accumulation, the movement of blood through the kidney, masses, malformations (congenital abnormalities), changes in size of the kidney or other structures, and obstructions, such as renal calculi. An ultrasound is usually done before a renal biopsy, and may be done with a needle biopsy to guide the placement of the needle. Patient preparation includes drinking two 8-ounce glasses of water one hour before the examination to ensure that the bladder is full. The patient should be reminded not to urinate before the ultrasound. The patient usually remains in a supine position throughout the procedure but may be asked to turn to the side. No special precautions are necessary post-procedure.

Genitourinary Procedures and Interventions

Procedures for Insertion and Removal of Urinary Catheter

Procedure for **inserting and removing a urinary catheter**:

1. Gather supplies (included in a urinary catheter insertion kit), perform hand hygiene, place a waterproof pad under the patient, and ensure that the light source is adequate to view the urinary meatus.
2. Place females in supine position with knees flexed and males in supine position.
3. Apply gloves and wash the perineal area with facility provided cleanser (sometimes included in the outside of the urinary catheter kit) and allow to dry.
4. Remove gloves and wash hands.
5. Using aseptic technique, place the catheter kit between the patient's legs, open the kit touching only the corners of the drape that wraps around the kit.
6. Apply sterile gloves.
7. Apply sterile drapes to the patient.
8. Following the steps provided with the kit, place the lubricant into the appropriate section of tray, remove the catheter from its plastic and place the tip into the lubricant, and pour iodine over the three cleansing swabs (if they do not come impregnated with iodine already). Attach the 10 cc syringe (filled with sterile water) to the appropriate port of the catheter.
9. Cleanse the urethral meatus with the iodine impregnated swabs.
10. Using the nondominant hand, hold the penis or open the labia to observe the urethral meatus. This hand now becomes "dirty" and cannot be used to touch the catheter.
11. Using the dominant hand, insert catheter with the drainage end attached to the collection bag. Insert until urine flows freely, advancing a little further after that point.
12. Inflate the balloon using the 10 cc sterile water syringe, and ensure the catheter is secure.
13. Secure the catheter to the patient's leg and hang the collection bag below the level of the patient. Secure any tubing to the bed and ensure no kinking is present.

Removal: Straight catheter—remove by pulling out slowly. To remove indwelling catheter, deflate the balloon using the appropriate port and gently pull the catheter out.

Renal Dialysis

Peritoneal Dialysis

Renal dialysis is used primarily for those who have progressed from renal insufficiency to uremia with end-stage renal disease (ESRD). It may also be temporarily for acute conditions. People can be maintained on dialysis, but there are many complications associated with dialysis, so many people are considered for renal transplantation. There are a number of different approaches to **peritoneal dialysis:**

- **Peritoneal dialysis:** An indwelling catheter is inserted surgically into the peritoneal cavity with a subcutaneous tunnel and a Dacron cuff to prevent infection. Sterile dialysate solution is slowly instilled through gravity, remains for a prescribed length of time, and is then drained and discarded.
- **Continuous ambulatory peritoneal dialysis:** A series of exchange cycles is repeated 24 hours a day.
- **Continuous cyclic peritoneal dialysis:** A prolonged period of retaining fluid occurs during the day with drainage at night.

Peritoneal dialysis may be used for those who want to be more independent, don't live near a dialysis center, or want fewer dietary restrictions.

Hemodialysis

Hemodialysis, the most common type of dialysis, is used for both short-term dialysis and long-term for those with ESRD. Treatments are usually done 3 times weekly for 3-4 hours or daily dialysis with treatment either during the night or in short daily periods. Hemodialysis is often done for those who can't manage peritoneal dialysis or who live near a dialysis center, but it does interfere with work or school attendance and requires strict dietary and fluid restrictions between treatments. Short daily dialysis allows more independence, and increased costs may be offset by lower morbidity. A vascular access device, such as a catheter, fistula, or graft, must be established for hemodialysis, and heparin is used to prevent clotting. With hemodialysis, blood is circulated outside of the body through a dialyzer (a synthetic semipermeable membrane), which filters the blood. There are many different types of dialyzers. High flux dialyzers use a highly permeable membrane that shortens the duration of treatment and decreases the need for heparin.

Continuous Renal Replacement Therapy

Continuous renal replacement therapy (**CCRT**) circulates the blood by hydrostatic pressure through a semipermeable membrane. It is used in critical care and can be instituted quickly:

- **Continuous arteriovenous hemofiltration** (CAVH) circulates blood from an artery (usually the femoral) to a hemofilter using only arterial pressure and not a blood pump. The filtered blood is then returned to the patient's venous system, often with added fluids to offset those lost. Only the fluid is filtered.
- **Continuous arteriovenous hemodialysis** (CAVHD) is similar to CAVH except that dialysate circulates on one side of the semipermeable membrane to increase the clearance of urea.

- **Continuous venovenous hemofiltration** (CVVH) pumps blood through a double-lumen venous catheter to a hemofilter, which returns the blood to the patient in the same catheter. It provides continuous slow removal of fluid, is better tolerated with unstable patients, and doesn't require arterial access.
- **Continuous venovenous hemodialysis** is similar to CVVH but uses a dialysate to increase the clearance of uremic toxins.

Dialysis Complications

There are many **complications** associated with dialysis, especially when used for long-term treatment:

- **Hemodialysis**: Long-term use promotes atherosclerosis and cardiovascular disease. Anemia and fatigue are common, as are infections related to access devices or contamination of equipment. Some experience hypotension and muscle cramping during treatment. Dysrhythmias may occur. Some may exhibit dialysis disequilibrium from cerebral fluid shifts, causing headaches, nausea and vomiting, and alterations of consciousness.
- **Peritoneal dialysis:** Most complications are minor, but it can lead to peritonitis, which requires removal of the catheter if antibiotic therapy is not successful in clearing the infection within 4 days. There may be leakage of the dialysate around the catheter. Bleeding may occur, especially in females who are menstruating as blood is pulled from the uterus through the fallopian tubes. Abdominal hernias may occur with long use. Some may have anorexia from the feeling of fullness or a sweet taste in the mouth from the absorption of glucose.

Radical Nephrectomy

Radical nephrectomy is done for adenocarcinoma of the kidney, which may be associated with paraneoplastic syndromes, and, because this type of cancer is associated with smoking, patients may have underlying coronary artery or respiratory disease. Some patients have erythrocytosis, but many are anemic and may require transfusions in preparation for surgery to increase hemoglobin to >10 g/dL. Surgery is done under endotracheal general anesthesia with an anterior subcostal, flank, or thoracoabdominal (preferred for large tumors) incision. The kidney and its adrenal gland with surrounding fat and fascia are removed together. Blood loss may be extensive because the tumors tend to be vascular and large, requiring multiple transfusions. However, controlled hypotension should be limited to brief periods because it may impair renal function. Mannitol is given prior to dissection. Continual direct arterial pressure monitoring and central venous cannulation must be done.

Nephron-sparing surgery (partial nephrectomy), often by laparoscopy, may be done if the renal cell carcinoma is <4 cm diameter. Postoperative analgesia and pulmonary hygiene are essential.

Reducing Infection Risks Associated with Urinary Catheters

Strategies for reducing infection risks associated with **urinary catheters** include:

- Using **aseptic technique** for both the straight and indwelling catheter insertion.
- **Limiting catheter use** by establishing protocols for use, duration, and removal; training staff; issuing reminders to physicians; using straight catheterizations rather than indwelling; using ultrasound to scan the bladder; and using condom catheters.
- Utilizing **closed-drainage systems** for indwelling catheters.
- **Avoiding irrigation** unless required for diagnosis or treatment.

- Using **sampling port** for specimens rather than disconnecting catheter and tubing.
- Maintaining **proper urinary flow** by proper positioning, securing of tubing and drainage bag, and keeping the drainage bag below the level of the bladder.
- **Changing catheters** only when medically needed.
- **Cleansing external meatal area** gently each day, manipulating the catheter as little as possible.
- Avoiding placing catheterized patients adjacent to those infected or colonized with antibiotic-resistant bacteria to reduce **cross-contamination.**

Respiratory Interventions and Procedures

Non-Invasive Ventilation

Nasal Cannula

A **nasal cannula** can be used to deliver supplemental oxygen to a patient, but it is only useful for flow rates ≤6 L/min as higher rates are drying of the nasal passages. As it is not an airtight system, some ambient air is breathed in as well so oxygen concentration ranges from about 24-44%. The nasal cannula does not allow for control of respiratory rate, so the patient must be able to breathe independently.

Non-Rebreather Mask

A **non-rebreather mask** can be used to deliver higher concentrations (60-90%) of oxygen to those patients who are able to breathe independently. The mask fits over the nose and mouth and is secured by an elastic strap. A 1.5 L reservoir bag is attached and connects to an oxygen source. The bag is inflated to about 1 liter at a rate of 8-15 L/min before the mask is applied as the patient breathes from this reservoir. A one-way exhalation valve prevents most exhaled air from being rebreathed.

Non-Invasive Positive Pressure Ventilators

Non-invasive positive pressure ventilators provide air through a tight-fitting nasal or face mask, usually pressure cycled, avoiding the need for intubation and reducing the danger of hospital-acquired infection and mortality rates. It can be used for acute respiratory failure and pulmonary edema. There are 2 types of non-invasive positive pressure ventilators:

- **CPAP (Continuous positive airway pressure)** provides a steady stream of pressurized air throughout both inspiration and expiration. CPAP improves breathing by decreasing preload for patients with congestive heart failure. It reduces the effort required for breathing by increasing residual volume and improving gas exchange.
- **Bi-PAP (Bi-level positive airway pressure)** provides a steady stream of pressurized air as CPAP but it senses inspiratory effort and increases pressure during inspiration. Bi-PAP pressures for inspiration and expiration can be set independently. Machines can be programmed with a backup rate to ensure a set number of respirations per minute.

**NEVER place a patient in wrist restraints while wearing these devices. If the patient vomits, they need to be able to remove the mask to prevent aspiration.*

Face Mask

Ensuring that a **face mask** (Ambu bag) is the correct fit and type is important for adequate ventilation, oxygenation, and prevention of aspiration. Difficulties in management of face mask ventilation relate to risk factors: >55 years, obesity, beard, edentulous, and history of snoring. In some cases, if dentures are adhered well, they may be left in place during induction. The face mask is applied by lifting the mandible (jaw thrust) to the mask and avoiding pressure on soft tissue. Oral or nasal airways may be used, ensuring that the distal end is at the angle of the mandible. There are a number of steps to prevent mask airway leaks:

- Increasing or decreasing the amount of air to the mask to allow better seal
- Securing the mask with both hands while another person ventilates
- Accommodating a large nose by using the mask upside down
- Utilizing a laryngeal mask airway if excessive beard prevents seal

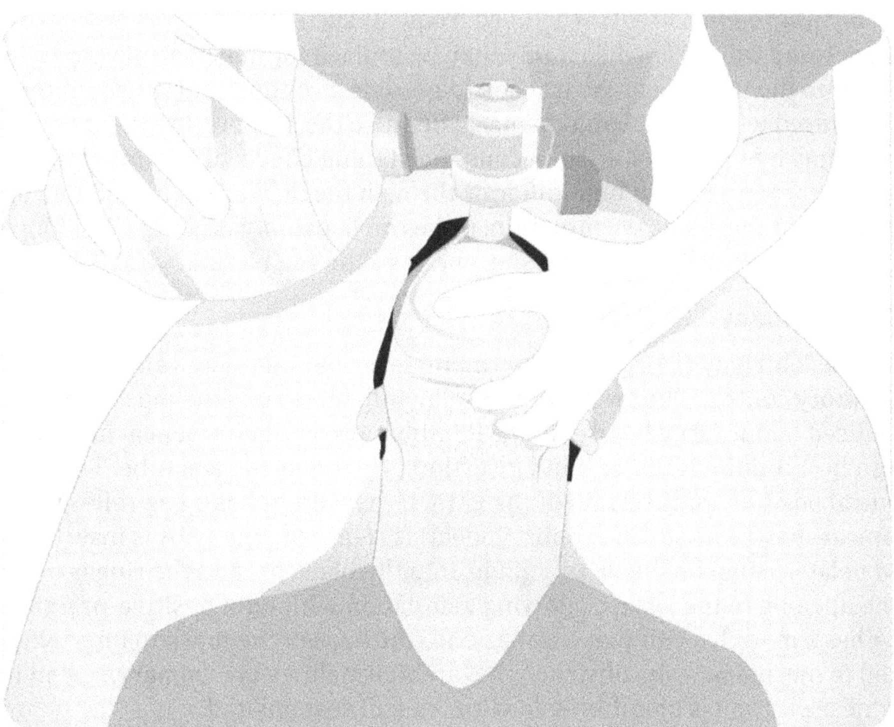

High and Low Flow Oxygen Delivery

High flow oxygen delivery devices provide oxygen at flow rates higher than the patient's inspiratory flow rate at specific medium to high FiO_2, up to 100%. However, a flow of 100% oxygen actually provides only 60-80% FiO_2 to the patient because the patient also breathes in some room air, diluting the oxygen. The actual amount of oxygen received depends on the type of interface or mask. Additionally, the flow rate is actually less than the inspiratory flow rate upon actual delivery. High flow oxygen delivery is usually not used in the sleep center. Humidification is usually required because the high flow is drying.

Low flow oxygen delivery devices provide 100% oxygen at flow rates lower than the patient's inspiratory flow rate, but the oxygen mixes with room air, so the FiO_2 varies. Humidification is usually only required if flow rate is >3L/min. Much oxygen is wasted with exhalation, so a number of different devices to conserve oxygen are available. Interfaces include transtracheal catheters and cannulae with reservoirs.

Airway Devices

Oropharyngeal, Nasopharyngeal, and Tracheostomy Tubes

Airways are used to establish a patent airway and facilitate respirations:

- **Oropharyngeal**: This plastic airway curves over the tongue and creates space between the mouth and the posterior pharynx. It is used for anesthetized or unconscious patients to keep tongue and epiglottis from blocking the airway.
- **Nasopharyngeal** (trumpet): This smaller flexible airway is more commonly used in conscious patients and is inserted through one nostril, extending to the nasopharynx. It is commonly utilized in patients who need frequent suctioning.
- **Tracheostomy tubes**: Tracheostomy may be utilized for mechanical ventilation. Tubes are inserted into the opening in the trachea to provide a conduit and maintain the opening. The tube is secured with ties around the neck. Because the air entering the lungs through the tracheostomy bypasses the warming and moistening effects of the upper airway, air is humidified through a room humidifier or through the delivery of humidified air through a special mask or mechanical ventilation. If the tracheostomy is going to be long-term, eventually a stoma will form at the site, and the tube can be removed.

Laryngeal Mask Airway

The **laryngeal-mask airway** (LMA) is an intermediate airway allowing ventilation but not complete respiratory control. The LMA consists of an inflatable cuff (the mask) with a connecting tube. It may be used temporarily before tracheal intubation or when tracheal intubation can't be done. It can also be a conduit for later blind insertion of an endotracheal tube. The head and neck must be in neutral position for insertion of the LMA. If the patient has a gag reflex, conscious sedation or topical anesthesia (deep oropharyngeal) is required. The LMA is inserted by sliding along the hard palate, using the finger as a guide, into the pharynx, and the ring is inflated to create a seal about the opening to the larynx, allowing ventilation with mild positive-pressure. The ProSeal® LMA has a modified cuff that extends onto the back of the mask to improve seal. LMA is contraindicated in morbid obesity, obstructions or abnormalities of oropharynx, and non-fasting patients, as some aspiration is possible even with the cuff seal inflated.

Esophageal-Tracheal Combitube®

The **esophageal tracheal Combitube®** (ETC) is an intermediate airway that contains two lumens and can be inserted into either the trachea or the esophagus (≤91%). The twin-lumen tube has a proximal cuff providing a seal of the oropharynx and a distal cuff providing a seal about the distal tube. Prior to insertion, the Combitube® cuffs should be checked for leaks (15 mL of air into distal and 85 mL of air into proximal). The patient should be non-responsive and with absent gag reflex with head in neutral position. The tube is passed along the tongue and into the pharynx, utilizing markings on the tube (black guidelines) to determine depth by aligning the ETC with the upper incisors or alveolar ridge. Once in place the distal cuff is inflated (10-15 mL) and then placement in the trachea or esophagus should be determined, so the proper lumen for ventilation can be used. The proximal cuff is inflated (usually to 50-75 mL) and ventilation begun. A capnogram should be used to confirm ventilation.

Mechanical Ventilation

Endotracheal Intubation

Endotracheal intubation is often necessary with respiratory failure for control of hypoxemia, hypercapnia, hypoventilation, and/or obstructed airway. Equipment should be assembled and tubes and connections checked for air leaks with a 10 mL syringe. The mouth and/or nose should be cleaned of secretions and suctioned if necessary. The patient should be supine with the patient's head level with the lower sternum of the clinician. With orotracheal/endotracheal intubation, the clinician holds the laryngoscope (in left hand) and inserts it into right corner of mouth, the epiglottis is lifted and the larynx exposed. A thin flexible intubation stylet may be used and the endotracheal tube (ETT) (in right hand) is inserted through the vocal cords and into the trachea, cuff inflated to minimal air leak (10 mL initially until patient stabilizes), and placement confirmed through capnometry or esophageal detection devices. The correct depth of insertion is verified: 21 cm (female), 23 cm (male). After insertion, the tube is secured.

Review Video: Mechanical Ventilation
Visit mometrix.com/academy and enter code: 679637

Rapid Sequence Intubation (RSI)

Rapid sequence intubation (RSI) is the simultaneous giving of a sedative and a paralytic in order to facilitate emergency intubation and is considered to be the standard of care for emergency airway management (except in patients with anticipated difficult intubation or in those with contraindications to sedatives/paralytics).

Initial preparation includes inserting 2 IV lines and establishing cardiac monitoring, oximetry, and capnography. The patient should be preoxygenated (100%) for at least 3 minutes, but without pressure ventilation that may cause aspiration of stomach contents. Procedure includes:

- **Induction agent**: Thiopental, ketamine, etomidate, propofol
- **Paralysis**: Succinylcholine, rocuronium, other NMBAs
- **Sellick's maneuver** (pressure applied externally with thumb and index finger to cricoid) to close off the esophagus and prevent aspiration
- **Suction** to clear mouth if necessary
- **Laryngoscopy** to visual vocal cords
- **EET** inserted, cuff inflated, and ETT secured

Proper placement verified by capnometer or capnograph. Breath sounds should be auscultated. Post intubation chest x-ray to assess depth of tube and check for any trauma or issue. Induction agents and use of additional sedation may vary from one institution to another, but the primary goal is to safely anesthetize and intubate while preventing regurgitation of stomach contents.

Confirming Correct Placement of Endotracheal Tubes

There are a number of methods to confirm correct placement of **endotracheal tubes**. Clinical assessment alone is not adequate.

- **Capnometry** utilizes an end-tidal CO_2 ($ETCO_2$) detector that measures the concentration of CO_2 in expired air, usually through pH sensitive paper that changes color (commonly purple to yellow). The capnometer is attached to the ETT and a bag-valve-mask (BVM) ventilator is also attached. The patient is provided 6 ventilations and the CO_2 concentration is checked.
- **Capnography** is attached to the ETT and provides a waveform graph, showing the varying concentrations of CO_2 in real time throughout each ventilation (with increased CO_2 on expiration) and can indicate changes in respiratory status.

- **Esophageal detection devices** fit over the end of the ETT so that a large syringe can be used to attempt to aspirate. If the ETT is in the esophagus, the walls collapse on aspiration and resistance occurs, whereas the syringe fills with air if the ETT is in the trachea. A self-inflating bulb (Ellik® device) may also be used.
- **Chest X-ray** provides visual confirmation of placement.

Ventilator Management

There are many types of ventilators now in use, and the specific directions for each type must be followed carefully, but there are general principles that apply to all **ventilator management**. The following should be monitored:

- **Type of ventilation:** Volume-cycled, pressure-cycled, negative-pressure, HFJV, HFOV, CPAP, Bi-PAP
- **Control mode**: Controlled ventilation, assisted ventilation, synchronized intermittent mandatory (allows spontaneous breaths between ventilator-controlled inhalation/exhalation), positive end-expiratory pressure (PEEP), CPAP, Bi-PAP
- **Tidal volume** (TV) range should be set in relation to respiratory rate
- **Inspiratory-expiratory ratio** (I:E) usually ranges from 1:2-1:5, but may vary
- **Respiratory rate** will depend upon TV and $PaCO_2$ target
- **Fraction of inspired oxygen** (FiO_2) [percentage of oxygen in the inspired air], usually ranging from 21-100%, usually maintained <40% to avoid toxicity
- **Sensitivity** determines the effort needed to trigger inspiration
- **Pressure** controls the pressure exerted in delivering TV
- **Rate of flow** controls the L/min speed of TV

High Frequency Jet Ventilation

High frequency jet ventilation (HFJV) (Life Pulse®) directs a high velocity stream of air into the lungs in a long spiraling spike that forces carbon dioxide against the walls, penetrating dead space and providing gas exchange by using small tidal volumes of 1-3 mL/kg, much smaller than with conventional mechanical ventilation. Because the jet stream technology is effective for short distances, the valve and pressure transducer must be placed by the person's head. Inhalation is controlled while expiration is passive, but the rate of respiration is up to 11 per second ("panting" respirations). HFJV may be used in conjunction with low-pressure conventional ventilation to increase flow to alveoli. HFJV reduces barotrauma because of the low tidal volume and low pressure. HFJV is used for numerous conditions, including evolving chronic lung disease, pulmonary interstitial emphysema, bronchopulmonary dysplasia, and hypoxemic respiratory failure. It reduces mean airway pressure (MAP) and the oxygenation index. Treatment with HFJV may reduce the need for ECMO.

High Frequency Oscillatory Ventilation

High frequency oscillatory ventilation (HFOV) provides pressurized ventilation with tidal volumes approximately equal to dead space at about 150 breaths per minutes (BPM). Pressure is usually higher with HFOV than HFJV in order to maintain expansion of the alveoli and to keep the airway open during gas exchange. Oxygenation is regulated separately. HFOV has both an active inspiration and expiration, so the respiratory cycle is completely controlled. HFOV reduces pulmonary vascular resistance and improves ventilation-perfusion matching and oxygenation without injuring the lung, reducing the risk of barotrauma. HFOV is used for respiratory distress syndrome, persistent pulmonary hypertension, more commonly for infants and children, but there is increasing interest in using HFOV with adults because of the smaller tidal volume that prevents overinflation of the lungs and atelectasis of those with ARDS.

Positive Pressure Ventilators

Positive pressure ventilators assist respiration by applying pressure directly to the airway, inflating the lungs, forcing expansion of the alveoli, and facilitating gas exchange. Generally, endotracheal intubation or tracheostomy is necessary to maintain positive pressure ventilation for extended periods. There are 3 basic kinds of positive pressure ventilators:

- **Pressure cycled:** This type of ventilation is usually used for short-term treatment in adolescents or adults. The IPPB machine is the most common type. This delivers a flow of air to a preset pressure and then cycles off. Airway resistance or changes in compliance can affect volume of air and may compromise ventilation.
- **Time cycled**: This type of ventilation regulates the volume of air the patient receives by controlling the length of inspiration and the flow rate.
- **Volume cycled**: This type of ventilation provides a preset flow of pressurized air during inspiration and then cycles off and allows passive expiration, providing a fairly consistent volume of air.

Tracheostomy

Tracheostomy, surgical tracheal opening, may be utilized for mechanical ventilation. Tracheostomy tubes are inserted directly into an opening in the trachea to provide a conduit and maintain the opening. Tracheostomy tubes are usually silastic or plastic, and may have permanent of disposable inner cannulas. The tube is secured with ties around the neck. Because the air entering the lungs through the tracheostomy bypasses the warming and moistening effects of the upper airway, air is humidified through a room humidifier or through delivery of humidified air through a special mask or mechanical ventilation. The patient with a tracheostomy must have continuous monitoring of vital signs and respiratory status to ensure patency of tracheostomy. The inner cannula should be cleaned/replaced regularly (every 8-24 hours and PRN). Regular suctioning is needed, especially initially, to remove secretions:

- Suction catheter should be 50% the size of the tracheostomy tube to allow ventilation during suctioning.
- Vacuum pressure: 80-100 mmHg
- Catheter should only be inserted ≤0.5 cm beyond tube to avoid damage to tissues or perforation.
- Catheter should be inserted without suction and intermittent suction on withdrawal.

Ventilation-Induced Lung Injury

Ventilation-induced lung injury (VILI) is damage caused by mechanical ventilation. It is common in acute distress syndrome (ARDS) but can affect any mechanically ventilated patient. VILI comprises 4 interrelated elements:

- **Barotrauma**: Damage to the lung caused by excessive pressure
- **Volutrauma**: Alveolar damage related to high tidal volume ventilation
- **Atelectotrauma**: Injury caused by repetitive forced opening and closing of alveoli
- **Biotrauma**: Inflammatory response

In VILI, essentially the increased pressure and tidal volume over-distends the alveoli, which rupture, and air moves into the interstitial tissue resulting in pulmonary interstitial emphysema. With continued ventilation, the air in the interstitium moves into the subcutaneous tissue and may result in pneumopericardium and pneumomediastinum, or rupture the pleural sac which can cause tension pneumothorax and mediastinal shift, which can cause respiratory failure and cardiac arrest.

VILI has caused a change in ventilation procedures with lower tidal volumes and pressures used as well as newer forms of ventilation, HFJV and HFOV, preferred to traditional mechanical ventilation for many patients.

Preventing Complications from Ventilators

Methods to **prevent complications from mechanical ventilation ("ventilator bundle")** include:

- Elevate patient's head and chest to 30° to prevent aspiration and ventilation-associated pneumonia.
- Reposition patient every 2 hours.
- Provide DVT prophylaxis, such as external compression support and/or heparin (5000 u sq 2-3 times daily).
- Administer famotidine or pantoprazole PO/IV daily to prevent gastrointestinal stress-ulcers/bleeding.
- Decrease and eliminate sedation/analgesia as soon as possible—regular sedation vacations to assess neurological status.
- Follow careful protocols for pressure settings to prevent barotrauma. Tidal volumes are usually maintained at 8-12 mL/kg PBW (per AACN guidelines), but in incidences of high probability of ARDS, volumes should be less (6 mL/kg) to avoid lung injury.
- Monitor for pneumothorax or evidence of barotrauma.
- Conduct nutritional assessment (including lab tests) to prevent malnutrition.
- Monitor intake and output carefully and administer IV fluids to prevent dehydration.
- Do daily spontaneous breathing trials and discontinue ventilation as soon as possible.

Ventilator Weaning

Ventilator weaning has 3 phases: Changing settings of the ventilator to allow the patient to demonstrate the ability to breath on their own (standby mode), extubation, and finally removal of supportive oxygen. Criteria for ventilator weaning include:

- Vital capacity 10-15 mL/kg
- Maximum (negative) inspiratory pressure of at least -20 cmH_2O
- Tidal volume (TV) of 7-9 mL/kg
- Minute ventilation of about 6L/min (Respiratory rate x TV)
- Rapid shallow breathing index <100 breaths/min/L
- PaO_2 >60 mmHg
- FiO_2 <40%

If these criteria are met and the patient passes a spontaneous breathing trial (SBT), then extubation can be done. Various protocols are followed in weaning patients off of ventilators, including the use of intermittent mandatory ventilation (IMV) and synchronized intermittent mandatory ventilation (SIMV), which can be used with pressure support ventilation (PSV).

Criteria for oxygen weaning:

- FiO_2 reduced until PaO_2 70-100 mmHg on room air
- Supplemental O_2 necessary with PaO_2<70 mmHg (Medicare requires PaO_2 55 mmHg for reimbursement for home oxygen use)

Spontaneous Breathing Trial as Preparation for Extubation

A **spontaneous breathing trial** (SBT) is when a patient is taken off mechanical ventilation while remaining intubated (usually by changing the ventilator settings to CPAP) for a short period of time to assess readiness to extubate. SBT should be used prior to extubating a patient if the patient is not agitated and has no evidence of myocardial ischemia or increased ICP. The patient should exhibit some spontaneous triggering of respirations and should not be receiving large doses of vasopressor or inotropic agent. SpO_2 should be ≥88% with FiO_2 of 0.50 and PEEP at 7.5 cmH_2O prior to the SBT. The SBT should be done in the morning for a prescribed period (usually 30-120 minutes). The ventilator rate is adjusted to 0 and pressure support decreased to 0–7. The SBT should be discontinued if the following occur:

- Respiratory rate >35 or <8 for at least 5 minutes
- Mental status changes
- SpO_2 <88% for >15 minutes
- Respiratory distress (HR >130 BPM or <60 BPM, marked dyspnea, diaphoresis, increased use of accessory respiratory muscles, respiratory arrest)

Patients who pass the SBT have an 85-90% chance of breathing successfully after extubation. Patients who repeatedly fail daily SBT may require tracheostomy.

Failure to Wean from Mechanical Ventilation

Failure to wean from mechanical ventilation can occur in approximately 20-30% of ventilated patients. Many factors affect a patient's ability to wean from mechanical ventilation including physical, psychological and situational factors. Before discontinuation of ventilation can be considered, the patient must be able to protect his/her airway, be hemodynamically stable and have resolution of the clinical problem that initiated the need for mechanical ventilation. Weaning protocols use clinical criteria such as oxygen saturation, blood pressure, respiratory rate, and tidal volume to determine the patient's tolerance of lessening mechanical ventilator support. Failure to wean is demonstrated by multiple daily spontaneous breathing trial failures or the need for reintubation within 48 hours of extubation. Failure to resolve the clinical problem(s) that initiated mechanical ventilation, insufficient ventilator drive, respiratory muscle weakness, co-morbidities, and/or the development of new clinical problems (e.g., infection) may contribute to the inability to wean.

Signs and symptoms: Decreased tidal volume, increased respiratory rate, increased $PaCO_2$, oxygen desaturation, anxiety, diaphoresis, fatigue, changes in blood pressure or heart rate, mental status changes, and hemodynamic changes.

Treatment: The initial treatment strategy for patients who experience a dysfunctional ventilator weaning response is identification and treatment of the underlying cause(s) of the weaning failure. In addition, other treatment strategies may include psychological preparation of the patient for further weaning attempts, readiness testing and respiratory muscle training.

Sedation/Analgesia with Mechanical Ventilation

Patients intubated for mechanical ventilation are usually given **sedation and/or analgesia** initially, but medications should be reduced and given in boluses rather than with continuous IV drip with a goal of stopping sedation as it prolongs ventilation time. Typical sedatives include midazolam, propofol, and lorazepam. Narcotic analgesics include fentanyl and morphine sulfate. Uses of sedation include:

- Controlling agitation and excessive movement that may interfere with ventilation
- Reduce pain and discomfort associated with ventilation
- Control respiratory distress

Triglyceride levels must be checked periodically if propofol is administered for more than 24–48 hours. Neuromuscular blocking agents are rarely used because they may cause long-term weakness and increase length of ventilation although they may be indicated in some cases, such as with excessive shivering or cardiac arrest. Many patients are able to tolerate mechanical ventilation without sedation, and sedation should always be decreased to the minimal amount necessary as excess sedation may delay extubation. An ideal level of sedation will keep the patient calm and compliant with the ventilator but still alert and able to follow commands.

Conscious Sedation

Conscious sedation is used to decrease sensations of pain and awareness caused by a surgical or invasive procedure, such a biopsy, chest tube insertion, fracture repair, and endoscopy. It is also used during presurgical preparations, such as insertion of central lines, catheters, and use of cooling blankets. Conscious sedation uses a combination of analgesia and sedation so that patients can remain responsive and follow verbal cues but have a brief amnesia preventing recall of the procedures. The patient must be monitored carefully, including pulse oximetry, during this type of sedation. The most commonly used drugs include:

- Midazolam (Versed®): This is a short-acting water-soluble sedative, with onset of 1-5 minutes, peaking in 30, and duration usually about 1 hour (up to 6 hours).
- Fentanyl: This is a short-acting opioid with immediate onset, peaking in 10-15 minutes and with a duration of about 20-45 minutes. Monitor respiratory function.

The fentanyl/midazolam combination provides both sedation and pain control. Conscious sedation usually requires 6 hours fasting prior to administration.

Therapeutic Gases

Carbon dioxide is a potent stimulator of respirations, but it is rarely used therapeutically because it can depress respirations if hypercarbia or respiratory acidosis is present. CO_2 may be administered at times as part of anesthesia, but it is most commonly used for insufflation for laparoscopic/endoscopic procedures.

Nitric oxide (NO) is used as a pulmonary vessel dilator to improve oxygenation by decreasing pulmonary artery pressure and pulmonary vascular resistance. NO is FDA-approved for use for neonatal PPH but is sometimes used for adults, although studies have not shown it an effective treatment for ARDS. NO should be delivered at 0.1-50 ppm to avoid toxicity that can occur over 50 ppm. Toxic reactions include methemoglobinemia and platelet inhibition with resultant bleeding.

Heliox is helium mixed with oxygen that is used to reduce airway resistance during mechanical ventilation and for pulmonary function tests. Heliox may also be used to treat respiratory obstruction and is used during laser surgery on the airway because it readily conducts heat away from the surgical site, reducing tissue damage. Heliox is sometimes used for COPD patients as it increases hyperventilation and reduces carbon dioxide levels.

Thoracentesis

A **thoracentesis** (aspiration of fluid or air from pleural space) is done to make a diagnosis, relieve pressure on the lung caused by pleural effusion, or instill medications. A chest x-ray is done prior to the procedure. A sedative may be given. The patient is in a sitting position, leaning onto a padded bedside stand, straddling a chair with head supported on the back of the chair, or lying on the opposite side with the head of the bed elevated 30-45° to ensure that fluid remains at the base. The patient should avoid coughing or moving during the procedure. The chest x-ray or ultrasound determines needle placement. After a local anesthetic is administered, a needle (with an attached 20-mL syringe and 3-way stopcock with tubing and a receptacle) is advanced intercostally into the pleural space. Fluid is drained, collected, examined, and measured. The needle is removed and a pressure dressing applied. A chest x-ray is done to ensure there is no pneumothorax. The patient is monitored for cough, dyspnea, and hypoxemia.

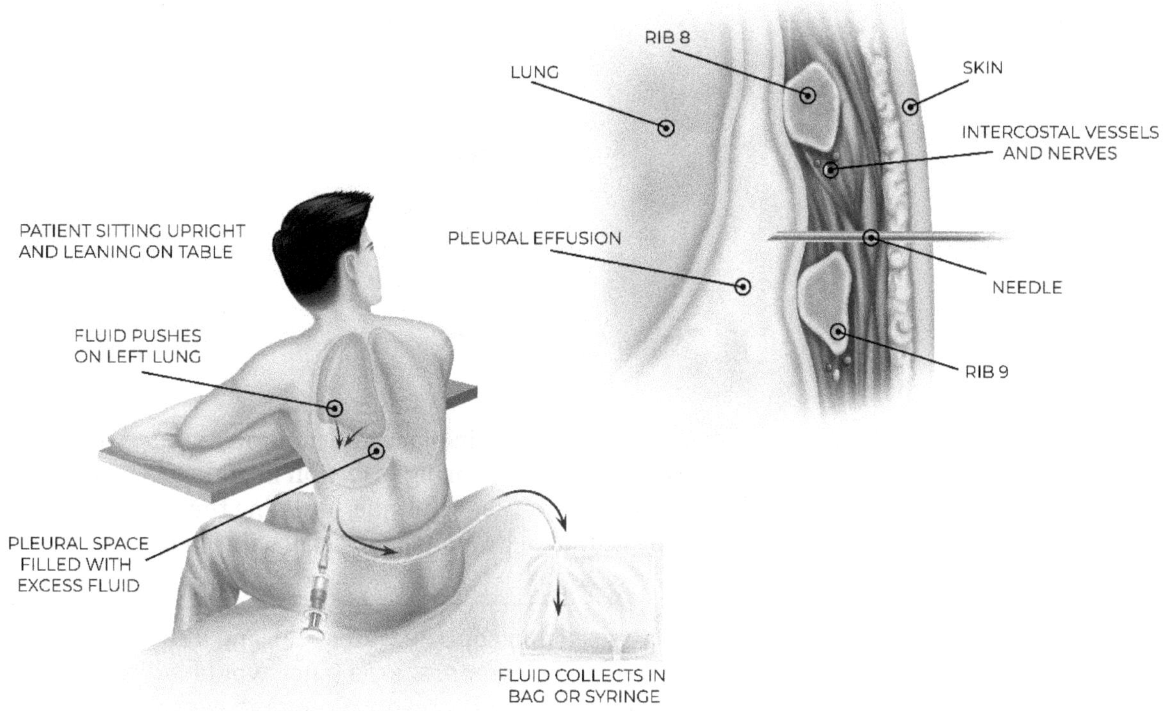

Bronchoscopy

Bronchoscopy utilizes a thin, flexible fiberoptic bronchoscope to inspect the larynx, trachea, and bronchi for diagnostic purposes. It is also used to collect specimens, obtain biopsies, remove foreign bodies or secretions, treat atelectasis, and to excise lesions. The patient is in supine position during the procedure. The Mallampati classification may be used to determine difficulty of airway. The patient receives local anesthesia to the nares (lidocaine gel) and oropharynx (lidocaine gel, spray, or nebulizer), and usually receives a benzodiazepine (commonly midazolam or lorazepam), an opioid (fentanyl or meperidine), or propofol. Medications are usually given in small incremental doses throughout the procedure and may be combined. Over-sedation may cause physiologic depression, but undersedation may result in recall and agitation with sympathetic activation. The tube is advanced through the nares and down the trachea to the bronchi. Airway patency, respiratory rate, and oxygen saturation must be constantly monitored. Complications can include bleeding, arrhythmias, obstruction, laryngospasm, and respiratory failure.

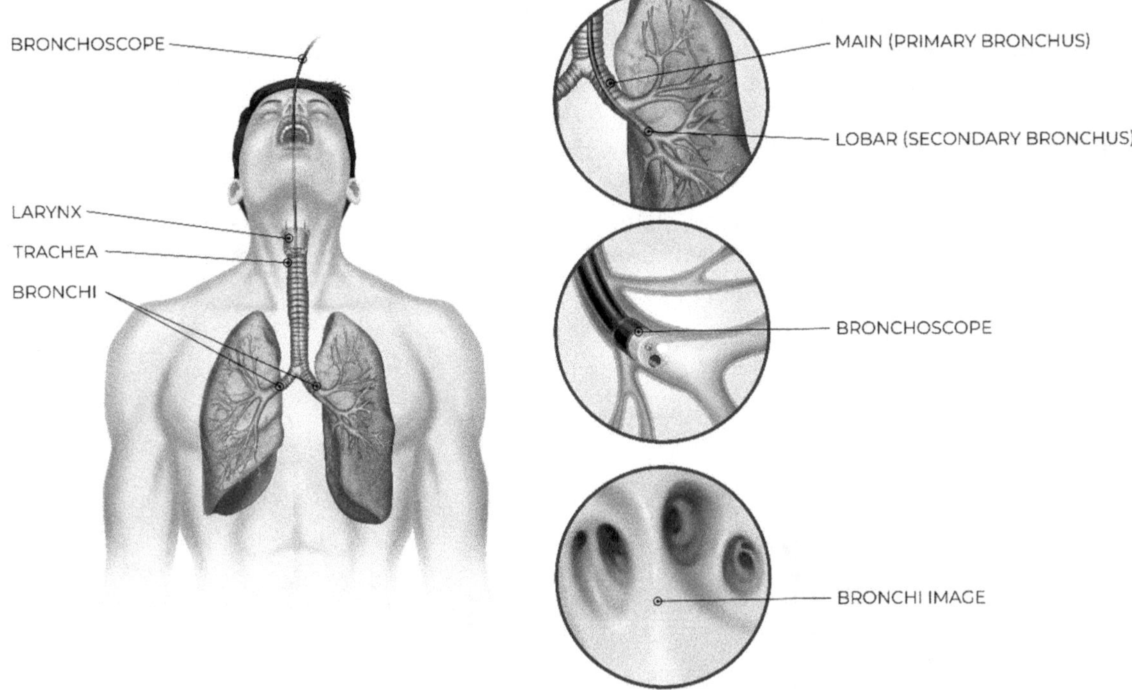

Chest Tubes

Chest tubes with a closed drainage system are usually left in place after thoracic surgery or pneumothorax to drain air or fluid. Nursing interventions during insertion include ensuring the patient receives adequate pain control, attending to sterile technique, assisting the physician with suturing as needed, attaching the tube to the chest tube drainage device, placing an occlusive dressing, and confirming placement.

Chest tube drainage systems have 3 major parts: suction control, water seal, and a chamber for collection. The system should have no bubbling in the water seal area (such would indicate a leak), but a subtle rise and fall of the water seal corresponding with respirations, and gentle bubbling in the suction control chamber.

Nursing interventions after chest tube is in place: in most circumstances, report drainage >100 mL/hr, assess tubing after position changes for occlusion, maintain sterile dressing, avoid stripping the tubing, and assessing the insertion site for drainage or crepitus, the tubing, the patency of the entire system, and the output (including color, amount, and any other traits). The nurse should be knowledgeable about specimen collection, replacing the system, and dealing with clots.

Thoracic Surgery

Lung Volume Reduction

Lung volume reduction surgery (LVRS) usually involves removing about 20-35% of lung tissue that is not functioning adequately in order to reduce the lung size so that the lungs work more effectively. This procedure is most commonly used with adult emphysematous COPD patients. In adults, surgery is usually bilateral; however, some patients are not candidates for bilateral surgery because of cardiac disease or emphysema affecting only one lung. Unilateral surgery has been shown to be effective. Surgical removal of part of the lung improves ventilation and gas exchange and does not require the immunosuppressant therapy required for lung transplantation. Studies have shown that those with low risk for the surgery and with emphysematous changes in the upper lobes can benefit from the surgery, but high-risk patients with more widespread emphysematous changes have increased mortality rates. The surgery may be done through an open-chest thoracotomy or through a less invasive video-assisted thoracotomy.

Pneumonectomy

Pneumonectomy is the surgical removal of one of the lungs. There are 2 surgical procedures:

- **Simple**: removal of just the lung
- **Extrapleural**: removal not only of the lung but also part of the diaphragm on the affected side and the pericardium on that same side

During the operative procedure, much care must be taken to prevent contamination of the remaining lung, including the use of bronchus blockers or prone position during surgery.

Removal of the lung is indicated for a number of conditions, including:

- Cancerous lesions (the most common reason for surgery)
- Severe bronchiectasis from chronic suppurative pneumonia, resulting in dilation of terminal bronchioles
- Severe hypoplasia
- Unilateral lung destruction with pulmonary hypertension
- Pulmonary hemorrhage
- Lobar emphysema
- Chronic pulmonary infections with destruction of lung tissue

Because the lung capacity is reduced, persistent shortness of breath may occur with exertion even many months after surgery.

Lobectomy and Other Procedures to Remove Partial Lung Tissue

Lobectomy removes one or more lobes of a lung (which has 2 on the left and 3 on the right) and is usually done for lesions or trauma that is confined to one lobe, such as tubercular lesions, abscesses or cysts, cancer (usually non-small cell in early stages), traumatic injury, or bronchiectasis. Surgery is usually done through an open thoracotomy or video-assisted thoracotomy. Complications can include hemorrhage, post-operative infection with or without abscess formation, and pneumothorax. Usually 1-2 chest tubes are left in place in the immediate post-surgical period to remove air and/or fluid.

- **Segmental resection** removes a bronchovascular segment and is used for small lesions in the periphery, bronchiectasis or congenital cysts or blebs.
- **Wedge resection** removes a small wedged-shape portion of the lung tissue and is used for small peripheral lesions, granulomas, or blebs.
- **Bronchoplastic (sleeve) reconstruction** removes part of bronchus and lung tissue with reanastomosis of bronchus and is used for small lesions of the carina or bronchus.

Respiratory Pharmacology

Pharmacological Agents Used for Asthma

Numerous **pharmacological agents** are used for control of asthma, some that are long-acting to prevent attacks and others that are short-acting to provide relief for acute episodes. Listed with each are the standard med and dosage used for urgent care:

- **β-Adrenergic agonists** include both long-acting and short-acting preparations used for relaxation of smooth muscles and bronchodilation, reducing edema, and aiding clearance of mucus. Medications include salmeterol (Serevent), sustained-release albuterol (Volmax ER®) and short-acting albuterol (Proventil®), and levalbuterol (Xopenex®). Albuterol 2.5-5.0 mg every 20 minutes, 3 doses by nebulizer.
- **Anticholinergics** aid in preventing bronchial constriction and potentiate the bronchodilating action of β-Adrenergic agonists. The most commonly used medication is ipratropium bromide (Atrovent®) 500 mcg every 20 minutes, 3 doses by nebulizer.
- **Corticosteroids** provide anti-inflammatory action by inhibiting immune responses and decreasing edema, mucus, and hyper-responsiveness. Because of numerous side effects, glucocorticosteroids are usually administered orally or parenterally for ≤5 days (prednisone, prednisolone, methylprednisolone) and then switched to inhaled steroids. If a person receives glucocorticoids for more than 5 days, then dosages are tapered. Methylprednisolone 60-125 mg IV is the standard dose for respiratory failure. The Global Initiative for Asthma (GINA) recommends daily inhaled corticosteroids for all individuals with severe asthma to reduce the risk of exacerbations.
- **Methylxanthines** are used to improve pulmonary function and decrease the need for mechanical ventilation. Medications include aminophylline and theophylline.
- **Magnesium sulfate** is used to relax smooth muscles and decrease inflammation. If administered intravenously, it must be given slowly to prevent hypotension and bradycardia. When inhaled, it potentiates the action of albuterol. Standard dosage: 2 g (8 mmol), 1 dose by IV over 20 minutes.
- **Heliox** (helium-oxygen) is administered to decrease airway resistance with airway obstruction, thereby decreasing respiratory effort. Heliox improves oxygenation of those on mechanical ventilation.
- **Leukotriene inhibitors** are used to inhibit inflammation and bronchospasm for long-term management. Medications include montelukast (Singulair®).

Additional Pulmonary Pharmacology

There is a wide range of agents used for **pulmonary pharmacology**, depending upon the type and degree of pulmonary disease. Agents include:

- **Opioid analgesics:** Used to provide both pain relief and sedation for those on mechanical ventilation to reduce sympathetic response. Medications may include fentanyl (Sublimaze®) or morphine sulfate (MS Contin®).
- **Neuromuscular blockers:** Used for induced paralysis of those who have not responded adequately to sedation, especially for intubation and mechanical ventilation. Medications may include pancuronium (Pavulon®) and vecuronium (Norcuron®). However, there is controversy about the use of such blockers, as induced paralysis has been linked to increased mortality rates, sensory hearing loss (pancuronium), atelectasis, and ventilation-perfusion mismatch.

- **Human B-type natriuretic peptides:** Used to reduce pulmonary capillary wedge pressure. Medications include nesiritide (Natrecor®).
- **Surfactants**: Reduces surface tension to prevent the collapse of alveoli. Beractant (Survanta®) is derived from bovine lung tissue and calfactant (Infasurf®) from calf lung tissue. They are administered as inhalants.
- **Alkalinizers**: Used to treat metabolic acidosis and reduce pulmonary vascular resistance by achieving an alkaline pH. Medications include sodium bicarbonate and tromethamine (THAM).
- **Pulmonary vasodilator (inhaled nitric oxide):** Used to relax the vascular muscles and produce pulmonary vasodilation. Some studies show it reduces the need for extracorporeal membrane oxygenation (ECMO).
- **Methylxanthines:** Used to stimulate muscle contractions of the chest and stimulate respirations. Medications include aminophylline (Aminophylline®), caffeine citrate (Cafcit®), and doxapram (Dopram®).
- **Diuretics**: Used to reduce pulmonary edema. Medications include loop diuretics such as furosemide (Lasix®) and metolazone (Mykrox®).
- **Nitrates**: Used for vasodilation to reduce preload and afterload, which in turn reduces myocardial need for oxygen. Medications include nitroglycerin (Nitro-Bid®) and nitroprusside sodium (Nitropress®).
- **Antibiotics**: Used for treatment of respiratory infections, including pneumonia. Medications are used according to the pathogenic agent and may include macrolides such as azithromycin (Zithromax®) and erythromycin (E-Mycin®).
- **Antimycobacterials**: Used for treatment of TB and other mycobacterial diseases. Medications include isoniazid (Laniazid®, Nydrazid®), ethambutol (Myambutol®), rifampin (Rifadin®), streptomycin sulfate, and pyrazinamide.
- **Antivirals**: Used to inhibit replication of a virus early in a viral infection. Effectiveness decreases as time passes because the replication process has already begun. Medications include ribavirin (Virazole®) and zanamivir (Relenza®).

Integumentary Procedures and Interventions

Wound VACs

Wound vacuum-assisted closure (wound VAC) (AKA negative pressure wound therapy) uses subatmospheric (negative) pressure with a suction unit and a semi-occlusion vapor-permeable dressing. The suction reduces periwound and interstitial edema, decompressing vessels, improving circulation, stimulating production of new cells, and decreasing colonization of bacteria. Wound VAC also increases the rate of granulation and re-epithelialization to hasten healing. The wound must be debrided of necrotic tissue prior to treatment. Wound VAC is used for a variety of difficult-to-heal wounds, especially those that show less than 30% healing in 4 weeks of post-debridement treatment or those with excessive exudate, including chronic stage II and IV pressure ulcers, skin flaps, diabetic ulcer, acute wounds, burns, surgical wound, and those with dehiscence and nonresponsive arterial and venous ulcers. Contraindications include:

- Wound malignancy.
- Untreated osteomyelitis.
- Exposed blood vessels or organs.
- Non-enteric, unexplored fistulas.

Nonadherent porous foam is cut to fit and cover the wound and is secured with occlusive transparent film with an opening cut to accommodate the drainage tube, which is attached to a suction canister in a closed system. The pressure should be set between 75 and 125 psi and the dressing changed 2 to 3 times weekly.

Biological Wound Debridement with Maggots

Medical maggots are applied to the open wound; periwound tissue must be protected:

- A **wound pattern** is transferred onto a hydrocolloid pad, an opening is cut, and a pad is applied to the skin with the wound exposed. The pattern is used to cut an opening in a semi-permeable film for an outer dressing.
- Maggots are wiped from the container with a saline-dampened 2x2 **gauze** (about 5-10 maggots per cm^2 wound size). The gauze is loosely packed into the wound.
- A porous **mesh** (*Creature Comfort*) is placed over the wound and secured to the hydrocolloid with tape or glue, creating a maggot cage.
- **Transparent film** is placed over the hydrocolloid, making sure that the cutout area is over the cage so that the maggots have air and drainage can escape. Saline-dampened gauze is placed loosely over the cage.
- **Dry gauze** is used for the outer dressing and changed every 4-8 hours as needed.

Maggots are wiped from the wound after 48 hours and the wound is **irrigated** with normal saline.

Pressure Reduction Surfaces

Pressure reduction surfaces redistribute pressure to prevent pressure ulcers and reduce shear and friction. There are various types of support surfaces for beds, examining tables, operating tables, and chairs. Functions of pressure reduction surfaces include temperature control, moisture control, and friction/shear control. General use guidelines include:

- Pressure redistribution support surfaces should be used for patients with stage II, III, and IV ulcers, as well as for those that are at-risk for developing pressure ulcers.
- Chairs should have gel or air support surfaces to redistribute pressure for chair bound patients, critically ill patients, or those who cannot move independently.
- Support surface material should provide at least an inch of support under areas to be protected when in use to prevent bottoming out. (Check by placing hand palm-up under the overlay below the pressure point.)
- Static support surfaces are appropriate for patients who can change position without increasing pressure to an ulcer.
- Dynamic support surfaces are needed for those who need assistance to move or when static pressure devices provide less than an inch of support.

Integumentary Pharmacology

Topical Anesthetics for Wound Pain

There are numerous different types of pain medications that may be used to control pain from wounds, including **topical anesthetics**:

- **Lidocaine 2-4%** is frequently used during debridement or dressing changes. Lidocaine is useful only superficially and may take 15-30 minutes before it is effective.
- **Eutectic Mixture of Local Anesthetics (EMLA Cream)** provides good pain control. The wound is first cleansed and then the cream is applied thickly (1/4 inch) extending about 1/2 inch past the wound to the periwound tissue. The wound is then covered with plastic wrap, which is secured and left in place for about 20 minutes. The wrapped time may be extended to 45-60 minutes if necessary, to completely numb the tissue. The tissue should remain numb for about 1 hour after the plastic wrap is removed, allowing time for the wound to be cleansed, debrided, and/or redressed.

Regional Anesthesia for Wound Pain

Regional anesthesia (injectable subcutaneous and perineural medications) is administered locally about the wound or as nerve blocks. Medications include lidocaine, bupivacaine, and tetracaine in solution. Epinephrine is sometimes added to increase vasoconstriction and reduce bleeding, although it is avoided in distal areas of the limbs (hands and feet) to prevent ischemia.

- **Field blockade** involves injecting the anesthetic into the periwound tissue or into the wound margins. The effect may be decreased by inflammation. The effects last for limited periods of time.
- **Regional nerve blocks** may involve single injections, the effects of which are limited in duration but can provide pain relief for treatments. Techniques that use continuous catheter infusions are longer lasting and can be controlled more precisely. Blocks may involve nerves proximal to affected areas, such as peripheral nerve blocks, or large nerve blocks near the spinal cord, such as percutaneous lumbar sympathetic blocks (LSB). Long-term blocks may use alcohol-based medications to permanently inactivate the nerves.

Musculoskeletal Procedures and Interventions

Monitoring Devices for Extremity Compartment Syndrome

Signs of **extremity compartment syndrome** include the 5 P's: (1) pain that is severe and out of proportion to injury, (2) paresthesia, (3) pallor, (4) paresis, and (5) pulse deficit. Pressure is typically measured with a device specially intended for measurement although it can also be measured by attaching a manometer to a needle and syringe. The procedure with the Stryker intercompartmental pressure monitor device includes:

- First, the skin is cleansed with antiseptic and a local anesthetic administered.
- The pressure monitor device (or similar) contains a 3 mL syringe, a chamber and needle that connect to the syringe, and a pressure monitor into which the syringe is placed.
- Air is purged from the chamber and needle with the saline.
- The syringe is placed into the pressure monitoring device.
- The device is turned on, zeroed automatically by pressing the "zero" button.

- The needle is inserted into the compartment.
- Once the needle is inserted, about 0.3 mL of NS is injected and the device automatically records the compartment pressure. If the compartment pressure is over 30 mmHg, a fasciotomy is usually needed.

Pelvic Stabilizer

Pelvic stabilizers are used to prevent excessive bleeding associated with pelvic fractures, to maintain the bones in the correct position, and to prevent further damage. Maintaining pressure and reducing the fracture often reduces bleeding. Various methods of stabilizing the pelvis may be employed, including the sheet wrap method in which a sheet is folded, center under the patient, wrapped tightly about the pelvis, and secured. The pneumatic anti-shock garment (PASG) is indicated for hypovolemic shock, and hypotension associated with and for stabilization of pelvic and bilateral femur fractures. PASG is contraindicated with respiratory distress, pulmonary edema, pregnancy (after the first trimester), heart failure, myocardial infarction, stroke, evisceration, abdominal or leg impalement, head injuries, and uncontrolled bleeding above the garment. Another device is the SAM pelvic sling, which has a wide band that fits under and about the pelvis and lateral hips and a belt anteriorly that allows adjustment.

Immobilization Devices

Immobilization devices include:

- **Cervical collar**: Support the head to prevent spinal cord injury with suspected injury to cervical vertebrae.
- **Cervical extrication splints**: Short board used to immobilize and protect the head and neck during extrication.
- **Backboards**: Used to immobilize the spine to prevent further injury to spinal cord. Both long and short spine boards are available in a number of different shapes and sizes.
- **Full-body splints** (such as vacuum mattress splint): Provide cushioned support to maintain body alignment.
- **Various types of splints for extremities**: Include rigid (should be padded), non-rigid (moldable), traction, and air (pneumatic devices) as well as the use of blankets, rolled towels, sheets, and pillows to maintain position. Traction splints are used for fractured femurs to keep bones in position.
- **Pneumatic anti-shock garment** (PASG): Provides pressure on lower extremities and abdomen and is used to control hemorrhage and shock to prevent pooling of blood in extremities and return blood to general circulation. Often used for pelvic fractures, but may increase risk of internal hemorrhage.

Spinal Immobilization

Spinal immobilization, once a standard for trauma patients, has been shown to have little effect and in some cases may cause harm. Because of these findings, spinal immobilization with backboard is now recommended only for patients with neurological complaints, such as numbness, tingling, weakness, paralysis, pain or tenderness in the spine, spinal deformity, blunt trauma associated with alterations of consciousness, and high energy injuries associated with drugs/alcohol, inability of the patient to communicate, and/or distracting injury. Cervical collars for cervical spine immobilization are to be utilized for trauma based on the NEXUS criteria or Canadian

C-spine rules (CCR). According to **NEXUS criteria**, a patient who exhibits all of the following does not require a cervical collar:

- Alert and stable
- No intoxication
- No midline tenderness of the spine
- No distracting injury
- No neurological deficit

Spinal immobilization should be continued for the shortest time possible, so imaging, such as CT, should be carried out upon admission. Cervical collars are applied while the head is supported in neutral position, and the patient is logrolled onto a backboard and strapped in place.

IMMOBILIZATION OF FRACTURES AND DISLOCATIONS

Immobilization techniques for fractures and dislocations include:

- **Cast**: Plaster and fiberglass casts are applied after reduction to ensure that the bone is correctly aligned. Cast should be placed over several layers of padding that extends slightly beyond the cast ends. Cast material, such as plaster, should NOT be immersed in hot water but water slightly above room temperature (70 °F).
- **Splint**: Plaster splints use 12 or more layers of plaster measured to the correct length and then several layers of padding (longer and wider than splint should be measured and cut). The plaster splint is submerged in water to saturate, removed, laid on a flat surface, and massaged to fuse the layers. The padding is laid on top, and the splint is positioned and wrapped with gauze to hold it in place. While setting the splint, position can be maintained by holding it in place with the palm of the hand (not the fingers). After setting, the splint may be wrapped by elastic compression bandages.

AMPUTATION CARE

IMMEDIATE INTERVENTIONS FOR TRAUMATIC AMPUTATION

Amputations may be partial or complete. The amputated limb should be treated initially as though it could be reattached or revascularized. Single digits, except the thumb, are often not reattached. Initial treatment includes stabilizing patient and stopping bleeding by applying a proximal blood pressure cuff proximal to injury 30 mmHg above systolic for <30 minutes. Instruments, such as clamps and hemostats, should be avoided. Other treatment includes:

- Tetanus prophylaxis
- Analgesia
- Prophylactic antibiotics may be needed
- Irrigation of stump with NS (not antiseptics) if contaminated
- Splint and elevate stump, with saline-moistened sterile dressing in place
- Neurovascular examinations of stump

The Allen test should be done to determine arterial injury if digits are amputated. In the Allen test, both the radial and ulnar artery are compressed and the patient is asked to clench the hand repeatedly until it blanches, and then one artery is released, and the tissue on that side should flush. Then the test is repeated again, releasing the other artery.

Care of Amputated Part Prior to Reattachment or Revascularization

The **amputated part** should be cooled to 4 °C to extend the time of viability and decrease damage from ischemia. (Single digits and lower limbs are not usually reattached, but the limbs should be treated as though they will until determination is made, especially for children.) The part should be reattached within 6 hours if possible but up to 24 hours if properly cooled. Initial care of amputated part includes:

- Removal of jewelry
- Irrigation with NS to remove debris or contamination
- Part stored wrapped in saline moistened dressing but NOT immersed in saline or hypotonic solution
- Minimal handling to prevent tissue damage
- Cool by placing wrapped part in sealed plastic bag and immersing the bag in ice water (1:1 ice to water), but avoid freezing the part

If the amputation is partial, treatment is similar but NS wrapped part is splinted and ice packs or commercial cold packs are applied over area that is devascularized.

Tourniquets

Tourniquets are used to control hemorrhage in an extremity and should be applied immediately with arterial bleeds or if pressure does not stop bleeding. Commonly used tourniquets include adjustable bands that are tightened and secured and then include a windlass handle twisted until blood flow stops and the handle is secured. Another type is a wide elastic band that is stretched, wrapped about the extremity tightly a number of times and secured. Blood pressure cuffs may also be used to apply pressure if standard tourniquets are not available. Regardless of the type, the tourniquet should be placed as high on the extremity as possible (avoiding joints), and the date and time of placement should be documented (on the tourniquet if possible). Tourniquets may be contraindicated with DVT, Reynaud's disease, crushing injuries, sickle cell disease, severe peripheral arterial disease, and open lower extremity fractures. Risks include damage to muscles, nerves, and vessels as well as increased risk of amputation. However, the first priority is always to prevent exsanguination.

Psychosocial Procedures and Interventions

Behavior Modification

Behavior modification is a type of systematic therapy that works toward the goal of replacing **maladaptive behaviors** with **positive behaviors.** This type of therapy can be utilized with individuals, groups, or entire communities. The hope of this approach is to get rid of the unwanted behaviors by utilizing positive reinforcement directed toward the desired behaviors. After experiencing **positive reinforcement**, the participant will want to repeat the good behaviors to gain the reward. These new behaviors will then become habits over time and will replace the old behaviors. This type of therapy can be very effective with eating disorders, smoking cessation, or addictions.

Cognitive-Behavioral Therapy

Cognitive-Behavioral Therapy (CBT) focuses on the impact that thoughts have on behavior and feelings, encouraging the individual to use the power of rational thought to alter perceptions. CBT centers on the concept of unlearning previous behaviors and learning new ones, questioning behaviors, and doing homework. This approach to counseling is usually short-term, about 12-20 sessions. The first sessions obtain a history, middle sessions focus on the problems, and the last sessions review and reinforce newly learned habits and thought patterns. Individuals are assigned homework during the sessions to practice new ways of thinking and to develop new coping strategies. The therapist helps the individual identify goals and then find ways to achieve those goals. CBT acknowledges that all problems cannot be resolved, but one can deal differently with problems. The therapist asks questions to determine the individual's areas of concern and encourages the individual to question his or her own motivations and needs. CBT is goal-centered, so each counseling session is structured toward a particular goal, such as coping techniques.

Aaron Beck's Cognitive Therapy

Aaron Beck discovered that during psychotherapy patients often had a second set of thoughts while undergoing free association. Beck called these **automatic thoughts**, which were labeled and interpreted, according to a personal set of rules. Beck called dysfunctional automatic thoughts **cognitive disorders**. Beck identified a triad of negative thoughts regarding the self, environment, and world. The key concepts in **Aaron Beck's cognitive therapy** include the following:

- **Therapist/patient relationship**: Therapy is a collaborative partnership. The goal of therapy is determined together. The therapist encourages the patient to disagree when appropriate.
- **Process of therapy**: The therapist explains the following: one's perception of reality is not reality. The interpretation of sensory input depends on cognitive processes. The patient is taught to recognize maladaptive ideation, identifying the following: observable behavior, underlying motivation, his or her thoughts and beliefs. The patient practices distancing the maladaptive thoughts, explores his or her conclusions, and tests them against reality.
- **Conclusions**: The patient makes the rules less extreme and absolute, drops false rules, and substitutes adaptive rules.

Recovery Model

The **Recovery Model** approach to mental health shifts control of treatment options to the **patient** rather than the physician deciding the plan of care. This has been effective in those patients who have the capacity to make decisions to allow them to be more independent and take a more active role in the decision-making regarding their treatment plan. The goal of this model is to allow the patient to be more **autonomous** so that they may achieve the ultimate goals of gaining employment, finding housing, and living independently. The more independent the patient can become, the more they progress to making independent decisions about the treatment of their mental health issues. This model is not appropriate for those patients who are so incapacitated by their illness that they do not understand they are ill. The amount of independence and decision-making that is turned over to the patient should increase as they become more stable.

Acceptance Commitment Therapy

Acceptance commitment therapy (ACT) approaches behavioral change from a different perspective than conventional CBT. Patients are encouraged to examine their thought processes (**cognitive defusion**) when undergoing episodes of anxiety or depression. They identify a thought, such as, "People think I am ugly," and then analyze whether or not this is true, listing evidence, and then evaluating whether or not the anxiety is decreased after this evaluation process. Eventually, this process becomes automatic, eliminating the need to write everything down. Mindfulness is a basic concept of ACT, and patients are encouraged to examine their values and control those things that are under their control, such as their facial expression or actions. ACT represents (A) **accepting** reactions, (C) **choosing** a direction, and (T) **taking** action to effect change.

Single-Session Therapy

Single-session therapy is the **most frequent form of counseling** because individuals often attend only one session for various reasons even if more are advised. Individuals may not have insurance or believe that one session is sufficient. Sessions typically last 1 hour. The goal is to identify a problem and reach a solution in one session. The therapist serves as a facilitator to motivate the individual to view the problem as part of a pattern that can be changed and to identify a solution. The therapist may use a wide range of techniques that culminates in a **plan for the individual** (e.g., homework exercises) so the individual can begin to make changes.

Solution-Focused Therapy

Solution-focused therapy aims to differentiate methods that are effective from those that are not, and to identify areas of strengths so they can be used in problem solving. The premise of solution-focused therapy is that change is possible but that the individual must identify problems and deal with them in the real world. This therapy is based on questioning to help the individual establish goals and find solutions to problems:

- **Pre-session**: The patient is asked about any differences he or she noted after making the appointment and coming to the first session.
- **Miracle**: The patient is asked if any miracles occurred or if any problems were solved, including what, if anything, was different and how this difference affected relationships.
- **Exception**: The patient is asked if any small changes were noted and if there were any problems that no longer seemed problematic and how that manifested.
- **Scaling**: The patient is asked to evaluate the problem on a 1–10 scale and then to determine how to increase the rating.
- **Coping**: The patient is asked about how he or she is managing.

Trauma-Informed Care

Trauma-informed care acts on the premise that many individuals have experienced some sort of trauma, and therefore every patient should be approached with sensitivity and care. Traumatic events are deeply individualized, and what may have been traumatic to one individual, may not be to the next. Withholding judgment of what qualifies as trauma is imperative for the psychiatric-mental health nurse.

The five elements of trauma-informed care include the following:

- **Safety**: Ensuring that the patient feels emotionally and physically safe must be the first priority in order to create a conducive environment for treatment.
- **Choice**: Treatment cannot be forced and must honor the individual's right to choose.
- **Collaboration**: The patient and the nurse must work collaboratively through shared decision-making.
- **Trustworthiness**: The patient must trust the nurse in order for treatment to be effective. Trustworthiness can be established by communicating what is happening and what will happen next to the patient.
- **Empowerment**: Empower the patient with tools to cope on their own so that their recovery extends outside the walls of treatment.

Psychiatric and Mental Health Programs

A variety of **psychiatric and mental health programs** are available and should be evaluated, according to the needs of the individual patient.

- **Inpatient programs** provide a secure environment and comprehensive care, often with psychologists, psychiatrists, occupational therapists, social workers, and other allied health personnel. Programs may be tailored to one specific type of patient (e.g., criminally insane, substance abusers) or to a general population. They may offer short-term or long-term care.
- **Outpatient programs** provide assessment and treatment, such as group therapy, cognitive-behavioral therapy, and family therapy. Programs may be community-based, targeting specific groups of people, such as alcoholics or the homeless.
- **Partial/day hospitalization programs** provide daily inpatient care during prescribed hours (e.g., 8 a.m. to 3 p.m.) as well as outpatient services. The stay is usually short-term (1–2 weeks) and may serve as a transition from inpatient to outpatient care.

Nonviolent Crisis Intervention and De-Escalation Techniques

Nonviolent crisis intervention and de-escalation techniques begin with self-awareness because the normal response to aggression is a stress response (freezing, fight/flight, fear). The nurse must control these responses in order to deal with the situation. The nurse should recognize signs of impending conflict (clenched fists, and sudden change in tone of voice or body stance, and change in eye contact). Steps include:

- Maintain social distance (≥12 feet) if possible and stay at the same level as the person (sitting or standing).
- Speak in a quiet calm tone of voice, limiting eye contact and avoiding changes in voice tone, facial expression, and gestures (especially avoid pointing or waving a finger at the person).
- Ask the person's name (if necessary) and use the name when addressing the person.
- Validate the person by acknowledging their issue: "I can see that you are angry about the changes in your treatment."
- Show empathy without being judgmental: "I'm sorry you are upset."
- Ignore questions that are challenging and avoid arguing.
- Practice active listening by paraphrasing and clarifying.
- Assist the person to explore options and the results of those options: "What is it that you would like to do?"

Physical Restraints

Restraints are used to restrict movement and activity when other methods of controlling patient behavior have failed and there is a risk of harm to the patient or others. There are two primary types of restraints: violent (behavioral) and non-violent (clinical). Violent restraints are more commonly used in the psychiatric unit or when individuals exhibit aggressive behavior. More commonly, non-violent restraints are used to ensure that the individual does not interfere with safe care. Non-violent restraints are commonly used in the confused elderly or intubated patient to prevent pulling out lines/removing equipment. The federal government and the Joint Commission have issued strict guidelines for temporary restraints or those not part of standard care (such as post-surgical restraint):

- Each facility must have a written policy and restraints are only used when ordered by a physician (usually require written/signed order every 24hrs and within 4 hours of restraint initiation).

- An assessment must be completed frequently, including circulation, toileting, and nutritional needs (generally every 1-2 hours).
- All alternative methods should be tried before applying a restraint and the least restrictive effective restraint should be used.
- A nurse must remove the restraint, assess, and document findings at least every 2 hours, every hour for violent restraints.

Key: Least restrictive option for the least amount of time.

CHEMICAL RESTRAINTS

Chemical restraints involve the use of pharmacological sedatives to manage an individual's behavior problems. This type of restraint is indicated only when severe agitation/violence puts the patient at risk for injury to themselves or others. Chemical restraints inhibit the individuals' physical movements, making their behavior more manageable. It is important to realize that medication used on an ongoing basis as part of treatment is not legally considered a chemical restraint, even though the medications may be the same. There is little consensus about the use of chemical restraints, although benzodiazepines and antipsychotics are frequently used to control severe agitation (haloperidol, lorazepam, etc.). Oral medications should be tried first before injections, as oral medication is less coercive. It is important for the nurse to realize that chemical restraints are used as a last resort when other measures (such as de-escalation and environmental modification) have failed and there is an immediate risk of harm to the patient or others.

Psychosocial Pharmacology

ANTIPSYCHOTIC MEDICATIONS

FIRST-GENERATION

There are a variety of **first-generation antipsychotics** available, though their use is becoming less prominent now that atypical antipsychotic agents are available. Some first-generation antipsychotics include:

- Chlorpromazine (Thorazine®)
- Thioridazine hydrochloride (Mellaril®)
- Haloperidol (Haldol®)
- Pimozide (Orap®)
- Fluphenazine hydrochloride (Prolixin®)
- Molindone hydrochloride (Moban®)
- Trifluoperazine hydrochloride (Stelazine®).

Possible side effects include photosensitivity, sexual dysfunction, dry mouth, dry eyes, nasal congestion, blurred vision, constipation, urinary retention, exacerbation of narrow-angle glaucoma, various cardiac effects, extrapyramidal effects, dyskinesia, sedation, cognitive dulling, amenorrhea, menstrual irregularities, hyperglycemia or hypoglycemia, increased appetite, and weight gain. The most common extrapyramidal symptom caused by antipsychotic agents is tardive dyskinesia, in which clients are unable to control their movements, such as tics, lip-smacking, and eye blinking. The extrapyramidal system is a group of neural connections outside of the medulla that control movement. **Extrapyramidal effects** are the result of drug influence on the extrapyramidal system and include:

- Akinesia (inability to start movement)
- Akathisia (inability to stop movement)
- Dystonia (extreme and uncontrolled muscle contraction, torticollis, flexing, and twisting)

Second-Generation

Second-generation antipsychotics (SGAs), also called atypical antipsychotics, are used for bipolar disorders, schizophrenia, and psychosis and include aripiprazole (Abilify®), clozapine (Clozaril®), olanzapine (Zyprexa®), quetiapine (Seroquel®), risperidone (Risperdal®), and ziprasidone (Geodon®). Females report more side effects than males, but the recommended doses for males and females are identical. Women were underrepresented when SGAs were clinically tested, because researchers feared teratogenic effects on fetuses:

- Side effects include constipation, increased appetite, weight gain, urinary retention, various sexual side effects, increased prolactin, menstrual irregularities, increased risk of diabetes mellitus, decreased blood pressure, dizziness, agranulocytosis, and leucopenia.
- Atypical antipsychotics may interact with fluvoxamine, phenytoin, carbamazepine, barbiturates, nicotine, ketoconazole, phenytoin, rifampin, and glucocorticoids.
- The use of atypical antipsychotic agents correlates with significant weight gain. Overweight and obese clients are likely to develop insulin resistance and glucose intolerance, which may lead to diabetes mellitus. Data show clozapine and olanzapine as the greatest offenders. Ziprasidone seems to present the lowest risk.

Review Video: Anti-Psychotic Drugs: Clozapine, Haloperidol, Etc.
Visit mometrix.com/academy and enter code: 369601

Antidepressants

Indications for Treatment with Antidepressant

The main **indicator** for use of an antidepressant is simply **depression**. This can be further expanded to include major depression, atypical depression, and anxiety disorders. Depression-type symptoms commonly include loss of interest in usual or pleasurable activities, decreased levels of energy, having a depressed mood, decreased ability to concentrate, loss of appetite, or suicidal thoughts. Antidepressants are also commonly used to treat **anxiety disorders** that include panic attacks, obsessive-compulsive disorder (OCD), social phobias, and post-traumatic stress disorder. They may also be beneficial in treating chronic pain syndromes, premenstrual syndrome, insomnia, attention deficit hyperactivity disorder, or bed-wetting.

SSRIs

Selective serotonin reuptake inhibitors (SSRIs) prevent the reuptake of serotonin at the presynaptic membrane. This increases the amount of serotonin in the synapse for neurotransmission. This class of antidepressants has been shown to reduce depression and anxiety symptoms. Common side effects are usually short in duration and include headache, GI upset, and sexual dysfunction. They do not cause significant anticholinergic, cardiovascular, or significant patient sedation side effects. Examples of SSRIs include citalopram (Celexa), escitalopram (Lexapro), fluoxetine (Prozac), Fluvoxamine (Luvox), paroxetine (Paxil), and sertraline (Zoloft). These drugs are not highly lethal in overdose.

Monitoring

SSRI monitoring includes the following:

- Monitor for increased depression and suicidal ideation, especially in adolescents.
- Inform patients of the following:
    - Smoking decreases effectiveness.
    - Fatal reactions may occur with monoamine oxidase inhibitors.
    - Taking SSRIs with benzodiazepines or alcohol has an additive effect.
    - Some drugs, such as citalopram, may increase the effects of β-blockers and warfarin.
- Avoid cimetidine, which is prescribed for ulcers and gastroesophageal reflux disease, and St. John's wort.
- Inform patients of possible decreased libido and sexual functioning.
- Monitor for insomnia and gastrointestinal upset.

Tricyclic Antidepressants

Tricyclic antidepressants not only block the reuptake of serotonin and norepinephrine, they also act to block muscarinic cholinergic receptors, histamine H1 receptors, and alpha1 noradrenergic receptors. These receptors do not affect depression symptoms, but their blockade is implicated in some of the side effects associated with tricyclics. The blockade of the muscarinic receptors produces anticholinergic side effects such as dry mouth, blurred vision, constipation, urinary retention, and tachycardia. The blockade of the histamine receptors is associated with drowsiness, low blood pressure, and weight gain. The alpha1 noradrenergic receptor blocking action produces the side effects associated with orthostatic hypotension, vertigo, and some memory disturbances.

Mechanism of Action and Necessary Evaluations

Most of the tricyclic antidepressants have very similar mechanisms of action and side effects. Although their exact **mechanism of action** is unknown, they are believed to act to inhibit the reuptake of both serotonin and norepinephrine. These drugs have a high **first-pass rate of metabolism** and are excreted by the kidneys. A complete **physical and history** should be obtained before starting a patient on tricyclic drugs. Because this class of antidepressants can cause death with an overdose, an initial **suicide risk assessment** must be obtained, and continued assessments for this risk are necessary. This class of drug can cause a prolongation in the electrical conduction of the heart. Therefore, a **baseline ECG** should be performed in children, young teenagers, anyone with cardiac electrical conduction problems, and adults over age 40.

Monitoring

Tricyclics monitoring includes the following:

- Observe for toxicity.
- Inform patients not to take with monoamine oxidase inhibitors.
- Observe for decreased therapeutic response to hypertensives (e.g., clonidine, guanethidine).
- Monitor other medications; the patient should avoid other central nervous system depressants, including alcohol. Some medications potentiate the effects of tricyclics, including bupropion, cimetidine, haloperidol, selective serotonin reuptake inhibitors, and valproic acid.
- Inform the patient to avoid prolonged exposure to sunlight or sunlamps.
- Administer major dosage of the drug at bedtime if the patient experiences drowsiness.
- Monitor for sedation, cardiac arrhythmias, insomnia, gastrointestinal upset, and weight gain.

MAOIs

The **mechanism of action** for monoamine oxidase inhibitors (MAOIs) is exactly what their name indicates. These drugs act to inhibit the enzyme **monoamine oxidase (MAO)**. There are actually two of these enzymes, **MAO-A** and **MAO-B**, and this class of medication inhibits both. These enzymes act to metabolize serotonin and norepinephrine. By inhibiting the production of these enzymes, there are increased levels of **serotonin** and **norepinephrine** available for neurotransmission. Medications that selectively inhibit MAO-B have no antidepressant effects and can be used to treat disease processes such as Parkinson's.

Side Effects

Side effects associated with the use of **monoamine oxidase inhibitors (MAOIs)** are similar to antipsychotic medications. They can include symptoms such as GI upset, vertigo, headaches, sleep disturbances, sexual dysfunction, dry mouth, visual disturbances, constipation, peripheral edema, urinary hesitancy, weakness, increased weight, or orthostatic hypotension. The elderly population is at greatest risk for problems with **orthostatic hypotension** and should have lying, sitting, and standing blood pressure checks to monitor for this side effect. Orthostatic hypotension can lead to injuries related to falls, such as fractures. The most dangerous side effect can be an extreme **elevation in blood pressure** or **hypertensive crisis**. Hypertension can develop due to the presence of increased levels of **tyramine**. These levels increase because **monoamine oxidase**, which normally metabolizes tyramine, is inhibited. Increased levels of tyramine produce a vasoconstrictive response by the body that leads to increased blood pressure. Symptoms associated with hypertensive crisis can include severe occipital headache, palpitations, chest pain, diaphoresis, nausea and vomiting, flushed face, or dilated pupils. Complications associated with hypertensive crisis include hemorrhagic stroke, severe headache, or death. It is vital that patients receive in-depth education about the symptoms of hypertension, the need for close monitoring of blood pressure, and methods for sustaining a low-tyramine diet.

Diet Restrictions

Monoamine oxidase inhibitors can lead to increased levels of **tyramine** in the nerve cell. These increased levels can lead to a dangerous and possibly fatal increase in **blood pressure**. Certain **foods that contain tyramine** should be avoided to help prevent hypertensive episodes. Foods high in tyramine include strong or aged cheeses, cured meats, smoked or processed meats, pickled or fermented foods, sauces, such as soy or teriyaki sauce, soybeans, snow peas or broad beans, dried or overripe fruits, meat tenderizers, products containing monosodium glutamate, yeast-extract spreads, alcoholic beverages, and improperly stored foods or spoiled foods.

Anti-Anxiety Medications

Benzodiazepines

Benzodiazepines are the most commonly prescribed medications for **anxiety**. Some of the more commonly prescribed include chlordiazepoxide, lorazepam, diazepam, flurazepam, and triazolam. Benzodiazepines act to enhance the neurotransmitter **GABA**. This neurotransmitter inhibits the firing rate of neurons and therefore leads to a decline in anxiety symptoms. Indications for their use can include anxiety, insomnia disorders, alcohol withdrawal, seizure control, skeletal muscle spasticity, or agitation. They can also be utilized to reduce the anxiety symptoms preoperatively or before any other type of medical procedure such as cardiac catheterization or colonoscopy. This class of drug is also the treatment of choice for alcohol withdrawal.

Side Effects

There are several common **side effects** associated with the use of benzodiazepines. One of the most common is the effect of **drowsiness**. Patients should be advised to use caution when operating motor vehicles or machinery. Activity will help decrease this effect. Other side effects include feelings of detachment, irritability, emotional lability, GI upset, dependency, or development of tolerance. The elderly population is at high risk for the development of **dizziness** or **cognitive impairment**, which places them at high risk for falls with associated injuries. When discontinuing a benzodiazepine after long-term use, the drug should be weaned off to prevent withdrawal side effects.

Treatment of Insomnia

Benzodiazepines are used to treat **insomnia** because of their **sedative-hypnotic effects**. There are three different types of insomnia, which include the inability to fall asleep, inability to stay asleep, or the combination of both. Many times, insomnia can be helped by a change in habits or talking about worries or stress the patient may be experiencing. When using a sedative-hypnotic to treat sleep disturbances, the medication should have rapid onset and allow the patient to wake up feeling refreshed instead of tired and groggy. When administered at bedtime, most benzodiazepines will produce a sleep-inducing effect and should be used on a short-term basis.

Use of Buspirone for Treatment of Anxiety

Due to the addictive potential of benzodiazepines, the use of **nonbenzodiazepines** to treat anxiety has increased. One of the most commonly used nonbenzodiazepine medications is the drug **buspirone**. This medication is highly effective in treating anxiety and its associated symptoms such as insomnia, poor concentration, tension, restlessness, irritability, and fatigue. Buspirone has no addiction potential, is not useful in alcohol withdrawal and seizures, and is not known to interact with other CNS depressants. Because it may take several weeks of continual use for the effects of this drug to be realized by the patient, it cannot be used on an as-needed basis. Buspirone does not increase depression symptoms and therefore is useful in treating anxiety associated with depression. Side effects associated with medication can include GI upset, dizziness, sleepiness, excitement, or headache.

Multisystem Procedures and Interventions

Thermoregulation in Critically Ill Patients

The hypothalamus, limbic system, lower brainstem, reticular formation, spinal cord, and sympathetic ganglia all play a role in the regulation of core temperature. The normal core body temperature of 35.5-37.5 °C is a narrow range which is frequently disrupted in the critically ill patient. **Impaired thermoregulation** can occur in patients with sepsis, brain or spinal cord trauma, stroke, and tumors of the central nervous system. Mild hypothermia is common during deep sedation. Hypothermia (core temperature of <35 °C) is associated with an increased risk of postoperative wound infections, blood loss, and adverse cardiovascular events. Hypothermia may occur in trauma patients, patients with sepsis, postoperative patients, and patients with severe burns. Hyperthermia (core temperature of >38 °C) may occur in systemic inflammatory response syndrome, malignant hyperthermia, heatstroke, neuroleptic malignant syndrome, and serotonin syndrome. Hyperpyrexia occurs when the core temperature exceeds 40 °C. Core temperatures exceeding 41.5 °C may be life-threatening.

Targeted Temperature Management

Targeted temperature management (previously referred to as therapeutic hypothermia) is used to reduce ischemic tissue damage associated with cardiac arrest, ischemic stroke, traumatic brain/spinal cord injury, neurogenic fever, and subsequent coma (3 on Glasgow scale). Reducing the body's temperature to below normal range has a neuroprotective effect by making cell membranes less permeable, thus reducing neurologic edema and damage. Hypothermia should be initiated immediately after an ischemic event if possible, but some benefit remains up to 6 hours. Hypothermia to 33 °C may be induced by cooled saline through a femoral catheter, reducing temperature 1.5-2.0 °C/hr by an electronic control unit. Hypothermic water blankets covering ≥80% of the body's surface can also lower body temperature. In some cases, both a femoral cooling catheter and a water blanket are used for rapid reduction of temperature. Rectal probes are used to measure core temperature, but Foley temperature catheters are more common. Desflurane or meperidine is given to reduce the shivering response. Hypothermia increases risk of bleeding (decreased clotting time), infection (due to impairing leukocyte function and introducing catheters), arrhythmias, hyperglycemia, and DVT. Rewarming is done slowly at 0.5-1.0 °C/hr. through warmed intravenous fluids, warm humidified air, and/or warming blanket. The warming process is a critical time, as it causes potassium to be moved from extracellular to intracellular spaces and the patient's electrolyte levels must be monitored regularly.

Continuous Temperature Monitoring

Continuous temperature monitoring may be carried out through various means:

- Pulmonary artery catheter (most accurate but generally not recommended because of invasiveness and potential for complications)
- Rectal or Foley temperature probes
- Skin probes
- Wearable Bluetooth monitors (patch applied to the skin), which transmit information to an external monitor or the patient's electronic health record. (For external temperature monitoring, the device must be applied properly and for the correct duration of time [e.g., the TempTraQ® wearable patch is applied in the underarm area and measures temperature for 72 hours].)

Indications for continuous temperature monitoring include:

- Skin flap transplantation—to assess perfusion
- Brain injury—to assess thermoregulation
- Therapeutic hypothermia—for cardiac arrest or post-cardiac surgery
- Malignant hyperthermia
- Immunocompromised patients—to assess for signs of infection
- Critically ill patients—at risk for temperature dysregulation

Fluid Resuscitation for Burn Injuries

Burn victims are at risk for hypovolemia and electrolyte imbalances because of loss of body fluids through burned areas. **Fluid resuscitation** is indicated with burns of 20% or more of total body surface area (TBSA) burned. Lactated Ringers IV solution is used instead of NS, which can lead to hypernatremia and hyperchloremia. The Parkland/Baxter formula is used to calculate the volume of LR solution needed:

$$\text{24 hour volume} = (\text{body weight [kg]}) \times (\text{TBSA burned [\%]}) \times (4\ \text{mL})$$

Example—70 kg adult with 36% TBSA burned:

$$\text{24 hour volume} = 70 \times 36 \times 4\ \text{mL} = 10{,}080\ \text{mL}$$

Half of the volume is administered over the first 8 hours and half over the next 16 hours. Using the preceding example, this patient will receive 5,040 mL each over the first 8 hours (rate = (5040/8) =

630 mL/hr), and over the following 16 hours (rate = (5040/16) = 315 mL/hr). Fluid intake should be sufficient to produce 30-50 mL of urine per hour. In the second 24 hours, fluid volume should be 1.5-2.0 times the normal maintenance values with crystalloid with appropriate electrolyte balance.

Permissive Hypotension

Permissive hypotension procedures allow the systolic blood pressure to fall low enough to prevent or control hemorrhage while still high enough to maintain perfusion. With trauma patients, this means restricting fluid resuscitation when active bleeding is occurring. While protocols vary, permissive hypotension usually includes systolic blood pressure no higher than 80 mmHg, although this may vary. For example, permissive hypotension with systolic blood pressure maintained at 80-100 mmHg may be indicated when massive transfusion protocols are activated. Permissive hypotension helps decrease some of the adverse effects associated with rapid and high-dose fluid resuscitation (emboli, coagulopathy, and hypothermia). However, the patient does remain at risk of hypoperfusion and must be monitored carefully. Permissive hypotension is generally contraindicated with brain or spinal cord injury, although studies are ongoing (and mostly conducted with animals) and some controversy remains about the use of permissive hypotension.

Sedation

Minimal Sedation

Minimal sedation includes local/topical anesthesia, peripheral nerve blocks, administration of <50% nitrogen oxide in oxygen by itself, or administration of one sedative or analgesic medication in a dosage that does not typically require supervision. The patient should be fully aware, able to respond appropriately to verbal and tactile stimulation, and able to maintain an airway independently, as these medications should not have cardiovascular or respiratory effects. The purpose of minimal sedation is to decrease perception of pain, relax the patient, and reduce fear. The patient's level of consciousness, sedation, and pain should be monitored throughout the procedure to ensure the dosage is adequate and the patient is not excessively sedated. Medications may include benzodiazepines (diazepam, lorazepam) and opioids (fentanyl, morphine, meperidine). Reversal agents (flumazenil, naloxone) should be available. Minimal sedation is often used during labor and delivery and for minor procedures, such as skin biopsies and removal of skin lesions.

Continuous vs. Intermittent Sedation

Sedation for critically ill patients may include:

- **Intermittent sedation** is that administered through IV push, so the expected duration is relatively short. Typical agents include benzodiazepines and opioids. Intermittent sedation is most often used for endoscopic procedures but is also sometimes used for patients who are on mechanical ventilation, especially if they have regular trials of weaning. Also, intermittent sedation is less likely to result in oversedation.
- **Continuous sedation** is that administered through a steady intravenous infusion to ensure longer-lasting sedation. Typical agents include opioids, midazolam, and propofol. Continuous sedation is more commonly used for patients on mechanical ventilation because it requires less intervention and maintains a steady blood level. Daily interruptions of continuous sedation may be carried out as a trial for weaning patients on mechanical ventilation.

With both intermittent sedation and continuous sedation, the patient's vital signs, respiratory status, temperature, and oxygen saturation should be monitored. Arousal scales (Richmond or Riker Agitation/Sedation Scales) should be utilized to assess arousal and to adjust sedation dosages.

Neuromuscular Blockade Agents

Neuromuscular blocker agents are used for induced paralysis of those who have not responded adequately to sedation, especially for intubation and mechanical ventilation. NMBAs do not produce unconsciousness, amnesia, or analgesia, therefore it is critical that they are administered *after* the patient has been adequately sedated. NMBAs include:

- **Depolarizing agents**: Succinylcholine. Risk for severe hyperkalemia after denervation injury persists for 7-10 days. Post-operative myalgia is common, and succinylcholine may trigger malignant hyperthermia and severe anaphylactic/anaphylactoid reactions.
- **Non-depolarizing agents**: Short-acting (mivacurium, rapacuronium), intermediate-acting (rocuronium, vecuronium, atracurium, cisatracurium), and long-acting (pancuronium, doxacurium, pipecuronium). Should be given for ≤2 days for those on ventilators because they may develop persistent quadriparesis. Most are not associated with malignant hyperthermia.

Eye lubricant should be applied every 2 hours and the eyes kept closed. Range of motion exercises should not extend beyond normal range because of the potential to damage joints. The patient must be repositioned frequently while paralyzed and on an adequate support surface. Pupil reactivity should be assessed every 1-4 hours to evaluate neurological status. Temperature should be monitored hourly if <36 °C or if placed under a cooling blanket because heat production is depressed. After cessation, the patient should be closely monitored to ensure that muscle function has returned to normal.

Moderate (Conscious) Sedation

The ASA sedation guidelines (2018) are intended for **moderate (conscious) sedation** used for procedures, such as colonoscopy. Steps include:

- **Pre-procedure evaluation**: Includes review of health records, physical examination and laboratory testing as indicated a few days or weeks prior to the procedure, and re-evaluating the patient again before the procedure.
- **Patient preparation**: Consult with a specialist if indicated, ensure the patient has informed consent and has been compliant with pre-procedure fasting, and insert intravenous line.
- **Patient monitoring**: LOC (every 5 minutes), oxygenation/ventilation (capnography, pulse oximetry), and hemodynamic with a designated person responsible for monitoring and recording.
- **Supplemental oxygen:** Use unless contraindicated by condition.
- **Emergency interventions**: Resuscitative equipment and reversal agents for opioids (naloxone) and benzodiazepines (Romazicon) must be present with a person trained in assessment and use available.
- **Sedatives**: Analgesics (opioids) and combinations of drugs as appropriate may be used (benzodiazepines and dexmedetomidine).
- **Sedative (propofol, ketamine, etomidate) and analgesics (local anesthetics, NSAIDs, and opioids) intended for general anesthesia**: Care must be consistent with that of general anesthesia and IV medications administered incrementally.
- **Recovery care**: Monitor oxygenation, ventilation, and circulation every 5-15 minutes.

Sedation Using Propofol

Sedation used for a drug-induced coma often includes **propofol**. Propofol is an IV non-opioid hypnotic anesthetic, the most common used for induction. It is also used for maintenance and postoperative sedation. Onset of action is rapid because of high lipid solubility, and propofol has a short distribution half-life and rapid clearance, so recovery is also fast. Propofol is metabolized by the liver, as well as through the lungs. Propofol decreases cerebral blood flow, metabolic rate of oxygen consumption, and ICP. Propofol causes vasodilation with resultant hypotension, but with bradycardia rather than tachycardia. Propofol is a respiratory depressant, resulting in apnea after induction and decreased tidal volume, respiratory rate, and hypoxic drive during maintenance. Propofol has antiemetic properties as well but does not produce analgesia.

Delayed Emergence

Delayed emergence (failure to emerge for 30-60 minutes after anesthesia ends) is more common in the elderly because of slowed metabolism of anesthetic agents but may have a variety of causes, such as drug overdose during surgery, overdose related to preinduction use of drugs or alcohol that potentiates intraoperative drugs. In this case, naloxone or flumazenil may be indicated if opioids or benzodiazepines are implicated. Physostigmine may also be used to reverse effects of some anesthetic agents. Hypothermia may also cause delay in emergence, especially core temperatures <33 °C, and may require forced-air warming blankets to increase the temperature. Other metabolic conditions, such as hypoglycemia or hyperglycemia, may also affect emergence. Patients suffering from delayed emergence must be evaluated for perioperative stroke, especially after neurological, cardiovascular, or cerebrovascular surgery. Metabolic disturbance may also delay emergence.

Postanesthetic Respiratory Complications

Postoperative respiratory complications are most common in the postanesthesia period, so monitoring of oxygen levels is critical to preventing hypoxemia:

- **Airway obstruction** may be partial or total. Partial obstruction is indicated by sonorous or wheezing respirations, and total by absence of breath sounds. Treatment includes supplemental oxygen, airway insertion, repositioning (jaw thrust), or succinylcholine and positive-pressure ventilation for laryngospasm. If edema of the glottis is causing obstruction, IV corticosteroids may be used.
- **Hypoventilation** ($PaCO_2$ >45 mmHg) is often mild but may cause respiratory acidosis. It is usually related to depression caused by anesthetic agents. A number of factors may slow emergence (hypothermia, overdose, metabolism) and cause hypoventilation. It may also be related to splinting because of pain, requiring additional pain management.
- **Hypoxemia** (mild is PaO_2 50-60 mmHg) is usually related to hypoventilation and/or increased right to left shunting and is usually treated with supplementary oxygen (30-60%) with or without positive airway pressure.

Postanesthetic Cardiovascular Complications

Cardiovascular complications after surgery are sometimes related to respiratory complications, which may need to be addressed as well. Complications include:

- **Hypotension** is most often mild and requires no specific treatment. It is most commonly caused by hypovolemia and is significant if BP falls 20-30% below the normal baseline. A bolus (100-250 mL IV colloid) is used to confirm hypovolemia. If severe, then medications such as vasopressors may be indicated. Hypotension may occur with pneumothorax, so careful respiratory assessment must be done.
- **Hypertension** usually occurs ≤30 minutes after surgery and is common in those with a history of hypertension. It may be secondary to hypoxemia or metabolic acidosis. Mild increases usually don't require treatment but medications may be used for moderate (β-adrenergic blockers) or severe (nitroprusside) increases.

- **Arrhythmias** usually relate to respiratory complications or effects of anesthetic agents. Bradycardia may relate to cholinesterase inhibitors, opioids, or propranolol. Tachycardia may relate to anticholinergics, β-agonists, and vagolytic drugs. Hypokalemia and hypomagnesemia may cause premature atrial and ventricular beats.

Pharmacologic Pain Management

WHO Pain Ladder

The WHO pain ladder was developed as an algorithm for treating pain through medications with progressively increasing potency. The approach can be used effectively with both adult and pediatric patients. Beginning with the least potent medication option, each step adds a stronger analgesic until optimum pain relief is reached.

The **WHO pain ladder** has three steps.

- **Step 1**: The patient is given a non-opioid medication which may be used alone or in conjunction with other adjuvant therapies.
- **Step 2**: If the patient reports no change in the pain level, mild- to moderate-level pain-relieving opioids are introduced along with adjuvants if they have not been previously introduced.
- **Step 3**: Uncontrolled pain is then treated with opioids for moderate to severe pain. Adjuvants may also be continued.

Scheduling of Pain Medications

For mild to moderate pain, patients may take **acetaminophen** alternating with an **NSAID** such as ibuprofen on a regularly scheduled basis or as needed (PRN) at the onset of pain or when pain is anticipated (such as before a dressing change). However, for severe chronic pain, long-acting **opioid pain medications**, such as time-released MS Contin, Duragesic, and OxyContin, should be given regularly around the clock, because these medications help not only control but also prevent pain. The patient should not skip a dose when free of pain, because this makes control more difficult when the pain recurs. In addition to **time-scheduled medications**, the patient may need **short-acting supplementary medications**, such as Percocet, to take on a PRN basis. When taking short-acting medications, the patient should take the medication at the onset of pain, before anticipated pain, or at the onset of increased pain, rather than waiting until the pain is severe, because the goal should always be to keep the pain under control.

Acetaminophen

Acetaminophen remains one of the safest analgesics for **long-term use**. It can be used to treat mild pain or as an adjuvant with other analgesics for more severe pain. Nonspecific musculoskeletal pain and osteoarthritis are particularly responsive to acetaminophen therapy. Acetaminophen also has a limited **anti-inflammatory nature**.

Acetaminophen should, however, be used cautiously in persons with altered liver or kidney function, as well as those with a history of significant alcohol use, regardless of liver function compromise. It should be dosed separately from any opioid analgesic, which should be given separately as well. This allows for individual titration of each drug to assess the individual needs and side effects separately.

NSAIDs

NSAIDs act by inhibiting the cyclooxygenase (COX) enzyme, which controls prostaglandin formation. COX-1 affects platelet clumping, gastric blood flow, and mucosal integrity. COX-2 affects pain, inflammation, and fever. COX-1 and 2 inhibitors include aspirin and ibuprofen. Ibuprofen has a lower occurrence of side effects, such as gastric bleeding, than aspirin does. A COX-2 inhibitor, such as Celebrex, must be used with caution due to increased cardiovascular risks when used for over 18 months. NSAIDs are useful for both arthritis and bone cancer pain and work well with opioids for relief of postoperative and other severe pain. NSAIDs may increase the effects of antiseizure drugs and warfarin. Smaller doses are needed if kidney function is impaired.

Local Anesthetic Pain Relief

Local anesthetics block neural conduction of pain through the application of the anesthetic directly to the nerve endings in the area of pain. It can be injected prior to minor surgery or suturing. It can be injected intercostally for thoracic or high abdominal surgeries. The addition of a vasoconstrictor prolongs effectiveness of the anesthetic. A cream containing local anesthetics (EMLA) can be rubbed on the skin to decrease pain from IV starts or lumbar punctures. It should be applied 60 to 90 minutes prior to the procedure. A lidocaine 5% patch is approved to relieve pain from postherpetic neuralgia. The patient applies up to 3 patches for 12 hours at a time. Local anesthetics can be applied via the use of an epidural catheter to provide pain control for surgery, childbirth, or postoperative pain control. Opioids can be infused along with the anesthetic agent. Patients using an epidural catheter for postoperative pain tend to ambulate sooner, suffer fewer complications as a result, and go home more quickly.

Opioids

Guidelines for Opioid Use

Opioid analgesic therapy is a widely used method of chronic pain control. By adhering to clinical guidelines, pain control can be safely optimized. **Intramuscular administration** should be used as a last resort except in the presence of a "pain emergency" when no other treatment is readily available. Such cases are rare since subcutaneous delivery is almost always an alternative. Noninvasive routes such as **transdermal** and **transmucosal**, which bypass the enteral route, are optimal for continuous pain control and are often effective in eliminating breakthrough pain as well. Changing from one opioid to another, or altering the delivery method, may become necessary under the assumption that incomplete cross-tolerance among opioids occurs. Changing analgesics or method of delivery may result in a decreased drug requirement. When altering opioid delivery regimens, use **morphine equivalents** as the common factor for all dose conversions. This method will help reduce medication errors. Side effects such as sedation, constipation, nausea, and myoclonus should be anticipated in every care plan, and require both prevention and treatment methods.

Side Effects of Opioid Analgesics

Examples of **opioid analgesics** are numerous and include morphine, hydromorphone, oxymorphone, methadone, meperidine, fentanyl, sufentanil, alfentanil, levorphanol, codeine, oxycodone, hydrocodone, propoxyphene, pentazocine, nalbuphine, and buprenorphine. Opioid analgesics have multiple effects on most of the organ systems of the body. Central nervous system (CNS) effects include respiratory depression, analgesia, euphoria, sedation, miosis, cough suppression, truncal rigidity, nausea, and vomiting. Cardiovascular effects are usually slight and include bradycardia, hypotension, reduced blood volume, and increased cerebral blood flow. Gastrointestinal effects can include constipation, decreased gastric motility, and decreased hydrochloric acid. Genitourinary effects are urinary retention and decreased renal function. Other effects are sweating, flushing, and histamine release with itching.

Opioid Use During Last Few Hours of Life

Assessment of pain continues in the **last hours of life**, and medication is adjusted according to assessment. Pain does not necessarily increase as death approaches. It can be assumed that if pain was present prior to loss of consciousness it will continue in the patient's unconscious state. It should be assessed for and treated accordingly. Research has confirmed that administering opioids at the end of life does not hasten nor prolong the dying process. The patient's **prior medication regimen** should be continued. However, adjustments may be made in consideration of reduced renal or hepatic clearance. The **route of administration** should also be assessed for appropriateness and adjusted as needed (e.g., loss of consciousness, inability to swallow).

Oral Transmucosal Fentanyl Citrate

Oral transmucosal fentanyl citrate consists of **fentanyl** on an oral applicator. The patient applies the dosage (starting at 200 mcg) to the **buccal mucosa** between the cheek and gum for rapid absorption and subsequent pain relief. This makes transmucosal fentanyl particularly useful for managing **breakthrough pain**. Pain relief generally begins within 5 minutes, but the patient should be instructed to wait 15 minutes after the previous dose has been completed before taking another dose. Swallowing even part of the dose rather than having it completely absorbed through the oral mucosa can affect the timing of pain relief onset. **Peak effect** occurs in 20 to 40 minutes with the total pain relief duration lasting 2 to 3 hours. Side effects can include somnolence, nausea, and dizziness. Consuming drinks such as coffee, tea, and juices that alter the oral secretion pH can also alter the absorption rate of transmucosal fentanyl.

Methadone

Methadone is useful for treating **severe or chronic pain** and may be particularly helpful in the presence of **neuropathic pain**. It has a long-acting pain relief factor for a lower cost than many comparable medications. However, the exact dosing ratios with morphine remain unclear within the available research. Metabolism of methadone can also be swayed (either increased or decreased) by many other medications normally taken by patients with chronic conditions. Methadone can also be used to treat opioid addiction. US law for the prescription of methadone for addiction in detoxification or maintenance programs requires a special license and patient enrollment. The words "for pain" need to be clearly stated in the prescription. Methadone can cause drowsiness, weakness, headache, nausea, vomiting, constipation, sweating, and flushing, as well as sedation, decreased respirations, or an irregular heart rate.

Oxycodone

Oxycodone, a synthetic formulation, is a long-acting opioid for **moderate to severe pain relief**. Side effects are similar to those of morphine. It has a similar pain relief ratio, with the possibility of less nausea and vomiting. Because if its **extended-release nature**, the medication cannot be cut or crushed for administration. Oxycodone does not carry any greater addiction risk than other types of opioids; however, public sensationalism related to this formulation may create hesitation for use among patient. Pharmacies may also limit the amount of this medication they will make available to an individual. Oxycodone should be used cautiously in patients with a history of hypothyroidism, Addison's disease, urethral stricture, prostatic hypertrophy, or lung or liver disease.

Hydromorphone

Hydromorphone is available as tablets, liquid, suppository, and parenteral formulations. It offers the advantage of being synthetic, allowing for its use in the presence of a true **morphine allergy**. It is also helpful when significant side effects have occurred in the past or pain has been inadequately controlled with other medications. It may also be useful for controlling cough. However, neurotoxicity may occur, particularly myoclonus, hyperalgesia, and seizures. It should also be used cautiously in the presence of kidney, liver, heart, and thyroid disease, seizure disorders, respiratory disease, prostatic hypertrophy, or urinary problems. Common *side effects* include dizziness, lightheadedness, drowsiness, upset stomach if taken without food, vomiting, and constipation.

Titration of Morphine for Pain Control

Morphine titration protocols vary according to the type of morphine used, the severity of pain, and the patient's tolerance:

Type	Peak	Duration (hours)
Short-acting	60 minutes	4-5
Long-acting	3-4 hours	8-24
IM	30-60 minutes	4-5
SQ	50-90 minutes	4-5
IV	20 minutes	4-5
Rectal	20-60 minutes	3-7

For example, **optimal dosage** is usually calculated by starting with short-acting oral morphine at 30 mg every 3 to 4 hours with doses increased by 25 to 50% for moderate pain or 50 to 100% for severe pain each time until the patient has at least 50% reduction in pain on a scale of 1 to 10 or a behavior scale. The dose may need to be reduced if excessive sedation occurs. Once the patient's pain is controlled on short-acting morphine and 24-hour dosage needs are calculated, the patient could be switched to extended-release. **Breakthrough pain** is usually treated with dosages that are 10% of the 24-hour dose. Dosages may be repeated or increased if there is inadequate relief of pain at the peak time. Increasing the dose prior to peak time will result in increased drowsiness.

Morphine Use for Chronic Cancer Pain

One advantage of morphine for chronic cancer pain is that it has no **ceiling dose**. As tolerance to the medication increases or the disease progresses in severity, the dose can be gradually increased to an infinite level. It is also available in many different forms for administration, including intravenous, intramuscular, immediate release, sustained release, long-acting, liquid oral preparations, and suppositories. Morphine is often used as the **equivalency standard** for other opioid analgesics. Common *side effects* of morphine include sedation, respiratory depression, itching, nausea, chronic spasms or twitching of muscle groups, and constipation. Constipation is experienced by all patients receiving opioids. This inevitability should be planned for and treated aggressively. Hallucinations are common when morphine is initiated. After the first few days, most patients will overcome the respiratory depression, nausea, itching, and extreme sedation as tolerance for the medication is developed.

Dosages for Morphine, Codeine, Hydromorphone, and Levorphanol

The dosages for both the enteral and parenteral routes of morphine, codeine, hydromorphone, and levorphanol are as follows:

- **Morphine**: Enteral dosage is 30 mg (available as continuous and sustained-release formulations to last 12 to 24 hours); parenteral dosage is 10 mg.
- **Codeine**: Enteral dosage is 200 mg (not generally recommended); parenteral dosage is 130 mg.

- **Hydromorphone**: Enteral dosage is 7.5 mg (available as a continuous-release formula lasting 24 hours); parenteral dosage is 1.5 mg.
- **Levorphanol**: In acute pain episodes, enteral dosage is 4 mg; parenteral dosage is 2 mg. For chronic pain, dosage is equivalent for both enteral and parenteral at 1 mg. Levorphanol has a long half-life, increasing the chances of dosage accumulation over time.

Adhering to the statement "If the gut works, use it," as much as 90 percent of all patients will at least start out able to use oral medications instead of other routes.

Calculation for Converting Medication Regimen Between Two Opioids

Calculate the current 24-hour drug dose, or the total amount given in a 24-hour period. Multiply the current 24-hour dose times the ratio of the 24-hour equivalent dose for the new drug over the 24-hour equivalent of the old drug. This calculation provides the **equivalent 24-hour dose** for the new drug. Divide the new dose amount by the number of doses to be provided during the day. This amount equals the new **target dosage**.

$$\text{current 24 hr dose} \times \frac{\text{new drug 24 hr equiv dose}}{\text{current drug 24 hr equiv dose}} = \text{new 24 hr dose}$$

$$\frac{\text{new 24 hr dose}}{\text{doses per day}} = \text{new target dosage}$$

Ketamine

Ketamine is a dissociative anesthetic that can provide pain relief as an alternate or complement to an opioid. The dissociative quality is an effective way to help the patient separate from the sensation of pain. Ketamine treatment begins with an initial bolus of 0.1 mg/kg IV. If there is no improvement, a second bolus with double the dosage is provided in 5 minutes. This can be repeated as needed. Boluses should be followed by a decrease in the patient's current opioid dose by 50% and an infusion of ketamine. **Infusion dosing** for ketamine is 0.015 mg/kg/min, or about 1 mg/min for a 70 kg person. If IV access cannot be attained, subcutaneous infusion is a possibility with dosing of 0.3 to 0.5 mg/kg. Consider concurrent treatment with a **benzodiazepine** to prevent hallucinations or frightful dreams and observe for increased secretions, as these are all possible side effects of ketamine. The secretions may be treated with glycopyrrolate, scopolamine, or atropine as needed.

Treating Breakthrough Pain

The three basic types of **breakthrough pain**, and their treatment measures are as follows:

- **Incident Pain**: Pain that can be specifically tied to an activity or event, such as a dressing change or physical therapy. These events can be anticipated and treated with a rapid-onset, short-acting analgesic just prior to the painful event.
- **Spontaneous Pain**: This type of pain is unpredictable and cannot be pinpointed to a relationship with any certain time or event. There is no way to anticipate spontaneous pain. In the presence of neuropathic pain, adjuvant therapy may be useful. Otherwise a rapid-onset, short-acting analgesic is used.
- **End-of-Dose Failure**: Pain that specifically occurs at the end of a routine analgesic dosing cycle when medication blood levels begin to taper off. Careful evaluation of end-of-dose failure can help prevent it sooner. It may indicate an increased dose tolerance and the need for medication dose alterations.

Treating Neuropathic Pain

Treatment options for **neuropathic pain** are often different from the methods used to treat other types of pain. The three drug classes most commonly used and proven effective for treating neuropathic pain are **anticonvulsants**, **anesthetics**, and **antidepressants**. Some are given on an as-needed basis, but most require consistent dosing with **24-hour symptom control**. Examples of the most common medications include amitriptyline, nortriptyline, duloxetine, gabapentin, topical lidocaine, opioids, and pregabalin. Medication choice is dependent on factors such as the type and progression of the disorder and the associated physical and emotional problems, such as nerve injury, muscle weakness or spasms, anxiety, depression, or sleep disturbances.

Treating Bone Pain

Treatment options for **bone pain** may depend on the causative agent related to the pain, such as the primary cancer site, severely weakened bones, or fractures. **Systemic treatment choices** include chemotherapy, radiation, and hormone therapy. **Hormone therapy** is used in the presence of estrogen and androgen receptors within the cancer cells. **Bisphosphonates**, such as ibandronate, zoledronate, and alendronate, may help strengthen the bones, slow damage, and prevent fractures; they can also help reduce pain. However, side effects can include fatigue, fever, nausea, vomiting, and anemia. **Surgery** may also be considered to remove cancerous cells or reinforce weakened areas of bone. **Opioids** and **NSAIDs/COX-2 inhibitors** are most often used for pain relief and need to be provided on a consistent basis.

Morphine combined with ibuprofen provides the benefit of a centrally acting opioid with a peripherally acting NSAID. Ibuprofen also acts as an effective adjuvant analgesic agent to enhance the relief provided by the opioid without increasing opioid side effects.

Measures Taken During Pain Crisis

During a pain crisis, assess for a change in the mechanism or location of the pain and attempt to differentiate between **terminal anxiety** or agitation and the **physical causes** of pain. Begin with a rapid increase in **opioid treatment**. If the pain is unresponsive to opioid titration, switching to **benzodiazepines**, such as diazepam and lorazepam, may produce a more effective response. If terminal symptoms remain unresponsive, assess for **drug absorption**. While invasive routes of medication delivery are generally avoided unless necessary, the only guaranteed route of drug delivery is the IV route. If there is any question about absorption, it is appropriate to establish parenteral access. IM delivery should be considered as a last resort. When all accessible resources have been exhausted, seek a pain management consultation as quickly as possible. Alternative methods of terminal pain control include radiotherapy, anesthetic, or neuroablative procedures.

Concerns Surrounding Use of Pain Medications with End-of-Life Patients

Common concerns surrounding the use of pain medications with end-of-life patients include:

- **Adequacy**: Patients are often concerned that medication may not be adequate to control pain and that chronic or breakthrough pain will occur. Patients may be concerned that if they take adequate pain medication, it will be less effective later when pain may be worse.
- **Sedation/Addiction**: Some patients and family members are concerned about the risks of addiction, and others may be concerned about the effects of the medication on the patient's cognition, as some patients may become confused, disoriented, or sedated, depending on the medication or dosage.

- **Adverse effects**: Nausea and vomiting may be almost as debilitating to a patient as the pain it is intended to alleviate. Constipation, a common adverse effect, may be very uncomfortable for a patient. Some medications may result in itching and others may cause myoclonus, both of which are uncomfortable for the patient.

Prescribing Controlled Substances to Patients with Advanced Illness and Addiction Challenges

In the presence of **addiction challenges**, it becomes important to choose a **long-acting opioid** that can facilitate around-the-clock dosing and minimize the need for short-term medications used for breakthrough doses. **Short-term medication** use should be very limited or eliminated entirely if possible. Whenever possible, **nondrug adjuvants** such as relaxation techniques, distraction, biofeedback, TNS, and therapeutic communication should be used in place of short-term medications. When short-term medication therapy is needed, a **nonopioid** is best. Limit the amount of medication available to the patient at any given time and monitor for compliance with pill counts and urine toxicology screens as necessary. In some instances, a referral to an addictions specialist is recommended.

Tolerance and Pseudotolerance

Tolerance is the adaptation of the body to continued exposure to a drug or chemical. The effects of the drug at the same level of exposure are minimized over time. Additional dosing is required to maintain the same outcomes.

Pseudotolerance is the misguided perception of the health care provider that a patient's need for increasing doses of a drug is due to the development of tolerance, when the reality is that disease progression or other factors are responsible for the increase in dosing needs.

Addiction and Pseudoaddiction

Addiction is a primary and constant neurobiologic disease with genetic, psychosocial, and environmental factors that create an obsessive and irrational need or preoccupation with a substance. Addictive behaviors include unrestricted, continued cravings, as well as compulsive and persistent use of a drug despite harmful experiences and side effects.

Pseudoaddiction is an assumption that the patient is addicted to a substance when in actuality the patient is not experiencing relief from the medication. It is prolonged, unrelieved pain that may be the result of undertreatment. This situation may lead the patient to become more aggressive in seeking medicated relief, thus resulting in the inappropriate "drug seeker" label.

Physical Dependence

Physical dependence occurs when the body adapts to a drug, requiring increasing dosages over time to gain the same effect, and withdrawal of that drug then will result in an **abstinence syndrome** (withdrawal). Physical dependence can be described as a form of **addiction.** While physical dependence was commonly thought of as being related to narcotic drugs (such as morphine, methadone, fentanyl), many different types of drugs may cause some degree of physical dependence. For example, abruptly stopping a beta-blocker may result in cardiac arrhythmias or cardiac arrest. Abruptly stopping SSRIs may result in severe depression and anxiety. Thus, when considering stopping a patient's drugs near the end of life, physical dependence must be considered as many drugs should be **tapered** to avoid withdrawal effects. Drugs that affect the **central nervous system**, such as ethanol, barbiturates, and benzodiazepines, pose considerable risk of dependence and may result in severe withdrawal symptoms.

Geriatric Pharmacology

Medication Considerations for Elderly Patients

An elderly patient has an increased chance of adverse effects from medications. Approximately 1/3 of hospitalizations that are related to side effects of drugs and 1/2 of drug-associated fatalities happen in patients that are at least 60 years of age. In the United States, expenses for prescriptions for elderly patients make up 30% of every prescription filled and 40–50% of non-prescription drugs. Elderly patients spend more than $3 billion annually on these medications. Most elderly individuals have at least one ongoing health condition, including arthritis, high blood pressure, heart problems, diabetes, or other conditions, often requiring more than one drug for treatment. There are more adverse drug reactions (ADR) amongst elderly patients, 10% of whom require hospitalization for treatment for the side effects. Frequently seen adverse reactions include edema, queasiness, vomiting, anorexia, vertigo, loose stools, infrequent and difficult stools, bewilderment, and urinary retention. Be careful not to misidentify these as another condition or symptom of aging.

Pharmacokinetics of Older Adults

Pharmacokinetics involves four steps: Absorption, distribution, metabolism and elimination. All of these steps are affected by the age of the patient as the organs involved degenerate from wear and tear:

1. **Absorption** of most drugs occurs in the small intestine. Drug absorption in older adults may be delayed or decreased due to decreased blood flow to the small intestine. This could change the blood levels of drugs achieved in the geriatric patient.
2. **Distribution** of the drug is altered due to a change in body composition. Elderly patients have decreased total body water and lean muscle mass. This relative increase in total body fat may increase the duration of action of lipid-soluble drugs.
3. Most drugs are **metabolized** by either the liver or the kidneys. Decreased function of these organs leads to delayed metabolism and elimination of certain medications.
4. **Renal function** and **elimination effectiveness** diminish with age, often decreasing the kidney's ability to remove toxins and medications from the body. For this reason, drugs may remain in the body longer, therefore requiring smaller doses among the elderly.

Beers Criteria

The **Beers Criteria**, also called the Beers List, identifies inappropriate medication use among older adults. The list is used to determine which medications are beneficial compared to those that impose risks for older adults. Because older adults are at risk of polypharmacy and inappropriate medication use, the Beers Criteria helps healthcare providers identify which medications are truly necessary and are in the patient's best interests to use. All medications that the patient takes are identified, and indications are given as to whether the medications should be avoided among those older than age 65. The recommendations are then rated for strength, and the quality of the research supporting the recommendations is identified.

Difficulties the Elderly Population May Encounter with Medication Use

Common **difficulties with medication use** amongst the elderly include:

- Overuse of prescription medications
- Medication adherence and compliance issues (e.g., providing incorrect or incomplete past medical history to the professional, or using medicine that is out of date, changing dose without practitioner's orders to do so)

- Misunderstanding of how the medicine is supposed to be used due to problems with comprehension, hearing, or proper education style
- Not remembering the reason, amount, or how often the drug should be used (may result in repeating the medicine when it has already been taken)
- Difficulty affording the medication
- Vision issues resulting in misreading the label and taking the wrong dosage
- Problems getting the bottle open, dealing with small pills, cutting pills in half, and using inhalers
- More than one medical worker or more than one pharmacy can lead to inadvertent redundancy of the same medication, as can using the generic and brand name of the same thing at the same time

Common Adverse Outcomes of Frequently Used Prescription Medications

Certain physical and psychological states may be an **adverse outcome** resulting from a prescribed medication:

- **Bewilderment:** Digoxin, cimetidine, dopamine agent, antihistamine, hypnotic, sedative, anticholinergic, anticonvulsant
- Anorexia: Digoxin
- **Low energy or weakness:** Diuretic, antidepressant, antihypertensive
- Absentmindedness: Barbiturate
- Difficult bowel movements: Anticholinergic
- **Loose stool:** Oral antacid
- **GI upset:** Iron, NSAID, salicylate, corticosteroid, estrogen, alcohol
- Ringing in the ears (tinnitus): Analgesic
- **Urinary retention:** Anticholinergic, alpha-agonist
- **Orthostatic low blood pressure:** Antihypertensive, sedative, diuretic, antidepressant
- **Depression:** Benzodiazepine
- **Vertigo:** Sedative, antihypertensive, anticonvulsant, diuretic

Adverse Outcomes of Histamine Blockers, Ibuprofen, and Beta-Blockers

Histamine blockers in the elderly can cause paradoxical central nervous system provocation that has an outcome of ataxia in this population. Antihistamines may cause problems with vision and walking, leading to falls, which may cause unforeseen hospital visits or require a nursing home. Antihistamines can also interfere with the effectiveness of other medications or enhance other medications' negative side effects.

Some elderly patients are already dealing with decreased renal functioning. **Ibuprofen** has the ability to worsen these issues leading to nephrosis, cirrhosis, and congestive heart failure.

If the patient is older, a **beta-blocker** is not a good option for treating hypertension due to their decreased beta-adrenergic receptor sensitivity for the elderly patient. Elderly patients need smaller amounts of calcium entry antagonists, ACE inhibitors, or diuretics. Too high a dose (in the elderly) will cause moodiness, impotence, weariness, and lessened ability to think clearly. Elderly patients are particularly prone to congestive heart failure and peripheral vascular insufficiency due to beta-adrenergic toxins.

Polypharmacy

Polypharmacy is a term used to describe inappropriate use of multiple medications at one time. It occurs when medications are taken that are not indicated, medications that have adverse interactions with one another are taken together, and patients take contraindicated medications. Polypharmacy is a common problem in the geriatric population. Most office visits result in new prescriptions being written and patients may accumulate many different medications in their home. Polypharmacy greatly increases the patient's risk of having an adverse drug reaction.

To manage polypharmacy and prevent complications, obtain a detailed drug history at each visit. This should include nonprescription medications and herbal remedies. Educating patients about the problem of polypharmacy is very important. This can occur in the clinician's office or with a community education program. Assist elderly patients with medication identification, recommending pill boxes to help the patient divide medications and minimize risks for medication misuse.

MASTER Rules for Rational Drug Therapy

Although drugs are often very useful and effective in treating illnesses, there is a point when it becomes dangerous to the patient. Drug resistance, drug interactions, and drug intolerances are all common problems, especially among elderly patients, because an iatrogenic illness can develop. For these reasons, it is important to limit drugs to only those that are absolutely necessary. To help the practitioner decide whether a drug should be used or not, they must remember the **MASTER rules**.

- **M** is for **minimizing** the number of drugs a patient is taking.
- **A** is for considering **alternate** treatments that may be as or more effective than using a drug.
- **S** is for **start** low and increase slowly. Only give the patient the minimum amount, and be careful when increasing doses.
- **T** is for **titration** of drugs; tailor the amount given over time to the individual patient.
- **E** is for **education** of the patient about the drugs he or she is taking.
- **R** is for **regular** reviewing of drugs and doses.

Alternative, Complementary, and Non-Pharmacologic Interventions

Complementary Therapy

Complementary therapies are often used, either alone or in conjunction with conventional medical treatment. These methods should be included if this is what the patient/family chooses, empowering the family to take control of their plan of care. Complementary therapies vary widely and most can easily be incorporated. The National Center for Complementary and Alternative Medicine recognizes the following:

- **Whole medical systems**: Chinese medicine (acupressure, acupuncture), naturopathic and homeopathic medicines, and Ayurveda
- **Mind-body medicine**: Prayer, artistic creation, music and dance therapy, biofeedback, focused relaxation, and visualization
- **Biological medicine**: Aromatherapy, herbs, plants, trees, vitamins and minerals, and dietary supplements
- **Manipulation**: Massage and spinal manipulation
- **Energy medicines**: Magnets, electric current, pulsed fields, Reiki, qi gong, and laying-on of the hands

Precautions

The use of **alternative and complementary therapies** should be thoroughly discussed by patients and their physician. Patients should be encouraged to use therapies that are shown to have a beneficial, complementary effect on conventional medical treatment. These therapies include the use of massage, superficial stimulation, relaxation, distraction, hypnosis, and guided imagery.

- Encourage patients to practice the techniques until they are proficient in their use to give them a chance to prove their value.
- Teach the patient how the therapies work to encourage the patient to believe in them to contribute to the placebo effect.
- Caution the patient against abandoning current medical treatment.
- Inform the patient of the high cost of alternate therapies that can divert needed funds and result in little or no benefit.
- Provide the patient with resources in the form of books, pamphlets, and informative websites that prove the results of scientific research so that they can evaluate alternative therapies for themselves.

Whole Medical Systems

Whole medical systems are different philosophies and methods of explaining and treating health and illness. Some systems include:

- **Homeopathic medicine**: This European system uses small amounts of diluted herbs and supplements to help the body to recover from disease by stimulating an immune response.
- **Naturopathic medicine**: This is a European system that uses various natural means (herbs, massage, acupuncture) to support the natural healing forces of the body.
- **Chinese medicine**: Centers on restoring the proper flow of life forces within the body to cure disease by using herbs, acupressure and acupuncture, and meditation.
- **Ayurveda**: This is an Indian system that tries to bring the spirit into harmony with the mind and body to treat disease via yoga, herbs, and massage.

Essential Oils and Cupping

Essential oils (concentrated oils from plants) are either inhaled (aromatherapy) or diluted and applied to the skin. Essential oils are believed to reduce stress, aid sleep, improve dermatitis, and aid digestion. Commonly used essential oils include eucalyptus, lavender, lemon, peppermint, rosemary, rose, and tea tree. Oils may cause skin irritation when applied to the skin.

Cupping is an ancient practice still used in Southeast Asia and the Middle East to reduce pain, promote healing, and improve circulation. With dry cupping, cups are heated by placing something flammable (such as paper or herbs) inside the cup and setting it on fire to heat the cup, which is then immediately placed on the back along the meridians (generally on both sides of the spine) to form a vacuum that draws blood to the skin and causes circular bruises believed to heal that part of the body. Wet cupping includes leaving the heated cup in place for three minutes, removing it, making small cuts in the skin, and then applying suction cups again to withdraw blood. Cupping should be avoided in children under 4 and limited to short periods in older children.

Acupuncture

Alternative systems of medical practice include acupuncture, homeopathy, and naturopathy. **Acupuncture**, an ancient Oriental practice, uses stainless steel or copper needles inserted into superficial skin layers at points where energy or life force called *qi* is believed to occur. The needles are supposed to restore balance and the flow of *qi*. The NIH has recognized the effectiveness of acupuncture for certain side effects of other cancer treatments, such as nausea, vomiting, and pain. However, there is no documented scientific evidence to support the principles expounded. Acupuncturists are certified through either formal coursework or apprenticeships, and there is also board certification in this area for physicians. The needles used are classified as class II, which means they have manufacturing and labeling requirements.

Herbal Remedies and Regulations

In the United States, most **herbal preparations** are classified as dietary supplements. That means that they are not subject to the same rigorous manufacturing, safety, efficacy, and control practices as pharmaceutical drugs. Herbal supplements are only governed by the Dietary Supplement and Health Education Act (DSHEA). As long as no specific disease treatment or curative claims are made, the supplement can be marketed without limitation and safety concerns must be pursued by the FDA after the fact. Nevertheless, some herbal remedies have been undergoing clinical trials in the U.S. to substantiate their health-enhancing or traditional/historical or international use claims. However, the focal point of these studies is still only on the effectiveness of the specific supplement. In Europe, there has been some movement toward greater regulation and licensing of herbal products, but not to the extent of formal drug regulations.

Toxicities Associated with Herbal Remedies

Use of herbal preparations has been associated with a variety of **toxicities**, primarily in categories such as cardiovascular problems, hypersensitivity reactions, disorientation, gastrointestinal problems, and liver malfunction. Because quality control measures are relatively lax for these remedies, contamination from infectious agents and toxic metals can potentially cause other side effects. Many of these herbal medicines **interact with conventional drugs**, thus altering their pharmacodynamics. For example, St. John's wort, which is primarily used for depressive disorders or as a sedative, interacts with a wide range of traditional pharmacologic agents and suppresses their levels in the bloodstream. Kava kava, made from dried roots of a type of pepper bush, is used as a sedative, but it also has been associated with hepatic failure and via interactions with several other drugs can actually induce a comatose state. Ginseng is an Asian remedy touted for its curative properties in a number of diseases. However, it can react with steroidal drugs and induce shaking and manic episodes. These are just a few examples of potential dangers.

Non-Pharmaceutical Pain Relief

Non-pharmaceutical methods to relieve pain that can be used exclusively or combined with medications include massage, heat, cold, electrical stimulation, distraction, relaxation, imagery, visualization, and music. Other **alternatives** or adjuncts to pain medication include hypnosis, magnets, acupuncture, acupressure, and therapeutic touch. Herbs, aromatherapy, reflexology, homeopathic medicine, and prayer may also be accepted by the patient. Any method that the patient feels may help that isn't harmful should be used to help get relief.

Mind-Body Medicine for Pain and Disease

Mind-body medicine (prayer, artistic creation, music and dance, biofeedback, relaxation, and visualization) can help distract people from pain or other symptoms if they are able to concentrate on the method. This can result in the transfer of less painful stimuli to the brain by stimulating the **descending control system**. These methods work if the patient can use them to create alternate sensations in the brain, but will not work if the patient is unable to concentrate due to intense pain.

Relaxation that occurs as a result of using these methods helps to reduce muscular tension that can make pain worse and reduces fatigue caused by chronic pain. Relaxation has been proven to be the most helpful after surgery. Postoperative patients report a greater feeling of control over their pain and tend to request fewer opioids to control pain. Biofeedback can help patients to recognize the feelings of both tension and relaxation and provide a way to indicate their success in managing muscle tension.

Use of Visualization

There are a number of methods used for **visualization** to reduce anxiety and promote healing. Some include audiotapes with guided imagery, such as self-hypnosis tapes, but the patient can be taught basic **techniques** that include:

- Sit or lie comfortably in a **quiet place** away from distractions.
- Concentrate on **breathing** while taking long slow breaths.
- **Close the eyes** to shut out distractions and create an image in the mind of the place or situation desired.
- Concentrate on that **image**, engaging as many senses as possible and imaging details.
- If the mind wanders, breathe deeply and **bring consciousness back** to the image or concentrate on breathing for a few moments and then return to the imagery.
- End with positive imagery.

Sometimes, patients are resistive at first or have a hard time maintaining focus, so **guiding** them through visualization for the first few times can be helpful.

Stimulation of the Skin to Reduce Pain

Skin, muscles, fascia, tendons, and the cornea contain **nociceptors** that are nerve endings that respond to painful stimuli. Massage, transcutaneous electrical nerve stimulation (TENS), heat and cold provide stimulation to other nerves that transfer only sensation, not pain. These signals block some of the transfer of the nociceptor impulses:

- **Massage** not only sends alternate sensation to the brain, but also results in relaxation that decreases the muscular tension that contributes to pain.
- **TENS** works well on incisional and neuromuscular pain by providing a gentle electrical stimulation that overrides the painful impulses from the area and may stimulate endorphins.
- **Heat therapy** increases blood flow and oxygen to promote healing and stimulates neural receptors, decreasing pain. Heat also helps loosen tense muscles that may be contributing to pain.
- **Cold therapy** decreases circulation and reduces production of chemicals related to inflammation, thereby reducing pain.

Temperature-Controlled Therapies

Methods of Heating and Cooling

There are a number of different ways to **heat** (thermotherapy) or **cool** (cryotherapy) for **healing**:

- **Conduction**: Conveyance of heat, cold, or electricity through direct contact with the skin, such as with hot baths, ice packs, and electrical stimulation.
- **Convection**: Indirect transmission of heat in a liquid or gas by circulation of heated particles, such as with whirlpools and paraffin soaks.
- **Conversion**: Heating that results from converting a form of energy into heat, such as with diathermy and ultrasound.

- **Evaporation**: Cooling caused by liquids that evaporate into gases on the skin with a resultant cooling effect, such as with perspiration or vapo-coolant sprays.
- **Radiation**: Heating that results from transfer of heat through light waves or rays, such as with infrared or ultraviolet light.

Shortwave Diathermy

Shortwave diathermy uses radio waves (27.12 MHz) to **increase the temperature in subcutaneous tissue** and is used along with passive and active range of motion exercises to **improve range** in painful conditions such as inflammation of the muscles, tendons, and bursae. The radio waves (eddy currents) are transmitted through a capacitor or inductor in a continuous or pulse waveform. Temperatures increase about 15 °C in fatty tissue and 4-6 °C in muscular tissue. Shortwave diathermy should not be used over any organs containing fluid, including the eyes, heart, head, or over pacemakers as the diathermy may disrupt the settings. Because this treatment may increase cardiac demand, it should be avoided in those with preexisting cardiac conditions and should not be used over malignancies. Additionally, it is contraindicated in areas of inflammation because heating the tissue increases inflammation. It cannot be used over prostheses as the metal may heat and damage tissue. Shortwave diathermy should avoid the epiphyses in children, as it may stimulate abnormal growth.

Microwave Diathermy

Microwave diathermy is used similarly to shortwave diathermy but has a lower rate of heat increase and penetrance so it is used for muscles and joints near the surface rather than deep muscles, such as the hip. Heat is created by **electromagnetic radiation** (9.15-14.50 MHz) and raises temperature in fatty tissues by about 10-12 °C and in muscular tissue by 3-4 °C. **Treatment** is usually given for 15-30 minutes per session and is followed by range of motion exercises (passive and active) to increase flexibility. Contraindications are similar to those of shortwave diathermy in that this treatment should not be used where increase in temperature may be detrimental, such as over organs containing fluid, areas of inflammation, and epiphyses of children. Additionally, it should not be used over prostheses or pacemakers and should be avoided in those with cardiac disease.

Superficial Heat

Superficial heat with externally applied heat sources penetrates only the superficial layers of the skin (1-2 cm after about 30 minutes), but it is believed to relax deeper muscles by reflex, decrease pain, and increase metabolisms (2-3 times for every 10 °C increase in skin temperature). Therapeutic temperature range is 40-45 °C. Superficial heat modalities include:

- **Moist heat packs** placed on the skin and secured by several layers of towels to provide insulation, applied for 15-30 minutes.
- **Paraffin baths** (52-54 °C) with the hand, foot, or elbow dipped 7 times, cooling between dippings, and then wrapping with plastic and towels for 20 minutes.
- **Fluidotherapy** uses hot-air warmed (38.8-47.8 °C) cellulose particles into which a hand or foot is submerged for 20-30 minutes.

Passive and active range of motion exercises are done after superficial heat treatment. Contraindications include cardiac disease, peripheral vascular disease, malignant tumor, bleeding, and acute inflammation.

Deep heat differs from superficial heat in that the heat is generated internally using ultrasound, short wave, and microwave diathermy rather than applied to the surface of the skin. Deep heating has penetrance to 3-5 cm.

Cryotherapy

Cryotherapy uses therapeutic cold treatment to cool the surface of the skin and underlying subcutaneous tissues in order to decrease blood flow, pain, and metabolism. Initially response to cold therapy causes **vasoconstriction** to occur within the first 15 minutes but if the tissues are cooled to -10 °C, then the body responds with **vasodilation**. Cryotherapy affects sensory response so the person will at first feel cold, which progresses to burning, aching, and finally to numbness and tingling. Treatment is usually given for 15-30 minutes. **Treatment modalities** include:

- **Ice packs** such as refrigerated gel packs (-5 °C) or plastic bags filled with water and ice chips are applied directly to the skin for 10-15 minutes for superficial cooling and 15-20 minutes for greater penetrance.
- A **towel dipped in ice and water slurry** is wrapped around limb to provide cold therapy, but this is best used only for emergency situations when ice packs are unavailable, as the towel must be changed frequently as the skin warms the towel rapidly.
- **Ice massage** is applied directly to the affected area for 5-10 minutes, usually rubbing the ice in circular motions on the skin surface. An ice massager is easily made by filled a paper cup with water and freezing it with a tongue depressor or Popsicle stick (to use as a handle) inserted into the center as the water starts to freeze. Then, the paper can be torn away from the bottom and sides when the ice is solid. Ice massage is often followed by friction massage.
- **Ice baths** (13-18 °C) are used for limbs, such as the lower leg, foot, or hand. The body part is immersed for 20 minutes.

Cryotherapy is usually followed by **active and passive exercises**. Contraindications include impaired circulation or sensation, cardiac disease, Raynaud's disease, and nerve trauma.

Whirlpool Baths

Whirlpool baths are used to increase **circulation** and promote **healing**. They are tubs with a turbine that mixes air with water, which is pressurized and flows into the tub water to create turbulence. Tubs are usually large enough to accommodate the full body although smaller limb-sized whirlpool tubs are available. Water temperature is 95-104 °F (adjusted for the individual) and should be deep enough to completely submerge the affected part. The body part should be cleaned with soap and water before immersion or a shower taken. If the full body is treated, then the patient should wear a swimming suit. During the whirlpool treatment, the muscles relax from the heat and **range of motion exercises** can be done while in the water. Typically, treatments last about 20 minutes, but the patient should be monitored, especially for the first 5 minutes, as some people become lightheaded and can lose consciousness.

Contrast Baths

Contrast baths (alternating hot and cold) are used in the sub-acute phase of healing (after edema begins to subside) for **strains and sprains**. It is believed that contrast baths increase the circulation and help to further decrease edema by a pumping action as the **vasoconstriction and vasodilation** alternate. Two containers are filled with water, one with hot and the other with cold. The hot water should be maintained at about 100-110 °F and the cold at 55-65 °F. The cycle begins and ends with immersion in cold water. Cold water immersions usually last about 1 minute and hot water immersions 4 minutes. Typically, the affected limb is immersed in the cold water for 1 minute, removed, and immediately immersed in hot water for 4 minutes. This cycle is repeated about 3-4 times.

THERAPEUTIC ULTRASOUND

Ultrasound treats soft-tissue injuries (such as myositis, bursitis, and tendinitis) with sound waves (frequency 0.8-3.0 MHz). Ultrasound utilizes a **piezoelectric crystal** that vibrates, producing sound waveforms, which are transmitted from the transducer through a gel substance into the tissue. The sound waves bounce off of the bone in an irregular pattern that causes an increase in temperature in the connective tissue, such as collagen fibers. Temperatures of the tissue may increase up to 43.5 °C, increasing metabolism in the area, neural conduction, as well as blood flow. Ultrasound is used to **decrease both contractures and scarring**. During treatment, the transducer passes in a circular motion about the skin surface, staying in contact with the gel medium. If a distal limb is submerged in water, the treatment is given with the head of the transducer 0.5-1 inch from the skin surface. Treatment is followed by range of motion exercises, passive and active. Contraindications are similar to other heat-producing modalities and include peripheral vascular disease, but ultrasound may be used over metal prostheses.

TENS

Transcutaneous electrical nerve stimulation (TENS) uses electrical stimulation to stimulate **peripheral sensory nerve fibers** to reduce acute or recurrent pain. TENS machines may be 2-lead or 4-lead and have adjustments for both frequency (1-20 Hz) and pulse width (50-300 microseconds, 10-50 mA). Stimulation can be intermittent or continuous. TENS units are small and battery-powered with wires and adhesive electrodes attached so that they can be worn while the person goes about usual activities. The positioning of the electrodes and the settings depend upon the site and type of injury, following guidelines provided by the manufacturer. The TENS machine can be used for a number of hours, but if used for days at a time, it will be less effective. TENS treatment is contraindicated with demand pacemakers and should not be used on the head or neck or over irritated skin.

Professional Role

Scope and Standards of Professional Practice

Advanced Practice Registered Nursing

Advanced practice registered nursing (APRN), according to the National Council of State Boards of Nursing (NCSBN), is acting as a nurse with a foundation on **information and proficiency** that was obtained in basic nursing school. This nurse has a license to be an RN and has completed and received a diploma from graduate school in an APRN program that has been accredited from a nationwide accrediting body. This nurse has up-to-date **certification** from a nationwide certification board to work in the proper APRN specialty.

Scope of Practice

The **scope of practice for the APRN** is dependent on each state and what the APRN in this position can do according to the Nurse Practice Act for that state. The scope provides **guidelines** instead of particular directives, which may be wide in range, depending on the state. Many times, the scope is founded on what is allowed legally both in the state and in the nation. The initial Scope of Practice for PNPs was created in 1983 by the National Association of Pediatric Nurse Practitioners, and has been updated multiple times since. The APRN's scope of practice is always changing and improving to meet the needs of the community, state, and country at large.

Credentials

Advanced practice registered nurses (APRN) are comprised of nurse anesthetists, nurse midwives, nurse practitioners, and clinical nurse specialists. These specialties must have proper **credentials** and take responsibility for the patient's care. Some other nurses who hold leadership responsibilities are not included under the term APRN. These nurses who are not included may have professional responsibilities but not in a clinical setting, such as teachers, administrators, or researchers, even though these nurses may have the same knowledge as an APRN. Someone that is not working in direct patient care with patients or in a family medical clinic cannot be considered an APRN.

Purposes of Credentials

Purposes of credentials for the APRN are to:

- Ensure there is accountability for proficient work.
- Authenticate that the practitioner has received the correct education, has a license, and is certified.
- Ensure that the local and national laws are followed.
- Recognize the growing scope for the APRN.
- Allow an avenue for patients to make a grievance.
- Ensure a responsibility to the community by making sure standards of practice are met.

RESPONSIBILITIES

Advanced practice registered nurse (APRN) **responsibilities** include but are not limited to the following:

- Evaluate the patient, produce and assess information; comprehend complex nursing practice and practice critical thinking.
- Assess many kinds of information; compile the differential diagnosis; determine proper medical care.
- Without supervision, determine how to handle difficult patient issues.
- Create a way to identify the condition, create objectives for the patient's medical management, and stipulate the medical routine or plan.
- Plan, modify and implement the medical plan. This includes prescribing and administering drugs that fall within the APRN's scope and specialty.
- Treat the patient's physical and mental condition.
- Maintain the privacy of the patient.
- Conduct care within a therapeutic environment.

CONSULTATION, REFERRAL, AND COORDINATION

As part of the **scope of practice**, the advanced practice nurse is able to provide and augment primary care to patients through a number of different services:

- **Consultation** services may include a variety of services, such as assessment of growth and development and risk factors, providing interventions, such as diet and exercise programs, and educating patients.
- **Referral services** include referring patients to physicians, such as orthopedic specialists, and to organizations or agencies, such as drug rehabilitation programs.
- **Coordination services,** with the nurse maintaining contact and receiving reports from referrals in order to provide an integrated plan of care, serves as a valuable service to patients, who often must deal with many different healthcare providers who have little or no contact with each other. This type of service can prevent unnecessary duplications of service but also ensure that findings are not overlooked.

PRESCRIPTION AND DIAGNOSTICS

Both **prescribing** medications and treatment and ordering **diagnostic** tests are within the scope of practice of nurse practitioners, but as with other aspects of practice, each state establishes how that will be carried out. Additionally, insurance reimbursement varies from one area to another and must be considered:

- **Prescription:** Terminology varies from state to state with nurse practitioners allowed to "furnish" or "prescribe" some types of medications. In some states they may do so independently; in others, they must be "supervised" by a physician under whose auspices they provide care to patients. The nurse practitioner should maintain a list of medications and consider cost-effectiveness when ordering medications.
- **Diagnostics:** Nurse practitioners can order laboratory, EKG, and radiographic tests for routine screening and health assessment as well as diagnosis based on assessment. There are limitations, depending upon the individual state nursing practice act.

Mission and Vision of the AACN

The **mission** of the AACN is as follows:

- The **American Association of Critical-Care Nurses (AACN)** provides and inspires leadership to establish work and care environments that are respectful, healing, and humane. The AACN's key to success is through its members. Therefore, the AACN is committed to providing the highest quality resources to maximize nurses' contribution to caring for critically ill patients and their families.

The **vision** of the AACN is as follows:

- The AACN is dedicated to creating a health care system driven by the needs of patients and families where critical care professionals make their optimal contribution.

Values Set Forth by the AACN

In addition to its mission and vision, the AACN has also published a **set of values** intended for all AACN members to uphold. These values state that the AACN member will:

- Be accountable for basing his or her practice on ethical actions and principles
- Advocate changes in the AACN organization that benefit patients and their families
- Practice with integrity, including honest communication, loyalty, and the honoring of promises and commitments
- Communicate and cultivate relationships with other AACN members
- Assume a leadership role, promoting strategic thinking, planning, and problem solving
- Meet or exceed all standards and expectations
- Remain a fair, impartial, and responsible leader
- Continue to make contributions through learning, questioning, and critical thinking
- Promote innovative thinking
- Remain committed and passionate about the organization, and inspire others to do the same

Standards of Professional Performance

The ANA and the AACN collaborated to publish a set of **standards of professional performance** for the ACNP as follows:

- **Standard I: Professional Practice** states that the ACNP will systematically evaluate the quality and effectiveness of his or her clinical practice in relation to institutional guidelines, professional practice standards, and laws and regulations.
- **Standard II: Education** states that the ACNP will maintain current knowledge in advanced nursing practice.
- **Standard III: Collaboration** states that the ACNP will collaborate with the patient, family, and other health care providers in the delivery of patient care.
- **Standard IV: Ethics** states that the ACNP will integrate ethical considerations into practice.
- **Standard V: Systems Thinking** states that the ACNP will develop and participate in organizational systems and processes to promote optimal patient outcomes.
- **Standard VI: Resource Utilization** states that the ACNP will consider factors related to safety, effectiveness, and cost in planning and delivering patient care.
- **Standard VII: Leadership** states that the ACNP will provide leadership in the practice setting and in the profession.

- **Standard VIII: Collegiality** states that the ACNP will promote a healthy work environment through the use of effective communication and respect for the individual.
- **Standard IX: Quality of Practice** states that the ACNP will continuously and systematically evaluate and enhance quality, safety and effectiveness of practice and the delivery of care across the continuum.
- **Standard X: Clinical Inquiry** states that the ACNP will participate in research and evidence-based care to expand the role of advanced nursing practice.

Standards of Clinical Practice

The ANA and the AACN have collaborated to provide published **standards of care** for the ACNP.

- **Standard I** states that the ACNP is responsible for collecting patient data through an **advanced assessment**.
- **Standard II** states that the ACNP is responsible for determining **differential diagnoses** by analyzing said data.
- **Standard III** states that the ACNP is responsible for **identifying expected outcomes** specific to the patient.
- **Standard IV** states that the ACNP is responsible for developing a **care plan** with specific interventions.
- **Standard V** states that the ACNP is responsible for **implementing patient interventions**.
- **Standard VI** states that the ACNP is responsible for **evaluating** the progress of the patient.

Areas of Competency

The **ACNP's Scope of Practice** identifies a number of areas in which the ACNP should be **competent**. The ACNP is expected to have an extensive working knowledge base, and he or she is also expected to have excellent communication skills. The ability to perform both a patient health history and a physical examination are central to the ACNP's scope of practice, as is the ability to both order and interpret laboratory tests and diagnostic procedures. In addition, the ACNP is expected to be able to perform certain invasive procedures, such as intensive wound care, to remove drains and staples, and to assist in surgical procedures. The ACNP is required to prescribe drugs and monitor the effects of those drugs during the course of treatment. The ACNP must be organized, enthusiastic, intuitive, inventive, and respectful towards patients, families, and other health care professionals.

ACNP's Role as Care Provider to High-Acuity Patients

The acute care nurse practitioner will encounter more high-acuity patients than the nurse practitioner that works in, say, a family medicine clinic. **High-acuity patients** are patients whose conditions are more critical, less stable, and require more attention; emergency departments, operating rooms, and intensive care units are areas of the hospital that see a high volume of high-acuity patients. The ANA and the AACN have established a set of components that comprise the **role** of the acute care nurse practitioner when working with high-acuity patients. The ACNP should include the following **components** in the workup of every high-acuity patient: a comprehensive health history, a comprehensive physical examination, a health risk profile and analysis, a differential diagnosis based on diagnostic reasoning, a therapeutic intervention plan, and consultation with health care providers in other specialties.

Health Care Policy and Systems

HEALTH POLICY

Health policy is the legal effort to make positive change in systemic health care and health care outcomes through a compilation of decisions, plans and actions made by representatives of the health care community in combination with local, state and federal government representatives. Often, the first step in health care policy efforts is to identify the goals and desired outcomes of new policy, then working backwards to formulate a plan and collect relevant needs that must be met in order for those goals to be attained.

Due to the inherently political nature of health policy, it is important that health care representatives commit to contributing to policy changes in the arenas they have deemed necessary from their work experience. Local politicians rely heavily on the expertise and knowledge of health care professionals to inform and guide policy change. The nurse has the unique skill set of working as a nurse, and also working as a clinical leader, which provides a critical dichotomy of insight that can be extremely valuable in addressing health policy change. Nurses have the opportunity to provide both hands on patient care and administrative duties, and often it is the miscommunication between these two entities that present challenges in policy formation. As a nurse it is a responsibility to contribute not only to change on the unit, but change in systemic policy to the benefit of patients and patient safety nationwide.

IMPACT OF SOCIAL, POLITICAL, REGULATORY, AND ECONOMIC FORCES ON DELIVERY OF CARE

The delivery of care is **impacted** by numerous forces:

- **Social forces** are increasing demand for access to treatment and medical services, both traditional and complementary. As society views equitable medical care as a right, then delivery of care must be available to all.
- **Political forces** affect medical care as the Federal and state governments increasingly become purchasers of medical care, imposing their guidelines and limitations on the medical system.
- **Regulatory forces** may be local, state, or Federal and can have a profound effect of delivery of care and services, differing from one state or region to another.
- **Economic forces**, such as managed care or cost-containment committees, try to contain costs to insurers and facilities by controlling access to and duration of treatment, and limiting products. Economic pressure is working to prevent duplication of services in a geographical area, and providers are creating networks to purchase supplies and equipment directly.

HEALTH IMPACT ASSESSMENT

Health impact assessment is a method of assessing the potential effects of a health policy or health program on the **overall health of the population** targeted by the policy or program. The purpose of health impact assessment is to maximize the benefits of health programs (in addition, of course, to minimizing the negative impact that the program may potentially have). There are typically 5 steps involved in the health impact assessment project. These steps include a **screening process** to ensure that the program is necessary or beneficial; **scoping**, which determines which population(s) will be impacted by the program; **identification and assessment** of all potential health impacts if the program is mandated; **decision making and recommendations** based on the assessment of potential impact; and **evaluation and monitoring**, which continues throughout the life of the program.

Nursing's Agenda for Health Care Reform from ANA (1991)

Nursing's Agenda for Health Care Reform encourages the development of health care that provides patients the ability to get to receive medical attention and help without excessive costs, and it encourages continual primary care. It fundamentally asks for **vital medical attention** to be accessible to everyone and for there to be a **reorganized health care system** that centers on patients, well-being and conditions so that they may get medical help in familiar and local places. It advocates providing for ongoing medical needs and insurance changes so that patients can use their coverage more easily. It asks for organizational assessment on public and private sectors regarding the use of resources, lowering expenses, and getting balanced and even reimbursement for each provider.

Health Care Delivery Systems

In the United States, **healthcare delivery systems** are traditionally fragmented, unique, and quite complex in nature. In contrast to the United States, most other countries in developed nations have national health insurance systems, which are commonly referred to as **universal access systems**. Such universal access systems are managed by the government and are funded by taxes. Healthcare delivery systems in the United States consist of subcategories such as managed care, military, vulnerable populations, and integrated service delivery. **Managed care healthcare delivery systems** are the predominant systems for the delivery of health care in the United States.

Managed Care Healthcare Delivery System

The **managed care healthcare delivery system** promotes efficiency by integrating all the basic functions of healthcare delivery and using management strategies to control healthcare service usage. Managed healthcare delivery systems also determine the **prices** of services and provider reimbursement. The government and employers primarily provide the financing for managed care systems. Managed care delivery systems act like insurance companies in that they use a contract health plan that is an agreement between the managed care system and the subscriber. Subscribers under a managed care delivery system are usually required to use selected healthcare providers.

Levels of Health Care

- **Acute care** is short-term medical treatment, usually in a hospital, for episodic illness or injury.
- **Long-term care** applies to major trauma patients or those with chronic and multiple medical, mental, and social problems who cannot take care of themselves.
- **Custodial care** is mainly for the purpose of assisting clients with their home personal care and does not necessarily require the provider to have specialized skills or training.
- **Intermediate care** applies to patients requiring more than custodial care and might require nursing supervision. Unless true skilled care is required, insurance companies group intermediate and custodial care under the same benefit guidelines.
- **Sub-acute care** is used for patients who are medically stable but still require active care from trained medical professionals. Treatments in this level include frequent or complex wound care, rehabilitation, complex intravenous therapy, and combination therapies. Patients are usually in an extended care facility (ECF), such as a nursing home or a **skilled nursing facility**.

Transitional Hospitals

Transitional hospitals are acute care facilities for patients that are medically stable and whose rehabilitation plan is too complex for an **extended care facility (ECF)**. Transitional hospitals that specialize in medically complex care do so at a lower cost than a traditional hospital because of their specialization. Some transitional hospitals supply only basic patient care, also at a lower cost than a traditional hospital. Examples of transitional hospitals are: burn or extensive wound care, hemodialysis, hospice, infectious disease management, intravenous (IV) medication therapies, neurobehavioral rehabilitation, pain control therapies, rehabilitation, total parenteral nutrition, and ventilator care/weaning from ventilators.

TELEHEALTH

Telehealth refers to the delivery of healthcare services to patients who are not physically present with the healthcare professional, usually due to remote location, disability, or pandemic (such as the recent outbreak of COVID-19). Telehealth can be delivered over a telephone, via email, or by video conference. The primary benefits of telehealth are that it allows for the extension of precious healthcare resources, lowers the overall cost of healthcare, and allows patients to receive healthcare who would not normally have access to it.

There are a number of **ways in which telehealth is useful** to healthcare professionals:

- Consultation with colleagues
- Patient interviews
- Monitor a patient's biometric values and assess their condition
- Evaluate diagnostic images which allows physicians to remotely view and evaluate these images even if they are located overseas (e.g., India)
- Evaluation of microscope slides and laboratory reports

Quality Improvement Processes

CONTINUOUS QUALITY IMPROVEMENT

Continuous quality improvement is a multidisciplinary management philosophy that can be applied to all aspects of an organization, whether related to such varied areas as the cardiac unit, purchasing, or human resources. The skills used for epidemiologic research (data collection, analysis, outcomes, action plans) are all applicable to the analysis of multiple types of events, because they are based on solid scientific methods. Multi-disciplinary planning can bring valuable insights from various perspectives, and strategies used in one context can often be applied to another. All staff, from housekeeping to supervising, must be alert to not only problems but also opportunities for improvement. Increasingly, departments must be concerned with cost-effectiveness as the costs of medical care continue to rise, so the quality professional in the cardiovascular unit is not in an isolated position in an institution but is just one part of the whole, facing similar concerns as those in other disciplines. Disciplines are often interrelated in their functions.

JURAN'S QUALITY IMPROVEMENT PROCESS

Joseph Juran's quality improvement process (QIP) is a 4-step method of change (focusing on quality control) which is based on a trilogy of concepts that includes quality planning, control, and improvement. The steps to the QIP process include the following:

1. **Defining** the project and organizing includes listing and prioritizing problems and identifying a team.
2. **Diagnosing** includes analyzing problems and then formulating theories related to cause by root cause analysis and test theories.

3. **Remediating** includes considering various alternative solutions and then designing and implementing specific solutions and controls while addressing institutional resistance to change. As causes of problems are identified and remediation instituted to remove the problems, the processes should improve.
4. **Holding** involves evaluating performance and monitoring the control system in order to maintain gains.

FOCUS Performance Improvement Model

Find, organize, clarify, uncover, start (FOCUS) is a performance improvement model used to facilitate change:

1. **Find**: Identifying a problem by looking at the organization and attempting to determine what isn't working well or what is wrong.
2. **Organize**: Identifying those people who have an understanding of the problem or process and creating a team to work on improving performance.
3. **Clarify**: Determining what is involved in solving the problem by utilizing brainstorming techniques, such as the Ishikawa diagram.
4. **Uncover**: Analyzing the situation to determine the reason the problem has arisen or that a process is unsuccessful.
5. **Start**: Determining where to begin in the change process.

FOCUS, by itself, is an incomplete process and is primarily used as a means to identify a problem rather than a means to find the solution. FOCUS is usually combined with PDCA (FOCUS-PDCA), so it becomes a 9-step process; however, beginning with FOCUS helps to narrow the focus, resulting in better outcomes.

Nurse's Involvement in Quality Improvement

The following are ways in which **nurses can be involved in quality improvement** in their facility:

- **Identify situations** in the nursing unit that require improvement and might benefit patient outcomes (cost containment, incident reporting, etc.) if changed.
- **Identify potential items** that can be measured to be able to test the problem or to be able to monitor patient outcomes.
- **Collect data** on those measurements and determine current patient outcomes.
- **Analyze the data** and identify procedures, methods, etc., that can be utilized to potentially make positive changes in patient outcomes, doing research if necessary.
- **Make recommendations for changes** to be implemented to determine the effect on patient outcomes.
- **Implement recommendations** after approval from administrative personnel.
- **Collect data** using the same measurements and determine if the changes improved patient outcomes or not.

Risk Management

Risk management attempts to prevent harm and legal liability by being proactive and by identifying a patient's **risk factors**. The patient is educated about these factors and ways that they can modify their behavior to decrease their risk. Treatments and interventions must be considered in terms of risk to the patient, and the patient must always know these risks in order to make healthcare decisions. Much can be done to avoid mistakes that put patients at risk. Patients should note medications and other aspects of their care so that they can help prevent mistakes. They should feel free to question care and to have their concerns heard and addressed. When mistakes are made, the actions taken to remedy the situation are very important. The physician should be made aware of the error immediately, and the patient notified according to hospital policy. Errors must be evaluated to determine how the process failed. Honesty and caring can help mitigate many errors.

Nursing Malpractice, Negligence, Unintentional Torts, and Intentional Torts

- **Malpractice** is unethical or improper actions or lack of proper action by the nurse that may or may not be related to a lack of skills that nurses should possess.
- **Negligence** is the failure to act as any other diligent nurse would have acted in the same situation.
- Negligence can lead to an **unintentional tort**. In this case, the patient must prove that the nurse had a duty to act, a duty proven via standards of care, and that the nurse failed in this duty and harm occurred to the patient as a result of this failure.
- **Intentional torts** differ in that the duty is assumed and the nurse breached this duty via assault and battery, invasion of privacy, slander, or false imprisonment of the patient.

Infection Control

Nosocomial Infections

Nosocomial infections are those that are healthcare-associated or hospital-acquired. The following is a list of common nosocomial infections.

- *Enterococci* infections include urinary infections, bacteremia, endocarditis as well as infections in wounds and the abdominal and pelvic areas.
- *Enterobacteriaceae* cause about half of the urinary tract infections and a quarter of the postoperative infections.
- *Escherichia coli* primarily causes urinary tract infections (especially related to catheters), diarrhea, and neonatal meningitis but it can also lead to pneumonia, and bacteremia (usually secondary to urinary infection).
- Group B β-hemolytic *Streptococci* (GBS) has increasingly been a cause of infections in neonatal units, causing pneumonia, meningitis, and sepsis. GBS infections may occur as wound infections after Caesarean sections, especially in those immunocompromised.
- *Staphylococcus aureus* is a major cause of nosocomial post-operative infections, both localized and systemic, and from indwelling tubes and devices.
- Methicillin-resistant *Staphylococcus aureus (MRSA)* is a common cause of surgical infections.
- *Clostridium difficile* causes more nosocomial diarrhea cases than any other microorganism.
- *Candida*, a yeast fungal pathogen, can overgrow and lead to mucocutaneous or cutaneous lesions and sepsis.
- *Aspergillus* spp., filamentous fungi, produce spores that become airborne and can invade the respiratory tract, causing pneumonia.

Catheter-Related Infections

Intravenous catheter-related infections are a significant cause of morbidity and mortality in the hospital setting. Usually, these infections are due to *Staphylococcus aureus*, *enterococcus*, or fungal infection such as *Candida*. These infections are important because they may progress and eventually lead to bacteremia, infective endocarditis, septic pulmonary emboli, septic shock, osteomyelitis, or superficial thrombophlebitis. Therefore, vigilance should be maintained to prevent these infections. The patient may exhibit fevers, chills, and discomfort around the catheter site. The site itself may show purulence or erythema. The subclavian vein is the preferred intravenous site and the femoral is the least-preferred site due to high infection rates. Infections are diagnosed with blood cultures and catheter tip cultures. Initial treatment includes removal of the catheter and antibiotic treatment. Antibiotics should be empiric at first, then directed toward culture results. Treatment duration should be 2 weeks at first, but 4-6 weeks if there is a complicated infection.

Infection Control Measures

Standard infection control measures are designed to prevent transmission of microbial substances between patients and/or medical providers. These measures are indicated for everyone and include frequent handwashing, gloves whenever bodily fluids are involved, and face shields and gowns when splashes are anticipated. For more advanced control with tuberculosis, SARS, vesicular rash disorders (such as VZV), and most recently COVID-19, **airborne precautions** should be instituted to prevent the spread of tiny droplets that can remain suspended in the air for days and travel throughout a hospital environment. Therefore, negative pressure rooms are essential, and providers and patients should wear high-efficiency N95 masks and be fitted in advance. For disorders such as influenza or other infections spread by droplets (spread by cough or sneeze) basic surgical masks should be worn (**droplet precautions**). For **contact precautions** in the setting of fecally-transmitted infection or vesicular rash diseases, gowns/gloves should be used and contact limited. White coats are not a substitute for proper gowning. In the case of a *Clostridium difficile* infection, contact precautions should be used in addition to washing hands with soap and water (rather than alcohol-based hand sanitizer) after patient contact.

Infection Control Plan

The **purpose of an infection control/surveillance plan** should be clearly outlined and may be multifaceted, including the following elements:

- **Decreasing rates of infection**: The primary purpose of a surveillance plan is to identify a means to decrease nosocomial infections, including a notification system and laboratory surveillance.
- **Evaluating infection control measures**: Surveillance can evaluate effectiveness of infection control measures. (Surgical checklists, handwashing, housekeeping, ventilation).
- **Establishing endemic threshold rates**: Establishing threshold rates can help to enact control measures to reduce rates.
- **Identifying outbreaks**: About 5-10% of infections occur in outbreaks, and comparing data with established endemic threshold rates can help to identify these outbreaks if analysis is done in a regular and timely manner.
- **Achieving staff compliance**: Objective evidence may convince staff to cooperate with infection control measures.
- **Meeting accreditation standards**: Some accreditation agencies require reports of infection rates.
- **Providing defense for malpractice suits**: Providing evidence that a facility is proactive in combating infections can decrease liability.
- **Comparing infection rates with other facilities**: Comparing data helps focus attention and resources.

Protocol for Needlestick Injury and Postexposure Prophylaxis

If the healthcare provider experiences a **needlestick injury**, the individual's initial response should be to irrigate the wound with soap and water. As soon as possible, the incident must be reported to a supervisor and steps taken according to established protocol. This may include testing and/or prophylaxis, depending on the patient's health history. In some cases, the patient may also be tested for communicable diseases, such as HIV, in order to determine the risk to the healthcare provider.

PEP (post-exposure prophylaxis) is available for exposure to HIV (human immunodeficiency virus) and hepatitis B virus (hepatis B immune globulin). However, no PEP is available for HCV (hepatitis C virus) although the CDC does provide a plan for management. PEP should be initiated within 72 hours of exposure. All testing and treatments associated with the needlestick injury must be provided free of cost at a hospital or medical facility.

Patient Safety

Joint Commission's Patient Safety Goals

The **Joint Commission** has a set of goals that impact **patient safety** for each type of healthcare facility. Within the hospital environment, there are several goals that pertain:

- Each facility must have a way to identify patients that will avoid errors of identification.
- Caregivers are to give careful, accurate communications about patients and their care so that mistakes are not made.
- A system to avoid medication errors must be in place.
- Medications must be reconciled when the patient moves from place to place within the hospital or is discharged to other caregivers.
- The risk of infection must be decreased so that patients are at less risk for hospital-related infections.
- The facility must have a fall prevention program and evaluate its effectiveness.

All patients and family must be encouraged to be active in their own care to help to avoid errors. They must also know how to make sure their concerns for safety of care are heard and acted upon.

Aspects of Patient Safety in the Hospital

Deliberate decisions by the health care providers/facility can help create an environment conducive for **patient safety.** Some of those aspects include:

- **Educating the patient on signaling staff**: The patient must be educated about the use of the call light, and the call light placed within easy reach. If the patient is unable to use the call light, then an alternative means of calling for help, such as a handheld bell, should be available. If the patient is unable to manage any type of signaling system, then the nurse should check on the patient at least every hour.
- **Protecting from falls and electrical hazards**: All clutter should be removed from floors and cords secured away from walkways. All electrical appliances should be checked to ensure they are working properly and have no frayed cords. Patients should be provided assistive devices, such as walkers, if necessary, to improve stability.
- **Making appropriate room assignments**: Patients with the greatest need for supervision should be placed closest to the nursing desk and within the line of sight whenever possible. In environments such as critical care, each nurse should be able to visualize their patient assignment from their nursing station.

Medication Errors

There are about 7,000 deaths yearly in the United States attributed to **medication errors.** Studies indicate that there are errors in 1 in 5 doses of medication given to patients in hospitals. Patient safety must be ensured with proper handling and administering of medications:

- **Avoid error-prone abbreviations or symbols**. The Joint Commission has established a list of abbreviations to avoid, but mistakes are frequent with other abbreviations as well. In many cases, abbreviations and symbols should be avoided altogether or restricted to a limited approved list.
- **Prevent errors due to illegible handwriting or unclear verbal orders**. Handwritten orders should be block printed to reduce chance of error; verbal orders should be repeated back to the physician.
- **Institute barcoding and scanners** that allow the patient's wristband and medications to be scanned for verification.
- **Provide lists of similarly-named medications** to educate staff.
- Establish an **institutional policy** for the administration of medications that includes protocols for verification of drug, dosage, and patient, as well as educating the patient about the medications.

Assessing Patients for Allergies

When assessing patients for **allergies** it's important to determine the type of symptoms they have, when the initial reaction occurred, and what type of treatment they have used in the past to manage this complication (including antihistamines). Allergies of particular interest include:

- **Food**: Ask patients about any specific foods that cause an adverse reaction as some foods may have cross-reactivity to latex (such as kiwi, papaya, avocado, and bananas), so patients may be at risk of developing latex allergy and should avoid contact with latex. Some medications may contain substances derived from food, such as eggs, fish, gelatin, lactose, and soy.
- **Latex**: Sensitivity to latex can result in mild reactions, such as itching and rash, to severe anaphylactic reactions, and is common among those with repeated contact with healthcare environments, such as those with spina bifida or multiple surgeries, so it should be suspected with these clients. While non-latex options are more readily available in most hospitals (non-latex gloves and Foley catheters, for instance), latex continues to be used in hospital materials, therefore this allergy must be assessed immediately upon arrival so that appropriate materials can be substituted if necessary.
- **Environmental**: The most common environmental allergies include pollens, dust mites, animals, cigarette smoke, cockroaches, and mold/mildew, so the nurse should be sure to ask about these as well as any other environmental allergies. Some patients are sensitive to strong colognes and perfumes, so the use of these are often regulated by hospital dress codes on units with immunocompromised patients.

NON-PHARMACOLOGIC PRESCRIPTION PRECAUTIONS

Some **non-pharmacologic prescriptions** may contribute to accident or injury, including the following:

- **Oxygen supplies**: Oxygen may be administered at the wrong level of liters (too much or too little), and the oxygen supply may be inadvertently obstructed or disconnected. Oxygen concentrators may not have backup batteries and may fail to function if electricity goes off. If people smoke around oxygen, this increases the risk of fires. Nasal cannulas and face masks that delivery oxygen, when used over prolonged periods of time, can cause pressure injuries, therefore appropriate assessment and skin care is also necessary.
- **Assistive devices**: If equipment, such as canes and walkers, are improperly fitted, they may increase risk of falls.
- **Dialysis equipment**: Contamination of equipment is always a concern and can result in peritonitis (peritoneal dialysis) and sepsis (hemodialysis). If the lines become separated, the client may exsanguinate.
- **Hot/Cold compresses**: If cold compresses are placed directly on the skin, they may damage the tissue, especially if left in place for too long. Hot compresses may cause burns if temperature is too high and may damage wounds if placed directly over them.

SEIZURE PRECAUTIONS

Seizure disorders are broadly categorized as partial seizures (which begin locally) or generalized seizures (which are bilateral and symmetrical and may be convulsive or non-convulsive):

- **Partial seizures** include *simple partial* (with motor, sensory, and/or autonomic symptoms but without impaired consciousness), *complex partial* (with cognitive, affective, psychosensory, and/or psychomotor symptoms, as well as impaired consciousness), or *partial secondarily generalized*.
- **Generalized seizures** include seizures that are bilateral and symmetric without local onset and may be convulsive or non-convulsive. These seizures include *tonic-clonic, tonic, clonic, absence* (petit mal), *atonic*, and *myoclonic seizures*, as well as *unclassified seizures*.

Seizure precautions are a standard set of safety protocol that ensure patient safety in those patients with a high risk or history of seizures. Generally, these precautions include padding the siderails, keeping the bed at the lowest position, and maintaining suctioning at the bedside Precautions also include ensuring privacy and providing supportive care in the event of a seizure, such as easing the patient to the floor and providing padding to protect the head. Side rails should be raised and pillow removed if the patient is in bed. The patient should be placed on one side with the head flexed so the tongue does not block the airway. The patient should *not* be restrained or a padded tongue-blade inserted between the teeth.

Research and Evidence-Based Practice

ELEMENTS OF RESEARCH

The following are **elements of research**:

- **Variable:** An entity that can be different within a population.
- **Independent variable:** The variable that the researchers change to evaluate its effect.
- **Dependent variable:** The variable that may be changed by alterations in the independent variable.
- **Hypothesis:** The proposed explanation to describe an expected outcome in a study.

- **Sample:** The selected population to be studied.
- **The experimental group:** The population within the sample that undergoes the treatment or intervention.
- **The control group:** The population within the sample that is not exposed to the treatment of intervention being evaluated.

The nurse must be taught and must understand the process of critical analysis and know how to conduct a survey of the literature. **Basic research concepts** include:

- **Survey of valid sources:** Information from a juried journal and an anonymous website or personal website are very different sources, and evaluating what constitutes a valid source of data is critical.
- **Evaluation of internal and external validity:** Internal validity shows a cause-and-effect relationship between two variables, with the cause occurring before the effect and no intervening variable. External validity occurs when results hold true in different environments and circumstances with different populations.
- **Sample selection and sample size:** Selection and size can have a huge impact on the results, but a sample that is too small may lack both internal and external validity. Selection may be so narrowly focused that the results can't be generalized to other groups.

Validity, Generalizability, and Replicability

Many research studies are most concerned with **internal validity** (adequate unbiased data properly collected and analyzed within the population studied), but studies that determine the efficacy of procedures or treatments, for example, should have **external validity** as well; that is, the results should be **generalizable** (true) for similar populations. **Replication** of the study under different circumstances and with different subjects and researchers should produce similar results. For various reasons, some people may be excluded from a study so that instead of randomized subjects, the subjects may be highly selected so when data is compared with another population in which there is less or more selection, results may be different. The selection of subjects, in this case, would interfere with external validity. Part of the design of a study should include considerations of whether or not it should have external validity or whether there is value for the institution based solely on internal validation.

Hypothesis

A **hypothesis** should be generated about the probable cause of the disease/infection based on the information available in laboratory and medical records, epidemiologic study, literature review, and expert opinion. For example, a hypothesis should include the infective agent, the likely source, and the mode of transmission: "Wound infections with *Staphylococcus aureus* were caused by reuse and inadequate sterilization of single-use irrigation syringes used during wound care in the ICU."

Hypothesis testing includes data analysis, laboratory findings, and outcomes of environmental testing. It usually includes case-control studies, with 2-4 controls picked for each case of infection. They may be matched according to age, sex, or other characteristics, but they are not infected at the time they are picked for the study. Cohort studies, whose controls are picked based on having or lacking exposure, may also be instituted. If the hypothesis cannot be supported, then a new hypothesis or different testing methods may be necessary.

Critical Reading

There are several steps to **critical reading** to evaluate research:

- **Consider the source** of the material. If it is in the popular press, it may have little validity compared to something published in a peer-reviewed journal.
- **Review the author's credentials** to determine if a person is an expert in the field of study.
- **Determine the thesis**, or the central claim of the research. It should be clearly stated.
- **Examine the organization** of the article, whether it is based on a particular theory, and the type of methodology used.
- **Review the evidence** to determine how it is used to support the main points. Look for statistical evidence and sample size to determine if the findings have wide applicability.
- **Evaluate** the overall article to determine if the information seems credible and useful and should be communicated to administration and/or staff.

Major Study Types Utilized in Statistical Analysis

When conducting research, the nurse should be aware of the **types of studies** available and when each type of study is appropriate and most reliable:

- **Case-control studies** are simple. They use pre-existing cases with and without the disorder of interest. For example, case-control studies may be done with mesothelioma and exposure to possible pleural irritants. These are good for rare diseases to determine cause and effect.
- **Cross-sectional studies** utilize a cross-section of data from the population and analyze variables at one time point. They are not good for determining cause and effect, but they are useful for correlating characteristics with disorders.
- **Cohort studies** follow a cohort of a population for a period of time and attempt to make a link with diseases. As in the previous example, researchers could follow a group exposed to asbestos and study the incidence of mesothelioma.
- **Randomized controlled trial** is the gold standard, with patients assigned to the control or experimental group. This is a difficult type of test to design and implement but very useful, as the data is often well-controlled. It is the most expensive type of study.

Bias in Research

Selection bias occurs when the method of selecting subjects results in a cohort that is not representative of the target population because of inherent error in design. For example, if all patients who develop urinary infections are evaluated per urine culture and sensitivities for microbial resistance, but only those patients with clinically-evident infections are included, a number of patients with sub-clinical infections may be missed, skewing the results. Selection bias is only a concern when participants in studies are specifically chosen. Many surveillance studies do not involve the selection of subjects.

Information bias occurs when there are errors in classification, so an estimate of association is incorrect. Non-differential misclassification occurs when there is similar misclassification of disease or exposure among both those who are diseased/exposed and those who are not. Differential misclassification occurs when there is a differing misclassification of disease or exposure among both those who are diseased/exposed and those who are not.

Qualitative and Quantitative Data

Both **qualitative and quantitative data** are used for analysis, but the focus is quite different:

- **Qualitative data**: Data are described verbally or graphically, and the results are subjective, depending upon observers to provide information. Interviews may be used as a tool to gather information, and the researcher's interpretation of data is important. Gathering this type of data can be time-intensive, and it can usually not be generalized to a larger population. This type of information gathering is often useful at the beginning of the design process for data collection.
- **Quantitative data**: Data are described in terms of numbers within a statistical format. This type of information gathering is done after the design of data collection is outlined, usually in later stages. Tools may include surveys, questionnaires, or other methods of obtaining numerical data. The researcher's role is objective.

Classes of Evidence-Based Practice

Evidence-based practice is treatment based on the best possible evidence, including a study of current research. Literature is searched to find evidence of the most effective treatments for specific diseases or injuries, and those treatments are then utilized to create clinical pathways that outline specific multi-departmental treatment protocols, including medications, treatments, and timelines. Evidence-based guidelines are often produced by specialty organizations that undertake the task of searching and analyzing literature to produce policies, procedures, and guidelines that become the standard of care for the disease. These guidelines are then used when a patient fits the disease criteria for that guideline.

Evidence-based nursing aims to improve the quality of nursing care by examining the reasons for all nursing practices and determining those that have the most positive outcomes. Evidence-based nursing focuses on the individual nurse utilizing evidence-based observations to influence decision-making.

Evidence-Based Practice Guidelines

The creation of **evidence-based practice guidelines** includes the following components:

- **Focus on the topic/methodology:** This includes outlining possible interventions and treatments for review, choosing patient populations and settings, and determining significant outcomes. Search boundaries (such as types of journals, types of studies, dates of studies) should be determined.
- **Evidence review:** This includes review of literature, critical analysis of studies, and summarizing of results, including pooled meta-analysis.
- **Expert judgment:** Recommendations based on personal experience from a number of experts may be utilized, especially if there is inadequate evidence based on review, but this subjective evidence should be explicitly acknowledged.
- **Policy considerations:** This includes cost-effectiveness, access to care, insurance coverage, availability of qualified staff, and legal implications.
- **Policy:** A written policy must be completed with recommendations. Common practice is to utilize letter guidelines, with "A" being the most highly recommended, usually based on the quality of supporting evidence.
- **Review:** The completed policy should be submitted to peers for review and comments before instituting the policy.

Critical Pathways

Clinical/critical pathway development is done by those involved in direct patient care. The pathway should require no additional staffing and cover the entire scope of an illness. Steps include:

1. Selection of patient group and diagnosis, procedures, or conditions, based on analysis of data and observations of wide variance in approach to treatment and prioritizing organization and patient needs.
2. Creation of interdisciplinary team of those involved in the process of care, including physicians to develop pathway.
3. Analysis of data including literature review and study of best practices to identify opportunities for quality improvement.
4. Identification of all categories of care, such as nutrition, medications, and nursing.
5. Discussion and reaching consensus.
6. Identifying the levels of care and number of days to be covered by the pathway.
7. Pilot testing and redesigning steps as indicated.
8. Educating staff about standards.
9. Monitoring and tracking variances in order to improve pathways.

Levels of Evidence in Evidence-Based Practice

Levels of evidence are categorized according to the scientific evidence available to support the recommendations, as well as existing state and federal laws. While recommendations are voluntary, they are often used as a basis for state and federal regulations.

- *Category IA* is well supported by evidence from experimental, clinical, or epidemiologic studies and is strongly recommended for implementation.
- *Category IB* has supporting evidence from some studies, has a good theoretical basis, and is strongly recommended for implementation.
- *Category IC* is required by state or federal regulations or is an industry standard.
- *Category II* is supported by suggestive clinical or epidemiologic studies, has a theoretical basis, and is suggested for implementation.
- *Category III* is supported by descriptive studies, such as comparisons, correlations, and case studies, and may be useful.
- *Category IV* is obtained from expert opinion or authorities only.
- *Unresolved* means there is no recommendation because of a lack of consensus or evidence.

Outcome Evaluation

Outcomes evaluation is an important component of evidence-based practice, which involves both internal and external research. All treatments are subjected to review to determine if they produce positive outcomes, and policies and protocols for outcomes evaluation should be in place. Outcomes evaluation includes the following:

- **Monitoring** over the course of treatment involves careful observation and record keeping that notes progress, with supporting laboratory and radiographic evidence as indicated by condition and treatment.
- **Evaluating** results includes reviewing records as well as current research to determine if outcomes are within acceptable parameters.
- **Sustaining** involves discontinuing treatment, but continuing to monitor and evaluate.

- **Improving** means to continue the treatment but with additions or modifications in order to improve outcomes.
- **Replacing** the treatment with a different treatment must be done if outcomes evaluation indicates that current treatment is ineffective.

Evidence-Based Nursing Interventions

Evidence-based nursing interventions enable nurses to provide high-quality patient care that is based upon research and knowledge, as opposed to giving care that is based upon tradition or information that is out of date. An evidence-based nursing approach is based on the integration of practical clinical experience with medical and clinical research; it utilizes proven clinical guidelines and assessment practices. **Evidence-based nursing interventions** allow nurses to make patient care decisions based on cutting-edge research that has been scientifically validated. Studies show that evidence-based nursing practice yields improved patient outcomes, enables nurses to practice up-to-date methods, improves nurse confidence and decision-making skills, and enhances Joint Commission standards.

Resources

There are numerous information **resources for evidence-base nursing interventions**. These resources include: evidence-based textbooks; databases such as CINAHL Plus, COCHRANE library, Mosby's Nursing Index, NursingConsult, and Nursing@Ovid; evidence-based nursing meta-sites such as the Academic Center for EBN, Joanna Briggs Institute, McGill University, ONS-EBN section, and EBN-University of Minnesota; online evidence-based nursing journals such as Clinical Nurse Specialist, Clinical Nursing Research, Evidence-Based Nursing, Journal of Nursing Care Quality, Journal of Advanced Nursing, Journal of Nursing Scholarship, Nurse Researcher, Nursing Research, Western Journal of Nursing Research, and Worldviews on Evidence-Based Nursing; and various online tutorials.

Obtaining Results of Research to Use in Evidence-Based Practice

When searching for **current evidence** in print and online literature, the nurse should look for **systematic reviews, analyses, and reports**. PUBMED lists all literature and can be searched for all published articles on a particular subject. These articles can be analyzed to determine treatments that have the best evidence of efficacy. Subject and methodological terms and clinical filters can be used to find necessary information, including specific medical subject heading (MH), subheading (SH), publication type (PT), and text word (TW). The nurse should also search the National Guideline Clearinghouse, Cochrane Databases, Agency for Healthcare Research and Quality, and US Preventive Services Task Force Recommendations for evidence and guidelines. When trials of a treatment provide evidence of effectiveness, the evidence is weighed for strength and confidence. Those that provide the strongest evidence of efficacy become recommendations and guidelines for use in the field. Research is also done on a smaller scale by specialists who publish in peer-reviewed journals their research results related to use of a particular intervention.

Educational Strategies and Health Literacy

Bandura's Theory of Social Learning

In the 1970s, Bandura proposed the **theory of social learning,** in which he posited that learning develops from observing, organizing, and rehearsing behavior that has been modeled. Bandura believed that people are more likely to adopt the behavior if they value the outcomes, if the outcomes have functional value, and if the person modeling the behavior is similar to the learner and is admired because of status. Behavior is the result of observation of behavioral, environmental, and cognitive interactions. There are **4 conditions required for modeling:**

- **Attention**: The degree of attention paid to modeling can depend on many variables (physical, social, and environmental).
- **Retention**: People's ability to retain models depends on symbolic coding, creating mental images, organizing thoughts, and rehearsing (mentally or physically).
- **Reproduction**: The ability to reproduce a model depends on physical and mental capabilities.
- **Motivation**: Motivation may derive from past performances, rewards, or vicarious modeling.

Transtheoretical Model of Change

The **Transtheoretical Model of Change** puts forth concepts applicable to the process of educating patients and their family members. The stages of the Transtheoretical Model of Change include the following:

1. The first stage is **precontemplation**. At this point, the patient is not aware of any need for a change in the health behavior.
2. In the next stage, **contemplation**, the patient begins to realize why the change may be necessary after recognizing that the health behavior in question is unhealthy and weighing the consequences of continuing this behavior.
3. During the stage of **preparation**, the patient imagines making the change at a future time, and starts to formulate a plan to do so.
4. The **action** stage occurs when the patient makes specific modifications in health behavior and begins to note the resulting positive changes.
5. During the **maintenance** stage, the patient is able to implement the change over time by utilizing strategies to prevent a return to previously unhealthy behaviors.
6. **Termination** is the stage at which a patient has incorporated the changed behavior into daily functioning, and the patient will not resume the previous unhealthy behavior.

Kurt Lewin

Force Field Analysis

Force field analysis was designed by Kurt Lewin, a social psychologist, to analyze both the driving forces and the restraining forces for change:

- **Driving forces** instigate and promote change, such as leaders, incentives, and competition.
- **Restraining forces** resist change, such as poor attitudes, hostility, inadequate equipment, or insufficient funds.

The educator can use this force field analysis diagram to discuss variables related to a proposed change in process:

- Write the proposed change in the center column.
- Brainstorm and list driving forces and opposed restraining forces. Score the forces. (When driving and restraining forces are in balance, this is a state of equilibrium or the status quo.)
- Discuss the value of the proposed change.
- Develop a plan to diminish or eliminate restraining forces.

Lewin's Model of Change Theory

Lewin's model of change theory may be used to help some patients make decisions for change. The nurse can educate the patient about the need for change and assist with making alterations in behavior or thoughts in order to better facilitate change; however, only the patient can truly implement the change permanently. Lewin's concept of change theory involves a three-part process:

- **Unfreezing** is the part of the model in which the patient becomes open to change, sees a need for it, and removes the boundaries inhibiting change.
- The patient then makes the **actual change** according to expected outcomes and goals.
- Finally, **refreezing** is the process of maintaining the change so that it becomes a habit, and one that the patient is likely to uphold for a long period of time.

Lewin's theory also involves either driving forces or restraining forces. Driving forces are those outside measures that support the change, while restraining forces inhibit success in implementing the change.

Principles of Adult Learning

Adults have a wealth of life and/or employment experiences. Their attitudes toward education may vary considerably. There are, however, some **principles of adult learning** and typical characteristics of adult learners that an instructor should consider when planning strategies for teaching parents, families, or staff.

- Practical and goal-oriented:
  - Provide overviews or summaries and examples.
  - Use collaborative discussions with problem-solving exercises.
  - Remain organized with the goal in mind.
- Self-directed:
  - Provide active involvement, asking for input.
  - Allow different options toward achieving the goal.
  - Give them responsibilities.
- Knowledgeable:
  - Show respect for their life experiences/ education.
  - Validate their knowledge and ask for feedback.
  - Relate new material to information with which they are familiar.
- Relevancy-oriented:
  - Explain how information will be applied.
  - Clearly identify objectives.

- Motivated:
    - Provide certificates of professional advancement and/or continuing education credit for staff when possible.

Learning Styles

Not all people are aware of their preferred **learning style.** A range of teaching materials and methods that relate to all three major learning preferences (visual, auditory, and kinesthetic) and that are appropriate for different ages should be available. Part of assessment for teaching involves choosing the right approach based on observation and feedback. Often presenting learners with different options gives a clue to their preferred learning style. Some people have a combined learning style.

Visual learners learn best by seeing and reading:

- Provide written directions, picture guides, or demonstrate procedures. Use charts and diagrams.
- Provide photos, videos.

Auditory learners learn best by listening and talking:

- Explain procedures while demonstrating and have the learner repeat.
- Plan extra time to discuss and answer questions.
- Provide audiotapes.

Kinesthetic learners learn best by handling, doing, and practicing:

- Provide hands-on experience throughout teaching.
- Encourage handling of supplies and equipment.
- Allow the learner to demonstrate.
- Minimize instructions and allow the person to explore equipment and procedures.

Bloom's Taxonomy

Bloom's taxonomy outlines behaviors that are necessary for learning and that can be applied to healthcare. The theory describes 3 types of learning.

Cognitive: Learning and gaining intellectual skills to master 6 categories of effective learning.

- Knowledge
- Comprehension
- Application
- Analysis
- Synthesis
- Evaluation

Affective: Recognizing 5 categories of feelings and values from simple to complex. This is slower to achieve than cognitive learning.

- **Receiving phenomena**: Accepting need to learn
- **Responding to phenomena**: Taking active part in care
- **Valuing**: Understanding value of becoming independent in care
- **Organizing values**: Understanding how surgery/treatment has improved life
- **Internalizing values**: Accepting condition as part of life, being consistent and self-reliant

Psychomotor: Mastering 7 categories of motor skills necessary for independence. This follows a progression from simple to complex.

- **Perception**: Uses sensory information to learn tasks
- **Set**: Shows willingness to perform tasks
- **Guided response**: Follows directions
- **Mechanism**: Does specific tasks
- **Complex overt response**: Displays competence in self-care
- **Adaptation**: Modifies procedures as needed
- **Origination**: Creatively deals with problems

Approaches to Teaching

There are many **approaches to teaching**, and the educator must prepare, present, and coordinate a wide range of educational workshops, lectures, discussions, and one-on-one instructions on any chosen topic. All types of classes will be needed, depending upon the purpose and material:

- **Educational workshops** are usually conducted with small groups, allowing for maximal participation. They are especially good for demonstrations and practice sessions.
- **Lectures** are often used for more academic or detailed information that may include questions and answers but limits discussion. An effective lecture should include some audiovisual support.
- **Discussions** are best with small groups so that people can actively participate. This is a good method for problem solving.
- **One-on-one instruction** is especially helpful for targeted instruction in procedures for individuals.
- **Online learning modules** are good for independent learners.

Participants should be asked to evaluate the presentations in the forms of surveys or suggestions, but ultimately the program is evaluated in terms of patient outcomes.

Teaching Techniques

There are many **teaching techniques** the nurse can utilize when educating patients. The nurse can demonstrate skills repeatedly when teaching and then allow the patient as much time as needed to practice the skill. The nurse should use equipment that will be available in the home and provide written instructions that can be referred to later if needed. Encouraging discussion of the information helps the patient understand and clarify. Discussion also allows the patient to vent emotions about the disease and the learning process, and to assimilate the information so that a change in behavior can result. Discussion provides feedback to the patient and encouragement to continue learning. Teaching groups of people may be appropriate when there are others who require the same information. The members can support each other with encouragement, empathy, and camaraderie, although some patients will not learn well in groups and will need individual teaching. Groups must be followed up with on an individual basis to give the chance to clarify information, to evaluate the level of learning and goal achievement, and to alter the learning plan as needed for each person.

Instruction Group Sizes

Both **one-on-one instruction and group instruction** have a place in patient/family education.

- **One-on-one instruction** is the most costly for an institution because it is time intensive. However, it allows the patient and family more interaction with the nurse instructor and allows them to have more control over the process by asking questions or having the instructor repeat explanations or demonstrations. One-on-one instruction is especially valuable when patients and families must learn particular skills, such as managing dialysis, or if confidentiality is important.
- **Group instruction** is the less costly because the needs of a number of people can be met at one time. Group presentations are more planned and usually scheduled for a particular time period (an hour, for example), so patients and families have less control. Questioning is usually more limited and may be done only at the end. Group instruction allows patients/families with similar health problems to interact. Group instruction is especially useful for general types of instruction, such as managing diet or other lifestyle issues.

Resources to Use When Teaching Patients and Their Families

Many hospitals that find the need to repeatedly teach the same information to patients and families prepare brochures or other written materials or teaching videos that are available for use. The nurse should review material first and make notes specific to the patient. The nurse should also watch the video with the patient and discuss it afterwards. Written materials can augment lecture and demonstrations and are useful for the patient to keep for later reference.

There are also commercial materials that can be used, provided by various drug or equipment companies. **Teaching resources** are available online from the National Institutes of Health and other reputable sources. The nurse can use these prepared materials whenever possible to save time for actual teaching but must remember to customize them to the patient. They help provide pictures, colors, and interesting features that keep the patient's interest in learning alive. There are also many books, groups, and websites that the patient should be made aware of for resources after discharge.

Readability

Studies have indicated that learning is more effective if oral presentations and/or demonstrations are supplemented with reading materials, such as handouts. **Readability** (the grade level of the material) is a concern because many patients and families may have limited English skills or low literacy, and it can be difficult for the nurse to assess people's reading level. The average American reads effectively at the 6th to 8th grade level (regardless of education achieved), but many health education materials have a much higher readability level. Additionally, research indicates that even people with much higher reading skills learn medical and health information most effectively when the material is presented at the 6th to 8th grade readability level. Therefore, patient education materials (and consent forms) should not be written at higher than 6th to 8th grade level. Readability index calculators are available on the internet to give an approximation of grade level and difficulty for those preparing materials without expertise in teaching reading.

Videos

Videos are a useful adjunct to teaching as they reduce the time needed for one-on-one instruction (increasing cost-effectiveness). Passive presentation of videos, such as in the waiting area, has little value, but focused viewing in which the nurse discusses the purpose of the video presentation prior to viewing and then is available for discussion after viewing can be very effective. Patients and/or families are often nervous about learning patient care and are unsure of their abilities, so they may not focus completely when the nurse is presenting information. Allowing the patients/families to watch a video demonstration or explanation first and allowing them to stop or review the video presentation can help them to grasp the fundamentals before they have to apply them, relieving some of the anxiety they may be experiencing. Videos are much more effective than written materials for those with low literacy or poor English skills. The nurse should always be available to answer questions and discuss the material after the patients/families finish viewing.

Learning Contract

In order to be compliant with a therapeutic regimen, the patient needs information about the disease, the purpose of medications and treatments, and side effects and complications to watch for. A written **learning contract** organizes this information into specific learning goals, demonstrates the importance of the information, and ensures that all pertinent information is taught. Others on the healthcare team can note patient progress and easily determine what to teach next. The patient has a written plan to follow as well.

The learning contract should take into consideration the patient's age, sex, cultural and religious values, and educational level achieved. One must consider the patient's financial status, socio-economic status, living situation, and support network. The complex nature of a therapeutic regimen combined with distracters such as side effects, pain, denial, and fear can weaken the patient's resolve to maintain compliance. One must evaluate the patient's attitudes towards healthcare, coping mechanisms, and motivation and provide reinforcement as needed.

Readiness to Learn

The patient/family's **readiness to learn** should be assessed because if they are not ready, instruction is of little value. Often readiness is indicated when the patient/family asks questions or shows and interest in procedures. There are a number of factors related to readiness to learn:

- **Physical factors:** There are a number of physical factors than can affect ability. Manual dexterity may be required to complete a task, and this varies by age and condition. Hearing or vision deficits may impact a person's ability to learn. Complex tasks may be too difficult for some because of weakness or cognitive impairment, and modifications of the environment may be needed. Health status, age, and gender may all impact the ability to learn.
- **Experience:** People's experience with learning can vary widely and is affected by their ability to cope with changes, their personal goals, motivation to learn, and cultural background. People may have widely divergent ideas about what constitutes illness and/or treatment. Lack of English skills may make learning difficult and prevent people from asking questions.
- **Mental/emotional status:** The external support system and internal motivation may impact readiness. Anxiety, fear, or depression about one's condition can make learning very difficult because the patient/family cannot focus on learning, so the nurse must spend time to reassure the patient/family and wait until they are emotionally more receptive.

- **Knowledge/education:** The knowledge base of the patient/family, their cognitive ability, and their learning styles all affect their readiness to learn. The nurse should always begin by assessing what knowledge the patient/family already has about their disease, condition, or treatment and then build form that base. People with little medical experience may lack knowledge of basic medical terminology, interfering with their ability and readiness to learn.

Educational Goals, Objectives, and Plans

Once a topic for performance improvement education has been chosen, then **goals**, **measurable objectives with strategies**, and **lesson plans** must be developed. A class should stay focused on one topic rather than trying to cover many. For example:

Goal: Increase compliance with hand hygiene standards in ICU.

Objectives:

- Develop series of posters and fliers by June 1.
- Observe 100% compliance with hand hygiene standards at 2 weeks, 1-month, and 2-month intervals after training is completed.

Strategies: Conduct 4 classes at different times over a one-week period, May 25-31.

- Place posters in all nursing units, staff rooms, and utility rooms by January 3.
- Develop a slide show presentation for class and provide online access to the presentation for all staff by May 25.
- Utilize handwashing kits.

Lesson plans: Discussion period: Why do we need 100% compliance?

- Slide show: The case for hand hygiene.
- Discussion: What did you learn?
- Demonstration and activities to show effectiveness.
- Handwashing technique.

Learner Outcomes

When the quality professional plans an educational offering, whether it be a class, an online module, a workshop, or educational materials, the professional should identify **learner outcomes,** which should be conveyed to the learners from the very beginning so that they are aware of the expectations. The subject matter of the educational material and the learner outcomes should be directly related. For example, if the quality professional is giving a class on decontamination of the environment, then a learner outcome might be: "Identify the difference between disinfectants and antiseptics." There may be one or multiple learner outcomes, but part of the assessment at the end of the learning experience should be to determine if, in fact, the learner outcomes have been achieved. A survey of whether or not the learners felt that they had achieved the learner outcomes can give valuable feedback and guidance to the quality professional.

Implementation and Evaluation of Teaching Plan

Implementation and evaluation of the teaching plan includes:

- Follow teaching plan but be flexible and alter plan to suit the patient's learning needs.
- Work with a healthcare team to follow the teaching plan and ensure consistency in teaching methods as well as coordinate efforts and take responsibility for altering the plan and evaluating learning to meet goals.
- Monitor patient's motivational level, encourage with positive feedback as needed, and record patient responses to teaching and changes in behaviors as a result of all teaching sessions.
- Use tools, such as checklists, rating scales, observed behavior, written tests, and the nature of the questions from the patient when evaluating the effectiveness of the teaching plan in reaching the patient's goals for learning.
- Evaluate the plan after each session and at the end.

Communicate information taught and patient learning to any home health or community nurses involved. They can then continue the patient's teaching by evaluating behavior in the home and continuing to address learning needs as they arise.

Evaluating Effectiveness of Education

Education, like all interventions, must be evaluated for **effectiveness**. Two determinants of effectiveness include:

- **Behavior modification** involves thorough observation and measurement, identifying behavior that needs to be changed and then planning and instituting interventions to modify that behavior. The nurse can use a variety of techniques, including demonstrations of appropriate behavior, reinforcement, and monitoring until new behavior is adopted consistently. This is especially important when longstanding procedures and habits of behavior are changed.
- **Compliance rates** are often determined by observation, which should be done at intervals and on multiple occasions, but with patients, this may depend on self-reports. Outcomes is another measure of compliance; that is, if education is intended to improve patient health and reduce risk factors and that occurs, it is a good indication that there is compliance. Compliance rates are calculated by determining the number of events/procedures and degree of compliance.

Teaching Elderly Patients

The **elderly patient's** level of functioning must be assessed before **teaching**. Cognitive abilities and mental functioning may be affected by illness and aging:

- Short-term memory loss can affect the amount of material retained.
- Concentration may be decreased.
- Reaction time is delayed.
- Color discrimination, general vision, and hearing may be decreased.

The nurse should **pace** the teaching accordingly and **tailor** materials for any deficits. Family should be present for teaching if possible, to help the patient to remember key points after discharge. Large print on non-glare paper that is easy to read should be used. The nurse should use color-coding cues only if colors are easily perceived. The learning environment must be quiet and comfortable with no distractions or interruptions.

- Repeat information numerous times and allow the patient as much practice time as needed.
- Use audio-visual aids to reinforce information given verbally.
- Face the patient when speaking and encourage him/her to use hearing devices if used.
- Make sure the lighting in the room is adequate.

Teaching Patients with Learning Disabilities

Determine the type of **learning disability** in order to design teaching:

- When a patient has a **visual problem**, the nurse should use **verbal teaching**, repeated several times as needed and record the session for the patient to hear later if possible or use prepared audiotapes or CDs containing the information. The patient should verbalize learning to show attainment of the learning goal.
- When **auditory perception** is a problem, learning materials should be **visual** with as few words as possible. Demonstration, role-playing, and practicing the procedure will be useful to the patient. Printed materials should employ pictures, and computer use can be useful.
- If the patient has an **expressive problem**, he/she needs time to process the input and to ask questions. **Hand gestures, demonstrations, and the senses** should be utilized for teaching when appropriate.

A developmental disability will require information presented in a format that is appropriate for the person's developmental level. The nurse should keep explanations simple, and use gestures, demonstrations, activities, and repetition to teach.

Teaching to Disabled Patients and Families

The **teaching of disabled patients** and their families begins with an assessment of the family's willingness and preparation for the heavy duty of care that will be required. The nurse must teach information about diseases or disabilities as well as medications, procedures, diet, and physical therapies. The patients must be taught to perform ADLs as well as possible and caregivers taught how to assist when needed:

- Give patients enough information to understand and manage the disabilities and to empower them with a sense of control and coping.
- Don't overwhelm them with information.
- Plan the teaching to provide information according to learning readiness and priorities but be flexible and change the plan if needed.
- Utilize checklists of skills to help keep track of all that has been learned.
- Give praise, continued feedback, support, and empathy with every teaching session.
- Provide resources that patients and family can use after discharge and refer to home health for continuing support and teaching.

Importance of Patient's Culture in Design of Teaching Plan

The nurse must always assess the individual's **cultural beliefs and values** and not assume that they are the same as the culture on a whole. These beliefs determine what information the patient feels that they can pursue. Teaching that conflicts with these beliefs will be rejected. The patient's perception of health and the healthcare system must be determined because a lack of confidence in the teacher can impair motivation to learn. The nurse must **assess the patient's beliefs** about the following to develop a personalized teaching plan:

- Body image, self-esteem
- Abilities and level of knowledge
- Principles of living
- Diet, activity, health practices
- Involvement of family and support persons
- Physical and mental health and disease
- Causes of disease
- Aging
- Gender issues
- Spirituality, customs, rituals, religious precepts

Relationship Development

Ethical Principles

Autonomy is the ethical principle that the individual has the right to make decisions about his or her own care. In the case of children or patients with dementia who cannot make autonomous decisions, parents or family members may serve as the legal decision maker. The nurse must keep the patient and/or family fully informed so that they can exercise their autonomy in informed decision-making.

Justice is the ethical principle that relates to the distribution of the limited resources of healthcare benefits to the members of society. These resources must be distributed fairly. This issue may arise if there is only one bed left and two sick patients. Justice comes into play in deciding which patient should stay and which should be transported or otherwise cared for. The decision should be made according to what is best or most just for the patients and not colored by personal bias.

Beneficence is an ethical principle that involves performing actions that are for the purpose of benefitting another person. In the care of a patient, any procedure or treatment should be done with the ultimate goal of benefitting the patient, and any actions that are not beneficial should be reconsidered. As conditions change, procedures need to be continually reevaluated to determine if they are still of benefit.

Nonmaleficence is an ethical principle that means healthcare workers should provide care in a manner that does not cause direct intentional harm to the patient:

- The actual act must be good or morally neutral.
- The intent must be only for a good effect.
- A bad effect cannot serve as the means to get to a good effect.
- A good effect must have more benefit than a bad effect has harm.

Nursing Code of Ethics

There is more interest in the **ethics** involved in healthcare due to technological advances that have made the prolongation of life, organ transplants, prenatal manipulation, and saving of premature infants possible, sometimes with poor outcomes. Couple these with healthcare's limited resources, and **ethical dilemmas** abound. Ethics is the study of **morality** as the value that controls actions. The American Nurses Association Code of Ethics contains nine statements defining **principles** the nurse can use when faced with moral and ethical problems. Nurses must be knowledgeable about the many ethical issues in healthcare and about the field of ethics in general. The nurse must help a patient to reveal their values and morals to the health care team so that the patient, family, and team can resolve moral issues pertaining to the patient's care. As part of the healthcare team, the nurse has a right to express personal values and moral concerns about medical issues.

Patient Rights and Responsibilities

Empowering patients and families to act as their own advocates requires they have a clear understanding of their **rights and responsibilities.** These should be given (in print form) and/or presented (audio/video) to patients and families on admission or as soon as possible:

- **Rights** should include competent, non-discriminatory medical care that respects privacy and allows participation in decisions about care and the right to refuse care. They should have clear understandable explanations of treatments, options, and conditions, including outcomes. They should be apprised of transfers, changes in care plan, and advance directives. They should have access to medical records information about charges.
- **Responsibilities** should include providing honest and thorough information about health issues and medical history. They should ask for clarification if they don't understand information that is provided to them, and they should follow the plan of care that is outlined or explain why that is not possible. They should treat staff and other patients with respect.

Informed Consent

Patients or guardians must provide **informed consent** for all treatment the patient receives. This includes a thorough explanation of all procedures and treatment and associated risks. Patients/guardians should be apprised of all options and allowed input on the type of treatments. Patients/guardians should be apprised of all reasonable risks and any complications that might be life threatening or increase morbidity. The American Medical Association has established guidelines for informed consent:

- Explanation of diagnosis.
- Nature and reason for treatment or procedure.
- Risks and benefits.
- Alternative options (regardless of cost or insurance coverage).
- Risks and benefits of alternative options.
- Risks and benefits of not having a treatment or procedure.
- Providing informed consent is a requirement of all states.

Note: A patient may waive their right to informed consent; if this is the case, the nurse should document the patient's refusal and proceed with the procedure. Also, informed consent is not necessary for procedures performed to save a life/limb in which the patient/family is unable to consent.

Confidentiality

Confidentiality is the obligation that is present in a professional-patient relationship. Nurses are under an obligation to protect the information they possess concerning the patient and family. Care should be taken to safeguard that information and provide the privacy that the family deserves. This is accomplished through the use of required passwords when family call for information about the patient and through the limitation of who is allowed to visit. There may be times when confidentiality must be broken to save the life of a patient, but those circumstances are rare. The nurse must make all efforts to safeguard patient records and identification. Computerized record keeping should be done in such a way that the screen is not visible to others, and paper records must be secured.

THERAPEUTIC COMMUNICATION

FACILITATING COMMUNICATION

Therapeutic communication begins with respect for the patient/family and the assumption that all communication, verbal and nonverbal, has meaning. Listening must be done empathetically. The following are some techniques that facilitate communication.

Introduction:

- Make a personal introduction and use the patient's name: "Mrs. Brown, I am Susan Williams, your nurse."

Encouragement:

- Use an open-ended opening statement: "Is there anything you'd like to discuss?"
- Acknowledge comments: "Yes," and "I understand."
- Allow silence and observe nonverbal behavior rather than trying to force conversation. Ask for clarification if statements are unclear.
- Reflect statements back (use sparingly): Patient: "I hate this hospital." Nurse: "You hate this hospital?"

Empathy:

- Make observations: "You are shaking," and "You seem worried."
- Recognize feelings:
    - Patient: "I want to go home."
    - Nurse: "It must be hard to be away from your home and family."
- Provide information as honestly and completely as possible about condition, treatment, and procedures and respond to the patient's questions and concerns.

Exploration:

- Verbally express implied messages:
    - Patient: "This treatment is too much trouble."
    - Nurse: "You think the treatment isn't helping you?"
- Explore a topic but allow the patient to terminate the discussion without further probing: "I'd like to hear how you feel about that."

Orientation:

- Indicate reality:
    - Patient: "Someone is screaming."
    - Nurse: "That sound was an ambulance siren."
- Comment on distortions without directly agreeing or disagreeing:
    - Patient: "That nurse promised I didn't have to walk again."
    - Nurse: "Really? That's surprising because the doctor ordered physical therapy twice a day."

Collaboration:

- Work together to achieve better results: "Maybe if we talk about this, we can figure out a way to make the treatment easier for you."

Validation:

- Seek validation: "Do you feel better now?" or "Did the medication help you breathe better?"

Avoiding Non-therapeutic Communication

While using therapeutic communication is important, it is equally important to avoid interjecting **non-therapeutic communication**, which can block effective communication. *Avoid the following:*

- Meaningless clichés: "Don't worry. Everything will be fine." "Isn't it a nice day?"
- Providing advice: "You should..." or "The best thing to do is...." It's better when patients ask for advice to provide facts and encourage the patient to reach a decision.
- Inappropriate approval that prevents the patient from expressing true feeling or concerns:
    - Patient: "I shouldn't cry about this."
    - Nurse: "That's right! You're an adult!"
- Asking for explanations of behavior that is not directly related to patient care and requires analysis and explanation of feelings: "Why are you upset?"
- Agreeing with rather than accepting and responding to patient's statements can make it difficult for the patient to change his or her statement or opinion later: "I agree with you," or "You are right."
- Making negative judgments: "You should stop arguing with the nurses."
- Devaluing the patient's feelings: "Everyone gets upset at times."
- Disagreeing directly: "That can't be true," or "I think you are wrong."
- Defending against criticism: "The doctor is not being rude; he's just very busy today."
- Changing the subject to avoid dealing with uncomfortable topics;
    - Patient: "I'm never going to get well."
    - Nurse: "Your family will be here in just a few minutes."
- Making inappropriate literal responses, even as a joke, especially if the patient is at all confused or having difficulty expressing ideas:
    - Patient: "There are bugs crawling under my skin."
    - Nurse: "I'll get some bug spray,"
- Challenging the patient to establish reality often just increases confusion and frustration:
    - "If you were dying, you wouldn't be able to yell and kick!"

Communicating with Patients with Disabilities

Guidelines for communicating with individuals with disabilities:

- Do not assume that the person with disabilities also has impaired cognition.
- Always treat the person with respect and dignity.
- Use first names with the patient if asked to do so, but start out formally as with any patient.
- Offer to shake hands even when a prosthesis is present.
- Be patient if communication is impaired.
- Offer assistance, but allow the patient to tell you what is helpful; otherwise don't assist.

- When a wheelchair is used, sit down so the patient does not have to strain their neck to speak with you.
- If providing directions, consider the obstacles that may be in the way and assist the person to find an appropriate way around them.

Communication with Patients with Cognitive Disabilities

The person with **cognitive disabilities** may be easily distracted, so **verbal communication** should be attempted in a quiet area:

- Address people with dignity and respect.
- Do not try to discuss abstract ideas but stick with concrete topics.
- Keep words and sentences very simple and try rephrasing when necessary. People may have difficulty in distinguishing your spoken words and deriving the meaning from them.
- Be very patient with people's attempts to speak to you since they may have difficulty in processing thoughts and changing them into spoken words.
- Use objects around you and gestures to illustrate your words since the patient may also use pointing and gesturing when unable to find the words to communicate with you. The person may prefer written communication, although some may be unable to read.
- Use touch to convey your regard during communication, as this is recognized by the patient as reassurance of your care and concern for them.
- Give a few instructions at a time as to not overwhelm them.

Communicating with Deaf or Hearing-Impaired Patients

Communicating with a person with **deafness** or **hearing impairment**:

- Try to communicate in a quiet environment if possible.
- Wave or touch the person to let him or her know you are trying to communicate.
- Determine the method the person uses to communicate: sign language, lip reading, hearing devices, or writing.
- Fingerspell or use some signs if able to do so.
- Address the person directly when you speak even though the person may be looking at an interpreter or your lips.
- Look at the person as the interpreter tells you what was said.
- Speak slowly so the interpreter can keep up with you.
- If the person reads lips, face the person and speak clearly and normally, using normal volume.
- If writing a communication, do not speak while writing.
- Do not be afraid to check that the person understands you, and ask questions if you do not understand the person.

Communication with People with Low Vision or Blindness

Communicating with a person with **low vision or blindness**:

- Greet the person with low vision or blindness, identifying yourself and others present.
- Always say goodbye when you are leaving.
- Alert the person to written communications, such as warning signs or printed notices.
- Face the person and touch briefly on the arm to let the person know you are speaking to him or her if you are in a group.
- Speak at normal loudness.

- Make any directions given specific in terms of the length of walk and obstacles, such as stairs.
- Use the position of hands on a clock face to give directions (potatoes at 3 o'clock) as well as using *right* or *left*.
- Mention sounds that the person may hear in transit or on arrival at a destination.
- Do not be afraid to use the word *see*, as the person will probably use it as well.

Communicating with a Patient on a Ventilator

When a patient **on a ventilator** is conscious, he or she may still be able to **communicate** by blinking, nodding, shaking the head, or pointing to a picture or word board:

- If the person is able to write, try to reposition the IV line to leave the dominant hand free to communicate.
- Discuss the need for communication with the physician and ask if a valve or an electric larynx can be used to permit speech.
- Help the patient practice lip reading of single words.
- Remember the patient's glasses or hearing aids when attempting to communicate.
- Enlist the aid of a speech therapist if there is frustration on the part of the patient and family due to communication difficulty.

Communicating with Persons with Speech Problems Due to a Stroke

Methods to communicate with stroke patients with speech problems:

- **Dysarthria**: Patients have problems forming the words to speak them aloud. Give them time to communicate, offer them a picture board or other means of communicating, and give encouragement to family members who are frustrated with the difficulty of trying to communicate.
- **Expressive aphasia**: The patients' efforts at speech come out garbled when they try to say sentences, but single words may be clear. Encourage the patients to try to write and to practice the sounds of the alphabet. Resist the urge to finish sentences for the patients.
- **Receptive aphasia**: The patients have a problem comprehending the speech they hear. Communicate in simple terms and speak slowly. Test comprehension of the written word as an alternative method of communication.
- **Global aphasia**: The patient has both receptive and expressive aphasia. Use simple, clear, slow speech augmented by pictures and gestures.

Communication Problems of Patients with Parkinson's Disease

Parkinson's disease causes problems with speaking in the majority (75-90%) of patients. The reason for this is not clear but may relate to increasing rigidity and changes in movement. Speech is often very low-pitched or hoarse, given in a monotone and with a soft voice. Speech production may decrease because of the effort required to speak. **Speech therapy** can develop exercises for the patient that can assist them in remembering to speak slowly and carefully, as patients are not always aware that their **communication** is impaired:

- Allow time for the patient to communicate, asking for repetition if you do not understand the message.
- Help family by teaching ways to facilitate communication with the patient and encouraging them to assist the patient to do the exercises provided by the therapist.
- If speech volume is very low, suggest amplification devices that can be obtained through speech therapy.

Communication with Patients with Psychiatric Problems

Persons with **psychiatric disorders** appreciate being addressed with respect, dignity, and honesty:

- Speak simply and clearly, repeating as necessary.
- Encourage patients to discuss their concerns regarding treatment and medications to improve compliance.
- Use good eye contact and be attentive to your body language messages.
- Be alert, but unless the person is known to be violent, try to relax and listen to them.
- Don't try to avoid words or phrases pertaining to psychiatric problems, but if you do say something inappropriate, apologize honestly to the patient.
- Offer patients outlets for their thoughts and feelings.
- Learn more about their disorder and ways to use therapeutic communication to help them with their problem, such as re-orienting them as needed.

Cultural Competence

Different cultures view health and illness from very different perspectives, and patients often come from a mix of many cultures, so the nurse must be not only accepting of cultural differences but must be sensitive and aware. There are a number of characteristics that are important for a nurse to have **cultural competence**:

- **Appreciating diversity**: This must be grounded in information about other cultures and understanding of their value systems.
- **Assessing own cultural perspectives**: Self-awareness is essential to understanding potential biases.
- **Understanding intercultural dynamics**: This must include understanding ways in which cultures cooperate, differ, communicate, and reach understanding.
- **Recognizing institutional culture**: Each institutional unit (hospital, clinic, office) has an inherent set of values that may be unwritten but is accepted by the staff.
- **Adapting patient service to diversity**: This is the culmination of cultural competence as it is the point of contact between cultures.

Religious Objections to Treatment

Jehovah's Witnesses

Jehovah's Witnesses have traditionally shunned transfusions and blood products as part of their religious beliefs. In 2004, the *Watchtower,* a Jehovah's Witness publication, presented a guide for members. When medical care indicates the need for blood transfusion or blood products and the patient and/or family members are practicing Jehovah's Witnesses, this may present a conflict. It's important to approach the patient/family with full information and reasons for the transfusion or blood components without being judgmental, allowing them to express their feelings. In fact, studies show that while adults often refuse transfusions for themselves, they frequently allow their children to receive blood products, so one should never assume that an individual would refuse blood products based on the religion alone. Jehovah's Witnesses can receive fractionated blood cells, thus allowing hemoglobin-based blood substitutes. The following guidelines are provided to church members:

Basic blood standards for Jehovah's Witnesses:

- **Not acceptable**: Whole blood: red cells, white cells, platelets, plasma.
- **Acceptable**: Fractions from red cells, white cells, platelets, and plasma.

Christian Scientists

Christian Science, a religion developed by Mary Baker Eddy in 1879, promotes the belief that sickness is most effectively treated through prayer alone. While Christian Scientists do not avoid all medical interventions, their beliefs are conservative regarding medical treatment. Most notably, Christian Scientists, for the most part, do not believe in vaccinations and may only agree to such if required by law, as they do acknowledge the importance of community health. They have widely appreciated the use of exemptions from mandatory vaccines, but as these exemptions have become more limited, religious leaders have given their members the right to decide upon vaccinations.

Cultural Characteristics

Hispanic Patients

Many areas of the country have large populations of Hispanics and Hispanic Americans. As always, it's important to recognize that cultural generalizations don't always apply to individuals. Recent immigrants, especially, have cultural needs that the nurse must understand:

- Many Hispanics are Catholic and may like the nurse to make arrangements for a priest to visit.
- Large extended families may come to visit to support the patient and family, so patients should receive clear explanations about how many visitors are allowed, but some flexibility may be required.
- Language barriers may exist as some may have limited or no English skills, so translation services should be available around the clock.
- Hispanic culture encourages outward expressions of emotions, so family may react strongly to news about a patient's condition, and people who are ill may expect some degree of pampering, so extra attention to the patient/family members may alleviate some of their anxiety.

Caring for Hispanic and Hispanic American patients requires understanding of cultural differences:

- Some immigrant Hispanics have very little formal education, so medical information may seem very complex and confusing, and they may not understand the implications or need for follow-up care.
- Hispanic culture perceives time with more flexibility than American culture, so if parents need to be present at a particular time, the nurse should specify the exact time (1:30 PM) and explain the reason rather than saying something more vague, such as "after lunch."
- People may appear to be unassertive or unable to make decisions when they are simply showing respect to the nurse by being deferent.
- In traditional families, the males make decisions, so a woman waits for the father or other males in the family to make decisions about treatment or care.
- Families may choose to use folk medicines instead of Western medical care or may combine the two.
- Children and young women are often sheltered and are taught to be respectful to adults, so they may not express their needs openly.

Middle Eastern Patients

There are considerable cultural differences among Middle Easterners, but religious beliefs about the segregation of males and females are common. It's important to remember that segregating the female is meant to protect her virtue. Female nurses have low status in many countries because they violate this segregation by touching male bodies, so parents may not trust or show respect for the nurse who is caring for their family member. Additionally, male patients may not want to be cared for by female nurses or doctors, and families may be very upset at a female being cared for by a male nurse or physician. When possible, these cultural traditions should be accommodated:

- In Middle Eastern countries, males make decisions, so issues for discussion or decision should be directed to males, such as the father or spouse, and males may be direct in stating what they want, sometimes appearing demanding.
- If a male nurse must care for a female patient, then the family should be advised that *personal care* (such as bathing) will be done by a female while the medical treatments will be done by the male nurse.

Caring for Middle Eastern patients requires understanding of cultural differences:

- Families may practice strict dietary restrictions, such as avoiding pork and requiring that animals be killed in a ritual manner, so vegetarian or kosher meals may be required.
- People may have language difficulties requiring a translator, and same-sex translators should be used if at all possible.
- Families may be accompanied by large extended families that want to be kept informed and whom patients consult before decisions are made.
- Most medical care is provided by female relatives, so educating the family about patient care should be directed at females (with female translators if necessary).
- Outward expressions of grief are considered as showing respect for the dead.
- Middle Eastern families often offer gifts to caregivers. Small gifts (candy) that can be shared should be accepted graciously, but for other gifts, the families should be advised graciously that accepting gifts is against hospital policy.
- Middle Easterners often require less personal space and may stand very close.

Asian Patients

There are considerable differences among different Asian populations, so cultural generalizations may not apply to all, but nurses caring for Asian patients should be aware of common cultural attitudes and behaviors:

- Nurses and doctors are viewed with respect, so traditional Asian families may expect the nurse to remain authoritative and to give directions and may not question, so the nurse should ensure that they understand by having them review material or give demonstrations and should provide explanations clearly, anticipating questions that the family might have but may not articulate.
- Disagreeing is considered impolite. "Yes" may only mean that the person is heard, not that they agree with the person. When asked if they understand, they may indicate that they do even when they clearly do not so as not to offend the nurse.
- Asians may avoid eye contact as an indication of respect. This is especially true of children in relation to adults and of younger adults in relation to elders.

Caring for Asian patients requires understanding of cultural differences:

- Patients/families may not show outward expressions of feelings/grief, sometimes appearing passive. They also avoid public displays of affection. This does not mean that they don't feel, just that they don't show their feelings.
- Families often hide illness and disabilities from others and may feel ashamed about illness.
- Terminal illness is often hidden from the patient, so families may not want patients to know they are dying or seriously ill.
- Families may use cupping, pinching, or applying pressure to injured areas, and this can leave bruises that may appear as abuse, so when bruises are found, the family should be questioned about alternative therapy before assumptions are made.
- Patients may be treated with traditional herbs.
- Families may need translators because of poor or no English skills.
- In traditional Asian families, males are authoritative and make the decisions.

Impact of Culture and Religion on Dietary Preferences

When performing a dietary assessment, the nurse should remember that culture and religion might dictate which foods and spices are used. The manner in which food is prepared, cooked, and served may also be specified. The utensils used at the meal as well as the persons who may eat together may be important. Mealtimes and required fasts should be determined. Holidays may be accompanied by particular foods. Alcohol (including extracts made with alcohol) and caffeine may be prohibited. The culture may also consider obesity a sign of affluence and success. The nurse should evaluate the foods that are eaten in light of the patient's medical condition. The patient may not wish to eat the usual hospital fare and may need to have a special diet prepared or food brought from home. The nurse can guide the patient and family to foods that are acceptable and within the patient's requirements for health.

Grief

Grief is an emotional response to a **loss** that begins at the time a loss is anticipated and continues on an individual timetable. While there are identifiable stages or tasks, it is not an orderly and predictable process. It involves overcoming anger, disbelief, guilt, and a myriad of related emotions. The grieving individual may move back and forth between stages or experience several emotions at any given time. Each person's grief response is unique to their own coping patterns, stress levels, age, gender, belief system, and previous experiences with loss.

Kubler-Ross's Five Stages of Grief

Kubler-Ross taught the medical and nursing community that the dying patient and family welcomes open, honest discussion of the dying process and felt that there were certain **stages** that patients and family go through. The stages may not occur in order, but may vary or some may be skipped. Stages include:

- **Denial**: The person denies the diagnosis and tries to pretend it isn't true. During this time, the person may seek a second opinion or alternative therapies. They may use denial until they are better able to emotionally cope with the reality of the disease or changes that need to be made. Patients may also wish to save family and friends from pain and worry. Both patients and family may use denial as a coping mechanism when they feel overwhelmed by the reality of the disease and threatened losses.
- **Anger**: The person is angry about the situation and may focus that rage on anyone.
- **Bargaining**: The person attempts to make deals with a higher power to secure a better outcome to their situation.
- **Depression**: The person anticipates the loss and the changes it will bring with a sense of sadness and grief.
- **Acceptance**: The person accepts the impending death and is ready to face it as it approaches. The patient may begin to withdraw from interests and family.

Review Video: Patient Treatment and Grief
Visit mometrix.com/academy and enter code: 648794

Anticipatory Grief

Anticipatory grief is the mental, social, and somatic reactions of an individual as they prepare themselves for a **perceived future loss**. The individual experiences a process of intellectual, emotional, and behavioral responses in order to modify their self-concept, based on their perception of what the potential loss will mean in their life. This process often takes place ahead of the actual loss, from the time the loss is first perceived until it is resolved as a reality for the individual. This process can also blend with past loss experiences. It is associated with the individual's perception of how life will be affected by the particular diagnosis as well as the impending death. Acknowledging this anticipatory grief allows family members to begin looking toward a changed future. Suppressing this anticipatory process may inhibit relationships with the ill individual and contribute to a more difficult grieving process at a later time. However, appropriate anticipatory grieving does not take the place of grief during the actual time of death.

Disenfranchised Grief

Disenfranchised grief occurs when the loss being experienced cannot be openly acknowledged, publicly mourned, or socially supported. Society and culture are partly responsible for an individual's response to a loss. There is a **social context** to grief; if a person incurring the loss will be putting himself or herself at risk if grief is expressed, disenfranchised grief occurs. The risk for disenfranchised grief is greatest among those whose relationship with the individual they lost was not known or regarded as significant. This is also the situation found among bereaved persons who are not recognized by society as capable of grief, such as young children, or needing to mourn, such as an ex-spouse or secret lover.

Grief vs. Depression

Normal **grief** is preoccupied with self-limiting to the loss itself. Emotional responses will vary and may include open expressions of anger. The individual may experience difficulty sleeping or vivid dreams, a lack of energy, and weight loss. Crying is evident and provides some relief of extreme emotions. The individual remains socially responsive and seeks reassurance from others.

Depression is marked by extensive periods of sadness and preoccupation often extending beyond 2 months. It is not limited to the single event. There is an absence of pleasure or anger and isolation from previous social support systems. The individual can experience extreme lethargy, weight loss, insomnia, or hypersomnia, and has no recollection of dreaming. Crying is absent or persistent and provides no relief of emotions. Professional intervention is required to relieve depression.

Loss

Loss is the blanket term used to denote the absence of a valued object, position, ability, attribute, or individual. The aspect of loss as it is associated with the death of an animal or person is a relatively new definition. Loss is an individualized and subjective experience depending on the **perceived attachment** between the individual and the missing aspect. This can range from little or no value of attachment to significant value. Loss also can be represented by the **withdrawal of a valued relationship** one had or would have had in the future. Depending on the unique and individual responses to the perception of loss and its significance, reactions to the loss will vary. Robinson and McKenna summarize the aspects of loss in three main attributes:

- Something has been removed.
- The item removed had value to that person.
- The response is individualized.

Mourning

Mourning is a public grief response for the death of a loved one. The various aspects of the mourning process are partially determined by **personal and cultural belief systems**. Kagawa-Singer defines mourning as "the social customs and cultural practices that follow a death." Durkheim expands this to include the following: "mourning is not a natural movement of private feelings wounded by a cruel loss; it is a duty imposed by the group." Mourning involves participation in religious and culturally appropriate customs and rituals designed to publicly acknowledge the loss. These rituals signify they are adjusting to the change in their relationships created by the loss, as well as mark the beginning of the reorganization and forward movement of their lives.

Bereavement

Bereavement is the emotional and mental state associated with having suffered a **personal loss**. It is the reactions of grief and sadness initiated by the loss of a loved one. Bereavement is a normal process of feeling deprived of something of value. The word bereave comes from the root "reave" meaning to plunder, spoil, or rob. It is recognized that the lost individual had value and a defining role in the surviving individual's life. Bereavement encompasses all the acts and emotions surrounding the feeling of loss for the individual. During this grieving period, there is an increased mortality risk. A **positive bereavement experience** means being able to recognize the significance of the loss while still recognizing the resilience and value of life.

Risk Factors Complicating Bereavement

The caregiver should assess for multiple **life crises** that take energy away from the grieving process. An important factor is the grieving individual's history with past grieving experiences. Assess for other recent, unresolved, or difficult losses that may need to be addressed before the individual can move toward resolution of the current loss. Age, mental health, substance abuse, extreme anger, anxiety, or dependence on the individual facing the end of life can add additional stressors and handicap natural coping mechanisms. Income strains, community support, outside and personal responsibilities, the absence of cultural and religious beliefs, the difficulty of the disease process, and age of the loved one lost can also present additional risk factors.

Nursing Interventions for Patients and Family Experiencing Loss and Grief

Loss is painful and frightening. Loss can occur through death or loss of health, self-esteem, or relationships. Loss can also occur from threats, such as fire, flood, theft, or severe weather. The severity of the loss, preparation for it, and the maturity, stability, and coping mechanisms of the person all affect the grieving process. Multiple losses and substance abuse can complicate grief and recovery. Previous life experience and cultural and religious beliefs can help in resolution of grief. Many emotions are triggered, and if the loss is not acknowledged, the person may become depressed or develop health problems. Nursing **interventions** for those experiencing **loss and grief** include:

- Teach patients to recognize symptoms, such as SOB, empty feelings in the chest or abdomen, deep sighing, lethargy, and weakness as signs of grief.
- Assist the patient and family to heal themselves by accepting the loss, recognizing the pain from it, making changes to adapt to and assimilate the loss, and moving toward new relationships and activity.
- Refer to groups or counseling for more intense support if needed.

Supporting Families and Patients as They Receive Bad News

It is best if the patient and family can **receive bad news** while being **supported** by a team that includes physicians, nurses, and social workers or clergy of their choice. However, the patient may not want family members or others to be present, and this should be respected.

- Provide privacy and ensure that there will be no interruptions.
- Provide seating for all participants.
- Do not provide too much information at once, as the opening statement may be all that the patient can comprehend at one time.
- Allow time for reactions before providing more information.
- Wait for the patient to signal the need for more information and then provide an honest answer in layman's terms. Information may not be absorbed and may need to be repeated as the patient and family are ready for it later after the initial conference.
- Use techniques of therapeutic communication. People may need others to sit and listen and provide comforting empathy many times before having a conversation about problem solving.

Spirituality

Spirituality provides a connection of the self to a higher power and a way of finding meaning in life experiences. It provides guidance for behavior and can help to clarify one's purpose in life. It can offer hope to those who are ill or facing loss and grief and can give comfort, support, and guidance. Spirituality is not always connected to a religion and is highly individualized. A person may lose faith and confidence in his/her spiritual beliefs during trying times:

- Ask patients about their spiritual beliefs.
- Listen attentively and do not offer opinions about their beliefs or share your own unless invited.
- Show respect for their views and offer to obtain spiritual support by calling a spiritual leader or setting up a spiritual ritual that has meaning for them.

This support can help them to regain their beliefs and endure illness by helping them to rise above their suffering and find meaning in this experience.

Palliative and Hospice Care

Palliative care attempts to make the rest of the patient's life as comfortable as possible by treating distressing symptoms to keep them controlled. It does not attempt to cure but only to control discomfort caused by the disease. Palliative care does not require terminal illness/prognosis and can be implemented for any patient with chronic disease and suffering.

Hospice care uses palliative care as it supports the patient and family through the dying process. Hospice teams support the daily needs of the patient and family and provide needed equipment, medical expertise, and medications to control symptoms. They offer spiritual, psychological, and social support to the patient and family as needed and desired. Assistance with end-of-life planning is given to help the patient and family accomplish goals important to them. Bereavement support is also given. The team consists of the attending physician, hospice physician advisor, nurses, social worker, clergy, hospice aides, and volunteers. Hospice care is given in the home when the patient has family who are willing to assume care with the assistance of the hospice team. Hospice care also occurs in hospice facilities, hospitals, and extended care facilities. To qualify for Hospice care, the patient must be deemed terminal and given a 6-month or less life expectancy by two separate physicians. Should the patient survive 6 months in hospice, they can be extended for two 90-day periods, and then an unlimited number of 60-day periods per physician order.

NP Acute Care Practice Test #1

1. Which of the following techniques should be used when interviewing an elderly woman?

a. Speak quickly to get through a focused assessment before the woman tires.
b. Speak in a quiet and calming tone so that the woman does not become agitated.
c. Speak loudly and clearly so that the woman can hear you.
d. Perform the entire interview in front of the primary caregiver.

2. A 77-year-old male patient has increasing dementia with short-term memory loss and symptoms that fluctuate frequently. The patient experiences visual hallucinations and exhibits muscle rigidity and tremors. These symptoms are characteristic of which type of non-Alzheimer's dementia?

a. Dementia with Lewy bodies
b. Frontotemporal dementia
c. Normal pressure hydrocephalus
d. Parkinson's dementia

3. What determines an APRN's right to write prescriptions?

a. Standards of Practice
b. The American Nursing Association
c. The state where the APRN is practicing
d. The Drug Enforcement Agency

4. A 40-year-old female hospitalized for severe exacerbation of asthma has been treated for 6 days with albuterol by small volume nebulizer, oral theophylline, and IV methylprednisolone. The patient's blood gases have stabilized. When discontinuing the IV steroid in preparation for discharge, the acute care nurse practitioner should order:

a. Inhaled steroid, such as Azmacort, only
b. Oral prednisone 20 mg daily for one week and then Azmacort
c. Oral prednisone in decreasing doses
d. Oral prednisone in decreasing doses and inhaled steroid, such as Azmacort

5. Which of the following statements about Medicaid is TRUE?

a. Everyone who falls below the federal poverty line is eligible to receive Medicaid.
b. The state is allowed to require that recipients pay a small copayment.
c. Recipients of Medicaid are not supposed to pay anything towards their medical care.
d. Though it is both a federal and state plan, only the state government is responsible for supervision of the program.

6. A woman complains of a history of nausea and burning, stabbing epigastric pain which is relieved for short periods by antacids or intake of food. The patient denies NSAID use but is a heavy smoker. A urea breath test is positive. Which of the following treatment protocols is most common?

a. Histamine-2 blocker plus bismuth plus tetracycline
b. Proton pump inhibitor only
c. Proton pump inhibitor plus tetracycline
d. Proton pump inhibitor plus clarithromycin and amoxicillin/metronidazole

7. A patient who receives multiple transfusions with citrated blood products must be monitored closely for:

a. Hyponatremia
b. Hypomagnesemia
c. Hypokalemia
d. Hypocalcemia

8. Negligence is:

a. Not acting in a way that a reasonable and prudent nurse would, resulting in harm to the patient
b. Acting in a way that is against the law, resulting in harm to the patient
c. Not taking the appropriate preventative measures that another nurse would, to the detriment of the patient
d. Not giving appropriate medical care to a patient

9. An incidence of which of the following conditions requires mandatory reporting to the CDC?

a. Influenza
b. Lyme disease
c. Hepatitis E
d. Methicillin-resistant Staphylococcus aureus infection

10. Which of the following arterial blood gas (ABG) findings is consistent with metabolic acidosis in an adult?

a. HCO_3 <22 mEq/L and pH < 7.35
b. HCO_3 >26 mEq/L and pH > 7.45
c. $PaCO_2$ 35-45 mmHg and $PaO_2 \geq 80$ mmHg
d. $PaCO_2 > 55$ mmHg and $PaO_2 < 60$ mmHg

11. A thin young adult comes into the emergency room with a sudden onset of right-sided chest pain and shortness of breath following a run. What do you suspect?

a. Myocardial infarction
b. Aortic dissection
c. Asthma flare
d. Spontaneous pneumothorax

12. A patient with severe type 1 diabetes mellitus refuses all treatment because of religious convictions. Which of the following is the most appropriate action?

a. Provide the patient with facts about the disease, treatments, and prognosis
b. Ask family members to intervene
c. Remind the patient that he will die without treatment
d. Refer the patient to a psychologist

13. A young woman presents in the emergency room with sudden shortness of breath, coughing, and slight chest pain. She is on the birth control pill and just returned home from a car trip several hours away. What tests should the practitioner order?

a. ABG, ECG, chest x-ray, and echocardiogram
b. CBC, pulmonary function test, stress test
c. ECG, cardiac enzymes, stress test
d. Sputum culture, CBC, pulmonary function test

14. When irrigating a wound, what wound irrigation pressure is needed to effectively cleanse the wound while avoiding trauma?

a. <4 psi
b. 20-30 psi
c. 10-15 psi
d. >15 psi

15. A thyroid panel comes back with the following results: elevated TSH, low free T4, and low free T3. What is the diagnosis?

a. Hyperthyroidism
b. Subclinical hypothyroidism
c. Primary hypothyroidism
d. Subclinical hyperthyroidism

16. When the nurse practitioner enters the room of a patient whose death is imminent, the daughter states, "I can't stay in the room when Dad dies! I can't stand the thought!" Which of the following is the best response?

a. "You will regret it if you don't."
b. "Your father would want you with him."
c. "I'll stay with him, and you can come and go as you feel comfortable."
d. "Is there someone else who can stay with him?"

17. A patient has chest pain, dyspnea, and hypotension. A 12-lead ECG shows atrial rates of 250 with regular ventricular rates of 100. P waves are saw-toothed (referred to as F waves), QRS shape and duration (0.04 to 0.11 seconds) is normal, PR interval is hard to calculate because of F waves, and the P:QRS ratio is 2-4:1. Which of the following diagnoses fits this profile?

a. Premature atrial contraction
b. Premature junctional contraction
c. Atrial fibrillation
d. Atrial flutter

18. What is the antibiotic of choice in a patient with syphilis, who reports an allergy to penicillin?

a. Doxycycline 100 mg PO BID x 14 days
b. Ofloxacin 400 mg PO BID x 14 days
c. Ceftriaxone 250 mg IM x 1 dose
d. Metronidazole 500 mg PO BID x 14 days

19. Which of the following communication approaches is most effective to facilitate communication with a patient who has global aphasia?

a. Speak slowly and clearly, facing the patient.
b. Use letter boards.
c. Ask yes/no questions.
d. Use pictures, diagrams, and gestures.

20. A 44-year-old obese woman recovering from a femoropopliteal bypass develops sudden onset of dyspnea with chest pain on inspiration, cough, and fever of 39°C. An S_4 gallop rhythm is present. The ECG shows tachycardia and nonspecific changes in ST and T waves. The most likely diagnosis is:

a. Myocardial infarction
b. Pulmonary embolism
c. Pneumonia
d. Sepsis

21. Which drug that is used for the treatment of coronary artery disease should be avoided in patients with asthma?

a. Spironolactone
b. Losartan
c. Propranolol
d. Captopril

22. When determining the burden of proof for acts of negligence, how would risk management classify willfully providing inadequate care while disregarding the safety and security of another?

a. Negligent conduct
b. Gross negligence
c. Contributory negligence
d. Comparative negligence

23. Which antibiotic should be avoided in patients taking theophylline?

a. Doxycycline
b. Erythromycin
c. Vancomycin
d. Penicillin

24. A 25-year-old patient with multiple fractures from an auto accident develops hypoxia, dyspnea, precordial chest pain, tachycardia, and thick milky sputum. Auscultation of the lungs shows crackles and wheezes. The patient complains of headache and has a fever of 40°C. Which of the following interventions should be done first?

a. High-flow oxygen
b. Corticosteroids (IV)
c. Vasopressors
d. Morphine

25. In patients taking valproic acid for seizure disorder, serum levels should be maintained at:

a. 50 to 100 mcg/mL
b. 20 to 80 mcg/mL
c. 10 to 20 mcg/mL
d. 4 to 12 mcg/mL

26. When the nurse practitioner is conducting medication reconciliation, the patient's list of current medications includes the following: Lasix®, metolazone, aminophylline, and doxapram. The nurse believes this list probably indicates:

a. Polypharmacy
b. Inaccurate reporting
c. Accurate reporting
d. Poor medical management

27. A patient is hospitalized for a myocardial infarction and exhibits increased preload, increased afterload, and decreased contractility with decreased cardiac output and increased systemic vascular resistance. BP is 84/40 and pulse 124 bpm, thready, and irregular. The patient has tachypnea, chest pain, basilar rales, and pallor. The most likely diagnosis is:

a. Cardiogenic shock
b. Pulmonary embolism
c. Heart failure
d. Atrial fibrillation

28. Which of the following sensory changes associated with aging has the most impact on older adults?

a. Hearing deficit
b. Vision deficit
c. Decreased taste and smell
d. Decreased sense of touch (vibration, temperature, pain)

29. An HIV-positive patient has experienced a recent drop in CD4 count to 190. She has developed a fever with general malaise and abdominal pain, and examination shows hepatosplenomegaly. Differential diagnoses should include:

a. Pneumocystis jiroveci pneumonia, bacterial pneumonia, and TB
b. Toxoplasmosis, herpes encephalitis, and CNS lymphoma
c. Histoplasmosis, Mycobacterium avium complex, and bacillary peliosis
d. TB, non-Hodgkin's lymphoma, and bacillary angiomatosis

30. With the Braden scale to assess risk for developing pressure sores, the patient scores 1 to 3 in all six assessment areas with a total score of 14. What is the patient's risk?

a. High risk, poor prognosis
b. Breakpoint for risk, moderate prognosis
c. Minimal risk, excellent prognosis
d. No risk

31. An 80-year-old male has had post-herpetic neuralgia for 11 months, but pain is increasingly intractable despite his taking 10 hydrocodone tablets daily. He has coronary stents in place and takes warfarin. The patient is weak, somnolent, and lethargic, and eats and sleeps poorly. Modifying his pain management should include:

a. Weaning patient from hydrocodone and starting gabapentin in slowly increasing doses
b. Discontinuing hydrocodone and starting morphine pump
c. Weaning patient from hydrocodone and starting biofeedback
d. Lowering the dose of hydrocodone and supplementing with NSAIDs

32. A 76-year-old male is recovering from surgery but exhibits sudden onset of confusion with fluctuating inattention, disorganized thinking, and altered level of consciousness. Which of the following assessment tools is most indicated?

a. Mini-mental state exam (MMSE)
b. Mini-Cog
c. Confusion assessment method (CAM)
d. Geriatric depression scale (GDS)

33. When forced expiratory volume in one second (FEV_1) is markedly more reduced than the reduction in forced vital capacity (FVC), the patient is probably experiencing:

a. Restriction of maximal lung expansion
b. Airway obstruction
c. Depressed respiratory center
d. Limitation in neurological impulses to the muscles of respiration

34. A 70-year-old female with Alzheimer's and a history of falls is admitted to the unit with pneumonitis after a seven-hour wait in the emergency department. The patient is agitated, restless, and repeatedly says "I'm hungry." The nurse's first priority should be to:

a. Assess diet needs and order food.
b. Institute a fall-prevention program.
c. Review all medications.
d. Assess cognitive abilities.

35. A patient with a score of 10 on the Glasgow coma scale is classified as:

a. Comatose
b. Severe head injury
c. Moderate head injury
d. Mild head injury

36. A patient's laboratory tests show that the TSH is 14 mU/mL, free T4 is 3.5 μg/dL and free T3 is 100 ng/dL. These findings indicate:

a. Normal values
b. Hypothyroidism
c. Hyperthyroidism
d. Hashimoto's thyroiditis

37. A patient with bone metastasis from prostate cancer is to be treated with zoledronic acid (Reclast®, Zometa®). Which laboratory test(s) must be done prior to initiating treatment?

a. Serum creatinine/creatinine clearance
b. Blood urea nitrogen (BUN)
c. Complete blood count (CBC)
d. Electrolyte panel

38. A 69-year-old female hospitalized for a fractured hip is being evaluated for comorbidities. The most common comorbidity for hospitalized patients ages 65 to 80 is:

a. Fluid and electrolyte imbalance
b. COPD
c. Anemia
d. Hypertension

39. A 45-year-old male has renal calculi. He has passed one stone, but ultrasound shows multiple stones present in the urinary tract. Stone analysis shows the stone is calcium-containing. In addition to analgesia and antispasmodics, which medication is indicated?

a. Indomethacin
b. Allopurinol and Vitamin B6
c. Alpha-mercato-propionyl-glycine (aMPG) and captopril
d. Hydrochlorothiazide

40. When prescribing an oral anti-diabetic agent for an older patient, the patient's initial dose should be

a. The same as the usual dose for a younger adult
b. 25% of the usual dose
c. 50% of the usual dose
d. 75% of the usual dose

41. A 56-year-old female has pain and swelling of the small joints of the hands and wrist. Which test(s) should the acute care nurse practitioner order to confirm a diagnosis of rheumatoid arthritis?

a. Rheumatoid factor (RF) and anti-citrullinated protein antibody (ACPA)
b. RF and erythrocyte sedimentation rate (ESR)
c. C-reactive protein (CRP) and RF
d. Synovial fluid analysis, ESR, and CRP

42. A 78-year-old patient is hospitalized with severe dehydration from influenza. Which type of precaution is indicated when caring for the patient?

a. Use personal protective equipment, including gown and gloves for all contact.
b. Wear a mask while caring for patient.
c. Wear a mask and gloves for all contact with patient.
d. Use a ≥N95 respirator while caring for patient.

43. A patient has a chronic leg ulcer covered with black eschar and is to have chemical debridement with collagenase. Preparation includes:

a. Thoroughly drying the eschar and surrounding skin
b. Applying topical antibiotic
c. Scrubbing the wound with hexachlorophene
d. Cross-hatching the upper layers of the eschar

44. A 36-year-old female was injured in a fall when drunk. CT shows contusion on the left side of the brain. The patient responds lethargically to verbal commands and shows some confusion and restlessness. Vital signs: BP 154/76, pulse 68, and respirations 28. Previous records indicate her normal BP was 128/70, pulse 76, and respirations 16. The change in VS is most likely an indication of:

a. Increasing intracranial pressure
b. Stress response
c. Ethanol intoxication
d. Delirium tremens

45. Which of the following is the best documentation of the behavior of a difficult patient?

a. "Patient is belligerent and uncooperative."
b. "Patient is spitting at nurses, throwing magazines, and refusing to get out of bed for therapy."
c. "Patient appears to dislike nurses and other care providers."
d. "Patient believes staff members are going to hurt her."

46. A 75-year-old male is receiving warfarin after the insertion of an aortic stent for aortic aneurysm. The patient states he usually takes a number of vitamins and herbal preparations. Which of the following should the patient avoid?

a. St. John's wort
b. Melatonin
c. Echinacea
d. Vitamin B complex

47. A retrospective attempt to determine the cause of an event, often a sentinel event such as an unexpected death, is the definition of:

a. A t-test
b. Regression analysis
c. Tracer methodology
d. Root cause analysis

48. A 72-year-old female on Medicare is being discharged home with a healing burn on her left arm that she is unable to care for independently because of arthritis. She requires dressing changes every 3 days. She depends on public transportation and walks with difficulty. The bus stop is two blocks from her house. Her 12-year-old granddaughter lives with her. The best solution is:

a. Transferring the patient to an extended care facility
b. Providing treatment on an outpatient basis at the hospital clinic
c. Teaching the woman's 12-year-old granddaughter to do the dressing changes
d. Making a referral to a home health agency to provide in-home care

49. If all patients who develop urinary infections with urinary catheters are evaluated per urine culture and sensitivities for microbial resistance, but only those patients with clinically evident infections are included, this is an example of:

a. Information bias
b. Selection bias
c. Compliance bias
d. Admission bias

50. A 68-year-old male has an asynchronous pacemaker and has been experiencing cardiac palpitations, headache, anxiety, general malaise, pain in the jaw and chest, and unexplained weakness with pulsations evident in the neck and abdomen. The most likely cause is:

a. Broken pacemaker wires
b. Dislodged pacemaker wires
c. Myocardial infarction
d. Pacemaker syndrome

51. A normally healthy male presents to the ER with complaints of productive cough and fever for the past three days. Chest x-rays reveals a small infiltrate in the right lower lobe. The most appropriate antibiotic therapy for this patient is:

a. Azithromycin 500 mg PO on day one, then 250 mg PO once daily for 4 days.
b. Ceftriaxone 1 g IM today, followed by doxycycline 100 mg PO twice daily for 10 days.
c. Amoxicillin 875 mg PO twice daily for 10 days.
d. No antibiotic therapy is necessary because the cause of these findings is most likely viral.

52. A pre-menopausal woman who has been treated for breast cancer is taking tamoxifen. She asks her nurse practitioner how long she will need to take this. The most appropriate answer is:

a. Two years following treatment of the cancer
b. Five years following treatment of the cancer
c. Seven years following treatment of the cancer
d. Ten years following treatment of the cancer

53. What is the rationale for initiating beta blocker therapy in a patient with congestive heart failure?

a. Beta blockers are contraindicated in patients with CHF.
b. Beta blockers will reduce catecholamine stimulation in patients with CHF.
c. Beta blockers will stimulate serotonin release to improve mood and decrease anxiety.
d. Beta blockers can help improve renal function.

54. A 54-year-old female is taking levothyroxine 0.125 mg daily. Her most recent labs show TSH increased at 8.1 and T4 decreased at 4.2. What is the most appropriate step to take next?

a. Continue the levothyroxine at the current dosage and recheck labs at her next follow-up.
b. Decrease the levothyroxine dosage to 0.1 mg daily and recheck labs in 6-8 weeks.
c. Increase the levothyroxine dosage to 0.137 mg daily and recheck labs in 6-8 weeks.
d. Increase the levothyroxine dosage to 0.3 mg daily and recheck labs in 6-8 weeks.

55. A contraindication for using gentamicin ear drops to treat otitis externa is:

a. Renal failure
b. A perforated ear drum
c. Liver failure
d. Hearing loss

56. Appropriate dosing of valacyclovir for treatment of a herpes zoster infection in a patient with normal kidney function is:

a. 1 g PO three times daily for 7 days
b. 500 mg PO twice daily for 10 days
c. 1 g PO twice daily for 10 days
d. 500 mg PO three times daily for 7 days

57. A 69-year-old male is taking Plavix for a history of coronary artery disease. His cardiac condition has been stable, but he requires treatment for GERD symptoms. The medication that is most appropriate to treat these symptoms is:

a. Nexium
b. Prilosec
c. Pepcid
d. Dexilant

58. A 52-year-old male is diagnosed with an uncomplicated UTI. The antibiotic that would be the least effective for this patient is:

a. Ciprofloxacin
b. Levofloxacin
c. Nitrofurantoin
d. Trimethoprim-sulfamethoxazole

59. A 42-year-old male with rheumatoid arthritis is beginning to develop increased symptoms with joint pain and deformity. His past medical history is significant for Hodgkins' lymphoma as a teenager and he has been in remission for 27 years. He is also being treated for hypertension and hypercholesterolemia, both well-controlled with medications. Based on his history, which factor is a contraindication for treatment with a biologic agent for his RA symptoms?

a. Age
b. History of lymphoma
c. Hypertension
d. Hypercholesterolemia

60. The pain reliever that would be the safest for treating arthritis knee pain in an elderly patient is:

a. Acetaminophen
b. Naproxen
c. Ibuprofen
d. Diclofenac

61. A 76-year-old female with mild dementia is brought in by her daughter for a routine appointment. Her daughter expresses interest in having her mother try one of the medications to "cure" her dementia. It is important she understand that:

a. The medications are very expensive and may not be covered by her insurance.
b. Frequent monitoring of blood tests is necessary if one of these medications is started.
c. There is no known cure for dementia and the medication will only temporarily improve the symptoms.
d. These medications are reserved for use in those patients with severe dementia.

62. In the patient with COPD, a long-acting bronchodilator should be used:

a. After prednisone has been given for at least 3 months and is not controlling the symptoms
b. As a first-line treatment
c. In nebulizer form only
d. When a short-acting inhaler is not adequate in controlling symptoms throughout the day

63. A 63-year-old female is seen for a dental abscess because she cannot get in with her Dentist for another week. Her past medical history is significant for a cardiac stent one year ago, hypothyroidism, hypertension, and hyperlipidemia. She is taking Plavix, levothyroxine, lisinopril, and atorvastatin. Based on her history, which antibiotic would be contraindicated?

a. Amoxicillin
b. Clarithromycin
c. Amoxicillin-clavulanate
d. Trimethoprim-sulfamethoxazole

64. During an annual physical of a 35-year-old female, small granulomatous nodules are seen in the bilateral conjunctivae. Based on that finding, further work-up should be done for:

a. Systemic lupus erythematosus
b. Multiple sclerosis
c. Rheumatoid arthritis
d. Sarcoidosis

65. Which adventitious lung sound is most often associated with congestive heart failure?

a. Rales
b. Wheezing
c. Stridor
d. There are no abnormal breath sounds associated with CHF.

66. Which heart murmur would most likely be associated with aortic stenosis?

a. A pansystolic murmur heard best over the left sternal border at the 4th-5th intercostal space
b. A mid-systolic murmur heard best over the right sternal border at the 1st-2nd intercostal space
c. A mid-systolic click with a crescendo-decrescendo murmur at the apex
d. A low-pitched and rumbling pan-diastolic murmur heard best at the apex

67. In the patient who comes in with complaints of a depression in the center of their fingernails and the edges curling up, the first test that should be done is:

a. A complete blood count
b. Renal function tests
c. A liver panel
d. A biopsy of the nail material

68. Which of the following patients are at most risk for developing an abdominal aortic aneurysm?

a. A 75-year-old female smoker with hypertension, well-controlled with medication
b. A 51-year-old male, non-smoker, with elevated LDL cholesterol
c. A 79-year-old male smoker with hypertension, hypercholesterolemia, and COPD
d. A 62-year-old male smoker with no chronic medical problems

69. According to the U.S. Preventive Services Task Force, the latest recommendation for routine PSA screening is:

a. It should be done every 5 years on men >40 years old.
b. It should be done annually on men >50 years old.
c. It should be done annually on men >60 years old.
d. It is not recommended.

70. A definitive diagnosis of Parkinson's disease is made with:

a. The presence of neurofibrillary tangles on brain MRI
b. The development of hallucinations and dementia-type symptoms
c. Frequent falls due to shuffling gait
d. The presence of at least two of the four main symptoms of Parkinson's disease

71. A 64-year-old male has type 2 diabetes that has not been well-controlled with metformin alone. His past medical history is significant for hypertension, hypercholesterolemia, congestive heart failure, and coronary artery disease. Which of the following medications would be contraindicated in this patient?

a. Byetta
b. Glipizide
c. Actos
d. Lantus insulin

72. The recommended treatment for chronic lymphocytic leukemia after initial diagnosis, is usually:

a. Chemotherapy
b. Radiation
c. Combination of chemotherapy and radiation
d. Continuing to monitor for progression of the disease

73. Most patients with plaque psoriasis are eligible candidates for treatment with a biologic if the disease is considered severe. All of the following are considered severe characteristics of psoriasis EXCEPT:

a. Thickened plaques that respond to topical treatments
b. Lesions covering more than 5-10% of the body
c. Significant psoriatic arthritis
d. Severe impact on quality of life

74. An elderly Orthodox Jewish man has died after suffering multiple strokes. The nurse practitioner knows that before his body is transported from the hospital:

a. All of the family members must come in his room one by one to pay their respects.
b. Any machines should be disconnected, but no tubes or probes should be removed from his body.
c. The body should be stripped and washed thoroughly.
d. He should be dressed in his regular clothes rather than a hospital gown.

75. The most common type of dementia is:

a. Lewy body dementia
b. Vascular dementia
c. Alzheimer's dementia
d. Dementia due to Parkinson's disease

76. What is the leading cause of accidental death in the United States?

a. Motor vehicle accidents
b. Drug overdose
c. Suicide
d. Other accidents in the home

77. Which of the following patients would be a candidate for a left ventricular assist device (LVAD)?

a. A 73-year-old male with chronic atrial fibrillation
b. A 55-year-old female with worsening mitral valve prolapse
c. A 62-year-old male with coronary artery disease who had 3 cardiac stents placed within the past year
d. A 57-year-old male with end-stage congestive heart failure undergoing evaluation for a heart transplant

78. Which recommendation from the U.S. Preventive Services Task Force regarding cervical cancer screening is true?

a. A Pap smear is recommended annually for all women age 30 to 75.
b. A Pap smear and HPV testing is recommended every 3 years for all women age 30 to 75.
c. A Pap smear is not recommended for women under the age of 21.
d. HPV testing should be done on all women, regardless of age, every 3 years.

79. A 52-year-old male is seen in the office for complaints of left great toe pain. He woke up this morning with the pain and rates his pain level as a 10/10. He denies any trauma. On exam, the left great toe is erythematous and edematous with significant pain with movement or palpation. The lab test that would be most appropriate at this time is:

a. A uric acid level
b. A chemistry panel
c. A complete blood count
d. No lab tests are available to diagnose this condition

80. What is the difference between palliative care and hospice care?

a. Palliative care is for inpatient end-of-life care, and hospice care is performed in the home.
b. Palliative care can be started at the time of diagnosis during treatment, and hospice care is started when the patient is not going to survive the illness and the end-of-life is nearing.
c. Palliative care can be provided by a patient's primary care provider, and hospice care is provided by a certified hospice care agency.
d. Palliative care specializes in only the different forms of therapy that a patient needs, and hospice care specializes in end-of-life comfort care.

81. The most accurate method of diagnosing temporal arteritis is:

a. MRI
b. Ultrasound
c. Biopsy of the temporal artery
d. Angiography

82. Which of the following patients would be most likely to show impairment on the Mini Mental Status Exam?

a. A 54-year-old female attorney with mild short-term memory impairment
b. A 62-year-old male college professor with moderate short-term memory impairment
c. A 57-year-old male engineer with very mild short-term memory impairment
d. A 67-year-old male, educated through grade 6, with moderate short-term memory impairment

83. A 63-year-old female develops a DVT and PE following knee replacement surgery. She has been transitioned from Heparin IV to Coumadin orally. The nurse practitioner is educating the patient and her family on dietary restrictions with Coumadin. The practitioner explains to them:

a. She can no longer eat any green vegetables because they will increase her vitamin K level, causing the blood to thicken.
b. She needs to avoid all citrus fruit because it will cause her blood to be too thin.
c. She needs to maintain a consistent diet with some vitamin K from leafy green vegetables, but no big fluctuations in vitamin K-rich foods.
d. She should avoid red meat because of the high iron content.

84. The formula used to calculate the dosage of enteral nutrition a patient receives daily is:

a. 25 kcal/kg/day plus 1.5 g protein/kg/day
b. 12.5 kcal/kg/day plus 1 g protein/kg/day
c. 30 kcal/kg/day plus 2 g protein/kg/day
d. 35 kcal/kg/day plus 3 g protein/kg/day

85. A 52-year-old obese male is seen for a routine medical checkup after several years without medical care. After review of screening labs, he is started on atorvastatin for hyperlipidemia and metformin for type 2 diabetes mellitus. His blood pressure was 188/100 in the office and he says it has been close to that when his wife has checked it at home. The most appropriate antihypertensive medication to start him on at this time would be:

a. Metoprolol
b. Lisinopril
c. Hydrochlorothiazide
d. Carvedilol

86. The modifiable risk factors used to calculate cardiac risk are:

a. Age, HDL cholesterol, LDL cholesterol, and smoking history
b. Gender, total cholesterol, blood pressure, and smoking history
c. Smoking history, HDL cholesterol, total cholesterol, and systolic blood pressure
d. Age, gender, LDL cholesterol, and HDL cholesterol

87. A 72-year-old male is seen for an exacerbation of COPD with low-grade fever. His current medications include lisinopril, simvastatin, timolol eye drops, albuterol inhaler, and Advair inhaler. One of the medications he should not receive for this exacerbation is:

a. Albuterol via nebulizer
b. Levaquin
c. Tessalon Perles
d. Prednisone

88. The EKG changes that are seen with severe hyperkalemia include:

a. Absent P waves, a prolonged PR segment, ST depression, and inverted T waves
b. Prolonged QRS, a bundle branch block, bradycardia, and a sine wave
c. Sinus tachycardia rhythm with ST segment elevation
d. Irregularly irregular rhythm with rate usually >120 and inverted T waves

89. An elderly female patient has a nasogastric drain. The results of her arterial blood gases are as follows: pH 7.5, HCO_3 29, pCO_2 37. Based on these values, which acid-base disorder has this patient developed?

a. Respiratory alkalosis
b. Respiratory acidosis
c. Metabolic alkalosis
d. Metabolic acidosis

90. The T-score the nurse practitioner would expect to see on the DEXA scan of an osteopenic female is:

a. -1.0 to -2.5
b. Less than -2.5
c. -1.0 to 1.0
d. 1.0 to 2.0

91. The nurse practitioner would expect the results of a pulmonary function test (PFT) in an asthmatic patient to be:

a. FEV1 90%, FVC 92%, FEV1/FVC 97%
b. FEV1 70%, FVC 83%, FEV1/FVC 84%
c. FEV1 94%, FVC 90%, FEV1/FVC 100%
d. FEV1 89%, FVC 84%, FEV1/FVC 104%

92. Regarding healthcare decision-making for the Hispanic patient, the nurse practitioner knows that:

a. The mother, or oldest female in the family, will be the primary decision maker.
b. The father, or oldest male in the family, will be the primary decision maker.
c. Medical decisions are made as a joint decision by all family members.
d. Medical decisions are primarily decided by the patient, regardless of age, with the support of the family.

93. In order for a patient with congestive heart failure to qualify for Hospice care, which of the following requirements must be met?

a. One or more hospitalizations for a CHF-related flare-up within the past year.
b. Symptoms are well-controlled with medications, but the patient is noncompliant and suffers frequent exacerbations because of the disease.
c. Along with CHF, there is a concomitant diagnosis of coronary artery disease or COPD.
d. The patient's ejection fraction is measured at <20% and there are symptoms at rest despite maximum medical treatment.

94. A geriatric patient with anemia is receiving a blood transfusion. The practitioner would be alerted to a possible transfusion reaction if the patient develops:

a. Dysuria
b. The hiccups
c. Ear pain
d. Tenderness at the IV site

95. The nurse practitioner has ordered a dopamine infusion for a patient in the ICU. Once it is completed, the effects from the medication should be gone:

a. Within 10 minutes
b. Within 1 hour
c. Within 4 hours
d. Within 12 hours

96. How much exercise is recommended for a relatively healthy 65-year-old patient?

a. At least 30 minutes of moderate aerobic exercise daily
b. At least 60 minutes of mild aerobic exercise daily
c. At least 150 minutes of moderate aerobic activity weekly
d. At least 60 minutes of moderate aerobic activity weekly

97. One of the differences in symptom presentation with Crohn's disease versus ulcerative colitis is:

a. Crohn's disease is more likely to cause rectal bleeding.
b. Crohn's disease is less likely to cause rectal bleeding.
c. Crohn's disease is more likely to cause occasional abdominal pain versus chronic pain with ulcerative colitis.
d. Crohn's disease is less likely to cause perianal symptoms such as fistulas and skin breakdown.

98. Current recommendations for screening mammography in women 75 years old and older state:

a. Annual mammography screening should be performed until it is deemed unnecessary due to other medical co-morbidities.
b. Screening mammography should be performed in this age group every 2 years.
c. Screening mammography is not recommended for women in this age group.
d. Annual mammography screening should be performed for all women until death or end-of-life issues are present.

99. A 59-year-old male is diagnosed with the flu. His wife, who is relatively healthy, is requesting a prescription for Tamiflu to take prophylactically. The best response to this is:

a. This is reasonable and you will write the prescription.
b. Routine prophylactic treatment of the flu is not recommended.
c. Under no circumstances are people treated prophylactically for the flu.
d. She would need an antibiotic to prevent getting the flu.

100. Which of the following antibiotics may cause an allergic response cross-reaction in a patient with a penicillin allergy?

a. Cefdinir
b. Azithromycin
c. Ciprofloxacin
d. Sulfamethoxazole

101. The nurse practitioner is entering dietary orders for an Orthodox Jewish patient being admitted to the medical floor. The practitioner knows the appropriate action is to:

a. Discuss the patient's diet with him or his family and ask if he would prefer a Kosher diet.
b. Order a regular diet.
c. Order a Kosher diet.
d. Do not order any specific diet because the family will bring in food prepared in their own kitchen.

102. When administering blood or blood products, which of the following is true?

a. A patient with A- blood can receive blood from a donor who is O- or O+.
b. A patient with A+ blood can receive blood from a donor who is AB+.
c. A patient with AB+ blood can receive blood from a donor of any blood type.
d. A patient with AB- blood can receive blood from a donor who is O+ or B+.

103. Why are albuterol and ipratropium (Duoneb) given together?

a. Adding ipratropium to the albuterol decreases the tremors that are often associated with albuterol.
b. The albuterol requires ipratropium be present to aid in absorption of the drug in the airway.
c. These two drugs are not available on their own, only as a combination medication.
d. They work together by causing dilation of the airway along with relaxation of the bronchial smooth muscle.

104. A patient with Lewy body dementia is started on Abilify to help with hallucinations. His wife has been giving him St. John's Wart and wants to continue to do so. She should be told that:

a. Since St. John's Wart is a natural, herbal remedy, it will be safe to take with the Abilify.
b. She should give him a half dose of the St. John's Wart while he is taking Abilify.
c. She should not give the St. John's Wart because it can decrease the drug level of the Abilify.
d. She should give him twice the prescribed dosage of Abilify if she is going to continue to give St. John's Wart.

105. The mineral that is often very low after the administration of intravenous Lasix is:

a. Calcium
b. Magnesium
c. Iron
d. Fluoride

106. A 72-year-old male has had a pacemaker for one year and has been doing very well. He and his wife are planning a trip to see their grandchildren and he is concerned that the security screening devices at the airport may interfere with his pacemaker. The best response is that:

a. He should not be within 10 feet of the electrical current that is emitted from the security x-ray devices.
b. He will need to carry the pacemaker identification card and instruct security that the handheld wands used for security clearance cannot be held directly over the implanted device.
c. He can be near the security equipment, but cannot walk through the traditional metal detectors.
d. There are no concerns with the equipment interacting with his pacemaker.

107. Which of the following would not be considered a restraint for a very restless patient who continues to try to remove IVs, oxygen, and other necessary medical equipment?

a. Mittens
b. Padded wrist bracelets that attach to the bed rail
c. A prn dose of a benzodiazepine
d. A Posey vest

108. When teaching tracheostomy care at home, it is important the caregivers understand:

a. Cleaning and changing the trach tube must be done under sterile conditions.
b. The trach tube can be reused after it has been cleaned properly.
c. The trach tube can only be changed by a Respiratory Therapist who will come to the home.
d. A new, sterile trach tube must be used each day.

109. When communicating with a non-English speaking patient and her family, it is best to:

a. Have another family member serve as an interpreter, if possible.
b. Improvise using pictures and video to teach the patient about their medical care.
c. Hold most of the conversation through an online translating program.
d. Arrange to have an interpreter familiar with medical terminology present.

110. The diet that would be most appropriate for the geriatric patient hospitalized with liver disease is:

a. Low sodium, high carbohydrate
b. High protein
c. Low carbohydrate, high protein
d. Non-dairy, high protein

111. The form of macular degeneration associated with deterioration of the central retina is:

a. Wet macular degeneration
b. Congenital macular degeneration
c. Dry macular degeneration
d. Acquired macular degeneration

112. One of the first signs of a urinary tract infection in an 86-year-old female patient is:

a. Dysuria
b. Confusion
c. Urinary frequency
d. Polydipsia

113. The medication that will require a dosage adjustment in the patient with renal failure is:

a. Lisinopril
b. Hydrochlorothiazide
c. Vitamin D
d. Ranitidine (Zantac)

114. What is the most common cause of ARDS, or acute respiratory distress syndrome?

a. Congestive heart failure
b. Sepsis
c. COPD
d. Malignant hypertension

115. A 67-year-old male presents to the clinic with complaints of vision changes causing some yellowish discoloration in his visual field. He has a past medical history of hypertension, coronary artery disease, and congestive heart failure. He is currently taking lisinopril, metoprolol, digoxin, and Plavix. Which of these medications is most likely causing his symptoms?

a. Plavix
b. Metoprolol
c. Digoxin
d. Lisinopril

116. Which of the following is an example of an iatrogenic condition?

a. A femur fracture following a motorcycle accident
b. A self-inflicted gunshot wound
c. Joint deformities due to rheumatoid arthritis
d. Hair loss following chemotherapy

117. A decubitus ulcer that has exposed adipose tissue and eschar present would be classified as:

a. Stage III
b. Stage II
c. Stage I
d. An unstageable ulcer

118. The level of care received by the patient who sees a cardiologist and is then admitted to the hospital for coronary artery bypass grafting is:

a. Primary care
b. Secondary care
c. Tertiary care
d. Terminal care

119. The most common cause of a small bowel obstruction in an elderly patient is:

a. Use of multiple pain medications
b. Frequent laxative use
c. History of past abdominal surgery
d. Uncontrolled diabetes mellitus

120. Which of the following is not normally examined when assessing a patient's functional status?

a. Learned activities of daily living
b. Basic activities of daily living
c. Intermediate activities of daily living
d. Advanced activities of daily living

121. For people without a personal history of colorectal cancer, the U.S. Preventive Services Task Force recommends regular screening consisting of annual fecal occult blood testing, along with sigmoidoscopy and colonoscopy every five and ten years, respectively, for adults ages:

a. 35-85
b. 40-65
c. 50-75
d. 65-85

122. Which of the following alternative therapies has been found to be helpful with relieving chronic low back pain?

a. Glucosamine/chondroitin supplements
b. Acupuncture
c. Laying on of hands
d. Gingko biloba herbal supplement

123. Of the following, the food that is most likely to cause a flare-up of gout is:

a. Broccoli
b. Oranges
c. Trout
d. Peanut butter

124. The most common cause of petechiae is:

a. Excessive straining
b. Endocarditis
c. Warfarin therapy
d. Thrombocytopenia

125. An 82-year-old male is seen for a laceration on his left hand. He builds sculptures out of scrap metal as a hobby and occasionally suffers a laceration. He is unsure when he last received a tetanus shot. The best medical advice to give him would be:

a. Tetanus shots are no longer necessary after the age of 75.
b. Tetanus has been eradicated in the U.S. and shots are no longer necessary.
c. Only major trauma or surgery requires a tetanus shot.
d. He should receive a tetanus shot today to reduce his risk of developing the disease.

126. The medication that is least likely to cause dysgeusia is:

a. Clarithromycin
b. Digoxin
c. Amlodipine
d. Amoxicillin

127. An 82-year-old male has been diagnosed with ischemic heart disease, and it is felt a coronary artery bypass graft (CABG) could help him. Which of the following would not be a contraindication to him undergoing this procedure?

a. Severe COPD
b. Severe CHF
c. His age
d. Current chemotherapy therapy for prostate cancer

128. Which of the following is true regarding the murmur heard with mitral valve prolapse?

a. It is best heard over the right sternal border.
b. It is louder when the patient is standing and decreases with squatting.
c. It is heard best during the diastolic phase.
d. It is associated with a loud carotid bruit.

129. The medical service that is covered under Medicare Part A is:

a. Durable medical equipment
b. Appointments with a primary care provider
c. Appointments with a specialist
d. Prescription drug coverage

130. Which of the following drugs would be least likely to help with the bradykinesia associated with Parkinson's disease?

a. Amantadine
b. Anticholinergics
c. Levodopa
d. MAOIs

131. A 65-year-old man has had chest pain that was diagnosed as angina. When taking his history, he tells the nurse that he is a heavy smoker, drinks alcohol daily, has a very poor diet, drinks a lot of caffeine every day, and does not exercise. What is the most important lifestyle change he should make?

a. Quit drinking alcohol
b. Quit smoking
c. Improve his diet
d. Start a regular exercise routine

132. If a patient is blind in his right eye, which of the following would be true?

a. A light shined in the opposite eye will cause both pupils to constrict.
b. A light shined in the blind eye will cause both pupils to dilate.
c. A light shined in the opposite eye will cause only that pupil to constrict.
d. A light shined in the blind eye will cause only the opposite pupil to dilate.

133. A 72-year-old male with type 2 diabetes mellitus is seen for irritation inside his mouth. On exam, he has white, cheese-like lesions in his mouth that can easily be scraped off with a tongue depressor. The most appropriate therapy for this is:

a. Acyclovir
b. Fluconazole
c. Penicillin
d. Prednisone

134. During a routine assessment, the nurse practitioner notices a patient has some dryness of his conjunctivae with white patches present there. This is indicative of a deficiency in vitamin:

a. A
b. B12
c. D
d. Niacin

135. A nurse practitioner sees a patient who would like to have a skin lesion removed. The lesion is on her upper arm, is 4 mm round with well-defined margins. She had noticed that it was black, but she thinks it has developed some purple discoloration recently. The best way to assess this would be:

a. Excisional biopsy
b. KOH prep
c. Punch biopsy
d. Wood's lamp assessment

136. A nurse practitioner is seeing a gentleman who underwent a total hip replacement 2 weeks ago. He has complaints of shortness of breath and pain in the lower leg in which he had the hip surgery. Which of the following studies is most appropriate for confirming your suspected diagnosis in this particular patient?

a. D-dimer serum test
b. P/V scintigraphy
c. Pulmonary angiogram
d. Spiral CT of the chest

137. A 75-year-old man is seen with complaints of dyspnea on exertion and bilateral ankle swelling. He has a history of hypertension and COPD, both of which have been well-controlled. On exam, he has 2 cm of JVD and 2+ pitting edema at the ankles. Which abnormal sound would the nurse practitioner expect to hear during his cardiac exam?

a. An ejection click
b. A thrill
c. S3
d. S4

138. Which of the following is indicative of right-sided heart failure?

a. Elevated jugular venous pressure
b. Hypotension
c. Interstitial edema on chest x-ray
d. Significant orthopnea

139. The diagnostic test of choice in a patient with coffee grounds emesis and dark tarry stools is:

a. Abdominal CT scan
b. Colonoscopy
c. Upper endoscopy
d. Upper GI series

140. Which of the following is true regarding an asymptomatic patient with a positive PPD test?

a. The patient has latent tuberculosis.
b. The patient is contagious.
c. Pharmacotherapy is not needed.
d. The patient should be in respiratory isolation.

141. A 65-year-old female has a long history of untreated hypercalcemia. The finding you would also expect to find is:

a. A DEXA score of 2.0
b. Decreased thirst
c. Shortness of breath
d. Nephrolithiasis

142. A 48-year-old male has abdominal obesity with a waist circumference of 45 inches. He is also being treated for hypertension, and his blood pressure is 142/90. The third finding that would confirm a diagnosis of metabolic syndrome is:

a. Fasting glucose of 98 mg/dL
b. HDL cholesterol 45 mg/dL
c. LDL cholesterol 120 mg/dL
d. Triglycerides 200 mg/dL

143. A patient has had GERD-type symptoms for a couple of months and tests positive for *Helicobacter pylori* infection. The treatment regimen consists of:

a. Amoxicillin, bismuth subsalicylate, and a proton pump inhibitor
b. Amoxicillin, clarithromycin, and a proton pump inhibitor
c. Clarithromycin, tetracycline, and bismuth subsalicylate
d. A proton pump inhibitor alone

144. Clinical pathways have been criticized as being potentially harmful to the patient because:

a. They increase the out of pocket medical expenses.
b. A patient may be discharged from the hospital earlier than they should be.
c. They do not allow for flexibility and individualizing a plan of care for the patient.
d. They may result in more medication errors.

145. The first basic principle of risk management is:

a. Risk analysis
b. Risk identification
c. Risk control
d. Risk financing

146. A 52-year-old female has been diagnosed with type 2 diabetes mellitus. When she returns for a follow-up, she is not able to repeat any of the information given at her previous appointment and she continues to have very high blood sugars at home. The most appropriate action at this time is to:

a. Give the written information again and stress how important it is for her to comply with the treatment plan.
b. Tell the patient's spouse that he needs to help her to comply with her treatment.
c. Refer her to some of the online resources available for controlling diabetes.
d. Try a different teaching approach that is more visual and hands-on and have her repeat back what she is taught in the office.

147. The 6 C's which are used to establish an effective therapeutic relationship with the patient and any caregivers are:

a. Consistency, collectivity, cause, critical thinking, co-management, and connection
b. Consideration, convincing, care, criticism, creation, and consistency
c. Communication, consistency, concomitant practices, cleverness, congeniality, and co-ownership
d. Care, commitment, compassion, courage, competence, and communication

148. When preparing a treatment plan for a patient, it is imperative that it include:

a. A very specific, refined goal that is to be reached
b. Multiple goals that will need to be reached
c. Measurable objectives for the identified goal
d. One measurable objective per identified goal

149. One of the benefits of adopting a patient- and family-centered plan of care is:

a. Relieving the burden on patients in making healthcare decisions and transferring that responsibility to the family instead
b. Increasing and improving communication between the staff, patients, and families
c. To decrease the amount of money spent on improving facilities
d. To increase the length of hospital stays to ensure that all members of the healthcare team are collaborating on a patient's care

150. When teaching a patient who has a hearing impairment, it is important to:

a. Face them directly so your face and lips are clearly visible to them.
b. Give them educational materials in print to take home and read on their own.
c. Have the patient be the only person receiving educational material so they can feel more involved in their treatment plan.
d. Discuss the treatment plan with the spouse or family so that they can communicate with the patient in the way that best suits his needs.

151. The Adult Gerontology Acute Care Nurse Practitioner functions as a patient advocate by:

a. Reporting any medication errors that occur involving the patient
b. Following the Clinical Pathway for the patient's diagnosis
c. Not sharing any personal information the patient has shared
d. Protecting the health, safety, and rights of the patient

152. A nurse practitioner receives a phone call from a local cardiologist's office requesting the discharge summary on a patient who was recently hospitalized whom the practitioner cared for. The best response is:

a. They must first fax over a release of information form signed by the patient.
b. It will be faxed right over to them.
c. They must ask the patient to obtain this for them.
d. The information must be mailed and cannot be faxed.

153. Using the patient-centered medical home model of healthcare delivery, the main person coordinating the patient's care is:

a. The primary care provider
b. The lead nurse within the primary care office
c. An assigned social worker
d. The patient coordinates their own care

154. A 59-year-old male is seen for complaints of a tremor in his right hand when he is at rest. On exam, he has a resting tremor, no arm movement when walking, and cog wheeling in the shoulders. The most likely diagnosis is:

a. Multiple sclerosis
b. Huntington's disease
c. Amyotrophic lateral sclerosis
d. Parkinson's disease

155. The medication with a mechanism of action of decreasing insulin resistance and increasing glucose utilization is:

a. Glipizide (Glucotrol)
b. Metformin (Glucophage)
c. Acarbose (Precose)
d. Pioglitazone (Actos)

156. On exam, a patient is found to have a systolic ejection murmur that is heard best at the right second intercostal space and radiating to the neck. Imaging shows a calcified, bicuspid aortic valve. Which of the following would be appropriate at this time?

a. Valve replacement surgery
b. Cardiac catheterization
c. Echocardiogram
d. Temporary valvuloplasty

157. Which of the following is more likely to occur in COPD due to emphysema as opposed to COPD due to bronchitis?

a. Dyspnea on exertion
b. Peripheral edema
c. Productive cough
d. Weight loss

158. A 74-year-old female is seen for weakness and shortness of breath that started this morning. An EKG is completed and shows ST elevation and Q waves in leads II, III, and aVF. The most likely diagnosis is:

a. Anterior wall infarction
b. Inferior wall infarction
c. Lateral wall infarction
d. Posterior wall infarction

159. For a patient diagnosed with schizophrenia, which of the following is usually an indicator of a better outcome with this disease?

a. Age of onset at 20 years old or older
b. Insidious onset of symptoms
c. Slow rate of progression of the illness
d. Low socioeconomic status

160. A patient is seen for complaints of low back pain that radiates into the thighs. An x-ray is completed and shows blurriness over the sacroiliac joints. Labs are completed and the HLA-B27 is positive. The demographic of this patient is most likely:

a. 62-year-old black female
b. 42-year-old white female
c. 17-year-old black male
d. 21-year-old white male

161. A 59-year-old female is seen for complaints of weakness and dyspnea for 2 days. Vital signs show a pulse of 42 bpm and BP of 162/50 mmHg. EKG shows irregularly spaced P waves with wide, slow QRS complexes. The most appropriate intervention for this patient at this time is:

a. IV atropine
b. IV fluid bolus
c. Synchronized cardioversion
d. Temporary pacemaker

162. A patient presents with complaints of general malaise and a throbbing headache over her left temple which has last lasted all day. On exam, the left temporal artery reveals a bounding palpable pulse and scalp tenderness. The most appropriate test to do at this time to confirm the diagnosis is:

a. Ultrasound of the temporal artery
b. Erythrocyte sedimentation rate
c. Temporal artery biopsy
d. Rheumatoid factor

163. In the patient with complaints of decreased hearing in the left ear due to impacted cerumen, what finding would the nurse practitioner expect to see on a Weber test?

a. Sound is heard longer through the air than through bone in the left ear.
b. Sound is heard longer through bone than through the air in the left ear.
c. Sound would lateralize to the left ear.
d. Sound would lateralize to the right ear.

164. The best option for treatment of osteoarthritis in the knees is:

a. Acetaminophen (Tylenol)
b. Naproxen (Naprosyn)
c. Capsaicin cream
d. Hydrocodone (Vicodin)

165. A 52-year-old male has started to play golf after several years of not playing. He has developed pain over the medial side of the right elbow. What would you expect to find on physical exam?

a. Bulging of the biceps muscle
b. Pain with a valgus stress of the elbow
c. Pain with resisted wrist extension
d. Pain with resisted wrist flexion

166. An anterior wall infarction is caused by occlusion of the:

a. Left anterior descending coronary artery
b. Right coronary artery
c. Left circumflex coronary artery
d. Left marginal coronary artery

167. An adult with asthma is using his inhaled daily steroid in addition to needing his inhaled short acting beta agonist. He is also woken up with wheezing a few times a month. Which of the following should be started at this time?

a. Inhaled long-acting beta agonist
b. Inhaled steroid plus a long-acting beta agonist
c. Nebulized short-acting beta agonist
d. Oral steroid on a tapering dose

168. A 65-year-old male with a history of coronary artery disease and hypertension presents with altered mental status for the past 2 hours. On exam, his BP is 220/120 mmHg and papilledema is seen on funduscopic exam. Which of the following should be started immediately?

a. Enalapril
b. Hydralazine
c. Labetalol
d. Nitroglycerin

169. The gold standard for diagnosing polymyositis is:

a. Serum antinuclear antibodies
b. Electromyography
c. Muscle biopsy
d. Serum aldolase level

170. A patient is in the critical care unit being treated for sepsis. On his second day of treatment, he develops hypokalemia that is not responding to potassium administration. Which other electrolyte abnormality should be looked for?

a. Hyperglycemia
b. Hypernatremia
c. Hypocalcemia
d. Hypomagnesemia

171. An Adult-Gerontology Acute Care Nurse Practitioner is working in the ER at a local hospital. At a social function, an acquaintance asks the NP how the daughter of a mutual friend is doing who was brought into the ER the day before with a broken arm. The most appropriate response is:

a. The patient is doing well and will be seeing Orthopedics.
b. To deny having seen the patient.
c. Tell her the patient was seen, but that her care can't discuss.
d. Explain to her that the care or prognosis of any patients cannot be discussed.

172. The ACO health care delivery model:

a. Is available under only certain health insurance plans
b. Was a failed attempt at streamlining patient care across the healthcare spectrum by organizing all aspects of care into one location
c. Focuses on the whole patient and requires all specialties and treatment modalities coordinate their treatment of the patient
d. Uses a traditional transaction-based reimbursement plan

173. The Adult Gerontology Acute Care Nurse Practitioner provides care for:

a. Young adult through geriatric patients
b. Adults age 40 years old and older
c. Patients from birth and older
d. Children and adults, age 10 years old and older

174. In order to obtain the certification to be an Adult Gerontology Acute Care Nurse Practitioner, the provider must have completed:

a. An LPN program, RN program, and an accredited Nurse Practitioner program
b. An RN program and an accredited Nurse Practitioner program
c. An accredited Nurse Practitioner program only
d. An LPN program and an RN program

175. The purpose of nursing informatics is to:

a. Streamline the communication process among health care providers
b. Form a database that can be used by nurses at all professional levels to promote networking
c. Utilize input from all levels of nursing care to formulate information technology resources to provide better care to patients
d. Integrate nursing science with analytics to communicate data and information

Answer Key and Explanations for Test #1

1. C: Speaking quickly or quietly may make it difficult for the woman to hear you. If possible, the interview should be performed outside of the presence of the primary caregiver so you can properly screen for elder abuse. If this is not possible, at least perform that part of the screening while the patient is alone. When interviewing an elderly woman, you should speak in a clear voice at an adequate volume, while facing the patient. Watch for signs that she is tiring or becoming stressed and adjust your technique accordingly, or take a break if necessary.

2. A: These symptoms are characteristic of dementia with Lewy bodies. Cognitive and physical decline is similar to Alzheimer's, but symptoms may fluctuate frequently. This form of dementia may include visual hallucinations, muscle rigidity, and tremors. Frontotemporal dementia may cause marked changes in personality and behavior and is characterized by difficulty using and understanding language. Normal pressure hydrocephalus is characterized by ataxia, memory loss, and urinary incontinence. Parkinson's dementia may involve impaired decision making and difficulty concentrating, learning new material, understanding complex language, and sequencing as well as inflexibility and short- or long-term memory loss.

3. C: The ability to write prescriptions is dictated by the scope of practice, which is set by the state in which the nurse is practicing.

4. D: Patients receiving oral or intravenous steroids should be prescribed oral prednisone in decreasing doses while initiating inhaled steroids. Severe episodes of asthma may occur with withdrawal of oral or IV steroids when switching to inhaled aerosol, so combining inhaled treatment with decreasing doses can help prevent adrenal suppression, which results in acute exacerbation of symptoms. Patients should use a metered-dose inhaler (MDI) with a reservoir device or a formulation with a spacing tube (such as Azmacort) and rinse the mouth thoroughly after inhaling to prevent thrush.

5. B: Medicaid is not always completely free for those who receive aid. Though they cannot bill recipients for medical care, the state is allowed by the federal government to charge a small co-pay. Not everyone who lives below the federal poverty guidelines will qualify for Medicaid. Medicaid is overseen by both the state and federal governments.

6. D: These symptoms are consistent with a duodenal ulcer, and the positive urea breath test indicates a *Helicobacter pylori* infection, which is usually treated with a proton pump inhibitor plus clarithromycin and amoxicillin/metronidazole. About 90% of duodenal ulcers are associated with an *H. pylori* infection. *H. pylori* weakens the mucosa and results in hypersecretion of gastric acid. Eating may increase pain with gastric ulcers but usually relieves pain with duodenal ulcers. Smoking increases the risk of peptic ulcer disease, and use of NSAIDs increases risk of serious complications, such as bleeding or perforation.

7. D: Patients who receive multiple transfusions with citrated blood products must be carefully monitored for hypocalcemia. Calcium is important for transmitting nerve impulses and regulating muscle contraction and relaxation, including the myocardium. Calcium activates enzymes that stimulate chemical reactions and has a role in coagulation of blood. Values include:

- Normal values: 8.2 to 10.2 mg/dL
- Hypocalcemia: <8.2 mg/dL. Critical value: <7 mg/dL
- Hypercalcemia: >10.2 mg/dL. Critical value: >12 mg/dL

Symptoms include tetany, tingling, seizures, altered mental status, and ventricular tachycardia. Treatment is calcium replacement and vitamin D.

8. A: The definition of negligence is a medical professional acting in a way that a reasonable person of the same education and skill level would not, and this action results in patient harm. Disloyalty, acting in an illegal manner, or not acting at all to prevent a patient from being harmed is called malpractice.

9. B: Lyme disease requires mandatory reporting while reporting of the other diseases is voluntary. The CDC maintains a reportable disease list, which is upgraded and revised as necessary and reissued July 1 of each year. Each state also maintains a reportable disease list, which may or may not be identical with that of the CDC, so the nurse must be familiar with all reportable disease requirements. Much data at the state and local level is confidential name-based information, but data collected at the CDC is without names or personal identifying information. Some states require reporting of hospital-acquired infections.

10. A: HCO_3 < 22 mEq/L and pH < 7.35 are consistent with metabolic acidosis, which may result from severe diarrhea, starvation, DKA, kidney failure, and aspirin toxicity. Symptoms may include headache, altered consciousness, agitation, lethargy, and coma. Cardiac dysrhythmias and Kussmaul respiration are common. Other readings:

- HCO_3 > 26 mEq/L and pH > 7.45 are consistent with metabolic alkalosis.
- $PaCO_2$ 35-45 mmHg and PaO_2 ≥ 80 mmHg are normal adult readings.
- $PaCO_2$ > 55 mmHg and PaO_2 < 60 mmHg are consistent with acute respiratory failure in a previously healthy adult.

11. D: Young, thin males are particularly prone to spontaneous pneumothorax, especially following exercise. Shortness of breath would not be present in patients having an aortic dissection, and chest pain would be on the left side if they were having an MI. Asthma generally does not cause chest pain.

12. A: Patients have a right to refuse treatment for religious or other personal reasons, so the most appropriate action is to simply provide the patient with factual information about the disease, treatments, and prognosis in a neutral manner, without trying to coerce or frighten the patient. In some cases, patients may change their minds when presented with information, but the nurse should remain supportive regardless of the patient's decision. Asking the family to intervene is not appropriate and refusal of treatment alone does not suggest the need for referral to a psychologist.

13. A: Given her history, the practitioner should immediately suspect that she has a pulmonary embolus, or a blood clot that passed into the lung tissue. The practitioner should also order an ABG to assess oxygenation, and an ECG and chest x-ray to rule out other causative conditions.

14. C: Wounds should be irrigated with pressures of 10 to 15 psi. An irrigation pressure of <4 psi does not adequately cleanse a wound, and pressures >15 psi can result in trauma to the wound, interfering with healing. A mechanical irrigation device is more effective for irrigation than a bulb syringe, which delivers about ≤2 psi. A 250 mL squeeze bottle supplies about 4.5 psi, adequate for low-pressure cleaning. A 35-mL syringe with a 19-gauge needle provides about 8 psi.

15. C: When the TSH is elevated, it is an indication that the thyroid is in a sluggish (i.e., hypothyroid) state and needs higher amounts of TSH to stimulate production of the thyroid hormones. In primary hypothyroidism, both levels of free T4 and free T3 are low. In cases of subclinical hypothyroidism, free T3 and free T4 are not affected, and their levels remain within the normal range.

16. C: The nurse practitioner should remain supportive and nonjudgmental. "I'll stay with him, and you can come and go as you feel comfortable" supports the daughter's stated desire while still leaving open the opportunity for her to spend time with her father during the death vigil. People react in very different ways to death, and many people have never seen a deceased person and may be very frightened. While many people find comfort in being with a dying friend or family member, this should never be imposed on anyone.

17. D:

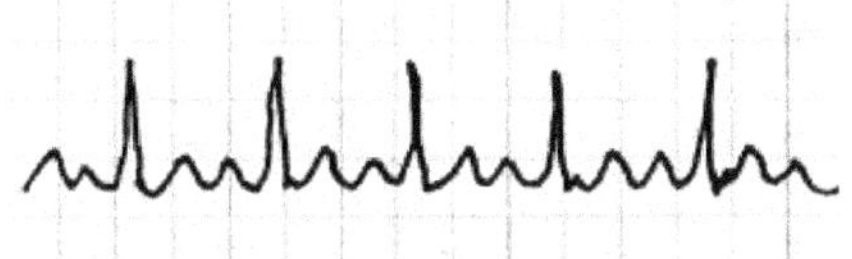

Atrial flutter (AF) occurs when the atrial rate is faster (usually 250-400 beats per minute) than the atrioventricular (AV) node conduction rate so not all of the beats are conducted into the ventricles (ventricular rate 75-150). The beats are effectively blocked at the AV node, preventing ventricular fibrillation although some extra ventricular impulses may go through. AF is caused by the same conditions that cause atrial fibrillation: coronary artery disease, valvular disease, pulmonary disease, heavy alcohol ingestion, and cardiac surgery. Treatment includes:

- Cardioversion if condition is unstable.
- Medications to slow ventricular rate and conduction through AV node: Cardizem®, Calan®.
- Medications to convert to sinus rhythm: Corvert®, Cardioquin®, Norpace®, Cordarone®.

18. A: Except for neurosyphilis, the primary treatment should be penicillin G 2.4 million units IM for one dose. In patients who are allergic to penicillin, the treatment of choice is doxycycline 100 mg PO twice a day for 14 days OR tetracycline 500 mg PO four times a day for 14 days. Pregnant patients are an exception; they should still be given penicillin after undergoing desensitization.

19. D: Aphasia is the loss of ability to use and/or understand written and spoken language because of damage to the speech center of the brain caused by brain tumors, brain injury, and stroke. Global aphasia is characterized by difficulty understanding and producing language in speaking, reading, and writing although patients may understand gestures. The nurse can use pictures, diagrams, and gestures to convey meaning. Picture charts are also useful. The speech pathologist should assess patients with aphasia and provide guidance in communicating with them.

20. B: Although symptoms of pulmonary embolism may vary widely depending on the size and location of the embolus, dyspnea, inspirational chest pain, cough, fever, S4 sound, tachycardia, and non-specific ECG changes in ST and T waves are common. Risk factors include obesity, recent surgery, history of deep vein thrombosis, and inactivity. Treatment includes oxygen, IV fluids, dobutamine for hypotension, analgesia for anxiety, and medications as indicated (digitalis, diuretic, antiarrhythmic). Intubation and mechanical ventilation may be required. Percutaneous filter may be placed in the inferior vena cava to prevent more emboli from reaching lungs.

21. C: Propranolol is a beta-blocker and reduces myocardial demand for oxygen. It also can cause bronchospasm and should be avoided in patients who have any form of bronchospastic disease, such as asthma.

22. B: Gross negligence. Negligence indicates that *proper care* has not been provided, based on established standards. *Reasonable care* uses rationale for decision-making in relation to providing care. Types of negligence:

- Negligent conduct indicates that an individual failed to provide reasonable care or to protect/assist another, based on standards and expertise.
- Gross negligence is willfully providing inadequate care while disregarding the safety and security of another.
- Contributory negligence involves the injured party contributing to his or her own harm.
- Comparative negligence attempts to determine what percentage amount of negligence is attributed to each individual involved.

23. B: Erythromycin lessens theophylline's effectiveness and should not be prescribed in a patient who is taking theophylline. Consider an alternate antibiotic.

24. A: These symptoms are consistent with fat embolism syndrome (FES), which may cause rapid acute pulmonary edema and ARDS, so the patient should be immediately provided with high-flow oxygen. Controlled-volume ventilation with positive end-expiratory pressure (PEEP) may be indicated to prevent/treat pulmonary edema. Corticosteroids may reduce inflammation of the lungs and reduce cerebral edema. Vasopressors prevent hypotension and interstitial pulmonary edema. Morphine with a benzodiazepine may be indicated for patients who require artificial ventilation.

25. A: The therapeutic serum levels for valproic acid is between 50 and 100 mcg/mL. Clonazepam therapeutic serum levels are between 20 and 80 ng/mL. Carbamazepine should be maintained at serum levels of 4 to 12 mcg/mL, and phenytoin should be maintained at serum levels of 10 to 20 mcg/mL.

26. A: Since Lasix® and metolazone are both diuretics and aminophylline and doxapram are both methylxanthines, this list probably indicates polypharmacy. Older adults are especially at risk for polypharmacy—taking too many drugs—because of taking the same drug under generic and brand names, taking drugs for one condition but contraindicated for another, and taking drugs that are not compatible. Reasons for polypharmacy include multiple prescriptions from different doctors; forgetfulness; confusion; failure to report current medications; the use of supplemental, over-the-counter, and herbal preparations in addition to prescribed medications; and failure of healthcare providers to adequately educate the patient.

27. A: These symptoms are consistent with cardiogenic shock. Cardiogenic shock has 3 characteristics: Increased preload, increased afterload, and decreased contractibility. Together these result in a decreased cardiac output and an increase in systemic vascular resistance (SVR) to compensate and protect vital organs. This results in an increase of afterload in the left ventricle with increased need for oxygen. As the cardiac output continues to decrease, tissue perfusion decreases, coronary artery perfusion decreases, fluid backs up, and the left ventricle fails to adequately pump the blood, resulting in pulmonary edema and right ventricular failure.

28. B: Older adults are most impacted by deteriorating vision (presbyopia, cataracts), which prevents them from reading and navigating safely. Most people older than 60 require glasses. People may be less sensitive to color differences (particularly blues and greens), and night vision decreases. Hearing impairment (impacted cerumen, presbycusis) may require periodic cleaning of the ears or hearing aids. Taste and smell usually remain fairly intact although smell of airborne chemicals may be less acute, and taste buds begin to atrophy around age 60, affecting the ability to taste sweet and salt especially. The sense of touch is usually somewhat reduced in older adults.

29. C: Fever, malaise, abdominal pain, and hepatosplenomegaly in an HIV-positive patient with CD4 count <200 may result from histoplasmosis, Mycobacterium avium complex, and bacillary peliosis. Fever, cough, and dyspnea may indicate Pneumocystis jiroveci pneumonia, bacterial pneumonia, and TB. Fever, headache, neck pain, and altered mental status may indicate toxoplasmosis, herpes encephalitis, and CNS lymphoma. Fever with asymmetric or unilateral lymphadenopathy may indicate TB, non-Hodgkin's lymphoma, and bacillary angiomatosis.

30. B: Breakpoint for risk, moderate prognosis. Six assessment areas include sensory perception, moisture, activity, mobility, usual nutrition pattern, and friction and sheer. The first four categories are scored from 1 (worst) to 4 (best) and the last category (friction and sheer) is scored from 1 to 3. The scores for all six items are totaled and a risk assigned according to the number.

- 23: (Best score) excellent prognosis, very minimal risk
- ≤16: Breakpoint for risk of pressure ulcer (will vary somewhat for different populations)
- 6: (Worst score) prognosis very poor, strong likelihood of developing pressure ulcers

31. A: Post-herpetic neuralgia is a chronic pain condition that responds poorly to opioids and is better treated with anticonvulsants, such as gabapentin. Tricyclic antidepressants are also used but may have severe side effects in the elderly. Because the patient has been on high doses of hydrocodone, he may experience withdrawal with abrupt discontinuation of the drug, so the dose should be decreased by one tablet every 2 to 3 days while gabapentin is started at a low dose and slowly increased to reduce incidence of side effects. Morphine pumps and NSAIDs are usually avoided with warfarin and are often ineffective.

32. C: CAM: Assesses development of delirium. Factors indicative of delirium include:

- Onset: Acute change in mental status.
- Attention: Inattentive, stable, or fluctuating.
- Thinking: Disorganized, rambling conversation, switching topics, illogical.
- Level of consciousness: Altered, ranging from alert to coma.
- Orientation: Disoriented (person, place, time).
- Memory: Impaired.
- Perceptual disturbances: Hallucinations, illusions.
- Psychomotor abnormalities: Agitation (tapping, picking, moving) or retardation (staring, not moving).
- Sleep-wake cycle: Awake at night and sleepy in the daytime.

MMSE and Mini-Cog are used to assess evidence of dementia or short-term memory loss, often associated with Alzheimer's disease. GDS is a self-assessment tool to identify older adults with depression.

33. B: Airway obstruction often results in FEV_1 that is more reduced than FVC because the air is trapped and cannot be readily expelled in one second. Normally, FEV_1 is about 80% of vital capacity with most of the remaining air expelled by 3 seconds (FEV_3). Proportional reduction of both FEV_1 and FVC indicate reduced lung expansion. Depression of respiratory centers results from anesthesia or sedation. Limitation in neurological impulses results from damage to the brain or spinal cord.

34. A: The first priority should be to attend to the patient's comfort needs by assessing diet needs, including food allergies, and ordering food. Because the patient has a history of falls, the nurse practitioner should institute a program of fall prevention, assessing the best methods to prevent injury to the patient. The nurse should then review all medications to ensure that no ongoing medical needs are overlooked, as patients may not provide full information in the emergency department. Cognitive abilities are best assessed when the patient is comfortable and rested.

35. C: A score of 10 on the Glasgow Coma Scale (GCS) indicates a moderate head injury. GCS measures the depth and duration of coma or impaired level of consciousness and is used for postoperative/brain injury assessment. The GCS measures three parameters—best eye response, best verbal response, and best motor response—with a total possible score that ranges from 3 to 15. Injuries/conditions are classified according to the total score:

- 3-8 coma
- ≥8 severe head injury
- 9-12 moderate head injury
- 13-15 mild head injury

36. B: These laboratory findings indicate hypothyroidism, which is characterized by increased TSH, decreased free T4, and normal free T3. Normal values for an older adult:

- TSH: 0.32-5.0 mIU/mL.
- Free T4: 4.5-12 µg/dL
- Free T3: 75-200 ng/dL.

Hyperthyroidism is characterized by decreased TSH (<0.30), increased free T4 and increased T3. Additional tests may be indicated for those with comorbidities and multiple medications. Thyroid autoantibody tests are used to help diagnose Hashimoto's thyroiditis.

37. A: Because zoledronic acid may result in decreased renal function in acute renal failure, a serum creatinine and calculation of creatinine clearance should be done before every dose. Zoledronic acid is contraindicated with creatinine clearance <35 mL/min or with severe renal impairment. Additional treatments are withheld if renal deterioration occurs and not resumed until creatinine is within 10% of baseline value. Normal CC values: Adult male: 97-137 mL/min: Adult female: 88-128 mL/min. During treatment, patients should receive calcium (500 mg) and vitamin D (400 IU) supplements daily unless the patient has hypercalcemia.

38. D: The most common comorbidities (with approximate percentages) for those hospitalized include:

Hypertension: 30%	CHF: 6%
COPD: 12%	Hypothyroidism: 6%
Diabetes: 12%	Depression/bipolar disorder: 5%
Fluid/electrolyte imbalance: 12%	Neurological disorder: 4%
Iron deficiency/anemia: 8%	Obesity: 4%

Comorbidities vary according to age. In those under 18 and over 80, fluid and electrolyte disorders from dehydration or excess fluids predominate while hypertension is most common for those over 18. Diabetes is the next most common disorder for those under 80.

39. D: Thiazides, such as hydrochlorothiazide, are indicated to increase reabsorption of calcium with calcium-containing renal calculi. Allopurinol and vitamin B6 are used with oxalate-containing stones. Alpha-mercato-propionyl-glycine (aMPG) and captopril are used with cystine-containing stones if increasing hydration and alkalinization is ineffective. Indomethacin is used with allopurinol to maintain uric acid levels. Alkalinizing agents, such as Polycitra and Allopurinol, are used with uric acid stones. Additional medications can include antibiotics if infection occurs. Some patients may require opioids, such as morphine, to control pain.

40. C: When prescribing an oral anti-diabetic agent for an older patient, the patient's initial dose should be 50% of the usual dose.

Problems associated with older adults and different types of drugs	
Anti-diabetics	Oral anti-diabetic agents should be started at 50% of the usual dose because of the danger of hypoglycemia. First generation drugs should be avoided. Glucotrol® has fewer side effects than Diabeta®.
Antidepressants	Antidepressants are associated with excess sedation, so typical doses are only 16-33% of a younger adult's dose. SSRIs are safest, but Prozac® should be avoided because it may cause anorexia, anxiety, and insomnia.
Anticoagulants	Anticoagulants may cause severe bleeding in those over 65. Warfarin should be used with care and at a lower dose if total protein or albumin concentration is low.

41. A: Tests for diagnosis of rheumatoid arthritis in the presence of joint involvement of the small joints (fingers, wrists) or large joints (elbows, hips, knees) includes primarily RF and ACPA. ESR and CRP may also show elevation but are less specific. Diagnosis is usually made if 4 of 7 positive symptoms for RA are present: morning stiffness >1 hour, ≥2 involved joints with involvement of wrists, or finger joints >6 weeks, bilateral and symmetrical involvement, presence of rheumatoid nodules, joint destruction on x-ray, and positive RF or ACPA.

42. B: Influenza requires droplet precautions, using a mask.

Contact	Use personal protective equipment (PPE), including gown and gloves, for all contacts with the patient or patient's immediate environment. Maintain patient in private room or >3 feet away from other patients.
Droplet	Use mask while caring for the patient. Maintain patient in a private room or >3 feet away from other patients with curtain separating them. Use patient mask if transporting patient from one area to another.
Airborne	Place patient in an airborne infection isolation room. Use ≥N95 respirators (or masks) while caring for patient.

43. D: Chemical debridement is used for chronic wounds (burns, ulcers) with necrotic tissue and eschar. However, the enzymes (collagenase and papain/urea) require a moist environment, so the eschar must be cross-hatched through the upper layers before the enzyme is administered. The pH must remain between 6 and 8 to prevent inactivation. Hexachlorophene, Burrow's solution, and heavy metal ions also inactivate the enzymes. Collagenase is applied one time daily, either directly to the wound for deep wounds or to gauze packing for shallow wounds.

44. A: These VS changes are consistent with increasing intracranial pressure. Typical findings include widened pulse pressure, with rising blood pressure and depressed heart rate. Because the patient is drunk, evaluating level of consciousness can be difficult, but lethargy, confusion, and restlessness are characteristic of increasing ICP. Stress response usually results in increased BP and pulse. Ethanol intoxication usually causes hypotension, bradycardia with arrhythmias, and respiratory depression. Delirium tremens includes tremors, tachycardia, and cardiac dysrhythmias.

45. B: "Patient is spitting at nurses, throwing magazines, and refusing to get out of bed for therapy" describes the patient's behavior without placing a value judgment ("belligerent and uncooperative"), which might indicate bias against the patient. The nurse should avoid interpreting behavior ("appears to dislike") or characterizing what's in a patient's mind ("Patient believes"). Patients, especially older adults or those who are confused, may behave in a difficult manner if they are afraid, in pain, or overwhelmed, so the nurse should attempt to find the reason for the behavior.

46. A: St. John's wort may interact with antibiotics, birth control pills, antidepressants, warfarin, anticonvulsants, MAO inhibitors, antivirals, immunosuppressants, and migraine drugs. Melatonin may interact with NSAIDS, antihypertensives, steroids, and anti-anxiety medications. Echinacea may interact with immunosuppressants and steroids. Vitamin B complex is safe to take with warfarin, as it does not affect the INR; however, multivitamins with vitamin K may. If patients take a multivitamin during warfarin therapy, they should do so daily and not intermittently so that intake of vitamin K does not fluctuate. Vitamin C should be limited to 500 mg daily and vitamin E to 400 IU daily.

47. D: Root cause analysis is a retrospective attempt to determine the cause of an event. Regression analysis compares the relationship between two variables to determine if the relationship correlates. T-test is used to analyze data to determine if there is a statistically significant difference in the means of two groups. The t-test looks at two sets of things that are similar, such as exercise in women over 65 with cancer and over 65 without cancer. Tracer methodology is a method that looks at the continuum of care a patient receives from admission to post-discharge.

48. D: The best solution is a referral to a home health agency to provide in-home care, as this ensures that the woman will receive skilled nursing care and be able to stay at home and supervise her granddaughter. A 12-year-old is too young for the responsibility of wound care. The patient's dependence on public transportation and difficulty walking precludes outpatient care. Home health care is a more cost-effective solution than transferring the patient to an extended care facility, which would leave the granddaughter without care. Medicare will not pay for extended hospital care for healing wounds.

49. B: This is an example of selection bias because those with catheters without clinically evident infections were excluded. The results are skewed because many patients may have subclinical infections. Information bias occurs when there are errors in classification, so an estimate of association is incorrect. Information bias may be non-differential or differential. Compliance bias occurs when adherence to protocol is inconsistent. Admission bias occurs when some groups, such as spinal cord injury patients, are omitted from the study.

50. D: These symptoms are consistent with pacemaker syndrome.

Mild	Pulsations evident in neck and abdomen. Cardiac palpitations. Headache and feeling of anxiety. General malaise and unexplained weakness. Pain or "fullness" in jaw, chest.
Moderate	Increasing dyspnea on exertion with accompanying orthopnea Dizziness, vertigo, increasing confusion. Feeling of choking.
Severe	Increasing pulmonary edema with dyspnea even at rest and crackling rales. Syncope. Heart failure.

51. A: The type of pneumonia that is most common in a person who is normally healthy is community-acquired pneumonia. Without any other co-morbidities present, the most appropriate treatment is with azithromycin. Clarithromycin and doxycycline are also options for treatment if there is an allergy to azithromycin.

52. D: The ATLAS trial evaluated the benefits of long-term tamoxifen treatment in thousands of women worldwide who had been treated for breast cancer. It was found that completing a ten-year treatment with tamoxifen provided longer survival rates and a lower repeat incidence of breast cancer.

53. B: Beta blockers have been shown to decrease catecholamine stimulation in patients with CHF. Catecholamine has been found to impair heart function by affecting ejection fraction, ventricular hypertrophy, and even contributing to cardiac muscle cell death. By decreasing the amount of catecholamine present, the heart is not subjected to the potential injury that can occur.

54. C: An increased TSH level and decreased T4 level would indicate mild hypothyroidism and her medication dosage should be increased. It is recommended that levothyroxine be increased in increments of 0.0125 to 0.025 mg and then have labs rechecked before adjusting the medication again.

55. B: Gentamicin ear drops should not be used if a perforated ear drum is present. This may cause systemic absorption of the medication which can increase the risk of ototoxicity and hearing loss. If indicated, oral medications should be used.

56. A: Valacyclovir (Valtrex) should be dosed at 1 g PO three times daily for 7 days for an acute outbreak of herpes zoster. This dose should be adjusted as appropriate for the patient suffering from renal insufficiency. Two other medications that can be used to treat this condition are Famvir and Zovirax.

57. D: Certain medications categorized as proton pump inhibitors (Nexium, Prilosec, Prevacid), can decrease the effectiveness of Plavix, which may cause an increased risk of cardiac events. They prevent full absorption of the medication. Dexilant is a PPI, but has been found to be safe when taken with Plavix.

58. C: Though it has been effective at treating urinary tract infections in females, nitrofurantoin has been shown to not be as effective in men due to low tissue concentrations of the drug. Nitrofurantoin has also been shown to not be effective at treating underlying prostatitis. Medications from the fluoroquinolone class and sulfa drugs are usually the best antibiotics to use, pending urine culture results.

59. B: The biologic agents used for treatment of rheumatoid arthritis pose an increased risk of lymphoma. Therefore, any patients with lymphoma or a history of lymphoma, cannot receive medications from this class. The CBC is routinely monitored in those patients who are taking a biologic agent.

60. A: Acetaminophen would be the safest due to its tolerability. The other medications listed are NSAIDs which pose the threat of GI bleed and increased risk of cardiovascular events. NSAIDs can be used in low doses for limited periods of time in this class of patients, but this should be monitored.

61. C: There is no known cure for dementia. Cholinesterase inhibitors have been proven to have some success with controlling some of the symptoms of dementia and in slowing down the progression of the disease. Unfortunately, the symptoms do continue to worsen with time.

62. D: Long-acting bronchodilators can be very effective at controlling the symptoms of COPD. When a patient is having to use their short-acting bronchodilator several times during the day, a long-acting medication should be considered to better control the symptoms and decrease the risk of exacerbations of the disease.

63. B: Clarithromycin can interfere with the efficacy of Plavix by decreasing its effectiveness. This could lead to an increased risk of blood clots. A different antibiotic should be chosen, when possible, for those patients who are taking Plavix for anticoagulation.

64. D: Sarcoidosis can cause chronic inflammation in the eyes that can cause granulomatous growths in the conjunctiva. Uveitis is another common ocular finding with this disease. Routine eye exams are necessary for patients with this disorder.

65. A: Rales develop with congestive heart failure due to fluid-filled alveoli in the lungs. Wheezing is normally seen with COPD due to airway constriction. Stridor is present with croup.

66. B: The murmur associated with aortic stenosis is best described as a mid-systolic ejection murmur. It is heard best over the righter, upper sternal border. An early peaking murmur is usually heard with a milder form of the disease while a late peaking murmur is usually heard when the aortic stenosis is more advanced.

67. A: Koilonychia, or "spooning," is most often associated with iron-deficiency anemia. The nails are very thin and may break or chip easily. This usually occurs when the anemia has been present for a lengthy amount of time. A CBC should be obtained to assess the severity of anemia.

68. C: Being of older age and male are the two biggest risk factors to developing an abdominal aortic aneurysm. Other risk factors include hypertension, COPD, smoking, and peripheral arterial disease.

69. D: It is no longer recommended that routine, annual PSA screening be performed. It has been found that this often leads to unnecessary prostate biopsy procedures and an increased risk of adverse outcomes from the biopsy. A digital rectal exam is still felt to be a helpful screening tool for prostate lesions.

70. D: The four main symptoms of Parkinson's disease are a tremor, bradykinesia, stiffness of the extremities or trunk, and postural instability causing frequent falls. At least two of these symptoms must be present in order to make a diagnosis of Parkinson's disease. There is not one, definitive test for Parkinson's disease. Rather, the diagnosis is made based on these clinical findings.

71. C: Actos has a black box warning for its risk of increasing the incidence of congestive heart failure. With there being multiple medications on the market to treat type 2 diabetes, it should be avoided with those patients who are known to have congestive heart failure.

72. D: Upon initial diagnosis, CLL is usually not treated with chemotherapy or radiation. The symptoms are monitored and treatment is reserved for later in the course of the disease. Early treatment has not been shown to prolong life or decrease the progression of the disease.

73. A: With severe psoriasis, topical treatments frequently are not strong enough to effectively decrease the lesions. For third party payment purposes, the failure of methotrexate to effectively control the symptoms of psoriasis is usually required for approval for treatment with a biologic drug.

74. B: Any tubes, including IV tubing, should be cut with the end still inserted in the body. It is Jewish tradition that the body be buried in its entirety, with as much of the blood and tissue left intact as possible. The funeral home will remove any devices or tubing while following Jewish law.

75. C: Alzheimer's dementia is the most common form of dementia today. According to the Alzheimer's Association, there are approximately 5.5 million people just in the United States who are living with Alzheimer's disease.

76. B: According to the American Society of Addiction Medicine, drug overdose is the leading cause of accidental death in the U.S. Of the more than 70,000 drug overdose-related deaths in 2017, 70% were due to overdose of opioids.

77. D: The LVAD was designed to function as a pump to assist the left ventricle with muscle contraction and increase cardiac output. It is used for patients waiting for a heart transplant and for those who are not a candidate for transplantation, but who will require the device long-term.

78. C: The current recommendations regarding cervical cancer screening state that Pap smears should be done every 3 years for women age 21 to 65. This can be lengthened to every 5 years with a Pap smear and HPV testing for women age 30 to 65. Screening is not recommended for women under the age of 21 or over the age of 65 if they have never had an abnormal Pap smear in the past.

79. A: Acute gout occurs when the body does not excrete enough uric acid and it accumulates within a joint space. A serum uric acid level is usually elevated with this condition. One way to prevent gout flare-ups is to eat a low-purine diet.

80. B: Palliative care is often utilized to offer a patient the extra care or therapy they need when faced with a chronic illness. Some palliative care patients will "graduate" from this and others may need to transition to hospice care as their chronic disease progresses.

81. C: Biopsy of the temporal artery is the most accurate method used to diagnose temporal arteritis. MRI may be helpful in identifying which segment of the artery is most affected, but it is not considered a standard of care at this time. Ultrasound and angiography are not considered reliable methods in which to diagnose the disease at this time.

82. D: The MMSE is used as a preliminary screening tool for determining whether a patient has some cognitive impairment, however, it does have its limitations. Patients over the age of 60 and those with a low education level have been shown to score lower on the test than others. Further testing and work up is indicated in order to make the diagnosis of dementia, so this should not be relied upon alone.

83. C: A common misconception in the dietary needs of patients taking Coumadin is that they are not allowed to eat leafy, green vegetables. This is not true. If they very rarely eat any of these types of vegetables, and suddenly greatly increase their intake of them, the INR level used to measure the therapeutic level of Coumadin will be decreased. The best advice is to continue with their normal diet without any great fluctuations in the amount of leafy greens they eat to maintain a consistent INR reading. Citrus fruits and red meat do not have an effect on the INR value.

84. A: Enteral nutrition is generally utilized before parenteral nutrition due to its lower risk of potential complications. The formula used to calculate the dosage of enteral nutrition a patient receives daily is 25 kcal/kg/day plus 1.5 g protein/kg/day. This is the formula used to maintain an adequate nutrition status for the patient. Insulin is usually necessary to help control glucose levels.

85. B: While all of these choices are adequate at lowering blood pressure, lisinopril would be the best choice because of its renal protection qualities. He has been diagnosed with type 2 diabetes and an ACE inhibitor is recommended for diabetics to help provide some protection from diabetes-associated renal insufficiency.

86. C: These are the modifiable risk factors used to calculate a patient's cardiac risk, which identifies whether they have an increased risk of a cardiovascular event occurring. Age and gender are not modifiable risk factors. Identifying those patients with an increased cardiac risk can help to implement a treatment plan to try to prevent the complications of cardiovascular disease.

87. D: In patients with glaucoma, prednisone orally and any steroid via eye drop should be avoided. These can cause an increase in intraocular pressure, which can worsen glaucoma symptoms. Patients receiving the steroid via an eye drop are going to be more likely to develop the increase in pressure.

88. B: Severe hyperkalemia is classified as a serum potassium level >7 mEq/L. When the potassium level is slightly elevated, tall and peaked T waves can be seen on EKG. As this worsens, the PR segment becomes longer and the P waves eventually disappear. Once severe, the changes listed here are present on EKG. If this continues to worsen, it will result in cardiac arrest.

89. C: Metabolic alkalosis will cause the arterial blood pH and bicarbonate levels to increase. Conversely, metabolic acidosis will cause arterial pH and bicarbonate levels to decrease. Respiratory acidosis will increase the arterial carbon dioxide level while decreasing the pH, and respiratory alkalosis will have the opposite results with a decrease in CO_2 level and an increased pH.

90. A: The T-score is the measure used with bone densitometry, or DEXA, scans to determine whether someone has adequate bone density, if they are osteopenic, or if they have osteoporosis. A T-score -1.0 or higher is considered normal. A T-score of -1.0 through -2.5 indicates osteopenia is present. A T-score of -2.5 or less indicates osteoporosis.

91. B: The FEV1 is the amount of air that can be exhaled within the first second after inhaling the maximum amount of air a person can inhale (the FVC). The normal range for the FEV1 and the FVC is 80-120%. The FEV1/FVC ratio is calculated and should be about 85%. A decrease in FEV1 and the FEV1/FVC ratio indicates asthma as a diagnosis.

92. B: Within the Hispanic culture, men are the primary decision makers and the leaders of the family. Men are usually the providers for the family and will often make the medical decisions for all family members.

93. D: In order for a CHF patient to qualify for hospice care, they must be suffering from chronic, debilitating symptoms of the disease despite being on maximum medical treatment. In addition to this, the ejection fraction should be less than or equal to 20%. Once these conditions are met, the patient is considered a candidate for hospice care.

94. D: One of the first signs that an acute intravascular hemolytic reaction is occurring is pain at the IV site. Other early signs include fever, chills, elevated heart rate, nausea, and dyspnea. This potentially life-threatening reaction usually occurs within 10 minutes of the beginning of the infusion of blood or blood products.

95. A: The half-life of dopamine is less than 2 minutes, so the total time in which the effects from the medication are seen is around 10 minutes. Dopamine is used to improve heart function, increase blood pressure, and increase renal perfusion.

96. C: At least 150 minutes of moderate aerobic activity is recommended for elderly patients weekly. This includes activities such as bike riding or walking. It is important to stress to patients that the whole body needs to be exercised and some strength training should also be performed to maintain joint and muscle health.

97. B: Crohn's disease is less likely to cause rectal bleeding, whereas rectal bleeding is more common with ulcerative colitis. This may be due, in part, to the location of the diseases within the GI tract. Crohn's disease can affect any portion of the GI tract from the mouth to the anus. Ulcerative colitis is confined to the colon.

98. C: According to the U. S. Preventive Services Task Force, routine screening mammography is not recommended in women 75 years old and older. It is felt that this age group may be more adversely affected by complications from over-diagnosing breast cancer. This population of patients are also at much greater risk of dying from other medical conditions rather than from any breast cancer that is detected.

99. B: The Centers for Disease Control does not recommend the routine use of antivirals for flu prophylaxis due to the risk of promoting viral resistance to the medication. Tamiflu is recommended for prophylactic therapy for those who are immunocompromised, those who could potentially suffer great complications if they were to contract the flu, and in a group living situation in which there is a flu outbreak. It is not recommended that anyone receive the prophylaxis treatment if they cannot be treated within 48 hours of their first exposure to the person who had the flu.

100. A: There is a 1% chance that a patient with a penicillin allergy may develop an allergic response to cefdinir, or other drugs in the cephalosporin class. The benefit of the cephalosporin with certain illnesses often outweighs the risk of developing a reaction. Unless there is no other choice, cephalosporins are avoided if the patient has had an anaphylactic reaction to medications in the penicillin class.

101. A: A Kosher diet is very specific in its guidelines regarding how and where foods are prepared, and which foods can be prepared together or must be kept separately. The best answer is to discuss this with the patient to make sure their dietary guidelines are followed. Most hospitals will have pre-made Kosher meals that can be heated to accommodate this diet.

102. C: A person with AB+ blood is considered a universal recipient because they can receive blood or blood products of any type. A universal donor would be a person with type O- blood. The most restricted recipient blood type is O- because those patients can only receive O- blood or blood products.

103. D: Ipratropium and albuterol can be given independent of each other, but they work well together to help with bronchospasm. The ipratropium works as an anticholinergic to dilate the airway while albuterol helps to relax the bronchial smooth muscle to prevent bronchospasm. They are both considered short-acting medications.

104. C: Even if a medication or supplement is natural or herbal, this does not necessarily mean that it is safe. St. John's Wart is a common herbal supplement given to help with symptoms of depression. It is relatively safe, but can be dangerous when given along with some prescription medications. It most commonly will affect the drug level or metabolism rate of certain prescription medications. In this case with Abilify, it will decrease the drug level of the prescription drug.

105. A: Calcium excretion is increased when a person receives Lasix. In the geriatric patient, this can affect bone density if it becomes severe. Calcium levels should be monitored and supplementation administered if necessary.

106. B: Airport security generally does not interfere with the function of an implanted pacemaker device. It is important to carry the identification card with the pacemaker information, but the metal in the device may or may not set off the security alarms. If airport personnel request a more thorough search, request a hand-patted exam. If a handheld metal detection device is used, advise them that it cannot be held directly over the pacemaker device for more than a second.

107. A: Mittens are not considered a restraint because they do not immobilize the hands or fingers. If they are tight and constrict movement, they would be considered a restraint. Mittens are used to prevent patients from picking, scratching, or grasping IV and oxygen lines and removing them.

108. B: Tracheostomy care can be taught to caregivers so this can be performed at home without having a Respiratory Therapist come to the home each day. The trach tube can be reused at home once it has been cleaned with soap and water and once mucus inside the tube has been cleaned out. In the hospital setting, trach care is done using aseptic technique to prevent contamination, but it is done under "clean" conditions at home.

109. D: Whenever possible, have an interpreter present in these types of situations, ideally one who has undergone some training in medical terminology. Using a family member is not ideal because without medical training a person will likely mistranslate medical terms and instructions. Online software may not be accurate and there is no way to verify that the terms and concepts are being interpreted appropriately.

110. A: Generally, patients dealing with liver disease need to decrease their sodium intake to help prevent swelling. Though some protein is needed in the diet, the majority of calories should come from carbohydrates, followed by fats, and then protein, which should be low.

111. C: There are two main types of macular degeneration: wet and dry. Wet macular degeneration involves formation of leaky blood vessels behind the retina. Dry macular degeneration occurs when there is wearing away of the center of the retina. Both forms can result in permanent blindness.

112. B: A urinary tract infection will usually cause dysuria, urinary frequency, and urinary urgency. These classic symptoms are usually not very pronounced, though, in the elderly population, especially those with underlying dementia, confusion is very common, along with other behavior changes.

113. D: Zantac is the only medication of these that will require a dosage adjustment in those patients with renal failure. Once the creatinine clearance becomes less than 50 mL/min., the dosage of Zantac needs to be decreased.

114. B: Sepsis is the most common cause of ARDS. Severe infection causes vascular instability within the lungs which leads to leakage of blood from the blood vessels to the lung tissue. This prevents adequate oxygenation of the blood and results in hypoxemia and multi-system organ failure due to poor perfusion.

115. C: One of the earliest signs of digoxin toxicity is a yellowish discoloration in vision, especially while looking at light. This is called xanthopsia. A digoxin level should be drawn and the normal range is 0.5-2 ng/mL.

116. D: An iatrogenic condition is caused as a result of any medication, treatment, procedure, or a combination thereof. This includes expected or adverse negative effects from a medication that is necessary to treat an illness. This is not necessarily a negative outcome, though, such as weight loss with some diabetic medications.

117. A: Stage I decubitus ulcers exhibit erythematous skin with no breakdown present. Stage II decubitus ulcers have a partial thickness skin loss with the dermis being visible. Stage III decubitus ulcers have a full thickness skin loss with exposed adipose tissue and sometimes eschar present.

118. B: Primary care is the care received by the primary care physician and is usually the first care a patient receives. Secondary care involves care from specialists and may involve services provided in a hospital. Tertiary care is the management and recovery from an acute or chronic illness that requires more intensive therapies. An example would be the services a patient receives at a skilled nurse facility following a total hip replacement.

119. C: Past abdominal surgeries can cause adhesions within the abdominal cavity. This has been found to be the most common cause of a small bowel obstruction due to the scar tissue affecting the motility of the small intestine. Frequent use of pain medications may also slow down GI motility, leading to constipation and small bowel obstruction, but this is not seen as often as adhesions as a cause for this condition.

120. A: Basic ADLs are those activities which are necessary for basic care. These include bathing, dressing, personal hygiene, and feeding oneself. Intermediate ADLs are more advanced activities, such as cooking, cleaning, driving, and managing medications. Advanced ADLs are the most advanced activities such as performing work duties, fulfilling family responsibilities, and participating in community activities.

121. C: According to the U.S. Preventive Services Task Force, it is recommended that adults age 50 through 75 undergo colorectal screening. It is recommended that a fecal occult blood test be performed every year with sigmoidoscopy every 5 years and colonoscopy every 10 years. These guidelines are for those patients who have not had a personal history of colorectal cancer.

122. B: Acupuncture is an ancient Chinese remedy that has been proven to help relieve some types of pain. The philosophy behind acupuncture is that the placement of very small needles helps to stimulate the central nervous system to release natural chemicals in the body that can help to decrease pain. It is also thought that acupuncture could help to release immune cells in the body.

123. C: A gout flare-up can be triggered by eating any foods which are high in purines. This includes meat, some seafood (such as trout), and any type of alcohol. Aged cheeses, shellfish, and processed foods are also known to be high in purines.

124. A: Prolonged straining that occurs with coughing, excessive vomiting, or weight lifting can cause the tiny surface capillaries to rupture, leading to the small, bruised-appearing lesions on the skin. These are especially evident on the face, neck, and chest.

125. D: Tetanus is caused by the *Clostridium tetani* spores that enter an open wound and mature into bacteria. This has a detrimental effect on the motor neurons which leads to severe muscle spasms. The spasms can be severe enough to break the underlying bones. A tetanus shot should be given every 10 years to prevent the disease from occurring.

126. D: Dysgeusia is a strong, foul taste in the mouth. This is often described as a metallic taste but can take different forms. Calcium channel blockers and some antibiotics, except for amoxicillin, are likely to cause this side effect.

127. C: Age alone is not a contraindication to undergoing a surgical procedure for ischemic heart disease. Given his other co-morbidities, however, this patient would not be a good surgical candidate.

128. B: The murmur associated with mitral valve stenosis is heard best over the apex of the heart while a patient is standing or performing a Valsalva maneuver. During those activities, the volume within the left ventricle is decreased, which makes the murmur worse. If the patient is squatting, there is an increase in venous return and diastolic filling which will hold the valve shut and decrease the murmur.

129. A: Medicare Part A covers the services available outside of a physician's office. This includes hospitalization, skilled nursing home care for the first 100 days after a 3-day hospital stay, hospice care, home care, and durable medical equipment. Medicare Part B covers the care provided within the physician's office.

130. B: Anticholinergic drugs can help with some of the rigidity seen with Parkinson's, but they do little to help with the bradykinesia. The side effects seen with this class of drugs can be more severe in elderly populations. The other medications listed are helpful with all of the symptoms of Parkinson's disease.

131. B: All of the choices are modifications that should be made to improve his general overall health, but smoking is the leading cause of cardiovascular death. He should work on all of these habits, but the smoking should go first.

132. A: As long as there is still sympathetic and parasympathetic nerve innervation, a light shined into the opposite eye will cause both pupils to constrict. If a light is shined into the blind eye, neither pupil will change.

133. B: Oral thrush lesions respond well to the antifungal fluconazole. Another option is to use nystatin in liquid form as a mouthwash.

134. A: A deficiency in vitamin A can cause xerosis, or dry conjunctivae, and the white patches are called Bitot's spots. The patient will often have problems with decreased vision at night. Vitamin A is found in foods rich in beta carotene, such as carrots.

135. A: With the discoloration present in this skin lesion, there is some concern for malignant melanoma. Excisional biopsy with clean margins is the preferred method for removing this lesion for it to be fully assessed. Though the ABCDs are always assessed with skin lesions, not all of the factors need to have negative findings in order for the skin lesion to be concerning.

136. D: A spiral CT of the chest is the most accurate, non-invasive assessment for a pulmonary embolism. The pulmonary angiogram is considered the gold standard to definitively diagnose, but it is invasive and has its risks. If there is a low probability of a pulmonary embolism, a D-dimer can be performed, and if it is negative, it will rule out the presence of an embolus.

137. C: An S3 is present when there is increased resistance in the ventricle as the atria are emptying. It is present with congestive heart failure. An S4 is the extra heart sound heard when there is increased resistance in the ventricle as the atria are contracting. An ejection click is heard with mitral valve prolapse or aortic stenosis. A thrill is felt when a harsh murmur is present.

138. A: Of these symptoms, only the elevated jugular venous pressure is seen in right-sided heart failure. All of the other symptoms listed are present with left-sided heart failure.

139. C: His symptoms sound more like the source of bleeding could be from the upper portion of the GI tract. Because of this, an upper endoscopy procedure would be best to visualize the esophagus, stomach, and duodenum. A colonoscopy is indicated when the lower GI tract needs further evaluation.

140. A: A positive PPD test indicates that the patient has been exposed to someone with tuberculosis, not that they have an active infection themselves. It is recommended that they be further evaluated with a chest x-ray and be treated with medications to prevent activation of the infection.

141. D: Hypercalcemia is due to hyperparathyroidism and can cause kidney stones. Most patients are asymptomatic, but some may have polyuria and polydipsia due to diabetes insipidus. With the elevated serum calcium level, there is decreased calcium in the bones which will affect the DEXA scan score, but this is usually less than -0.1.

142. D: Metabolic syndrome consists of central obesity (>40 inches in men, >35 inches in women), HDL <40 mg/dL in men and <50 mg/dL in women, and triglycerides >150 mg/dL. A diagnosis of metabolic syndrome means a patient is at greater risk for diabetes, heart disease, and stroke.

143. B: Amoxicillin, clarithromycin, and a proton pump inhibitor is the combination therapy necessary to treat *H. pylori* peptic ulcer disease. Metronidazole can be substituted for amoxicillin if the patient is allergic to amoxicillin. The patient may need to continue with the proton pump inhibitor after the treatment regimen is completed.

144. C: A clinical pathway is a structured plan of care for a specific diagnosis. The intent of this is to outline the steps to follow when caring for a patient, from admission to discharge. One criticism of this tool is that it does not allow for personalization of the patient's care and may result in negative outcomes if the appropriate care for the patient is delayed.

145. B: There are five basic principles of risk management, with identifying the potential risks within an organization as the first. Once those risks are identified, other steps can be taken to ensure the threat of risk is minimized.

146. D: Ensuring that the patient with diabetes understands the plan of care and the importance of managing the illness is imperative to prevent the complications of the disease. It is important to remember that everyone has different methods at which they learn the best. Many factors influence this, such as education level, socioeconomic status, cultural traditions, and age.

147. D: The 6 C's (care, commitment, compassion, courage, competence, and communication) work as a guideline which can be used to establish a therapeutic relationship with the patient. These work as a framework which can be used to develop a trusting relationship with open communication for the patient and caregivers.

148. C: The first step in implementing a treatment plan for a patient is to identify the main goal that is to be achieved. This should be broad and describe what is to be achieved with the program put into place. Once the goal is identified, measurable objectives should be listed to describe how the end goal is to be achieved. There are usually several objectives for each goal identified.

149. B: The patient- and family-centered care model was designed to open communication between patients, their family members who are helping to provide care, and the nursing and medical providers delivering care. It involves developing more effective communication with everyone involved in the patient's care with a common goal to improve the patient's outcome.

150. A: Having a patient with a hearing impairment offers the opportunity to utilize different forms of teaching. Some of these patients may have some degree of hearing acuity left, but most have learned to adapt and read lips. It is important to be aware of any distracting background noises and to face the patient directly so that your face and mouth are clearly visible. Remember not to turn away when talking or cover your mouth with your hand as that will make it difficult for the patient.

151. D: The Adult Gerontology Acute Care Nurse Practitioner functions as a patient advocate through many different actions, but the overall goal is to keep the patient safe and ensure they are receiving the highest quality of care possible. This can involve providing necessary education about a disease state or coordinating efforts with many providers for the patient to receive all of the necessary care they need.

152. B: According to HIPAA, information regarding the care of a patient can be shared with other members of the healthcare team without permission from the patient or patient representative. This information can be faxed over to the cardiologist's office.

153. A: The patient-centered medical home model utilizes the primary care provider as the main person coordinating all care for the patient. This way, specific specialties or other medical care that is needed can be delegated by one person.

154. D: These are the typical symptoms seen with Parkinson's disease. Multiple sclerosis presents with weakness, numbness, and paresis that is intermittent. Huntington's disease is genetically acquired and presents with flowing chorea movements and dementia. ALS begins with numbness and weakness in the lower extremities and speech difficulties.

155. D: Pioglitazone decreases insulin resistance and increases glucose utilization. Glipizide increases insulin secretion. Metformin lowers blood sugar levels by decreasing glucose production in the liver and increasing glucose utilization. Acarbose works by delaying the absorption of glucose.

156. B: Before any plans can be made for possible heart valve replacement surgery, further workup needs to be done to include a cardiac catheterization. Valve replacement surgery is performed only for symptomatic patients who are having shortness of breath, heart failure, or syncopal episodes due to the faulty valve. A valvuloplasty is less effective and has had high restenosis rates.

157. D: Weight loss is seen more commonly with emphysema. Dyspnea on exertion can be seen with either emphysema or bronchitis, but it is generally worse with bronchitis. Peripheral edema is more common with bronchitis. A productive cough is common with bronchitis while a dry cough is seen with emphysema.

158. B: EKG changes consistent with an infarct in the inferior wall are evident in leads II, III, and AVF. An anterior wall infarct is evident in leads I, AVL, and V2-V6. A lateral wall infarct is evident by ST depression, as opposed to ST elevation, in leads I, AVL, and V5-V6. Posterior wall infarcts also show ST depression except in leads V1-V3 where ST elevation is present.

159. A: A diagnosis at 20 years old or older is associated with a better outcome. An insidious onset in disease symptoms with a slow rate of progression of the disease are considered to be poorer outcomes. Being from a lower socioeconomic class is also associated with a poor outcome.

160. D: The symptoms, x-rays, and lab findings are most consistent with a diagnosis of ankylosing spondylitis. This disease is more common in males than females and it effects white people more often than black people. The age of onset is usually in the late teens or early 20s.

161. D: Her symptoms and EKG findings are consistent with a 3rd-degree heart block and a temporary pacemaker is necessary until a permanent unit can be surgically implanted. AV block will not respond to atropine. Cardioversion will not be helpful either because she has a functioning sinus node, but her ventricles are not responding appropriately.

162. C: The gold standard for diagnosing temporal arteritis is by temporal artery biopsy. This needs to be performed as soon as possible once the diagnosis is suspected and steroids should be started immediately to begin treatment. The rheumatoid factor is not relevant for this diagnosis and a sedimentation rate is too nonspecific to confirm diagnosis. An ultrasound will also not provide a definitive diagnosis of this condition.

163. C: Cerumen impaction will cause a conductive hearing loss. This would cause a Weber test to reveal lateralization of the sound to the left ear. With sensorineural hearing loss, air conduction is stronger than bone conduction in the affected test, which is called a Rinne's test.

164. B: NSAIDs (such as naproxen) have been proven to relieve pain due to osteoarthritis more efficiently than other medications. The anti-inflammatory action of this class of drugs helps to relieve the pain due to degenerative joint disease. While narcotics, such as hydrocodone, are effective at relieving pain, they are not the ideal choice for treating chronic arthritis pain.

165. D: His symptoms are consistent with medial epicondylitis. Pain can be reproduced with resisted wrist flexion. Pain on resisted wrist extension is seen with lateral epicondylitis. A biceps muscle bulge would be expected if the biceps muscle had ruptured. A posterior elbow impingement would be most likely to cause pain with a valgus stress of the elbow.

166. A: The left anterior descending artery supplies blood to the anterior wall of the left ventricle and the anterior two-thirds of the interventricular septum. The right coronary artery supplies the posterior heart and the AV node. The left circumflex artery supplies the posterolateral surface of the heart and the left marginal artery supplies the left lateral wall of the heart.

167. B: Based on his symptoms, this patient has moderate to persistent asthma and would benefit from a combination of an inhaled steroid along with a long-acting beta agonist (LABA). According to 2019 GINA recommendations, patients with mild to moderate asthma should use a daily inhaled steroid, as this has been shown to more effectively decrease asthma exacerbations than a short acting bronchodilator alone. If this regimen still results in asthma exacerbations, then the inhaled steroid with a LABA is the 2019 GINA recommendation. An oral steroid tapering dose is usually reserved for acute exacerbations of asthma symptoms.

168. C: Labetalol functions as a beta and alpha-blocker and is the most effective at lowering blood pressure quickly. Enalapril and hydralazine will lower blood pressure, but not as quickly or effectively as the labetalol in this situation. Nitroglycerin is used for patients with chest pain.

169. C: Polymyositis is a type of inflammatory myopathy in which only a biopsy of the involved muscle can be used to definitively diagnose the disease. It causes progressive proximal muscle weakness and the facial muscles are spared. The other test choices can be ordered, but their results will not definitively diagnose the condition.

170. D: Magnesium is necessary for potassium uptake and maintenance. If hypokalemia will not improve despite administration of potassium, this may be due to low levels of magnesium preventing the potassium from being used.

171. D: HIPAA regulations state that the care of a patient cannot be discussed to anyone without appropriate permission. This includes confirming or denying that the patient was seen at a specific healthcare facility. Most people understand this once it is explained to them.

172. C: The ACO, or Accountable Care Organization model, coordinates the efforts of all specialties and treatment modalities for the patient. The reimbursement plan varies, but there is extra incentive to address wellness and disease prevention.

173. A: The Adult-Gerontology Acute Care Nurse Practitioner cares for patients from adolescents through geriatrics. They do not care for pediatric patients.

174. B: In order to qualify to obtain the certification to be an Adult Gerontology Acute Care Nurse Practitioner, the provider must be an RN that has completed an accredited Nurse Practitioner program.

175. D: Nursing Informatics uses the data information and knowledge gathered to better inform those involved in patient care. The goal is to better inform not just those who make up the healthcare team, but to help to use the data gathered to provide better care for patients and to better inform patients of their care. Nursing Informatics is a growing field that has become more popular in recent years with the changing face of healthcare.

NP Acute Care Practice Test #2

1. Patients are especially at risk for neurogenic shock with spinal cord injuries at:

a. >T5
b. <T5
c. <L1
d. >L2

2. According to the Department of Health and Human Services' Healthy People 2030 initiative, the target goal for the percentage of people who receive the annual influenza vaccine is:

a. 50%
b. 60%
c. 70%
d. 80%

3. A long-time nurse, who is a member of a performance improvement committee, focuses exclusively on the needs of nursing staff and thinks that nursing concerns should be addressed before other concerns in the organization. The barrier to system change that this person exemplifies is:

a. Feelings of victimization
b. Relying on past experience
c. Failure to adapt
d. Identification with role rather than purpose

4. When analyzing data, the NP expects what percentage of data to fall within one standard deviation of the mean?

a. 33%
b. 68%
c. 95%
d. 99.7%

5. When auscultating the heart sounds of a 78-year-old male patient, the NP notes a third heart sound (S3) that persists when the patient sits up. This may be an indication of:

a. Normal physiologic heart sounds
b. Heart failure
c. Mitral stenosis
d. Hypothyroidism

6. A patient with a surgical site infection exhibits the following:

- Heart rate of 130 bpm, respiratory rate 24/min (tachycardia, tachypnea)
- Nausea and vomiting, confusion (altered mental status)
- Fever of 39 °C with shaking and chills
- WBC count 15,000 mm^3, $PaCO_2$ 30 mmHg (leukocytosis)

On the continuum of infection, this would be categorized as:

a. Systemic inflammatory response syndrome (SIRS)
b. Septicemia
c. Sepsis
d. Septic shock

7. If a patient is receiving 24 mg of intravenous (IV) morphine daily and is transitioning to oral morphine, what dosage of oral medication is needed?

a. 12 mg
b. 24 mg
c. 48 mg
d. 72 mg

8. Which of the following skin lesions is premalignant?

a. Actinic keratosis
b. Cherry angioma
c. Seborrheic keratosis
d. Senile lentigo

9. When conducting research, which type of sampling poses the greatest risk of bias?

a. Stratified random
b. Convenience
c. Purposive
d. Quota

10. In qualitative research, the three primary sources of data include interviews, observations, and:

a. Artifacts (records, documents, photos, and videos)
b. Meta-analysis of multiple randomized studies
c. Questionnaires
d. Biophysiological measures

11. A 16-year-old male patient has developed gynecomastia, which is causing the patient much anxiety. On examination, the NP notes small, firm testes, sparse body hair, long limbs, and feminine fat distribution. The NP recommends genetic testing to determine if the patient has:

a. Gonadal dysgenesis
b. Ovotestis
c. Klinefelter syndrome
d. Androgen insensitivity syndrome

12. In an emergent situation, a physician directs the NP to carry out an intervention that is outside of the individual's scope of practice. The most appropriate response is to:

a. Ignore the direction.
b. Carry out the intervention.
c. Ask if the physician will be legally liable.
d. Refuse to carry out the intervention.

13. In which phase of the cell cycle does DNA synthesis occur?

a. G1
b. S
c. G2
d. M

14. A patient presents with a plethoric, rounded ("moon") face, erythematous cheeks, prominent jowls, hirsutism, and acneiform rash on the chest. The NP recognizes these signs as being characteristic of:

a. Cushing's syndrome
b. Addison's disease
c. Scleroderma
d. Hypothyroidism

15. Which type of pressure facilitates the movement of fluid from the interstitial space into the capillaries?

a. Capillary hydrostatic pressure
b. Capillary oncotic pressure
c. Interstitial hydrostatic pressure
d. Interstitial oncotic pressure

16. A 50-year-old female complains of weight gain, fatigue, and constipation. Laboratory findings include thyroid-stimulating hormone (TSH) 22 μIU/mL, free T4 3.9 ng/dL, and serum cholesterol 269. On examination, the NP finds that the deep tendon reflexes are slow and that the thyroid gland is nontender but slightly enlarged. These findings are characteristic of:

a. Hyperthyroidism
b. Hypoparathyroidism
c. Secondary hypothyroidism
d. Primary hypothyroidism

17. A 40-year-old patient with positive *BRCA1* and *BRCA2* genes has a palpable mass in the right breast and is scheduled for a magnetic resonance imaging (MRI) scan. The MRI should be scheduled:

a. At any time during the menstrual cycle
b. On days 1–6 of the menstrual cycle
c. On days 7–14 of the menstrual cycle
d. On days 8–28 of the menstrual cycle

18. A patient receiving enteral feedings has developed diarrhea. What initial intervention is indicated?

a. Increase the rate of feeding.
b. Slow the rate of feeding.
c. Increase the fluid intake.
d. Monitor the blood glucose level.

19. If a patient receiving total parenteral nutrition (TPN) develops hyperammonemia and exhibits lethargy, a change in mental status, and asterixis, the most appropriate intervention is to:

a. Decrease the protein concentration of the formula.
b. Decrease the amino acids in the formula.
c. Hold the TPN feedings for 12 hours.
d. Decrease the lipid intake.

20. Which of the following antidepressants inhibits reuptake of norepinephrine and dopamine?

a. Citalopram (Celexa)
b. Venlafaxine (Effexor)
c. Nefazodone (Serzone)
d. Bupropion (Wellbutrin)

21. An 80-year-old patient is scheduled for an MRI with contrast because of an abdominal mass. What laboratory test must be carried out before the MRI?

a. Complete blood count (CBC)
b. Glucose
c. Basic metabolic panel
d. Serum creatinine

22. The NP notes that another healthcare provider is spending much more time catering to the needs of a famous patient while spending much less time with other patients. Which ethical principle is the person violating?

a. Veracity
b. Nonmaleficence
c. Fidelity
d. Justice

23. Which type of hypersensitivity response is associated with autoimmune thrombocytopenia?

a. Type I (immunoglobulin E-mediated)
b. Type II (tissue specific)
c. Type III (immune complex)
d. Type IV (cell mediated)

24. The NP approaches a patient in the emergency department to examine the patient for injuries incurred in an altercation. The patient screams obscenities, grabs items from the bedside table, and begins throwing them while climbing off the gurney. The most appropriate response is to:

a. Back out of the room and call for security.
b. Turn and run away.
c. Scream for security and help.
d. Tell the patient to calm down.

25. A 66-year-old patient with a history of hypertension and type 2 diabetes mellitus presents with complaints of increasing shortness of breath on exertion and paroxysmal nocturnal dyspnea. The patient's hemoglobin is 14.6 g/dL, and the hematocrit is 39%. Examination shows a blood pressure (BP) reading of 100/84, pulse of 112, respiratory rate of 28, 2+ pitting edema of the feet and ankles, rales and crackles throughout the lungs, decreased ventilation, and jugular venous distension 6 cm above the sternal angle. This profile is characteristic of:

a. Pleural effusion
b. Right-sided heart failure
c. Left-sided heart failure
d. Right- and left-sided heart failure

26. If a patient has a primary tumor in the prostate, the most likely sites for metastasis are:

a. Lungs and liver
b. Bones and liver
c. Lungs, liver, and brain
d. Lymphatics, lungs, and bones

27. If the NP is using the prioritize, question, recheck, self-reliance, and treat (PQRST) method of time management, the first task is to:

a. Develop a time frame for accomplishing tasks.
b. Identify tasks within personal control.
c. Make a list of tasks in the order of importance.
d. Make a list of available staff to delegate tasks to.

28. A 25-year-old male comes to the emergency department after experiencing a spider bite. Upon assessing the wound, it is determined that the spider bite most likely came from a black widow spider. Initial therapy for a black widow spider bite is:

a. Ice and elevation
b. Nonsteroidal anti-inflammatory drugs
c. Black widow spider (Latrodectus) antivenom
d. Calcium gluconate IV

29. If a study shows that 50% of patients who are advised to return to the emergency department for follow-up fail to do so, the most effective method of increasing compliance is likely to:

a. Send a letter to remind the patient.
b. Make a post-visit telephone call.
c. Emphasize the importance at the visit.
d. Email a reminder.

30. The first phase of nociceptive pain is:

a. Modulation
b. Transmission
c. Perception
d. Transduction

31. When examining a patient's eyes, the NP notes xerophthalmia and Bitot's spots (foamy plaques). These observations are indicative of which nutrient deficiency?

a. Niacin
b. Riboflavin
c. Vitamin A
d. Vitamin C

32. What waist circumference in female patients increases the risk for heart disease, diabetes mellitus, and metabolic syndrome?

a. >30 inches
b. >35 inches
c. >38 inches
d. >40 inches

33. A patient is admitted to the emergency department with multiple abrasions and injuries. The NP reviews the record of a previous admission that recorded that the patient had a "pattern of bruises and fractures." This indicates:

a. Defensive wounds on the arms and legs
b. Injuries in various stages of healing
c. Wounds in nonvisible areas
d. Multiple new injuries

34. When examining the heart rate of a 16-year-old patient, the NP notes that the heart rate increases during the peak of inspiration and slows during expiration. The rhythm is characterized as:

a. Respiratory sinus arrhythmia
b. Normal sinus rhythm
c. Sinus bradycardia
d. Sinus tachycardia

35. As part of quality improvement, the NP needs to collect and display data to establish priorities for problem solving. The most appropriate display tool is a:

a. Bar graph
b. Histogram
c. Pie chart
d. Pareto chart

36. On an electrocardiogram (ECG) tracing, which segment, complex, or interval represents ventricular depolarization and atrial repolarization?

a. P-R interval
b. QRS complex
c. ST segment
d. Q-T interval

37. When documenting the observation of undermining about a patient's pressure ulcer, the most appropriate description is:

a. "Undermining of 1 cm at the periphery of the RLQ of the wound."
b. "Undermining 1 cm × 5 cm."
c. "Undermining of 1 cm width extending from 3 o'clock to 5 o'clock."
d. "Undermining noted around a small portion of the wound."

38. The paraneoplastic syndrome associated with pancreatic adenocarcinoma is:

a. Nephrotic syndrome
b. Hypoglycemia
c. Polycythemia
d. Venous thrombosis

39. The NP notes that an unlicensed nursing assistant performing BP measurements routinely halts pressure descent and reinflates the cuff to double-check systolic BP. The NP recognizes that:

a. This is a good practice.
b. This may result in falsely high systolic readings.
c. This may result in falsely low systolic readings.
d. This may result in falsely high diastolic readings.

40. Which performance improvement model was developed to improve business practices and increase profits by eliminating "defects" in processes?

a. Six Sigma
b. Juran's quality improvement procedure
c. Focus, analyze, develop, and execute
d. Find, organize, clarify, uncover, and start

41. For a patient who has come to the emergency department with chronic hyperuricemia and recurrent severe attacks of gout, the target for treatment is a uric acid level of:

a. <5 mg/dL
b. <6 mg/dL
c. <7 mg/dL
d. <8 mg/dL

42. If an older adult takes atorvastatin to control cholesterol levels, what laboratory monitoring is recommended?

a. CBC
b. Basic metabolic panel
c. Liver function tests
d. Serum creatinine

43. A patient with bipolar disorder has stabilized on lithium after three dosage changes. Now that the patient is stabilized, how frequently should the patient have the serum lithium levels monitored?

a. Monthly
b. Every 3 months
c. Every 6 months
d. Every 12 months

44. A patient who speaks no English comes to the emergency department and appears to be in pain. The patient has brought his 8-year-old son to interpret. The NP should:

a. Arrange for a different interpreter.
b. Allow the 8-year-old to interpret.
c. Ask the 8-year-old questions to ensure that the child can interpret correctly.
d. Communicate with gestures and signs.

45. If the NP is applying electrodes for a 12-lead ECG, V1 is placed on the:

a. Right arm
b. Left arm
c. Left sternum, fourth intercostal space
d. Right sternum, fourth intercostal space

46. The NP is administering the National Institutes of Health (NIH) stroke scale to a patient with a suspected stroke in the intensive care unit (ICU). To assess part 5 (motor arm), the patient is in the supine position with an arm elevated to 45°. Drift is scored if the arm falls before:

a. 2 seconds
b. 5 seconds
c. 10 seconds
d. 20 seconds

47. A 50-year-old patient with abdominal pain and distension has a history of diverticulosis. Which imaging is the procedure of choice to verify a diagnosis of diverticulitis?

a. X-ray
b. Ultrasound
c. Computed tomography (CT) scan
d. Barium enema

48. An adolescent who is an avid basketball player comes to the emergency department with knee pain and swelling and is diagnosed with patellar tendinitis ("jumper's knee"). The initial recommended treatment is:

a. Ice, rest, modified activity, and physical therapy
b. Surgical repair
c. Corticosteroid injection to the joint, ice, rest, and modified activity
d. Hyaluronidase injection to the joint, rest, and physical therapy

49. A 15-year-old patient is on the unit in preparation for a spinal instrumentation and fusion for his severe scoliosis, being overseen by the NP. His curvature is currently 70°. What is the biggest risk factor from this severity of scoliosis?

a. Cardiovascular defects, particularly mitral regurgitation
b. Neurovascular injury
c. Poor perfusion to the lower extremities
d. Disrupted pulmonary functioning

50. If a patient complains that a nurse left the patient sitting on the bedside commode for 15 minutes, what type of risk event does this represent?

a. Serious incident
b. Service occurrence
c. Sentinel event
d. This is not a risk event

51. A 26-year-old patient with sickle cell disease is hospitalized for a vaso-occlusive pain crisis and has reached the established (postinfarctive) phase. This phase typically lasts for:

a. 1 day
b. 2–3 days
c. 4–5 days
d. 7–10 days

52. According to the American Thoracic Society, if using the 6-minute walk test to measure improvement in a patient's functional status, how many meters of improvement are necessary to ensure that the improvement is significant?

a. >40
b. >50
c. >60
d. >70

53. A patient receiving an antipsychotic has developed extrapyramidal effects (muscle spasms, restlessness, bradykinesia, tremor, and rigidity). Which medication is indicated?

a. Benztropine
b. Amitriptyline
c. Lorazepam
d. Haloperidol

54. A patient with type 2 diabetes mellitus has an Hgb A1c level of 8, which corresponds to a glucose level of approximately:

a. 120 mg/dL
b. 140 mg/dL
c. 160 mg/dL
d. 180 mg/dL

55. Long-term use of a proton pump inhibitor, such as omeprazole, should be avoided because of an increased risk of:

a. Hypermagnesemia
b. Fractures
c. Gastrointestinal (GI) hemorrhage
d. Escherichia coli enteritis

56. A patient is admitted to the ICU for bone pain, fatigue, severe weakness and numbness in the legs, increased thirst, and weight loss. Urinary testing is positive for Bence-Jones protein. This is a tumor marker for:

a. Multiple myeloma
b. Acute lymphoblastic leukemia
c. Hodgkin's lymphoma
d. Lung cancer

57. A patient is hospitalized in the ICU for a repeat exacerbation of stage III chronic obstructive pulmonary disease (COPD). Based on this staging, the NP expects that the patient's FEV1 will be:

a. >80% of predicted
b. 50–80% of predicted
c. 30–50% of predicted
d. <30% of predicted

58. The serotonin antagonist used to treat mild to moderate serotonin syndrome is:

a. Propranolol
b. Cyproheptadine
c. Dantrolene
d. Olanzapine

59. In evidence-based research, experimental designs include:

a. Correlational designs
b. Nonequivalent control group pretest–posttest
c. Time series designs
d. Two-group pretest–posttest

60. If the NP is a member of the quality improvement council and believes that the council needs to evaluate the overall processes in place for patients being hospitalized and treated, the most appropriate approach is to use:

a. Brainstorming
b. Root cause analysis
c. Tracer methodology
d. Force-field analysis

61. A frail 82-year-old patient seemed alert and responsive on admission before surgery, but, in the postoperative period, the patient exhibits fluctuating confusion, agitation, and combativeness and appears to have visual hallucinations. The most likely cause is:

a. Delirium
b. Impending stroke
c. Dementia
d. Hypersensitivity response to medications

62. A 70-year-old homeless male is brought to the emergency department after a fall. The patient reports long-term increasing weakness. On examination, the NP notes lymphadenopathy and hepatomegaly. The CBC shows a WBC count of 60,000 with 95% lymphocytes. The NP believes that these signs and symptoms are consistent with:

a. Sepsis
b. Hepatitis C
c. Liver abscess
d. Chronic lymphocytic leukemia

63. A patient at increased risk of a venous thromboembolic event undergoing hip fracture surgery is to receive dalteparin as a prophylaxis. The medication should be continued for at least:

a. 2 days
b. 5 days
c. 10 days
d. 14 days

64. A patient taking warfarin has a target international normalized ratio (INR) level of 2-3, but INR testing shows a level of 3.2. The most appropriate response is to:

a. Continue the warfarin at the same dosage but recheck within a week.
b. Hold warfarin for 1 day and resume at a 5–10% reduced dosage.
c. Hold warfarin for 1 day and resume at a 10–15% reduced dosage.
d. Hold warfarin and administer vitamin K antidote.

65. When examining an adolescent female patient, the NP notes that the patient has sparse, dark hair along the labia majora only and has small developing breasts. This is consistent with Tanner stage:

a. II
b. III
c. IV
d. V

66. A patient has been hospitalized with acute adrenal crisis because of inconsistent compliance with treatment for primary adrenal insufficiency (Addison's disease). Which one of the following questions exemplifies therapeutic questioning?

a. "Why did you fail to take your medication properly?"
b. "What did you do to cause an adrenal crisis?"
c. "What strategies do you use to treat your disease?"
d. "Did you forget to take your medication?"

67. A postsurgical patient has developed a cough. On examination, the NP notes that the tactile fremitus is decreased at the bases of both lungs, and the areas are dull to percussion. Breath and voice sounds are absent. These observations are consistent with:

a. Atelectasis
b. Lobar pneumonia
c. Bronchitis
d. Heart failure

68. A patient often delays dressing changes or refuses to cooperate and complains to the NP that dressing changes are too painful. The most appropriate response is:

a. "The dressing changes should be less painful each day."
b. "I'm sorry dressing changes are painful, but they are necessary for healing."
c. "Practice relaxation exercises during the dressing changes."
d. "Let's talk about this and figure out a way to make the dressing changes easier for you."

69. When referring a patient to another healthcare provider, the first issue that the NP should consider is:

a. Insurance coverage
b. Necessity
c. Expertise
d. Reciprocity

70. Assisting patients to navigate the healthcare system may include:

a. Charging insurance companies for services
b. Collaborating with others to provide patient care
c. Educating patients about the need for screening
d. Identifying patient candidates for a research project

71. A patient's heart rate is 82 with a regular rhythm, but pulsus alternans is evident with the force of alternating beats varying from large to small amplitude. This finding is consistent with:

a. Aortic valve regurgitation
b. Cardiac tamponade
c. Right ventricular failure
d. Left ventricular failure

72. When conducting a neurological exam, the NP notes that the patient has right unilateral weak contraction of the temporal and masseter muscles of the face and decreased pain sensation in that area. This suggests a lesion affecting cranial nerve:

a. III
b. IV
c. V
d. VI

73. A patient has an intention tremor present with activity, but it is absent at rest. This type of tremor is typical with:

a. Multiple sclerosis
b. Hyperthyroidism
c. Parkinson's disease
d. Anxiety

74. A patient with a history of *Helicobacter pylori* gastritis has taken long-term protein pump inhibitors. The patient is at increased risk for:

a. Iron deficiency anemia
b. Aplastic anemia
c. Folate deficiency anemia
d. Vitamin B12 (pernicious) anemia

75. A patient recently experienced bleeding from esophageal varices and is scheduled for band ligation. Which medication is also indicated to reduce the risk of rebleeding?

a. An angiotensin-converting enzyme (ACE) inhibitor (captopril)
b. An angiotensin II receptor blocker (ARB) (irbesartan)
c. An alpha-blocker (doxazosin)
d. A beta-blocker (propranolol)

76. Following a right nephrectomy, a patient complains of abdominal discomfort, distension, and nausea, although the abdomen is nontender to palpation. Bowel sounds are very minimal. The NP determines that the patient likely has:

a. Peritonitis
b. A small bowel obstruction
c. Paralytic ileus
d. A surgical site infection

77. A 70-year-old patient has been on long-term digoxin therapy. How often should serum digoxin levels be monitored?

a. Every 3 months
b. Every 6 months
c. Every 9 months
d. Every 12 months

78. Which of the following may cause serotonin syndrome in a patient taking selective serotonin reuptake inhibitors (SSRIs)?

a. Chamomile
b. Kava
c. Grapefruit
d. St. John's wort

79. If a patient with sickle cell disease is hospitalized with acute chest syndrome, packed red blood cell transfusions are administered to a target hemoglobin of:

a. 9 g/dL
b. 10 g/dL
c. 11 g/dL
d. 12 g/dL

80. A patient with a history of alcoholism and cirrhosis is admitted with upper GI bleeding and is vomiting bright-red blood. The emergent medication that is indicated before endoscopy is:

a. Octreotide
b. Omeprazole
c. Cefazolin
d. Ondansetron

81. If the average effective dose (ED_{50}) of a drug is 10 mg and the average lethal dose (LD_{50}) is 110 mg, the drug is:

a. Relatively unsafe
b. Somewhat unsafe
c. Somewhat safe
d. Relatively safe

82. A patient with chronic liver disease and ascites develops fever and abdominal pain. Paracentesis and examination of the ascitic fluid shows 95% neutrophils. The most likely diagnosis is:

a. Malignant ascites
b. Intestinal obstruction
c. Bacterial peritonitis
d. Acute hepatitis

83. A patient who has been experiencing abdominal discomfort passes maroon-colored stools. This suggests that bleeding is occurring in the:

a. Rectosigmoid area
b. Right colon or distal small intestine
c. Left colon
d. Stomach or proximal small intestine

84. A patient with moderately severe Alzheimer's disease underwent emergency surgery for bowel obstruction and in the postoperative period is extremely confused and continually tries to pull out IVs and tubes and climb out of bed. The intervention that is most appropriate is:

a. Administering haloperidol
b. Administering lorazepam
c. Applying physical restraints
d. Using a sitter

85. The hemodynamic status associated with septic shock is:

a. Massive vasoconstriction with increased capillary permeability
b. Massive vasoconstriction with decreased capillary permeability
c. Massive vasodilation with increased capillary permeability
d. Massive vasodilation with decreased capillary permeability

86. A population factor that can impact individual health is:

a. Family size
b. Climate extremes
c. Natural disasters
d. Environmental contamination

87. When prescribing medications for older adults, the NP should especially consult:

a. A physician
b. A pharmacist
c. The Beers Criteria for Potentially Inappropriate Medication Use in Older Adults
d. The Physicians' Desk Reference

88. When treating a patient for shock, the urinary output that is necessary to ensure adequate organ perfusion is:

a. >0.1–0.5 mL/kg/hr
b. >0.5–1.0 mL/kg/hr
c. >1.0–2.0 mL/kg/hr
d. >2.0–3.0 mL/kg/hr

89. A patient is diagnosed with class II hypovolemia, with a 15–30% volume loss. Indications that support this classification include:

a. Stable BP, tachycardia, and tachypnea
b. Essentially asymptomatic status
c. Hypotension, heart rate of 130 bpm
d. Altered mental status, heart rate of 146 bpm, hypotension

90. Which of the following is used to predict outcomes of treatment by accounting for various factors, such as age, gender, history of drinking, and history of smoking?

a. Risk stratification
b. Random variation
c. Proportionate sampling
d. Sampling distribution

91. The NP recognizes that hospital policy regarding a specific treatment is not in line with current evidence-based research. When implementing treatment, the NP should base the treatment on:

a. Evidence-based research
b. Hospital policy
c. Staff consensus
d. Personal treatment preference

92. A female patient's test results include:

- Fasting insulin 78%
- Fasting serum glucose 112 mg/dL
- Fasting triglycerides 160 mg/dL
- High-density lipoprotein 30 mg/dL
- Body mass index (BMI) 28, hip-to-waist ratio 1.0
- BP 138/88
- Uric acid 7.8 mg/dL

These results are consistent with:

a. Chronic gout
b. Type 1 diabetes mellitus
c. Type 2 diabetes mellitus
d. Metabolic syndrome

93. According to Joint Commission accreditation guidelines, patients hospitalized with acute myocardial infarction should receive aspirin within:

a. 1 hour
b. 6 hours
c. 12 hours
d. 24 hours

94. A 25-year-old male comes to the emergency department with complaints of yellow-green purulent urethral discharge and scrotal pain, consistent with gonorrhea. The recommended first-line treatment is:

a. Benzathine penicillin G 2.4 million units intramuscularly (IM), one dose
b. Ceftriaxone 500 mg, one dose
c. Metronidazole 2 g by mouth (po), one dose
d. Azithromycin 1 g po, one dose

95. When the NP is assessing a diabetic patient's sensory system in the lower extremities with sharp and dull points to test the ability to perceive a pinprick, how much time should elapse between each stimulus that is provided?

a. 0.5 second
b. 1 second
c. 2 seconds
d. 3 seconds

96. A patient is very disgruntled after waiting an hour for a procedure and states "I'm never coming to this hospital again." If the NP is using the connect, apologize, repair, and exceed (CARE) approach to calm the patient, the most appropriate initial response is:

a. "Tell me about the problem and how I can help."
b. "We had a number of unexpected emergencies."
c. "You have every right to be angry."
d. "I'm sorry. It's terrible that you've had to wait so long."

97. A patient tells the NP that she wants medication to lose weight. The NP informs the patient that these medications are recommended for patients with BMI of:

a. >26 or >24 with risk factors
b. >27 or >25 with risk factors
c. >30 or >27 with risk factors
d. >32 or >30 with risk factors

98. If a patient is being treated for a pressure ulcer, to promote healing, nutrient intake should include:

a. 30–40 kcal/kg/day and 1.0–1.5 g/kg/day of protein
b. 30–40 kcal/kg/day and 2.0–3.0 g/kg/day of protein
c. 20–30 kcal/kg/day and 1.0–1.5 g/kg/day of protein
d. 20–30 kcal/kg/day and 0.5–1.0 g/kg/day of protein

99. When a patient arrives at the emergency department with an ST segment elevation myocardial infarction, reperfusion should ideally be completed within:

a. 60 minutes
b. 90 minutes
c. 4 hours
d. 6 hours

100. When discharging a 35-year-old female patient who is receiving acitretin for severe psoriasis, it is important to include instructions about:

a. Dietary restrictions
b. The continuous use of two forms of contraception
c. The monitoring of vital signs
d. Limiting alcohol intake to one drink daily

101. When auscultating a patient's heart at the 5th intercostal space, left midclavicular line, the NP notes a murmur that has a high-pitched "blowing" sound that is more pronounced during expiration and when the patient is supine. The murmur radiates to the left axilla and back. This is characteristic of:

a. Tricuspid regurgitation
b. Pulmonic stenosis
c. Aortic stenosis
d. Mitral regurgitation

102. The normal pH of gastric fluids is:

a. 1.5–3.5
b. 5.0–6.0
c. 7.35–7.45
d. 7.8–8.0

103. If a patient with COPD experiences exertional dyspnea, this is generally an indication that the patient's FEV1 is at least:

a. 70% of the norm
b. 60% of the norm
c. 50% of the norm
d. 40% of the norm

104. The NP suspects that a patient's confusion is caused by delirium. Which assessment tool is indicated to verify this diagnosis?

a. Time and Change Test
b. Confusion Assessment Method
c. Mini-Cog
d. Trail Making Test

105. A patient comes to the emergency department with symptoms indicating possible appendicitis. The NP assesses for rebound tenderness (McBurney's sign) by:

a. Placing the patient on the left side with the patient's right upper leg flexed backward
b. Applying pressure in the right lower quadrant (RLQ) at a point two-thirds the distance from the navel to the right anterior superior iliac spine
c. Applying pressure in the left lower quadrant (LLQ) of the abdomen
d. Flexing the right knee to 90° and internally rotating the hip

106. A patient reports episodes of nausea and abdominal pain lasting 2-4 hours in the right upper quadrant (RUQ) and radiating to the right scapula after eating fatty foods or drinking alcohol. The NP recognizes that these symptoms are consistent with:

a. Gastroesophageal reflux disease
b. Cholecystitis
c. Appendicitis
d. Gastritis

107. The NP notes that a patient's hands are very pale, and the patient complains of feeling cold and numb. Slowly the hands become blue-tinged and painful and then erythematous and edematous with burning, throbbing pain. The NP recognizes these signs and symptoms as probable:

a. Raynaud's phenomenon
b. Lymphedema
c. Rheumatoid arthritis
d. Gout

108. A characteristic of chronic peripheral arterial disease includes:

a. Pain relieved by walking
b. Pain aggravated by prolonged standing
c. Deep muscle pain with onset gradual with exertion
d. Chronic aching pain that increases throughout the day

109. A patient has a small ulcer on the medial malleolus. The NP notes on examination that the patient has hemosiderosis on both lower legs. These findings suggest:

a. Venous stasis
b. Arterial insufficiency
c. Deep vein thrombophlebitis
d. Traumatic injury

110. An older patient with heart failure is admitted to the hospital. During the physical examination, the NP notes an approximately 5 cm pulsating mass palpable above the umbilicus and slightly to the left of midline. A harsh continuous murmur is noted. These findings indicate:

a. Pericarditis
b. Splenomegaly
c. Hydronephrosis
d. Aortic aneurysm

111. An 80-year-old patient comes to the emergency room with signs and symptoms of giant cell temporal arteritis: headache, scalp tenderness, diplopia, jaw claudication, and throat pain. The patient's erythrocyte sedimentation rate is markedly elevated. Emergent treatment should include:

a. Corticosteroids
b. Antibiotics
c. Antiviral medications
d. Muscle relaxants

112. A patient comes to the emergency department and reports that he is a heroin addict and has shared needles with a person 2 days previously and just learned that the person is HIV positive. The NP recommends that:

a. The patient should immediately begins postexposure prophylaxis (PEP).
b. The patient should enter rehabilitation for heroin use.
c. The patient should come in for testing in 10 days to assess the need for PEP.
d. The patient should stop using heroin before beginning PEP.

113. The variety of hepatitis that poses the greatest risk of becoming a chronic disease is:

a. Hepatitis A
b. Hepatitis B
c. Hepatitis C
d. Hepatitis D

114. A patient is brought to the emergency room after fainting in a shopping mall. The patient reports having frequent dizzy spells. The ECG shows the following tracing, consistent with:

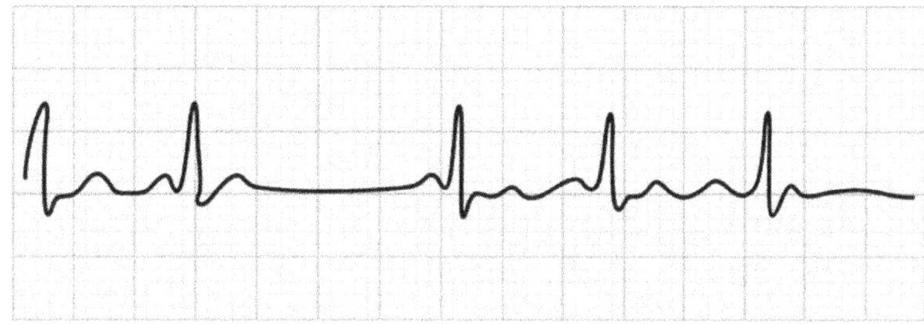

a. Right bundle branch block
b. Left bundle branch block
c. Third-degree AV block
d. Sinus pause

115. If an organ enlarges because the number of cells increase, this is referred to as:

a. Hypertrophy
b. Hyperplasia
c. Dysplasia
d. Metaplasia

116. According to a paramedic, a patient enroute to the emergency department after a motor vehicle accident has a Glasgow coma scale score of 7. The NP expects, based on this score, that the patient's condition is:

a. Mild
b. Moderate
c. Severe
d. Comatose

117. If a patient reports that he is allergic to penicillin, the NP should be aware that the patient may have cross sensitivity to:

a. Cephalosporins
b. Tetracyclines
c. Aminoglycosides
d. Macrolides

118. Considering membrane transport, the movement of a solute molecule from an area of greater solute concentration to one of lesser concentration is:

a. Filtration
b. Osmosis
c. Diffusion
d. Evaporation

119. A patient who has been noncompliant with treatment for epilepsy is hospitalized with generalized tonic-clonic status epilepticus. After IV access is established, the patient initially receives a 50 mL bolus of 50% dextrose, but seizures still persist in 5 minutes. The first-line treatment next administered is:

a. Valproic acid
b. Fosphenytoin
c. Phenytoin
d. Lorazepam

120. When applying trending analysis to a control chart, seven or more consecutive data points all above or all below the mean is referred to as a:

a. Trend
b. Run
c. Cycle
d. Astronomical value

121. When a problem arises in a medical context, the first step to resolve the problem is to:

a. Collect data.
b. Consider reasons for the actions.
c. Define the issue.
d. Make a decision.

122. In an elderly patient, the presenting symptom of an acute myocardial infarction (MI) is often:

a. Dyspnea
b. Diaphoresis
c. Heartburn
d. Chest pain

123. A patient received a blunt abdominal injury during a motor vehicle accident and is hypotensive and complains of diffuse abdominal pain. The NP notes ecchymosis around the umbilicus (positive Cullen's sign), which indicates:

a. Ruptured kidney
b. Ruptured bowel
c. Liver laceration
d. Ruptured spleen

124. If the NP participates in a pay for performance (P4P) value-based contract with an insurance company, this means that the NP:

a. Receives the same monthly payment each month
b. May receive less pay for negative outcomes and more pay for positive outcomes
c. Is expected to cut costs of care
d. Receives higher pay as additional certifications are acquired

125. A patient is hospitalized with acute alcohol-induced pancreatitis. The primary treatment is:

a. Supportive
b. Antibiotics
c. Corticosteroids
d. Infliximab

126. Which of the following is an example of an external trigger that may indicate the need for further analysis?

a. Sentinel events
b. Benchmarks
c. Performance rate
d. Rate change

127. If an adolescent patient is admitted with benzodiazepine-induced coma and severe respiratory depression after a suicide attempt with stolen drugs, the most appropriate emergent treatment is:

a. Supportive care
b. Fomepizole
c. Naloxone
d. Flumazenil

128. The leading cause of acute liver failure is:

a. Alcoholism
b. Antituberculosis drugs
c. Acetaminophen toxicity
d. Fatty liver of pregnancy

129. When preparing educational materials for patients, the NP uses the Fog Formula to determine the readability level. For readability, calculations are based on the number of:

a. Words per sentence/independent clause and three-syllable (or greater) words
b. Words per sentence and dependent clauses
c. Dependent and independent clauses
d. Words per sentence only

130. Which type of measurement is vulnerable to measurement error?

a. Direct measures (such as with a scale or tape measure)
b. Indirect measures (concepts, ideas)
c. Measures of nominal data
d. All types of measurement

131. For burn patients, electrolyte imbalance may be life-threatening if burns cover more than:

a. 10% of body surface area (BSA)
b. 20% of BSA
c. 30% of BSA
d. 40% of BSA

132. If a patient was exposed to burning plastic in a factory fire and is suspected of having cyanide poisoning, the most appropriate treatment is:

a. Hyperbaric oxygen treatment
b. Diazepam
c. Hydroxocobalamin
d. Sodium bicarbonate

133. The NP is serving as a preceptor for a newly graduated NP who is in a probationary period at work. The primary goal of the preceptor is to:

a. Prepare the nurse to assume full responsibility.
b. Ensure that the nurse is competent.
c. Identify areas of weakness in nursing practice.
d. Report observations to nursing administration.

134. A research study that focuses on a particular group of people who were exposed to a toxin in a work environment in order to determine causality would be classified as a:

a. Population-based study
b. Prospective cohort study
c. Retrospective control study
d. Retrospective cohort study

135. A patient taking metoprolol for hypertension has developed severe muscle pains and is switching to irbesartan. The NP should advise the patient to:

a. Immediately stop the metoprolol and begin irbesartan.
b. Decrease the dosage of metoprolol over 1–2 weeks and then start irbesartan.
c. Start irbesartan immediately and continue metoprolol in reduced dosages for 2 weeks.
d. Immediately stop the metoprolol, wait 2 days, and then start the irbesartan.

136. A core concept of Continuous Quality Improvement is that problems relate to:

a. Individuals
b. Administration
c. Processes
d. Market forces

137. Angina that lasts for less than 5 minutes and results from atherosclerotic lesions obstructing greater than 75% of the lumen of the affected coronary artery is classified as:

a. Angina decubitus
b. Unstable angina
c. Variant (Prinzmetal's) angina
d. Stable angina

138. A 20-year-old is admitted with sudden onset (<12 hours) of headache, nuchal rigidity, fever, and altered mental status. The NP suspects bacterial meningitis. The most appropriate initial intervention is to:

a. Administer empiric antibiotics.
b. Administer prednisone.
c. Carry out a lumbar puncture.
d. Schedule stat CT and lumbar puncture.

139. In a research study, manipulation refers to:

a. Altering data
b. Outcomes
c. The treatment
d. The control

140. The government agency that regulates the protection of human subjects and requires any researcher involving individuals in research to obtain informed consent in language that is understandable is:

a. CDC
b. OSHA
c. FDA
d. CMS

141. If using the HOPE mnemonic to guide spiritual assessment, the H stands for:

a. Health considerations
b. Sources of hope
c. Belief in Heaven
d. Help resources

142. The NP uses the PERSON method to carry out a physical health assessment. The last element, N, refers to:

a. Notable
b. Nature
c. Nervous system
d. Nutrition

143. When treating hypertension in a male African-American patient, which type of drug is generally avoided?

a. Beta-blockers
b. Calcium channel blockers
c. ARBs
d. ACE inhibitors

144. If the NP wants to effect changes in public health policy, the most effective method is to:

a. Write letters to Congress.
b. Carry out clinical research.
c. Participate in national healthcare organizations.
d. Talk to peers about the need for change.

145. The primary purpose in using the SBAR method of handoff and transition of care is:

a. Patient safety
b. Time savings
c. Liability reduction
d. Convenience

146. According to Peplau's four levels of anxiety, if a patient speaks rapidly in a high pitch and experiences muscle tension, diaphoresis, rapid pounding pulse, headache, dry mouth, gastrointestinal upset, and frequent urination and the patient's perceptual field narrows to a specific task, the level of anxiety is:

a. Mild
b. Moderate
c. Severe
d. Panic

147. A patient was hospitalized with a stroke for 4 days and then transferred to a skilled nursing facility (SNF) for 20 days. The patient was then discharged home but was readmitted to an acute hospital 62 days later because of another stroke. After 3 days of hospitalization, the patient was transferred to the same SNF. What is the maximum number of days that Medicare will cover in the SNF?

a. 0
b. 20
c. 80
d. 100

148. The NP is using the CAGE tool to assess a patient's risk of alcohol abuse. The patient answers "yes" to one out of four questions. This represents:

a. A possible drinking problem
b. A mild drinking problem
c. A moderate drinking problem
d. No drinking problem

149. An older patient is admitted to an acute hospital from an SNF because of a stroke. The NP notes that the transfer document indicates that the patient has a score of 14 out of 23 on the Braden scale for predicting the risk of developing pressure ulcers. This indicates:

a. No current risk
b. Minimal risk
c. Risk of pressure ulcer
d. Strong likelihood of developing a pressure ulcer

150. The NP is writing nursing diagnoses for a patient with end-stage COPD. According to Maslow's hierarchy of needs, which nursing diagnosis would have priority?

a. Risk for aspiration
b. Latex allergy response
c. Risk for loneliness
d. Defensive coping

151. If a patient with a gunshot wound has tattooing and stippling about the entry wound, this indicates that the injury resulted from a(n):

a. Distant range
b. Indeterminate distance range
c. Intermediate distance range
d. Contact range

152. Considering vulnerable populations, what unique problems should the NP expect may be identified for homeless individuals?

a. Risk for falls and aspiration
b. Lice, malnutrition, substance abuse, psychiatric condition
c. Posttraumatic stress disorder, substance abuse
d. Injuries, chronic illness, infections

153. The NP is preparing to educate an ICU patient regarding the importance of the annual influenza vaccine and to then offer it to the patient if they choose to receive it. This is an example of:

a. Primary prevention
b. Secondary prevention
c. Tertiary prevention
d. Quaternary prevention

154. The NP is serving on the cost-containment committee, which is considering a request by the radiology department. The cost to repair a current CT scanner is $70,000. The cost to buy a similar refurbished one is $120,000, and the cost of a new, updated scanner is $1.5 million. What should the committee recommend?

a. Repair the scanner.
b. Buy the refurbished scanner.
c. Buy the new scanner.
d. Do a cost analysis before a decision is made.

155. A patient is to have IV antibiotics for 48 hours before switching to oral antibiotics. Which type of IV access is indicated?

a. Short peripheral catheter (SPC)
b. Midline peripheral catheter
c. Butterfly needle
d. Peripherally inserted central catheter

156. In an emergent situation, the NP must start an intraosseous infusion for an adult patient using the Fast1 Intraosseous Infusion System. The intraosseous needle should be inserted into the:

a. Medial malleolus
b. Proximal tibia
c. Sternum
d. Proximal humerus

157. If a patient's arterial blood pH is greater than 7.45, partial pressure of carbon dioxide is less than 35 mmHg, and serum bicarbonate is decreased, this is indicative of:

a. Respiratory acidosis
b. Respiratory alkalosis
c. Metabolic acidosis
d. Metabolic alkalosis

158. The type of necrosis that results from ischemia of neurons and glial cells in the central nervous system is:

a. Liquefactive
b. Coagulative
c. Caseous
d. Fat

159. A pregnant patient needs an infusion of a drug whose dosage is based on body weight. The patient's prepregnancy weight was 125 lb/57 kg, but her current weight at 6 months of gestation is 137 lb/62 kg. What weight should the patient's dosage be based on?

a. 125 lb/57 kg
b. 131 lb/59 kg
c. 137 lb/62 kg
d. 142 lb/64 kg

160. Drugs that are administered orally are primarily absorbed in the:

a. Esophagus
b. Stomach
c. Small intestines
d. Large intestines

161. The type of cell that serves as the primary defense against parasites is:

a. Natural killer cells
b. Neutrophils
c. Monocytes
d. Eosinophils

162. A patient's ECG shows a slightly peaked P wave, slightly prolonged PR interval, ST depression, shallow T wave, and prominent U wave. The electrolyte imbalance associated with these findings is:

a. Hypokalemia
b. Hyperkalemia
c. Hypochloremia
d. Hyperchloremia

163. The type of immune response that involves antibodies binding to antigens on infective agents (primarily bacteria and viruses) is referred to as:

a. Cell-mediated immunity
b. Humoral immunity
c. Active acquired immunity
d. Passive acquired immunity

164. A patient developed a sudden onset of severe retrosternal chest pain that increases with respirations and when lying down in a supine position. The patient has a low-grade fever and sinus tachycardia. On auscultation, the NP notes a friction rub at the cardiac apex and left sternal border. These signs and symptoms are consistent with:

a. Myocardial infarction
b. Aortic stenosis
c. Pericarditis
d. Myocarditis

165. The NP is monitoring the capnography of a patient with severe asthma. The monitor shows a sloped "shark fin" waveform with loss of plateau. This indicates:

a. Normal ventilation
b. Obstruction
c. Hypoventilation
d. Hyperventilation

166. The NP is examining a patient with a traumatic brain injury. The patient's pupils are in midposition, slightly dilated (5 mm), and fixed. This indicates:

a. Damage to the midbrain
b. Severe anoxia
c. Damage to the hypothalamus
d. Drug-induced brain damage (cocaine, amphetamines)

167. A patient is to be discharged with a referral to hospice. How long may a patient be cared for under the Medicare hospice benefit?

a. Two 90-day periods
b. Two 90-day periods and one 60-day period
c. Two 60-day periods
d. Two 90-day periods and unlimited 60-day periods

168. The spouse of a patient with end-stage liver disease is distraught, cries frequently, and tells the NP that she has no appetite, no patience, and is sleeping poorly. The stage of grief (Kübler-Ross) that the spouse is experiencing is:

a. Denial
b. Depression
c. Anger
d. Acceptance

169. A patient complains of increasing shortness of breath, weight gain of 7 pounds in the past week, and increased abdominal girth. The patient's abdomen in the supine position is large, and the skin is taut with an everted umbilicus. Both flanks are bulging. Bowel sounds are normal over the intestines but diminished over lateral areas. Tympany is noted at the center of the abdomen, but the sound is dull over the bulging areas. These findings are consistent with:

a. Obesity
b. Trapped air/gas
c. Ascites
d. Fecal impaction

170. When using the Doppler stethoscope to find the patient's ankle-brachial index, the NP finds that the systolic arm pressure is 146 and the systolic ankle pressure is 122, resulting in an ankle-brachial index score of 0.84. This indicates:

a. A normal finding
b. Mild claudication
c. Severe claudication
d. Ischemia

171. The type of gait that is associated with alcohol or barbiturate effects on the brain is:

a. Waddling
b. Scissors
c. Steppage
d. Cerebellar ataxia

172. A patient with hemophilia B has developed major bleeding after an injury. What treatment is indicated to control the bleeding?

a. Factor IX product
b. Desmopressin
c. Factor VIII product
d. Fresh frozen plasma

173. If a patient with severe rheumatoid arthritis is being discharged on methotrexate, the discharge instructions should include the need to avoid:

a. Foods high in purines
b. Exposure to sunlight
c. All alcoholic beverages
d. Dairy products

174. A 35-year-old patient has responded only to SSRIs for depression but has developed erectile dysfunction and an inability to reach orgasm, resulting in a suicide attempt. Which SSRI is likely to cause the highest rate of sexual dysfunction?

a. Sertraline
b. Fluoxetine
c. Paroxetine
d. Citalopram

175. A 65-year-old patient has mild hypertension in the range of 140/90. A typical first-line therapy is:

a. Hydrochlorothiazide
b. Furosemide
c. Terazosin
d. Metoprolol

Answer Key and Explanations for Test #2

1. A: Patients are especially at risk for neurogenic shock with spinal cord injuries >T5, which blocks sympathetic outflow. Without sympathetic outflow, vagal innervation is not opposed, resulting in the typical symptoms of hypotension, bradycardia, and vasodilation. This results in a loss of vascular tone so that venous return is impaired, causing venous pooling. Patients may be hypothermic with no sweating below the injury level. The volume of blood is adequate with neurogenic shock, but the body cannot sustain perfusion.

2. C: According to the Department of Health and Human Services' Healthy People 2030 initiative, the target goal for the amount of people who receive the annual influenza vaccine is 70%. Currently, about 49% of people are vaccinated annually. The CDC recommends that people 6 months of age and older receive annual vaccinations by October of each year. Flu season typically begins in October and peaks from December to February but may persist through the spring. The flu vaccine does not protect against the coronavirus.

3. D: If a long-time nurse, who is a member of a performance improvement committee, focuses exclusively on the needs of nursing staff and thinks that nursing concerns should be addressed before other concerns in the organization, the barrier to system change that this person exemplifies is identification with role rather than purpose. The person views organizational needs from the perspective of the person's role in the system and is not able to step outside of preconceived ideas to view situations holistically or to accept the roles of others.

4. B: When analyzing data, the NP expects 68% of data to fall within one standard deviation of the mean, 95% of data to fall within two standard deviations of the mean, and 99.7% to fall within three standard deviations of the mean. The 68-95-99.7 rule represents the normal distribution of data. Outliers are the data that lie outside of the normal distribution. Outliers alter the mean but have little effect on the median or mode.

5. B: A third heart sound (S3) in a 78-year-old male patient that persists when he sits up may be an indication of heart failure. S3 is normally heard in children and young adults, although it disappears if the person sits up. However, it is usually abnormal if found after age 35, but it may occasionally persist until age 40 in females. S3 (also referred to as a ventricular gallop) is often an early sign of heart failure.

6. C: A patient with a surgical site infection exhibits:

- Heart rate of 130 bpm, respiratory rate 24/min (tachycardia, tachypnea)
- Nausea and vomiting, confusion (altered mental status)
- Fever of 39 °C with shaking and chills
- WBC count 15,000 mm^3, $PaCO_2$ 30 mmHg (leukocytosis)

On the continuum of infection, this would be categorized as sepsis because it involves systemic inflammatory response syndrome and a widespread systemic response to the infection.

7. D: If a patient is receiving 24 mg of IV morphine daily and is transitioning to oral morphine, the dosage of oral medication that is needed is 72 mg. IV medication is readily absorbed, and the entire dose is active. However, oral medication is absorbed more slowly and less completely, so the ratio of IV to oral morphine is 1:3: 24 mg × 3 = 72 mg. Equianalgesic tables are available because the ratio may vary from one drug to another. For example, the ratio for hydromorphone is 1:5.

8. A: Actinic keratoses are premalignant lesions, which should be removed before they evolve to cancerous lesions. Different procedures may be used:

- Surgical: chemical peel, cryosurgery, laser removal, and curettage and desiccation
- Photodynamic therapy
- Topical therapy: 5FUO, diclofenac + hyaluronic acid, imiquimod, and ingenol mebutate

Cherry angioma, seborrheic keratosis, and senile lentigo are all benign lesions; however, if there is a sudden occurrence of multiple cherry angiomas in one area, in rare cases this can indicate an internal malignancy.

9. B: When conducting research, convenience sampling (a type of nonprobability sampling) poses the greatest risk of bias because it allows all available subjects to participate, so the sample may not represent the target population. Nonprobability sampling does not require randomization and also includes quota sampling and purposive sampling. Probability sampling requires randomization and includes simple random sampling, stratified random sampling, cluster sampling, and systematic random sampling.

10. A: In qualitative research, the three primary sources of data include interviews (one-to-one, in-depth), observations (carried out directly), and artifacts (records, documents, photos, and videos). Data analysis in qualitative research is generally subjective and focuses on a narrative rather than on numbers. The primary sources of data for quantitative research include questionnaires, observation, scales, and biophysiological measures.

11. C: If a 16-year-old male patient has developed gynecomastia and the NP notes small, firm testes, sparse body hair, long limbs, and feminine fat distribution, the NP should recommend genetic testing to determine if the patient has Klinefelter syndrome. Klinefelter syndrome results from a sporadic genetic mutation in which a male is born with an extra X chromosome (XXY), resulting in some degree of feminization and infertility.

12. D: If, in an emergent situation, a physician directs the NP to carry out an intervention that is outside of the individual's scope of practice, the most appropriate response is to refuse to carry out the intervention by pointing out that the individual's license limits the scope of practice. In this case, the physician and the NP (as well as the hospital) would be legally liable for complications that resulted from the intervention.

13. B: DNA synthesis occurs in the S phase of the cell cycle. Phases of the cell cycle are listed as follows:

- G1: RNA and protein synthesis take place.
- S: DNA synthesis takes place.
- G2: DNA synthesis is complete, and the mitotic spindle forms.
- M: Mitosis takes place with cell replication.
- G0: This is the resting (inactive) phase.

Most cell cycle-specific agents target the S phase or the M phase of the cell cycle. Cell cycle-nonspecific agents are longer acting and unrelated to the cell cycle.

14. A: If a patient presents with a plethoric, rounded ("moon") face, erythematous cheeks, prominent jowls, hirsutism, and acneiform rash on the chest, the NP recognizes these signs as being characteristic of Cushing's syndrome. Cushing's syndrome most commonly occurs as the result of steroid therapy, such as for patients with COPD or rheumatoid arthritis, but it may also occur with adrenal or pituitary tumors that increase cortisol levels.

15. C: Interstitial hydrostatic pressure facilitates the movement of fluid from the interstitial space into the capillaries. Interstitial oncotic pressure attracts fluid from the capillaries into the interstitial space. Capillary hydrostatic pressure facilitates the movement of fluid from the capillaries to the interstitial space. Capillary oncotic pressure attracts fluid from the interstitial space into the capillaries.

16. D: If a 50-year-old female complains of weight gain, fatigue, and constipation and laboratory findings include TSH 22 μIU/mL, free T4 3.9 ng/dL, and serum cholesterol 269 and a physical examination shows that the deep tendon reflexes are slow and the thyroid gland is nontender but slightly enlarged, these findings are characteristic of primary hypothyroidism, in which the TSH level increases to stimulate production of T4 but the T4 level remains low.

17. C: If a 40-year-old patient with positive *BRCA1* and *BRCA2* genes has a palpable mass in the right breast and is scheduled for an MRI, the MRI should be scheduled on days 7–14 of the menstrual cycle because hormonal changes make the breast tissue best visualized during that time period. Because the MRI is more sensitive than the mammogram, it can identify smaller lesions and better identify invasive malignancies.

18. B: If a patient receiving enteral feedings develops diarrhea, the initial intervention is to slow the rate of feeding or use a continuous drip because diarrhea is a response to rapid feeding. Medications should also be evaluated because some, such as antibiotics, may cause diarrhea. The tubing should be changed every 24 hours, and formula should be disposed of after 8 hours to reduce the risk of contamination. If diarrhea persists, a formula change, such as increasing the fiber content, may be necessary.

19. A: If a patient receiving TPN develops hyperammonemia and exhibits lethargy, a change in mental status, and asterixis (hand flapping and tremors), the most appropriate intervention is to decrease the protein concentration of the formula. The patient should also be evaluated for hepatic insufficiency because hyperammonemia may occur with cirrhosis of the liver. Amino acids are decreased if the patient develops azotemia. Lipid intake is decreased with hyperlipidemia, and it is increased for essential fatty acid deficiency.

20. D: Bupropion (Wellbutrin) is an antidepressant that inhibits reuptake of the neurotransmitters norepinephrine and dopamine. If a medication inhibits reuptake, this means that, after neurotransmitters are released to send messages from one nerve cell to another, instead of the neurotransmitter being reabsorbed, it temporarily remains in the synapse. Different kinds of reuptake inhibitors target different neurotransmitters; for example, SSRIs target serotonin reuptake and SNRIs target serotonin and norepinephrine.

21. D: If an 80-year-old patient is scheduled for an MRI with contrast because of an abdominal mass, the laboratory test that must be carried out before the MRI is serum creatinine. Gadolinium contrast is contraindicated for patients older than age 70 or those with diabetes mellitus with an abnormal serum creatinine because it increases the risk of developing nephrogenic systemic fibrosis. The serum creatinine level along with the age, race, and gender are used to calculate the estimated glomerular filtration rate. An estimated glomerular filtration rate of <30 is a contraindication to the use of gadolinium contrast.

22. D: If the NP notes that another healthcare provider is spending much more time catering to the needs of a famous patient while spending much less time with other patients, the ethical principle that the person is violating is justice. Justice relates to fairness and the distribution of the limited resources of healthcare benefits to the members of society. The expectation is that healthcare providers will provide equitable care to all patients, and fame should not be a deciding factor.

23. B: A type II (tissue-specific) hypersensitivity reaction is associated with autoimmune thrombocytopenia, specifically targeting platelet cells. Other type II reactions include hemolysis associated with drug allergies and hemolytic disease of the newborn. Cell destruction occurs by antibodies and complement, by phagocytosis with macrophages, by toxic products produced by neutrophils, by antibody-dependent cell-mediated cytotoxicity, and by antibody-associated cell malfunction.

24. A: If a patient is screaming obscenities and grabbing items from the bedside table and throwing them while climbing off the gurney, then the most appropriate response is to back out of the room and call for security. As a standard procedure, if a patient exhibits behavior that indicates the potential for violence (tense expression, swearing, anger, rapid speech, delusions, or a history of violence), security should be alerted before anyone approaches that patient.

25. D: The profile of a 66-year-old patient with a history of hypertension and type 2 diabetes mellitus who presents with complaints of increasing shortness of breath on exertion and paroxysmal nocturnal dyspnea and examination shows a BP of 100/84, pulse of 112, respiratory rate of 28, 2+ pitting edema of the feet and ankles, rales and crackles throughout the lungs, decreased ventilation, and jugular venous distension 6 cm above the sternal angle is characteristic of right- and left-sided heart failure. The patient's hemoglobin is normal, but the hematocrit is slightly low because of the dilutional effect of fluid retention.

26. B: If a patient has a primary tumor in the prostate, the most likely sites for metastasis are the bones (especially the lumbar spine) and the liver. Cancers metastasize by spreading through lymphatics and blood and usually spread first regionally and then to more distant sites. Most cancer cells that spread from the primary site do not form tumors because the conditions must be optimal for them to do so. The cells have to survive during transit, attach, grow, and begin angiogenesis.

27. C: If the NP is using the PQRST method of time management, the first task is to make a list of tasks in the order of importance, keeping in mind the tasks that must be done at a specific time and that emergencies may occur and will take precedence. Once the list is created, then questioning takes place to determine the most effective way to complete the tasks, following by rechecking. Self-reliance includes identifying those tasks within personal control and tasks in the control of others. Finally, the treat step includes planning time for breaks and time off as well as educational opportunities.

28. A: Initial therapy for a black widow spider bite is ice and elevation because many spider bites do not involve envenomation. The patient must be monitored for at least 24 hours. Envenomation grades are as follows:

- Grade 1 (mild): No pain or stabbing pain. Fang marks with a pale area surrounded by an erythematous ring.
- Grade 2 (moderate): Severe muscle pain, cramps, pain in the upper chest or abdomen (depending on the bite site), normal vital signs, and weakness.
- Grade 3 (severe): Hypertension, arrhythmias, headache, anxiety, generalized pain, pruritis, chills, nausea and vomiting, dyspnea, salivation, shock, and eventually coma.

Treatments include opioids, nitroprusside, tetanus toxoid/immune globulin, calcium gluconate (for muscle cramps) and Latrodectus antivenom (for severe envenomation).

29. B: If a study shows that 50% of patients who are advised to return to the emergency department for follow-up fail to do so, the most effective method of increasing compliance is likely to make a post-visit telephone call. The call allows the NP to connect personally with the patient, to show concern, and to obtain an update on the patient's condition as well as to remind the patient to make a follow-up visit.

30. D: Nociceptive pain progresses through the following phases:

- Phase 1—Transduction: The stimulus occurs in the periphery, and neurotransmitters are released, carrying the pain impulse to the spinal cord.
- Phase 2—Transmission: The pain impulse moves from the spinal cord to the brain, through the thalamus, and to higher cortical areas.
- Phase 3—Perception: The impulse is perceived as a painful sensation.
- Phase 4—Modulation: The perception of pain is inhibited.

31. C: If, when examining a patient's eyes, the NP notes xerophthalmia (dry eyes) and Bitot's spots (foamy plaques), these observations are indicative of vitamin A nutrient deficiency. Keratomalacia may also be present. Pale conjunctivae indicate a deficiency of iron, vitamin B6, or vitamin B12. Red conjunctivae indicate riboflavin deficiency, and blepharitis indicates vitamin B complex or biotin deficiency.

32. B: A waist circumference of greater than 35 inches in females increases the risk for heart disease, diabetes mellitus, and metabolic syndrome. The same risks hold true for males with a waist circumference greater than 40 inches. The waist-hip ratio (waist circumference divided by hip circumference) may also be used to assess risk. A waist-hip ratio of greater than 0.8 for females and greater than 1.0 for males indicates upper body obesity and an increased risk of obesity-associated disorders.

33. B: If a patient is admitted to the emergency department with multiple abrasions and injuries, and the NP reviews the record of a previous admission that recorded that the patient had a "pattern of bruises and fractures," this indicates injuries in various stages of healing. This type of injury typically indicates long-term and ongoing physical abuse. Injuries should be carefully documented, and the patient's report concerning the injuries should be documented verbatim. If policy permits, photographs of the injuries should be taken.

34. A: A heart rate that increases during the peak of inspiration and slows during expiration is characterized as respiratory sinus arrhythmia. Respiratory sinus arrhythmia is a benign finding that is most common in childhood but may persist for some individuals. Respiratory sinus arrhythmia may prolong the P-P interval to greater than 0.16 seconds.

35. D: If, as part of quality improvement, the NP needs to collect and display data to establish priorities for problem solving, the most appropriate display tool is the Pareto chart. The Pareto chart helps to demonstrate the frequency of problems and their effects. The Pareto principle states that 80% of outcomes result from 20% of inputs. Plotting data on the Pareto chart helps to identify the 20% that should have priority in problem solving.

36. B: On an ECG tracing, the complex that represents ventricular depolarization and atrial repolarization is the QRS complex. Contraction occurs with ventricular depolarization. The duration of the QRS complex is typically 0.06-0.10 second. If conduction is impaired, the QRS complex may be prolonged.

37. C: When documenting the observation of undermining about a patient's pressure ulcer, the most appropriate description is "Undermining of 1 cm width extending from 3 o'clock to 5 o'clock." If the undermining is open, then measuring is usually done by inserting a sterile swab. If it is not open, then the extent of undermining may be estimated by palpation because the tissue will feel spongy. Undermining develops when damage occurs under intact tissue.

38. D: The paraneoplastic syndrome associated with pancreatic adenocarcinoma is venous thrombosis (Trousseau phenomenon). Patients develop recurrent and migrating episodes of thrombophlebitis. This syndrome can also occur with gastric and lung adenocarcinoma. Adenocarcinomas produce mucin compounds that result in activation and aggregation of thrombocytes. With venous thrombosis, emboli occur frequently and may cause pulmonary embolism or stroke.

39. D: If the NP notes that an unlicensed nursing assistant performing BP measurements routinely halts pressure descent and reinflates the cuff to double-check the systolic BP, the NP recognizes that this may increase congestion in the veins and result in falsely high diastolic readings. This is an opportunity for teaching because the NP is responsible for delegated tasks.

40. A: Six Sigma is a performance improvement model developed to improve business practices and increase profits by eliminating "defects" in processes. This program focuses on continuous improvement with the customer's perception as key, so that the customer defines what is critical to quality. Two different types of improvement projects may be used: define, measure, analyze, improve, and control for existing processes or products that need improvement and define, measure, analyze, design, and verify for the development of new high-quality processes or products.

41. B: For a patient who has come to the emergency department with chronic hyperuricemia and recurrent severe attacks of gout, the target for treatment is a level of <6 mg/dL. Gout occurs when uric acid crystalizes in the joints, tendons, or bursa, resulting in inflammation, swelling, and severe pain. Uric acid is the end product of the metabolism of purines, found in meats and some vegetables. Normal values for uric acid vary by age, but for adults 19 and older, the normal value for males is 4–8 mg/dL and for females it is 2.5–7 mg/dL. Treatment may include nonsteroidal anti-inflammatory drugs, colchicine, allopurinol, and/or corticosteroids.

42. C: If an older adult takes atorvastatin (or other statins) to control cholesterol levels, the laboratory monitoring that is recommended is liver function tests. The tests should be taken before beginning treatment with the statin, at 12 weeks, and then every 6 months for the duration of the treatment. Borderline elevations are clinically insignificant, but statins have the potential for causing liver damage, especially at high doses. However, some authorities question the necessity of routine testing.

43. B: If a patient with bipolar disorder has stabilized on lithium after three dosage changes, the patient should continue to have serum lithium levels monitored every 3 months. Lithium has a very narrow therapeutic window, and patients can develop severe toxic reactions. Therapeutic values range from 0.8–1.0 mmol/L (although some patients may need slightly lower or higher levels). Toxic reactions may occur at 1.3–1.4 mmol/L. Initial symptoms of toxicity may include nausea, vomiting, diarrhea, weakness, tremors, muscle twitching, and incoordination advancing to altered mental status, agitation, tinnitus, oliguria, hypotension, and death.

44. A: If a patient who speaks no English comes to the emergency department and appears to be in pain and has brought his 8-year-old son to interpret, the NP should arrange for a different interpreter. In emergency situations, sometimes family members may interpret, but children should never do so because they lack the necessary vocabulary and health literacy to interpret accurately and interpreting changes the family dynamics. Also, the patient may withhold information from the child.

45. D: V1 is placed on the right sternum, fourth intercostal space. There are four limb electrodes: RA, LA, RL, LL. Place the electrodes avoiding heavily muscled areas and bony prominences. The six precordial electrodes are placed as follows:

- V1—Right sternum, fourth intercostal space.
- V2—Left sternum, fourth intercostal space.
- V3—Halfway between V2 and V4.
- V4—Midclavicular line, fifth intercostal space.
- V5—In line with V4 at the anterior axillary line.
- V6—In line with V4 and V5 at the midaxillary line.

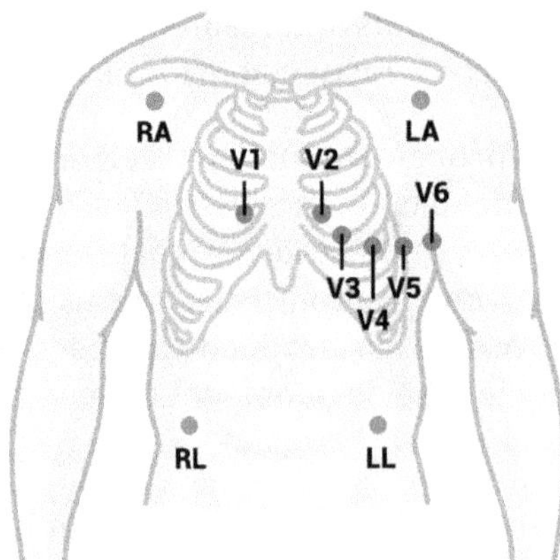

46. C: If the NP is administering the NIH stroke scale to a patient with suspected stroke in the ICU and is assessing part 5 (motor arm) with the patient in the supine position with an arm elevated to 45°, drift is scored if the arm falls before 10 seconds. The NIH stroke scale has 11 parts: level of consciousness, best gaze, visual, facial palsy, motor arm, motor leg, limb ataxia, sensory, best language, dysarthria, and extinction and inattention (formerly neglect).

47. C: If a 50-year-old patient has abdominal pain and distension and a history of diverticulosis, the imaging that is the procedure of choice to verify a diagnosis of diverticulitis is the CT scan. Mild cases usually respond to antibiotic therapy (ciprofloxacin 500 mg two times a day and metronidazole 250 mg three times a day), but patients with more severe disease may need bowel rest and IV fluids in addition to antibiotics. In case of perforation or obstruction, surgical intervention is indicated.

48. A: If an adolescent who is an avid basketball player comes to the emergency department with knee pain and swelling and is diagnosed with patellar tendinitis ("jumper's knee"), the recommended initial treatment is ice, rest, modified activity, and physical therapy. If conservative treatment is ineffective and pain and inflammation persist, then more invasive procedures may be considered: corticosteroid injections, platelet-rich plasma injections, or oscillating needle procedures. Surgical repair is rarely indicated. Patellar tendinitis affects the patellar tendon that connects the patella and the tibia.

49. D: A 15-year-old patient is recovering from spinal instrumentation and fusion for scoliosis. Surgical intervention is indicated for scoliosis when the curvature reaches a magnitude of 40° or greater. Once the curvature exceeds 40°, it usually continues to progress, and a curvature of 70° can seriously impact pulmonary function during adulthood. Fusion is avoided as long as possible in young children who are still growing. Alternatives include casting, bracing, and growth-modulating surgical procedures.

50. B: If a patient complains that a nurse left the patient sitting on the bedside commode for 15 minutes, the type of risk event that this represents is a service occurrence. No injury occurred, even though the patient was inconvenienced. Other service occurrences may include minor property/equipment damage or service interruption. A serious incident is one that may result in minor injuries or loss of or severe damage to equipment. A sentinel event results in death or serious injury, such as a medication error that resulted in death.

51. C: If a 26-year-old patient with sickle cell disease is hospitalized for a vaso-occlusive pain crisis and has reached the established (postinfarctive) phase, this phase typically lasts for 4–5 days. Phases:

- Prodromal: 1–4 days, numbness, aching, paresthesia.
- Initial (infarctive): 1–2 days, severe pain, fever, anxiety, lack of appetite.
- Established (postinfarctive): 4–5 days, severe pain with swelling, joint pain, joint effusions, and leukocytosis.
- Resolving (postcrisis): 1–2 days, gradual reduction in pain.

52. D: According to the American Thoracic Society, if using the 6-minute walk test to measure improvement in a patient's functional status, it is necessary to have greater than 70 meters of improvement to ensure that the improvement is significant. To test, a 30-meter length (such as in a long hallway) should be marked at the beginning and end (with cones if possible) and the patient is asked to walk the length, back and forth, at a comfortable pace for 6 minutes. Chairs should be placed at both ends in case the patient needs to rest, and the patient must be observed carefully.

53. A: If a patient receiving an antipsychotic has developed extrapyramidal effects (muscle spasms, restlessness, bradykinesia, tremor, and rigidity), the medication that is indicated is benztropine (Cogentin), although it is not used with tardive dyskinesia, so it's important to differentiate the disorders. The dosage of the benztropine must be reduced slowly rather than abruptly stopped, and older adults are more prone to adverse effects. Patients receiving benztropine may experience anhidrosis, dry mouth, and urinary retention. Patients should avoid strenuous activities because of the risk of overheating.

54. D: If a patient with type 2 diabetes mellitus has an Hgb A1c level of 8, this corresponds to a glucose level of approximately 180 mg/dL. The A1c to glucose levels are as follows:

A1c	Glucose (mg/dL)
4	50
5	80
6	115
7	150
8	180
9	215

55. B: Long-term use of a proton pump inhibitor, such as omeprazole, should be avoided because of an increased risk of fractures. Other possible adverse effects include an increased risk of hypergastrinemia, pneumonia, hypomagnesemia, vitamin B_{12} deficiency, dementia, *Clostridium difficile* infection, subacute cutaneous lupus erythematosus, and acute interstitial nephritis. Patients should be advised to avoid taking over-the-counter proton pump inhibitors for longer than 2 weeks unless advised to do so by a healthcare provider who is monitoring the patient.

56. A: If a patient is admitted for bone pain, fatigue, severe weakness and numbness in the legs, increased thirst, weight loss, and urinary testing is positive for Bence-Jones protein, the symptoms and the test results are consistent with multiple myeloma, a malignancy of the bones. The average age of onset is 70. M protein levels are monitored because multiple myeloma causes plasma cells to produce an excess of M proteins and abnormal light chain proteins.

57. C: If a patient is hospitalized for a repeat exacerbation of stage III COPD, the NP expects that the patient's FEV1 will be 30–50% of the predicted level. The stages of COPD are as follows:

Stage	FEV1	Symptoms
I	>80%	May have chronic cough, sputum.
II	50–80%	Exertional dyspnea, may have cough. Sputum.
III	30–50%	Increased dyspnea, wheezing, cough, fatigue, reduced exercise tolerance, frequent exacerbations.
IV	<30% (<50%)	Dyspnea at rest, increased functional impairment, hypoxemia, hypercapnia, lung hyperventilation. (Note: FEV1 may be <50% with chronic respiratory failure.)

58. B: The serotonin antagonist used to treat mild to moderate serotonin syndrome is cyproheptadine, which is an H1-blocking antihistamine that also blocks serotonin receptors. Dosage is typically 4–8 mg orally at the onset of symptoms with relief usually evident within 2 hours. Serotonin syndrome is caused by excessive levels of serotonin. Signs of serotonin syndrome include confusion, tachycardia, hypertension, diaphoresis, agitation, muscle twitching and rigidity, and diarrhea.

59. D: In evidence-based research, experimental designs include the two-group pretest–posttest. Experimental designs are indicated when showing evidence of cause and effect is important. The elements that must be included in an experimental design are randomization, control, and manipulation. Other types of experimental designs include two-group posttest, multiple experimental groups, crossover designs, factorial designs, and Solomon four-group design.

60. C: If the NP is a member of the quality improvement council and believes that the council needs to evaluate the overall processes in place for patients being hospitalized and treated, the most appropriate approach is to use tracer methodology. Tracer methodology looks at the continuum of care that a patient receives from admission to postdischarge. A patient is selected to be "traced" with the medical record serving as a guide.

61. A: If a frail 82-year-old patient seemed alert and responsive on admission before surgery, but, in the postoperative period, the patient exhibits fluctuating confusion, agitation, and combativeness and appears to have visual hallucinations, the most likely cause is delirium. Delirium occurs in 10–40% of older adults who are hospitalized and may result from drugs, infection, trauma, surgery, and untreated pain. Medications to reduce symptoms include trazodone, lorazepam, and haloperidol.

62. D: If a 70-year-old homeless male is brought to the emergency department after a fall, and the patient reports long-term increasing weakness and, on examination, the NP notes lymphadenopathy and hepatomegaly and the CBC shows a WBC count of 60,000 with 95% lymphocytes, these signs and symptoms are consistent with chronic lymphocytic leukemia. This disease is slowly progressing, and the average age at diagnosis is 70 (rarely occurring before age 50).

63. C: If a patient at increased risk of a venous thromboembolic event undergoing hip fracture surgery is to receive dalteparin as prophylaxis, the medication should be continued for at least 10 days. If the patient is at high risk, then treatment may be continued for up to 30 days. The initial dose is 2,500 units subcutaneously within 2 hours before surgery and a second 2,500-unit dose 4-8 hours after surgery with subsequent daily doses of 5,000 units subcutaneously. Dalteparin is an anticoagulant in the class of low-molecular-weight heparin.

64. A: If a patient taking warfarin has a target INR level of 2-3, but INR testing shows a level of 3.2, the most appropriate response is to continue the warfarin at the same dosage but recheck within a week. The dosage is not changed unless a pattern of increased INR emerges. If the INR increases to 3.21–3.69 and remains elevated, then the dosage may be decreased by 5–10%. If the INR reaches 3.7–4.99, warfarin is withheld for 1 day and the dosage is reduced by 10–15%. For 5.9-8.9, warfarin is held until the INR stabilizes and then restarted at a 10–15% reduced dosage. Vitamin K antidote is recommended for INR levels of ≥9.

65. B: This patient is demonstrating signs of Tanner stage III development. Stages for females are as follows:

Stage	Breasts	Pubic hair
I	Only the nipples are raised above the chest	None
II	Breast budding	Soft and downy, along the labia majora
III	Breast and areolas enlarge	Sparse, dark hair along the labia majora
IV	Areolas and nipples enlarge, may form secondary elevations	Heavy, coarse pubic hair along the labia majora
V	Full breast, pigmented areolas, projecting nipples	Adult distribution of pubic hair

66. C: If a patient has been hospitalized with acute adrenal crisis because of inconsistent compliance with treatment for primary adrenal insufficiency (Addison's disease), an example of therapeutic questioning is "What strategies do you use to treat your disease?" It's important to avoid yes/no questions and to focus on information questions but without indicating that the patient is to blame because the patient may become defensive. "Why" questions should be avoided if possible.

67. A: If a postsurgical patient has developed a cough, and the NP notes that the tactile fremitus is decreased at the bases of both lungs, the areas are dull to percussion, and breath and voice sounds are absent, these observations are consistent with atelectasis. Atelectasis occurs when the alveoli don't properly inflate or become filled with fluids so that part of the lung partially or completely collapses. Preventive measures include deep breathing and coughing exercises, use of an incentive spirometer, and early ambulation.

68. D: If a patient often delays dressing changes or refuses to cooperate and complains to the NP that dressing changes are too painful, the most appropriate response is "Let's talk about this and figure out a way to make the dressing changes easier for you." Encouraging collaboration may help the patient to feel more in control, and the patient's input may help to find a solution to the problem.

69. B: When referring a patient to another healthcare provider, the first issue that the NP should consider is necessity. A referral may be indicated if the patient's needs are outside of the NP's scope of practice or field of expertise and if the NP cannot provide adequate assessment and treatment for the patient's condition. The healthcare provider must often be selected from healthcare providers participating in the patient's healthcare plan.

70. C: Assisting patients to navigate the healthcare system may include educating patients about the need for screening. Other steps include:

- Explaining diagnoses and treatments
- Providing information about health insurance policies/costs
- Using translators when necessary
- Assisting patients with referrals
- Providing patients with necessary medical records
- Encouraging patients to have advance directives
- Providing and explaining a list of patient's rights and explaining rights to privacy and confidentiality
- Answering questions completely

71. D: If a patient's heart rate is 82 (in the normal range) and the rhythm is regular, but pulsus alternans is evident with the force of alternating beats varying from large to small amplitude, this finding is consistent with left ventricular failure, and the prognosis is poor. Left ventricular failure associated with pulsus alternans may be caused by coronary artery disease, dilated cardiomyopathy, hypertension, or aortic stenosis. Treatment includes identifying and treating the underlying cause, such as through aortic valve replacement.

72. C: If, when conducting a neurological exam, the NP notes that the patient has right unilateral weak contraction of the temporal and masseter muscles of the face and decreased pain sensation in that area, this suggests a lesion affecting cranial nerve V, the trigeminal nerve.

I	Olfactory	VII	Facial
II	Optic	VII	Vestibulocochlear
III	Oculomotor	VIII	Glossopharyngeal
IV	Trochlear	X	Vagus
V	Trigeminal	XI	Accessory
VI	Abducens	XII	Hypoglossal

73. A: If a patient has an intention tremor present with activity but it is absent at rest, this type of tremor is typical with multiple sclerosis. Static/resting tremors are the opposite: prominent at rest and absent with voluntary movement. This type of tremor ("pill rolling") is common with Parkinson's disease. Postural tremors occur when a patient is holding a posture (such as when holding out a hand) and is typically a fine rapid tremor. This type of tremor is associated with hyperthyroidism and anxiety.

74. D: If a patient with a history of *H. pylori* gastritis has taken long-term protein pump inhibitors, the patient is at an increased risk for vitamin B12 (pernicious) anemia. Protein pump inhibitors, such as omeprazole, suppress the production of gastric acids, changing the acidity, and this can affect the absorption of vitamin B12. Because the body requires vitamin B12 to produce red blood cells, a decrease in vitamin B12 can lead to anemia. Patients may develop nausea, loss of appetite, diarrhea or constipation, and hepatomegaly. A smooth, very red tongue is an indication of vitamin B12 deficiency.

75. D: If a patient recently experienced bleeding from esophageal varices and is scheduled for band ligation, the medication that is also indicated to reduce the risk of rebleeding is the beta-blocker propranolol. Combination therapy has been shown to be more effective than either therapy alone. However, up to about a third of patients with cirrhosis cannot tolerate beta-blockers. If used, propranolol is usually initiated at 20 mg two times a day with the dosage increased every 1–2 weeks until a 25% reduction in heart rate (or to 55–60 bpm) as long as the patient can tolerate the drug and the systolic BP remains >90 mmHg.

76. C: If, following a right nephrectomy, a patient complains of abdominal discomfort, distension, and nausea although the abdomen is nontender to palpation and bowel sounds are minimal, the patient likely has paralytic ileus. Restricting oral intake, then gradually increasing it is usually effective as is encouraging early ambulation and movement. Paralytic ileus typically resolves within 2–3 days with supportive care, which may include insertion of a rectal tube. Decreasing opioids may help to resolve paralytic ileus. Nasogastric tubes are generally not recommended unless the patient develops severe vomiting.

77. B: A 70-year-old patient that has been on long-term digoxin therapy should have serum digoxin levels monitored every 6 months. Blood should be drawn during the trough (never the peak), preferably 12–24 hours after the last dose of medication but at least 6 hours. Therapeutic levels range from 0.8–2.0 ng/mL with toxicity occurring at levels greater than 2.4 ng/mL, although some patients may exhibit toxic reactions at lower levels. The risk of toxicity increases if the patient is hypokalemic.

78. D: The herbal supplement that may cause serotonin syndrome in a patient taking SSRIs is St. John's wort. This herbal therapy is an over-the-counter preparation used to treat mild depression and anxiety, but it may interact with numerous drugs, usually decreasing their effectiveness, although with some drugs, such as SSRIs, St. John's wort may cause a toxic reaction. Women of childbearing age should be warned that St. John's wort can reduce the effectiveness of oral contraceptives.

79. B: If a patient with sickle cell disease is hospitalized with acute chest syndrome, packed red blood cell transfusions are administered to a target hemoglobin of 10 g/dL. Patients with sickle cell disease are chronically anemic. Other treatments include IV fluids, antibiotics, analgesia, L-glutamine, bronchodilators, and oxygen. Acute chest syndrome results from obstruction of vessels in the lungs by sickled red blood cells. Other processes may include atelectasis, fat embolism (from necrosis of bone marrow), thromboembolism, and infection.

80. A: If a patient with a history of alcoholism and cirrhosis is admitted with upper GI bleeding and is vomiting bright-red blood, the emergent medication that is indicated before endoscopy is octreotide, given by a 100 mcg bolus followed by continuous infusion of 50–100 mcg per hour. Octreotide decreases portal BP, and splanchnic blood flow and is indicated if liver disease and/or portal hypertension is suspected in the presence of upper GI bleeding.

81. D: If the average effective dose (ED_{50}) of a drug is 10 mg and the average lethal dose (LD_{50}) is 110 mg, the drug is relatively safe (no drug is 100% safe) because the ED_{50} is a much lower dosage than the LD_{50} (a high therapeutic index), so there is little chance that a patient will receive a lethal dose. If the ED_{50} and LD_{50} are close (a low therapeutic index), then administration carries a greater risk. Drugs with a low therapeutic index include digoxin, lithium, aminoglycosides, cyclosporine, warfarin, carbamazepine, phenytoin, phenobarbital, theophylline, digitalis glycosides, flecainide, and rifampin.

82. C: If a patient with chronic liver disease and ascites develops fever and abdominal pain, and paracentesis and examination of the ascitic fluid shows 95% neutrophils, the most likely diagnosis is bacterial peritonitis, which may be caused by enteric bacteria translocating across the gut wall or from bacteremia originating at another site. Typically, with bacterial peritonitis, laboratory studies show that the neutrophils are greater than 50–70% and may be 100%. Treatment is often with a third-generation cephalosporin. Recurrence is common within 1 year, so ongoing antibiotic prophylaxis is indicated.

83. B: If a patient who has been experiencing abdominal discomfort passes maroon-colored stools, this suggests that bleeding is occurring in the right colon or distal small intestine. Bright-red blood usually indicates bleeding from the left colon, whereas brown stool mixed or streaked with bright-red blood indicates bleeding in the rectosigmoid area. Melena (black, tarry stool) occurs when bleeding is proximal to the ligament of Treitz, which is the suspensory muscle of the duodenum.

84. D: If a patient with moderately severe Alzheimer's disease underwent emergency surgery for bowel obstruction and in the postoperative period is extremely confused and continually tries to pull out IVs and tubes and climb out of bed, the intervention that is most appropriate is using a sitter. Restraining a patient with Alzheimer's almost always causes increased agitation and combativeness, and medications to calm patients are often ineffective. A calm presence to comfort and reassure the patient is often the best approach. If sitters are not available in the hospital, then sometimes family members are willing to sit with the patient.

85. C: The hemodynamic status associated with septic shock is massive vasodilation with increased capillary permeability. Septic shock is a form of distributive shock. Septic shock is most often associated with Gram-negative (60–70%) or Gram-positive bacteria (often associated with indwelling catheters). Gram-negative bacteria release endotoxins, and Gram-positive bacteria release exotoxins, which cause vascular inflammation and vasodilation. Septic shock manifests as early stage (flushing, fever, and chills) and late stage (hypotension, tachycardia, tachypnea, and altered mental status).

86. A: Population and global environmental factors may impact individual health:

- Population factors: Family size (the average family size has decreased, leaving fewer family members to assist), aging population (increased demand for services), population movement (family members are often widespread and not available to help), and unemployment/retirement (a loss of income impacts the ability to pay for care).
- Global environmental factors: Natural disasters, climate extremes, and smog/environmental contamination.

87. C: When prescribing medications for older adults, the NP should especially consult the Beers Criteria for Potentially Inappropriate Medication Use in Older Adults. These criteria list medications that those older than age 65 should avoid because of potential problems, such as adverse effects and risk of falls. These criteria also include information about medications that should be used with caution, changes in dosage needed with impaired kidney function, and medicine interactions.

88. B: When treating a patient for shock, the urinary output that is necessary to ensure adequate organ perfusion is greater than 0.5–1.0 mL/kg/hr. This is slightly lower than the normal urinary output, which usually ranges from 1.0–2.0 mL/kg/hr because the body prioritizes organ perfusion over peripheral perfusion. Other indications of perfusion, such as BP, heart rate, and capillary refill time, may vary depending on the patient's overall condition, so they cannot be relied upon exclusively to assess perfusion.

89. A: If a patient is diagnosed with class II hypovolemia, with a 15–30% volume loss, indications that support this classification include stable BP, tachycardia, and tachypnea. Classes of volume loss are described as follows:

- Class 1: ≤15% volume loss, essentially asymptomatic
- Class 2: as above
- Class 3: 30–40% volume loss, BP falling, heart rate >120 bpm, oliguria, and altered mental status
- Class 4: >40% volume loss, hypotension, heart rate >140 bpm, narrowed pulse pressure, altered mental status, piloerection, cold clammy skin, mottled skin, and cyanosis

90. A: Risk stratification, an important element of data analysis, is used to predict outcomes of treatment by accounting for various factors such as age, gender, history of drinking, and history of smoking. These are factors that place the individual at greater risk. Risk stratification involves statistical adjustment to account for confounding issues (things that confuse data outcomes) and differences in risk factors.

91. B: If the NP recognizes that hospital policy regarding a specific treatment is not in line with current evidence-based research, when implementing treatment, the NP should base the treatment on hospital policy for legal reasons and in recognition that evidence-based research may not be generalizable to all situations. However, the NP should take steps to change the policy if it is appropriate to do so.

92. D: A female patient with the following test results meets the criteria for metabolic syndrome:

- Fasting insulin 78% (indicated insulin resistance)
- Fasting serum glucose 112 mg/dL (elevated)
- Fasting triglycerides 160 mg/dL (elevated)
- High-density lipoprotein 30 mg/dL (low)
- BMI 28, hip-to-waist ratio 1.0 (obese)
- BP 138/88 (elevated)
- Uric acid 7.8 mg/dL (elevated)

93. D: According to Joint Commission accreditation guidelines, patients hospitalized with acute myocardial infarction should receive aspirin within 24 hours. Aspirin reduces the risk of adverse effects and death by up to 20%. Long-term aspirin therapy (usually low dose) is recommended on discharge for prevention unless contraindications (such as taking warfarin, under 18 years of age, under hospice care, the patient has aspirin sensitivity) are present.

94. B: If a 25-year-old male comes to the emergency department with complaints of yellow-green purulent urethral discharge and scrotal pain, consistent with gonorrhea, the recommended first-line treatment is ceftriaxone.

STD	Treatment	Frequency
Gonorrhea	Ceftriaxone 500 mg IM	One time
Syphilis	Benzathine penicillin G 2.4 million units IM	One time
Trichomoniasis	Metronidazole 2 g po	One time
Chlamydia	Azithromycin 1 g po	One time

95. C: The pinprick test is used to determine the patient's ability to perceive pain and pressure. Both a sharp point and a dull point should be used for assessment, and the patient is asked to indicate when the stimulus is felt and to report if it is dull or sharp. At least 2 seconds should elapse between each stimulus because summation may occur if stimuli are too close together. With summation, a number of consecutive stimuli are perceived by the patient to be one large stimulus.

96. A: If a patient is very disgruntled after waiting an hour for a procedure and states "I'm never coming to this hospital again," and the NP is using the CARE approach to calm the patient, the most appropriate initial response is "Tell me about the problem and how I can help." It's important to allow the person time to vent and express frustrations. The next step is to apologize for the inconvenience without making excuses or blaming anyone. The repair step involves finding a way to make things better, and the exceed step involves doing more than the patient expects.

97. C: If a patient tells the NP that she wants medication to lose weight, the NP should inform the patient that these medications are recommended for patients with BMI of >30 or >27 with risk factors (such as type 2 diabetes mellitus). Patients should try to lose weight through diet and exercise before taking medications to suppress the appetite or to inhibit absorption of fats because of the adverse effects associated with the medications.

98. A: If a patient is being treated for a pressure ulcer, to promote healing, nutrient intake should include 30–40 kcal/kg/day and 1.0–1.5 g/kg/day of protein. Fluid intake should be 1-2 liters daily because dehydration impairs healing. Patients should be turned at least every 2 hours, and positioning devices should be used. The head of the bed should be maintained at <30° when the patient is side-lying or supine, and time in a chair should be limited.

99. B: When a patient arrives at the emergency department with an ST elevation myocardial infarction, reperfusion should ideally be completed within 90 minutes to reduce morbidity and mortality. Reperfusion may be done with fibrinolytics (such as streptokinase, alteplase, and reteplase) or mechanically through percutaneous coronary intervention. In older adults especially, fibrinolytic treatment increases the risk of intracranial hemorrhage. Fibrinolytic therapy should be done within 6 hours of the onset of symptoms.

100. B: When discharging a 35-year-old female patient who is receiving acitretin for severe psoriasis, it is important to include instructions about the continuous use of two forms of contraception because acitretin is teratogenic. Before beginning treatment, patients must have two negative pregnancy tests and are required to have regular pregnancy tests during treatment and must continue to use two forms of birth control until 3 years after discontinuing the medication. Patients may not consume any alcohol or food or medicine that contains alcohol during treatment.

101. D: If, when auscultating a patient's heart at the 5th intercostal space, left midclavicular line, the NP notes a murmur that has a high-pitched blowing sound that is more pronounced during expiration and when the patient is supine, and the murmur radiates to the left axilla and back, this is characteristic of mitral regurgitation. Mitral regurgitation may occur with chronic rheumatic fever, acute bacterial endocarditis, mitral valve prolapse, and papillary muscled rupture.

102. A: Normal pH values are as follows:

1.5–3.5	Gastric fluids
4.5–8	Urine
6.6 +/− 0.3	Feces
7.31–7.41	Venous blood
7.35–7.45	Arterial blood
7.33–7.52	Cerebrospinal fluid

103. C: If a patient with COPD experiences exertional dyspnea, this is generally an indication that the patient's FEV1 is at least 50% of the norm. In the early stages of COPD, patients may be essentially asymptomatic or may experience dyspnea primarily during episodes of bronchitis over a number of years until gradually the FEV1 falls to the point that the patient becomes dyspneic on exertion without bronchitis and then without exertion. The three primary symptoms of COPD are exertional dyspnea, cough, and sputum production.

104. B: If the NP suspects that a patient's confusion is caused by delirium, the assessment tool that is indicated to verify this diagnosis is the Confusion Assessment Method. This tool covers nine factors: onset, attention, thinking, level of consciousness, orientation, memory, perceptual disturbances, psychomotor abnormalities, and sleep-wake cycle. The Time and Change Test and the Trail Making Test are used to assess dementia. The Mini-Cog is a short assessment tool that is used to assess cognitive function in older adults, particularly with regard to dementia.

105. B: If a patient comes to the emergency department with symptoms indicating possible appendicitis, the NP assesses for rebound tenderness (McBurney's sign) by applying pressure in the RLQ at a point two-thirds the distance from the navel to the right anterior superior iliac spine. If the appendix is inflamed, this should cause severe pain. Other signs of appendicitis are as follows:

- Psoas: Place the patient on the left side with the right upper leg flexed backward. Pain causes the knee to flex toward the abdomen.
- Rovsing's sign: Apply pressure to the LLQ. Pain is felt in the RLQ.
- Obturator: Flex the right knee to 90° and internally rotate the hip. This causes pain.

106. B: A patient reports episodes of nausea and abdominal pain lasting 2–4 hours in the RUQ and radiating to the right scapula after eating fatty foods or drinking alcohol. The NP recognizes that these symptoms are consistent with cholecystitis. A positive Murphy's sign is also indicative of cholecystitis. This is tested by asking the patient to breathe out, place the hand over the area of the gallbladder (below the right costal margin) and then ask the patient to breathe in. If positive, this causes pain and the patient briefly holds the breath.

107. A: If the NP notes that a patient's hands are very pale, and the patient complains of feeling cold and numb with the hands slowly becoming blue-tinged and painful and then erythematous and edematous with burning, throbbing pain, the NP recognizes these signs and symptoms as probable Raynaud's phenomenon. The "red, white, and blue" signs occur when cold or stress causes circulatory impairment (white) and then blood slowly returns (blue) and then returns fully to dilated capillaries (red).

108. C: A characteristic of chronic peripheral arterial disease includes deep muscle pain with onset gradual with exertion. Pain is usually in the calf but may involve other areas of the lower leg and foot (dorsum). Pain may involve intermittent claudication (cramping, numbness, tingling, feeling of coldness) and is aggravated by activity and elevation. Pain is often relieved by standing for 1–2 minutes. Risk factors include older age, hypertension, diabetes, obesity, vascular disease, and hypercholesterolemia.

109. A: If a patient has a small ulcer on the medial malleolus, and the NP notes on examination that the patient has hemosiderosis on both lower legs, this finding suggests venous stasis. With venous stasis, the increased pressure in the veins causes red blood cells to leak out of the veins and into the tissues where the red blood cells break down and leave hemosiderin (iron) in the tissues, resulting in brownish discoloration.

110. D: A harsh continuous murmur and an approximately 5 cm pulsating mass palpable above the umbilicus, slightly to the left of midline, indicate an aortic aneurysm. Most abdominal aortic aneurysms extend to the umbilicus. Femoral pulses generally remain, but the force of the pulses is decreased. The aortic aneurysm is typically asymptomatic unless it ruptures. Repair (surgical, endovascular) is usually done for aneurysms greater than 5 cm.

111. A: If an 80-year-old patient comes to the emergency room with signs and symptoms of giant cell temporal arteritis (headache, scalp tenderness, diplopia, jaw claudication, and throat pain), and the patient's erythrocyte sedimentation rate is markedly elevated, emergent treatment should include corticosteroids. The typical dosage is 60 mg of prednisone daily. If loss of vision has occurred, treatment rarely effects improvement. Low-dose aspirin is usually given with the corticosteroid to reduce the risk of vision loss or stroke. A biopsy should be done as soon as possible, but treatment should not be delayed for the biopsy because of the risk of blindness.

112. A: If a patient comes to the emergency department and reports that he is a heroin addict and has shared needles with a person 2 days previously and just learned that the person is HIV positive, the NP should recommend that the patient immediately begin PEP, which should begin within 72 hours of exposure. PEP currently consists of three drugs: a combination of tenofovir with emtricitabine and raltegravir or dolutegravir. Although the patient should be provided information about rehabilitation, PEP is more critical.

113. C: The variety of hepatitis that poses the greatest risk of becoming a chronic disease is hepatitis C, which accounts for up to 70% of chronic cases with 75% of acute hepatitis C becoming chronic. Hepatitis B becomes chronic in only 5% to 10% of cases. Hepatitis A does not have a chronic form. Hepatitis D has acute and chronic forms, but the prevalence is much lower because hepatitis D occurs only as a coinfection with hepatitis B. Incidence of hepatitis D is rare in the United States because of decreased rates of hepatitis B.

114. D: This ECG tracing is consistent with sinus pause, which occurs when the sinus node fails to function properly to stimulate heart contractions and the P wave, so there is a pause on the ECG recording that may persist for a few seconds to a few minutes. During the sinus pause, the P wave, QRS complex, and PR and QRS intervals are all absent. P: the QRS ratio is 1:1, and the rhythm is irregular. The pulse rate may vary widely, usually from 60-100. Patients frequently complain of dizziness or syncope.

115. B: If an organ enlarges because the number of cells increase, this is referred to as hyperplasia. With hypertrophy, the existing cells enlarge but don't increase in number. Dysplasia (a type of atypical hyperplasia) is characterized by cells of abnormal shape and size. With metaplasia, one mature cell of a specific type is replaced by a cell of a different type. Metaplasia may be reversible if the cause is identified.

116. D: A Glasgow coma scale score of 7 indicates that the patient is comatose.

Eye opening	4: Spontaneous 3: To verbal stimuli 2: To pain [not of face] 1: No response
Verbal	5: Oriented 4: Conversation is confused, but can answer questions 3: Uses inappropriate words 2: Speech is incomprehensible 1: No response
Motor	6: Moves on command 5: Moves purposefully to respond to pain 4: Withdraws in response to pain 3: Decorticate posturing (flexion) in response to pain 2: Decerebrate posturing (extension) in response to pain 1: No response

For classifying head injuries, mild is 13–15, moderate is 9–12, and severe is 8 or less. Additionally, any score of 8 or less is considered comatose.

117. A: If a patient reports that he is allergic to penicillin, the NP should be aware that the patient may have a cross sensitivity to cephalosporins. Up to 7% of those with an allergy to penicillin have this cross sensitivity, but if the person's allergic response is severe, cross sensitivity increases to 50%. The patient may also react to different drugs in the same family, such as amoxicillin. Cross sensitivity can also occur with the IV beta-lactam imipenem.

118. C: Considering membrane transport, the movement of a solute molecule from an area of greater concentration to one of lesser concentration is diffusion. The difference in concentration is the concentration gradient. The process of diffusion continues until equilibrium is achieved and the concentration is the same in both areas. The rate of diffusion is affected by differences in electrical potential, the size of the molecules (small molecules diffuse more quickly than large molecules), and the lipid solubility.

119. D: If a patient who has been noncompliant with treatment for epilepsy is hospitalized with generalized tonic-clonic status epilepticus, after IV access is established, the patient initially receives a 50 mL bolus of 50% dextrose (because hypoglycemia may induce status epilepticus) but seizures still persist in 5 minutes, the first-line treatment administered next is a benzodiazepine, typically lorazepam. If seizures persist, then an anticonvulsant, such as fosphenytoin, valproic acid, or phenytoin, is administered. Thiamine is added to the IV bolus if the patient is at risk for Wernicke's encephalopathy.

120. B: Seven or more consecutive data points that are all higher or lower than the mean is considered a run. Trending analysis terms include the following:

- Run (shift): ≥7 consecutive data points all above or all below the median (run chart) or mean (control chart).
- Trend: ≥7 consecutive data points in either ascending or descending order with ≥21 total data points or ≥6 with fewer than 21 total data points.
- Cycle: Up and down variation forming a sawtooth pattern with 14 successive data points, suggestive of a systemic effect on the data. If the trend is related to common cause variation, the variation may be demonstrated with 4–11 successive data points.
- Astronomical value: A data point unrelated to other points indicates a sentinel event or special cause variation.

121. C: When a problem arises in a medical context, the first step to resolve the problem is to define the issue through interviews and discussions with interested parties, such as patients, staff, and family members. The next step is to collect data, such as through interviewing additional individuals and reviewing documentation. Then the reasons for actions that led to the problem should be considered, and finally a decision is made in order to prevent recurrence of the problem.

122. A: In an elderly patient, the presenting symptom of an acute MI is often dyspnea. Chest pain associated with MI declines with age. Fewer than half of those age 80 experience chest pain, and many do not exhibit diaphoresis. About 40% have symptoms of acute heart failure. Patients frequently have other atypical symptoms, so MI is sometimes overlooked as a diagnosis. Older patients often have existing cardiovascular disease, so ECGs may be nondiagnostic.

123. D: If a patient received a blunt abdominal injury during a motor vehicle accident and is hypotensive and complains of diffuse abdominal pain and has ecchymosis around the umbilicus (positive Cullen's sign), this indicates bleeding from a ruptured spleen. The spleen is the most frequently injured solid organ in blunt trauma. Splenic injuries are classified according to the degree of injury:

7. Tear in splenic capsules or hematoma
8. Laceration of parenchyma (<3 cm)
9. Laceration of parenchyma (>3 cm)
10. Multiple lacerations of parenchyma or burst-type injury

124. B: If the NP participates in a P4P value-based contract with an insurance company, this means that the NP may receive less pay for negative outcomes and more pay for positive outcomes. P4P is a general term referring to programs that provide monetary incentives for hospitals and healthcare providers to improve the quality of care. P4P programs are usually based on four types of quality measures: performance, outcomes, patient satisfaction, and structures/technology.

125. A: If a patient is hospitalized with acute alcohol-induced pancreatitis, the primary treatment is supportive. Food and oral fluids are restricted initially, and IV fluids are provided. Analgesia usually includes opioids because of severe pain. If NPO status must be maintained for a prolonged period, then the patient may receive enteral (jejunal) feedings or TPN to maintain adequate nutrition. Alcohol-induced pancreatitis typically occurs after more than a dozen years of 8–10 drinks daily. The most important factor in preventing chronic pancreatitis is abstinence from alcohol.

126. B: A benchmark is an example of an external trigger that may indicate the need for further analysis. Benchmarking involves analyzing data from outside an institution, such as monitoring national rates of hospital-acquired infections and comparing them to internal rates. Other external triggers may include feedback from customers (patients, vendors, family, and community members), strategic planning initiatives, practice guidelines, and research findings. Internal triggers may include sentinel events, the performance rate, and rate change.

127. D: If an adolescent patient is admitted with benzodiazepine-induced coma and severe respiratory depression after a suicide attempt with stolen drugs, the emergent antidote is flumazenil because this patient is unlikely to be a chronic user, so the reversal agent can be safely used. If a patient is a chronic user, however, life-threatening withdrawal symptoms, including seizures, may occur. Flumazenil should also be avoided for patients who use multiple drugs.

128. C: The leading cause of acute liver failure is acetaminophen toxicity (45%) with 44% of those cases caused by intentional overdose. Toxicity occurs with dosage >140 mg/kg in one dose or >7.5g in 24 hours. Serum levels higher than 150 require an antidote:

- GI decontamination with activated charcoal (orally or nasogastrically) <24 hours
- Antidote: 72-hour N-acetylcysteine protocol includes 140 mg/kg initially and 70 mg/kg every 4 hours for 17 more doses (orally or IV)
- Supportive therapy

The antidote is most effective within 8 hours of ingestion but decreases hepatotoxicity even after more than 24 hours.

129. A: When preparing educational materials for patients and using the Fog Formula to determine readability, calculations are based on the number of words per sentence/independent clause and the number of three-syllable (or greater) words. Almost all readability formulas are based on these same things. Generally, the longer and more complex the sentence, the more difficult it is for those with low literacy to read it, and the same is true of long words.

130. D: All types of measurement are vulnerable to measurement error. Direct measures are usually the most accurate but can still produce error. For example, if a scale is not properly balanced, the result may be inaccurate. When considering measurement, one must take into account the true score (if no error existed), the recorded score (arrived at by observation), and the error score. In research, the true score is never achieved.

131. B: For burn patients, electrolyte imbalance may be life-threatening if burns cover more than 20% of BSA. The metabolic rate increases because the sympathetic nervous system stimulates the release of epinephrine and norepinephrine, which increases cardiac output and hastens the loss of fluids. Electrolytes are lost through exposed tissue resulting in hypophosphatemia, hypocalcemia, hyponatremia, and hyperkalemia. Fluid and electrolyte replacement is based on weight and the extent of burns using the Parkland formula: 4 mL/kg/wt × BSA per 24 hours.

132. C: If a patient was exposed to burning plastic in a factory fire and is suspected of having cyanide poisoning, the most appropriate treatment is hydroxocobalamin, which combines chemically with the cyanide and forms cyanocobalamin (vitamin B12), which is then excreted through the kidneys. Other antidotes that may be used include sodium nitrate and sodium thiosulfate (usually given in combination), but sodium nitrate has a higher risk of adverse effects than hydroxocobalamin.

133. A: If the NP is serving as a preceptor for a newly graduated NP who is in a probationary period at work, the primary goal of the preceptor is to prepare the nurse to assume full responsibility. The preceptor ensures that the new NP is fully oriented to the organization and nursing responsibilities through educating, coaching, supporting, and evaluating. The preceptor should be alert to performance issues and assist the new NP to improve performance.

134. D: A research study that focuses on a particular group of people who were exposed to a toxin in a work environment in order to determine causality would be classified as a retrospective cohort study. With this type of study, a group of people who experience a similar event are studied after the event to determine if the event affected health positively or negatively and compared to another group that did not experience the event. For example, the researcher may compare the original group with another group in a similar environment who were not exposed to the toxin.

135. B: If a patient taking metoprolol (a beta-blocker) for hypertension has developed severe muscle pains and is switching to irbesartan (a calcium-channel blocker), the NP should advise the patient to decrease the dosage of metoprolol over 1–2 weeks and then start irbesartan. Beta-blockers should not be stopped abruptly because this can cause exacerbation of angina or myocardial infarction. They must be withdrawn by slowly decreasing the dosage over a 1- to 2-week period.

136. C: A core concept of Continuous Quality Improvement is that problems relate to processes and variations in processes lead to variations in results. Other core concepts include:

- Quality and success are meeting or exceeding internal and external customers' needs and expectations.
- Change can be in small steps.

Continuous Quality Improvement emphasizes the organization and systems and processes within that organization rather than individuals and recognizes internal customers (staff) and external customers (patients) and uses data to improve processes.

137. D: Angina that lasts for less than 5 minutes and results from atherosclerotic lesions obstructing greater than 75% of the lumen of the affected coronary artery is classified as stable angina. Unstable angina usually lasts for more than 5 minutes and is less predictable and controllable. It may indicate rupture of an atherosclerotic plaque and the beginning of thrombus formation. Variant (Prinzmetal's) angina results from spasms of the coronary arteries, either associated with or without atherosclerotic plaques, and is often related to smoking, alcohol, or illicit stimulants. Angina decubitus is angina that occurs at night when the patient is recumbent.

138. A: If a 20-year-old patient is admitted with a sudden onset (<12 hours) of headache, nuchal rigidity, fever, and altered mental status, and the NP suspects bacterial meningitis, the most appropriate initial intervention is to administer empiric antibiotics, typically vancomycin with cefotaxime or ceftriaxone, before further testing because of the high risk of morbidity and mortality. A CT scan may be ordered if indicated. A lumbar puncture should be done as soon as possible. If infection with *Staphylococcus pneumoniae* is suspected; dexamethasone may be given 15–20 minutes before the antibiotic.

139. C: In a research study, manipulation refers to the treatment that is being provided. For example, one group of patients may have wound care with one type of occlusive dressing and another group may have treatment with a different type to determine which is more effective. In research, treatment variables (which are also the independent variables) are purposely manipulated in order to study causality (how cause leads to effect).

140. C: The government agency that regulates protection of human subjects and requires any researcher involving individuals in research to obtain informed consent in language that is understandable is the FDA, under the Code of Federal Regulations, Title 21, Volume 1. Informed consent must include an explanation of the research, the purpose, and the expected duration as well as a description of any potential risks. Potential benefits must be described, and possible alternative treatments should be explained. Any compensation to be provided must be outlined.

141. B: If using the HOPE mnemonic to guide spiritual assessment, the H stands for sources of hope.

H	Sources of hope	What are your sources of hope? What helps you cope with difficulties?
O	Organized religion	Do you participate in a religious/spiritual community? Does it comfort you?
P	Personal spirituality/practices	Do you have your own personal spiritual beliefs?
E	Effects on medical care/end-of-life issues	Does your health allow you do participate in practices that help you spiritually? Do you have religious-based restrictions or beliefs that may affect medical care?

142. D: The PERSON method of carrying out a physical health assessment focuses on functions and includes **P**sychosocial, **E**limination, **R**est/regulatory/reproductive, **S**afety, **O**xygenation, and **N**utrition. Other methods include the traditional head-to-toe exam and Gordon's functional health patterns, which includes (1) health perception/management, (2) nutritional/metabolic, (3) elimination, (4) activity/exercise, (5) cognitive and perceptual, (6) sleep/rest, (7) self-perception and concept, (8) role/relationship, (9) sexuality and reproductive, (10) coping/stress tolerance, and (11) value and belief.

143. A: When treating hypertension in a male African-American patient, the type of drug that is generally avoided is beta-blockers because they are less effective for African Americans than for other races. Additionally, African Americans tend to have better control of hypertension with two types of antihypertensive drugs rather than a single drug. Commonly used drug combinations include an ACE inhibitor or ARB and a calcium channel blocker or thiazide diuretic (long-acting).

144. C: If the NP wants to effect changes in public health policy, the most effective method is to participate in national healthcare organizations. Individuals usually have little power to bring about change on a national level, but much public health policy has been developed and promoted by national healthcare organizations. Members can often indicate an interest in serving on policy committees and can participate in organizational activities and studies.

145. A: The primary purpose in using the SBAR method of handoff and transition of care is patient safety. During handoff and transition of care, patients are particularly at risk because critical information may be forgotten or overlooked. SBAR:

- Situation: Name, age, overseeing physician, diagnosis
- Background: Brief medical history, comorbidities, review of lab tests, current therapy, IVs, vital signs, pain, special needs, educational needs, discharge plans
- Assessment: Review of systems, lines, tubes, and drains, completed tasks, needed tasks, future procedures
- Recommendations: Review plan of care, medications, precautions (restraints, falls), treatments, wound care

146. B: This patient is experiencing moderate anxiety. Peplau's four levels of anxiety are as follows:

11. Mild: Increased motivation, sharpened senses, enlarged perceptual field, hypersensitivity to sensory input, able to solve problems, learning effective. Possible gastrointestinal upset.
12. Moderate: Perceptual field narrows to a specific task; attention is selective. Speaks rapidly in a high pitch, and experiences muscle tension, diaphoresis, pounding pulse, headache, dry mouth, gastrointestinal upset, and frequent urination.
13. Severe: Perceptual field narrows; cannot complete tasks, solve problems, or learn effectively. Feels fear, dread, or horror; experiences multiple physiological symptoms.
14. Panic: Perceptual field focuses on self, does not respond to environmental stimuli, experiences perceptual distortions, unable to think rationally or recognize danger, and may be suicidal.

147. D: A patient was hospitalized with a stroke for 4 days and then transferred to an SNF for 20 days. Because the patient was hospitalized for at least 3 days, the patient was eligible for up to 100 days of SNF coverage. The patient was then discharged home but was readmitted to an acute hospital 62 days later because of another stroke. Because this is more than 60 days, the first benefit period ended. After 3 days of hospitalization, the patient was transferred to the same SNF. The patient had 3 qualifying days of hospitalization and is now eligible for up to another 100 days of SNF coverage.

148. A: If the NP is using the CAGE tool to assess a patient's risk of alcohol abuse and the patient answers "yes" to one out of four questions, this represents a possible drinking problem, whereas a "yes" answer on two or more questions indicates a drinking problem. The CAGE tool is as follows:

C	Cutting down	Do you think about trying to cut down on drinking?
A	Annoyed at criticism	Are people starting to criticize your drinking?
G	Guilty feeling	Do you feel guilty or try to hide your drinking?
E	Eye opener	Do you increasingly need a drink earlier in the day?

149. C: If an older patient has a score of 14 out of 23 on the Braden scale, this indicates that the patient has a risk of developing a pressure ulcer. The Braden scale for predicting risk of developing pressure sores scores six different areas with one to four points. The first four areas include sensory perception, moisture, activity, and mobility. The last two areas include usual nutrition pattern and friction and shear.

- 23: (Best score) excellent prognosis, very minimal risk
- ≤16: Breaking point for risk of pressure ulcer (varies somewhat for different populations)
- 6: (Worst score) prognosis is very poor; strong likelihood of developing pressure ulcers

150. A: According to Maslow's hierarchy of needs, the nursing diagnosis that would have priority is risk for aspiration. Hierarchy of needs:

1	Physiological (basic needs to sustain life—oxygen, food, fluids, sleep)	Risk for aspiration Deficient fluid volume Impaired spontaneous ventilation
2	Safety and security (physiological and psychological threats)	Verbal communication impaired Latex allergy response Death anxiety
3	Love/Belonging (support, caring, intimacy)	Risk for loneliness Anxiety Caregiver role strain
4	Self-esteem (sense of worth, respect, independence)	Defensive coping Disturbed body image Post-traumatic response
5	Self-actualization	Health-seeking behaviors Spiritual distress

151. C: If a patient with a gunshot wound has tattooing and stippling around the entry wound, this indicates that the injury resulted from an intermediate distance range. This means that the gun was not touching the patient's body but was close enough when discharged that gunpowder is driven into the skin surrounding the entry wound, discoloring the skin (tattooing) or causing punctate abrasions (stippling).

152. B: Considering vulnerable populations, the unique problems that the NP should expect may be identified for homeless individuals include lice because the homeless population may lack facilities to bathe or wash their clothes, malnutrition because of inadequate diet, substance abuse, and psychiatric conditions (affecting about one-third of the homeless population). Schizophrenia and bipolar disorder are especially common among the homeless population. Homeless patients may need referrals for psychiatric care and substance abuse, and discharge planning often requires the assistance of social services and housing authorities.

153. A: If the NP is preparing to educate an ICU patient about the importance of receiving the annual influenza vaccine, this is an example of primary prevention.

- Primary: Aims to prevent disease occurrence and may include educational campaigns (no smoking, use of seat belts, vaccinations).
- Secondary: Aims to identify and reduce health impacts (screening mammograms, BP checks).
- Tertiary: Aims to prevent/delay disease progression (support programs).
- Quaternary: Aims to protect the patient from treatment-induced complications, such as from overmedication or unnecessary testing/treatment.

154. D: If the NP is serving on the cost-containment committee, which is considering a request by the radiology department, and the cost to repair a current CT scanner is $70,000, the cost to buy a similar refurbished model is $120,000, and the cost of a new, updated scanner is $1.5 million, the committee should recommend that a cost analysis be done before a decision is made. Repeated repairs and downtown can be costly with older machines, and refurbished machines may not be as up to date as new machines. Sometimes, the most expensive option provides the best return on investment.

155. A: If a patient is to have IV antibiotics for 48 hours before switching to oral antibiotics, the type of IV access that is indicated is a short peripheral catheter (SPC). SPCs are used when infusions are needed for a few days with 96 hours usually being the maximum duration of the SPC, and the SPC is usually inserted into the hand, wrist, or forearm (avoiding areas of flexion). Most are made of polyurethane. SPCs are usually over-the-needle catheters with the catheter length being 7.5 cm. Gauges range from 15 (massive trauma) to 24 (small, fragile vessels). Fluids include isotonic fluids/drugs and fluids with pH values ranging from >5 to <9. Vesicants and IV solutions with >10% glucose should be avoided.

156. C: If, in an emergent situation, the NP must start an intraosseous infusion for an adult patient using the Fast1 Intraosseous Infusion System, the intraosseous needle should be inserted into the sternum (proximal area). The set automatically prevents insertion into the thoracic cavity. The infusion set can deliver up to 80 mL/min and can be used with patients 12 years and older. The Bone Injection Gun is another system that comes in an adult and a pediatric form. For adults using this system, the intraosseous needle is inserted into the proximal tibia or proximal humerus.

157. B: An arterial blood pH greater than 7.45, partial pressure of carbon dioxide ($PaCO_2$) is less than 35 mmHg, and decreased serum bicarbonate (HCO_3^-) is indicative of respiratory alkalosis.

Characteristics	Decreased $PaCO_2$ Normal or decreased serum bicarbonate (HCO_3^-) as kidneys conserve hydrogen and excrete HCO_3^- Increased pH
Symptoms	Vasoconstriction with decreased cerebral blood flow resulting in lightheadedness, alterations in mentation, and/or unconsciousness Numbness and tingling Tinnitus Tachycardia and dysrhythmias

158. A: Liquefactive necrosis is the type that results from ischemia of neurons and glial cells in the central nervous system. Coagulative necrosis results from hypoxia and primarily affects the kidneys, adrenal glands, and heart. Caseous necrosis results from pulmonary tuberculosis and is a combination of liquefactive and coagulative necrosis. Fat necrosis results from lipases (enzymes) that break down triglycerides to release fatty acids, which then combine with ions (calcium, sodium, magnesium) to form soap-like areas. Gangrenous necrosis results from severe hypoxia and infection, causing death of the tissue.

159. C: If a pregnant patient needs an infusion of a drug whose dosage is based on body weight and the patient's prepregnancy weight was 125 lb/57 kg but her current weight at 6 months of gestation is 137 lb/62 kg, the weight that the patient's dosage should be based on is the current weight of 137 lb/62 kg. Fluids should achieve euvolemia, so fluid excess should be avoided. If rehydrating the patient because of dehydration, thiamine should be administered before IV fluids containing glucose because of the increased risk of Wernicke encephalopathy.

160. C: Drugs that are administered orally are primarily absorbed in the small intestines. Absorption is determined to a great extent by surface area; the greater the surface area, the greater the absorption. The stomach is small, with a surface area of about 800 square centimeters. Because the small intestine is lined with villi, the actual surface area is about 25,000 square centimeters. Other factors that affect absorption include the lipid solubility, rate of dissolution, blood flow, and pH partitioning.

161. D: Eosinophils (a type of WBCs) serve as the immune system's primary defense against parasites. Eosinophils normally comprise 2–3% of WBCs. Eosinophils are a type of granulocyte and are also active in allergic reactions. The eosinophil's granules are not only toxic to other organisms but also to tissues. The granules act as a poison to invading parasites. Eosinophils are mildly phagocytic. Eosinophils also help regulate vascular mediators that are released from mast cells, reducing inflammation of wounds.

162. A: If a patient's ECG shows a slightly peaked P wave, slightly prolonged PR interval, ST depression, shallow T wave, and prominent U wave, the electrolyte imbalance associated with these findings is hypokalemia. Potassium is necessary for repolarization, so ventricular repolarization is delayed. This may cause various dysrhythmias, including AV block, sinus bradycardia, and paroxysmal atrial tachycardia. Mild hypokalemia is usually asymptomatic, but with increased loss, the patient may experience muscle weakness, loss of smooth muscle tone, and respiratory depression.

163. B: The type of immune response that involves antibodies (immunoglobulins) binding to antigens on infective agents (primarily bacteria and viruses) is referred to as humoral immunity. The immune response includes antibodies and T cells. The part of the response by antibodies provides humoral immunity, whereas the response by T cells provides cell-mediated immunity. T cells attack and kill cells (primarily viruses and cancerous cells) directly.

164. C: If a patient developed a sudden onset of severe retrosternal chest pain that increases with respirations and when lying down in a supine position, the patient has a low-grade fever and sinus tachycardia, and on auscultation the NP notes a friction rub at the cardiac apex and left sternal border, these signs and symptoms are consistent with pericarditis. Most cases are caused by viruses or are idiopathic, but pericarditis may also occur with myocardial infarctions, autoimmune disorders, uremia, or cardiac surgery.

165. B: If the NP is monitoring the capnography of a patient with severe asthma, and the monitor shows a sloped "shark fin" waveform with loss of plateau, this indicates obstruction. With the normal waveform, the line rises with exhalation, levels, and drops with inhalation. The point immediately before the drop (the end point of exhalation) is where the $EtCO_2$ is measured. Hyperventilation lowers the waveform and increases the number of waveforms, whereas hypoventilation raises the waveform but decreases the number.

166. A: If the NP is examining a patient with a traumatic brain injury and the patient's pupils are in midposition, slightly dilated (5 mm), and fixed, this indicates structural damage to the midbrain (mesencephalon). This part of the brain, located in the superior portion of the brainstem, is important for motor movement, especially of the eyes, and in processing auditory and visual stimuli. Damage may cause movement disorders, memory deficit, and impaired hearing and vision.

167. D: If a patient is to be discharged with a referral to hospice, the patient may be cared for under the Medicare hospice benefit for two 90-day periods and unlimited 60-day periods. On referral, the healthcare provider must certify that the patient's life expectancy is 6 months or fewer; however, after the two 90-day periods, the healthcare provider can continue to certify the same for 60-day periods because predicting the time of death is an imperfect science. For each 60-day certification, the healthcare provider must have a face-to-face visit with the patient.

168. B: If the spouse of a patient with end-stage liver disease is distraught, cries frequently, and tells the NP that she has no appetite, no patience, and is sleeping poorly, the stage of grief that the spouse is experiencing is depression. Kübler-Ross's five stages of grief include:

- Denial: Disbelieving, confused, stunned, detached, repeating questions.
- Anger: Directed inward (self-blame) or outward.
- Bargaining: If-then thinking (if I go to church, then I will heal). Trying to find a different outcome.
- Depression: Sad, withdrawn, tearful, crying but beginning to accept the loss.
- Acceptance: Resolution and acceptance.

169. C: This patient is showing symptoms of ascites. The following findings are consistent with ascites:

- Weight gain and increased abdominal girth
- Shortness of breath
- Abdomen is large, skin is taut, and the umbilicus is everted
- Flanks bulging (where fluid collects when the patient reclines)
- Tympany at the center of the abdomen but it is dull over fluid
- Normal bowel sounds but the sound is diminished over fluid

Ascites is most commonly associated with cirrhosis of the liver. Cirrhosis may be treated with sodium and fluid restriction, diuretics, and paracentesis.

170. B: Mild claudication. Ankle-brachial index scores:

>1.3	Abnormally high, may indicate calcification
1–1.2	Normal
0.70–0.95	Narrowing of one or more leg vessels; mild claudication
0.5–0.70	Moderate to severe, intermittent claudication with borderline perfusion; severe disease and ischemia occurring with scores less than 0.60
<0.50	Pain at rest; the limb is threatened
0.25	Critical, limb-threatening condition

171. D: Cerebellar ataxia is associated with alcohol or barbiturate effects on the brain. It is characterized by a wide-based, staggering gait with uncoordinated movements. This gait may also occur with cerebellar tumors and multiple sclerosis. Waddling occurs with weak hip girdle muscles, causing the opposite hip to drop when the person takes a step. The scissors gait is characterized by crossed knees and results from leg paraparesis or multiple sclerosis. Steppage gait, characterized by lifting the knee and foot high and slapping it down because of foot drop, results from lower motor neuron lesions.

172. A: If a patient with hemophilia B has developed major bleeding after an injury, the treatment that is indicated to control bleeding is factor IX product, usually administered for 3–10 days. There are three types of hemophilia: A (lacks clotting factor VIII), B (lacks clotting factor IX), and C (lacks factor XI). Types A and B are usually X-linked and affect only males, but type C (rarely found in the US) affects males and females. Symptoms of hemophilia include bleeding with trauma, unexplained bruises, joint pain, swelling, epistaxis, and spontaneous hemorrhage (often in joints).

173. B: If a patient with severe rheumatoid arthritis is being discharged on methotrexate, discharge instructions should include the need to avoid exposure to sunlight. The patient should be cautioned to wear sunscreen (preferably one with titanium dioxide or zinc oxide), sunglasses, and clothing that covers the arms and legs when in the sunlight and to try to stay in shady areas. Methotrexate causes radiation recall, a condition in which areas of the skin that have previously been sunburned develop a dermatitis.

174. C: The SSRI that is likely to cause the highest rate of sexual dysfunction is paroxetine. Sertraline and fluoxetine have the lowest incidence of sexual dysfunction. In some cases, administration of bupropion as an adjunct to the SSRI may reduce sexual dysfunction. SSRI use may result in sexual dysfunction in up to 65% of patients.

175. A: If a 65-year-old patient has mild hypertension in the range of 140/90, a typical first-line therapy is a thiazide diuretic, such as hydrochlorothiazide. Thiazide diuretics decrease BP by decreasing plasma volume and reducing peripheral vascular resistance; given alone, they control BP in approximately 50% of patients. Some patients may require additional medications, such as beta-blockers, ARBs, and ACE inhibitors. African Americans tend to respond better to two or more medications than to a single medication.

How to Overcome Test Anxiety

Just the thought of taking a test is enough to make most people a little nervous. A test is an important event that can have a long-term impact on your future, so it's important to take it seriously and it's natural to feel anxious about performing well. But just because anxiety is normal, that doesn't mean that it's helpful in test taking, or that you should simply accept it as part of your life. Anxiety can have a variety of effects. These effects can be mild, like making you feel slightly nervous, or severe, like blocking your ability to focus or remember even a simple detail.

If you experience test anxiety—whether severe or mild—it's important to know how to beat it. To discover this, first you need to understand what causes test anxiety.

Causes of Test Anxiety

While we often think of anxiety as an uncontrollable emotional state, it can actually be caused by simple, practical things. One of the most common causes of test anxiety is that a person does not feel adequately prepared for their test. This feeling can be the result of many different issues such as poor study habits or lack of organization, but the most common culprit is time management. Starting to study too late, failing to organize your study time to cover all of the material, or being distracted while you study will mean that you're not well prepared for the test. This may lead to cramming the night before, which will cause you to be physically and mentally exhausted for the test. Poor time management also contributes to feelings of stress, fear, and hopelessness as you realize you are not well prepared but don't know what to do about it.

Other times, test anxiety is not related to your preparation for the test but comes from unresolved fear. This may be a past failure on a test, or poor performance on tests in general. It may come from comparing yourself to others who seem to be performing better or from the stress of living up to expectations. Anxiety may be driven by fears of the future—how failure on this test would affect your educational and career goals. These fears are often completely irrational, but they can still negatively impact your test performance.

Review Video: 3 Reasons You Have Test Anxiety
Visit mometrix.com/academy and enter code: 428468

Elements of Test Anxiety

As mentioned earlier, test anxiety is considered to be an emotional state, but it has physical and mental components as well. Sometimes you may not even realize that you are suffering from test anxiety until you notice the physical symptoms. These can include trembling hands, rapid heartbeat, sweating, nausea, and tense muscles. Extreme anxiety may lead to fainting or vomiting. Obviously, any of these symptoms can have a negative impact on testing. It is important to recognize them as soon as they begin to occur so that you can address the problem before it damages your performance.

Review Video: 3 Ways to Tell You Have Test Anxiety
Visit mometrix.com/academy and enter code: 927847

The mental components of test anxiety include trouble focusing and inability to remember learned information. During a test, your mind is on high alert, which can help you recall information and stay focused for an extended period of time. However, anxiety interferes with your mind's natural processes, causing you to blank out, even on the questions you know well. The strain of testing during anxiety makes it difficult to stay focused, especially on a test that may take several hours. Extreme anxiety can take a huge mental toll, making it difficult not only to recall test information but even to understand the test questions or pull your thoughts together.

Review Video: How Test Anxiety Affects Memory
Visit mometrix.com/academy and enter code: 609003

Effects of Test Anxiety

Test anxiety is like a disease—if left untreated, it will get progressively worse. Anxiety leads to poor performance, and this reinforces the feelings of fear and failure, which in turn lead to poor performances on subsequent tests. It can grow from a mild nervousness to a crippling condition. If allowed to progress, test anxiety can have a big impact on your schooling, and consequently on your future.

Test anxiety can spread to other parts of your life. Anxiety on tests can become anxiety in any stressful situation, and blanking on a test can turn into panicking in a job situation. But fortunately, you don't have to let anxiety rule your testing and determine your grades. There are a number of relatively simple steps you can take to move past anxiety and function normally on a test and in the rest of life.

Review Video: How Test Anxiety Impacts Your Grades
Visit mometrix.com/academy and enter code: 939819

Physical Steps for Beating Test Anxiety

While test anxiety is a serious problem, the good news is that it can be overcome. It doesn't have to control your ability to think and remember information. While it may take time, you can begin taking steps today to beat anxiety.

Just as your first hint that you may be struggling with anxiety comes from the physical symptoms, the first step to treating it is also physical. Rest is crucial for having a clear, strong mind. If you are tired, it is much easier to give in to anxiety. But if you establish good sleep habits, your body and mind will be ready to perform optimally, without the strain of exhaustion. Additionally, sleeping well helps you to retain information better, so you're more likely to recall the answers when you see the test questions.

Getting good sleep means more than going to bed on time. It's important to allow your brain time to relax. Take study breaks from time to time so it doesn't get overworked, and don't study right before bed. Take time to rest your mind before trying to rest your body, or you may find it difficult to fall asleep.

Review Video: The Importance of Sleep for Your Brain
Visit mometrix.com/academy and enter code: 319338

Along with sleep, other aspects of physical health are important in preparing for a test. Good nutrition is vital for good brain function. Sugary foods and drinks may give a burst of energy but this burst is followed by a crash, both physically and emotionally. Instead, fuel your body with protein and vitamin-rich foods.

Also, drink plenty of water. Dehydration can lead to headaches and exhaustion, especially if your brain is already under stress from the rigors of the test. Particularly if your test is a long one, drink water during the breaks. And if possible, take an energy-boosting snack to eat between sections.

Review Video: How Diet Can Affect your Mood
Visit mometrix.com/academy and enter code: 624317

Along with sleep and diet, a third important part of physical health is exercise. Maintaining a steady workout schedule is helpful, but even taking 5-minute study breaks to walk can help get your blood pumping faster and clear your head. Exercise also releases endorphins, which contribute to a positive feeling and can help combat test anxiety.

When you nurture your physical health, you are also contributing to your mental health. If your body is healthy, your mind is much more likely to be healthy as well. So take time to rest, nourish your body with healthy food and water, and get moving as much as possible. Taking these physical steps will make you stronger and more able to take the mental steps necessary to overcome test anxiety.

Mental Steps for Beating Test Anxiety

Working on the mental side of test anxiety can be more challenging, but as with the physical side, there are clear steps you can take to overcome it. As mentioned earlier, test anxiety often stems from lack of preparation, so the obvious solution is to prepare for the test. Effective studying may be the most important weapon you have for beating test anxiety, but you can and should employ several other mental tools to combat fear.

First, boost your confidence by reminding yourself of past success—tests or projects that you aced. If you're putting as much effort into preparing for this test as you did for those, there's no reason you should expect to fail here. Work hard to prepare; then trust your preparation.

Second, surround yourself with encouraging people. It can be helpful to find a study group, but be sure that the people you're around will encourage a positive attitude. If you spend time with others who are anxious or cynical, this will only contribute to your own anxiety. Look for others who are motivated to study hard from a desire to succeed, not from a fear of failure.

Third, reward yourself. A test is physically and mentally tiring, even without anxiety, and it can be helpful to have something to look forward to. Plan an activity following the test, regardless of the outcome, such as going to a movie or getting ice cream.

When you are taking the test, if you find yourself beginning to feel anxious, remind yourself that you know the material. Visualize successfully completing the test. Then take a few deep, relaxing breaths and return to it. Work through the questions carefully but with confidence, knowing that you are capable of succeeding.

Developing a healthy mental approach to test taking will also aid in other areas of life. Test anxiety affects more than just the actual test—it can be damaging to your mental health and even contribute to depression. It's important to beat test anxiety before it becomes a problem for more than testing.

Review Video: Test Anxiety and Depression
Visit mometrix.com/academy and enter code: 904704

Study Strategy

Being prepared for the test is necessary to combat anxiety, but what does being prepared look like? You may study for hours on end and still not feel prepared. What you need is a strategy for test prep. The next few pages outline our recommended steps to help you plan out and conquer the challenge of preparation.

Step 1: Scope Out the Test

Learn everything you can about the format (multiple choice, essay, etc.) and what will be on the test. Gather any study materials, course outlines, or sample exams that may be available. Not only will this help you to prepare, but knowing what to expect can help to alleviate test anxiety.

Step 2: Map Out the Material

Look through the textbook or study guide and make note of how many chapters or sections it has. Then divide these over the time you have. For example, if a book has 15 chapters and you have five days to study, you need to cover three chapters each day. Even better, if you have the time, leave an extra day at the end for overall review after you have gone through the material in depth.

If time is limited, you may need to prioritize the material. Look through it and make note of which sections you think you already have a good grasp on, and which need review. While you are studying, skim quickly through the familiar sections and take more time on the challenging parts. Write out your plan so you don't get lost as you go. Having a written plan also helps you feel more in control of the study, so anxiety is less likely to arise from feeling overwhelmed at the amount to cover.

Step 3: Gather Your Tools

Decide what study method works best for you. Do you prefer to highlight in the book as you study and then go back over the highlighted portions? Or do you type out notes of the important information? Or is it helpful to make flashcards that you can carry with you? Assemble the pens, index cards, highlighters, post-it notes, and any other materials you may need so you won't be distracted by getting up to find things while you study.

If you're having a hard time retaining the information or organizing your notes, experiment with different methods. For example, try color-coding by subject with colored pens, highlighters, or post-it notes. If you learn better by hearing, try recording yourself reading your notes so you can listen while in the car, working out, or simply sitting at your desk. Ask a friend to quiz you from your flashcards, or try teaching someone the material to solidify it in your mind.

Step 4: Create Your Environment

It's important to avoid distractions while you study. This includes both the obvious distractions like visitors and the subtle distractions like an uncomfortable chair (or a too-comfortable couch that makes you want to fall asleep). Set up the best study environment possible: good lighting and a comfortable work area. If background music helps you focus, you may want to turn it on, but otherwise keep the room quiet. If you are using a computer to take notes, be sure you don't have any other windows open, especially applications like social media, games, or anything else that could distract you. Silence your phone and turn off notifications. Be sure to keep water close by so you stay hydrated while you study (but avoid unhealthy drinks and snacks).

Also, take into account the best time of day to study. Are you freshest first thing in the morning? Try to set aside some time then to work through the material. Is your mind clearer in the afternoon or evening? Schedule your study session then. Another method is to study at the same time of day that you will take the test, so that your brain gets used to working on the material at that time and will be ready to focus at test time.

Step 5: Study!

Once you have done all the study preparation, it's time to settle into the actual studying. Sit down, take a few moments to settle your mind so you can focus, and begin to follow your study plan. Don't give in to distractions or let yourself procrastinate. This is your time to prepare so you'll be ready to fearlessly approach the test. Make the most of the time and stay focused.

Of course, you don't want to burn out. If you study too long you may find that you're not retaining the information very well. Take regular study breaks. For example, taking five minutes out of every hour to walk briskly, breathing deeply and swinging your arms, can help your mind stay fresh.

As you get to the end of each chapter or section, it's a good idea to do a quick review. Remind yourself of what you learned and work on any difficult parts. When you feel that you've mastered the material, move on to the next part. At the end of your study session, briefly skim through your notes again.

But while review is helpful, cramming last minute is NOT. If at all possible, work ahead so that you won't need to fit all your study into the last day. Cramming overloads your brain with more information than it can process and retain, and your tired mind may struggle to recall even previously learned information when it is overwhelmed with last-minute study. Also, the urgent nature of cramming and the stress placed on your brain contribute to anxiety. You'll be more likely to go to the test feeling unprepared and having trouble thinking clearly.

So don't cram, and don't stay up late before the test, even just to review your notes at a leisurely pace. Your brain needs rest more than it needs to go over the information again. In fact, plan to finish your studies by noon or early afternoon the day before the test. Give your brain the rest of the day to relax or focus on other things, and get a good night's sleep. Then you will be fresh for the test and better able to recall what you've studied.

Step 6: Take a practice test

Many courses offer sample tests, either online or in the study materials. This is an excellent resource to check whether you have mastered the material, as well as to prepare for the test format and environment.

Check the test format ahead of time: the number of questions, the type (multiple choice, free response, etc.), and the time limit. Then create a plan for working through them. For example, if you have 30 minutes to take a 60-question test, your limit is 30 seconds per question. Spend less time on the questions you know well so that you can take more time on the difficult ones.

If you have time to take several practice tests, take the first one open book, with no time limit. Work through the questions at your own pace and make sure you fully understand them. Gradually work up to taking a test under test conditions: sit at a desk with all study materials put away and set a timer. Pace yourself to make sure you finish the test with time to spare and go back to check your answers if you have time.

After each test, check your answers. On the questions you missed, be sure you understand why you missed them. Did you misread the question (tests can use tricky wording)? Did you forget the information? Or was it something you hadn't learned? Go back and study any shaky areas that the practice tests reveal.

Taking these tests not only helps with your grade, but also aids in combating test anxiety. If you're already used to the test conditions, you're less likely to worry about it, and working through tests until you're scoring well gives you a confidence boost. Go through the practice tests until you feel comfortable, and then you can go into the test knowing that you're ready for it.

Test Tips

On test day, you should be confident, knowing that you've prepared well and are ready to answer the questions. But aside from preparation, there are several test day strategies you can employ to maximize your performance.

First, as stated before, get a good night's sleep the night before the test (and for several nights before that, if possible). Go into the test with a fresh, alert mind rather than staying up late to study.

Try not to change too much about your normal routine on the day of the test. It's important to eat a nutritious breakfast, but if you normally don't eat breakfast at all, consider eating just a protein bar. If you're a coffee drinker, go ahead and have your normal coffee. Just make sure you time it so that the caffeine doesn't wear off right in the middle of your test. Avoid sugary beverages, and drink enough water to stay hydrated but not so much that you need a restroom break 10 minutes into the test. If your test isn't first thing in the morning, consider going for a walk or doing a light workout before the test to get your blood flowing.

Allow yourself enough time to get ready, and leave for the test with plenty of time to spare so you won't have the anxiety of scrambling to arrive in time. Another reason to be early is to select a good seat. It's helpful to sit away from doors and windows, which can be distracting. Find a good seat, get out your supplies, and settle your mind before the test begins.

When the test begins, start by going over the instructions carefully, even if you already know what to expect. Make sure you avoid any careless mistakes by following the directions.

Then begin working through the questions, pacing yourself as you've practiced. If you're not sure on an answer, don't spend too much time on it, and don't let it shake your confidence. Either skip it and come back later, or eliminate as many wrong answers as possible and guess among the remaining ones. Don't dwell on these questions as you continue—put them out of your mind and focus on what lies ahead.

Be sure to read all of the answer choices, even if you're sure the first one is the right answer. Sometimes you'll find a better one if you keep reading. But don't second-guess yourself if you do immediately know the answer. Your gut instinct is usually right. Don't let test anxiety rob you of the information you know.

If you have time at the end of the test (and if the test format allows), go back and review your answers. Be cautious about changing any, since your first instinct tends to be correct, but make sure you didn't misread any of the questions or accidentally mark the wrong answer choice. Look over any you skipped and make an educated guess.

At the end, leave the test feeling confident. You've done your best, so don't waste time worrying about your performance or wishing you could change anything. Instead, celebrate the successful completion of this test. And finally, use this test to learn how to deal with anxiety even better next time.

Review Video: 5 Tips to Beat Test Anxiety
Visit mometrix.com/academy and enter code: 570656

Important Qualification

Not all anxiety is created equal. If your test anxiety is causing major issues in your life beyond the classroom or testing center, or if you are experiencing troubling physical symptoms related to your anxiety, it may be a sign of a serious physiological or psychological condition. If this sounds like your situation, we strongly encourage you to seek professional help.

Thank You

We at Mometrix would like to extend our heartfelt thanks to you, our friend and patron, for allowing us to play a part in your journey. It is a privilege to serve people from all walks of life who are unified in their commitment to building the best future they can for themselves.

The preparation you devote to these important testing milestones may be the most valuable educational opportunity you have for making a real difference in your life. We encourage you to put your heart into it—that feeling of succeeding, overcoming, and yes, conquering will be well worth the hours you've invested.

We want to hear your story, your struggles and your successes, and if you see any opportunities for us to improve our materials so we can help others even more effectively in the future, please share that with us as well. **The team at Mometrix would be absolutely thrilled to hear from you!** So please, send us an email (support@mometrix.com) and let's stay in touch.

If you'd like some additional help, check out these other resources we offer for your exam: http://mometrixflashcards.com/NP

Additional Bonus Material

Due to our efforts to try to keep this book to a manageable length, we've created a link that will give you access to all of your additional bonus material.

Please visit http://www.mometrix.com/bonus948/npadgeracutec to access the information.

CPSIA information can be obtained
at www.ICGtesting.com
Printed in the USA
BVHW011817270222
630184BV00012B/444